BIOSENSORS FOR HEALTH, ENVIRONMENT AND BIOSECURITY

Edited by **Pier Andrea Serra**

INTECHOPEN.COM

Biosensors for Health, Environment and Biosecurity
Edited by Pier Andrea Serra

CBS, Edition **2016**

Published by InTech

Janeza Trdine 9, 51000 Rijeka, Croatia

Publishing Process Manager Mirna Cvijic

Technical Editor Teodora Smiljanic

Cover Designer InTech Design Team

Additional hard copies can be obtained from orders@intechopen.com

Biosensors for Health, Environment and Biosecurity, Edited by Pier Andrea Serra
p. cm.
ISBN 978-953-307-443-6

INTECH

open science | open minds

Contents

Preface

A biosensor is defined as a detecting device that combines a transducer with a biologically sensitive and selective component. When a specific target molecule interacts with the biological component, a signal is produced, at transducer level, proportional to the concentration of the substance. Therefore biosensors can measure compounds present in the environment, chemical processes, food and human body at low cost if compared with traditional analytical techniques.

This book covers a wide range of aspects and issues related to biosensor technology, bringing together researchers from 16 different countries. The book consists of 24 chapters written by 76 authors and divided in three sections. The first section, entitled Biosensors Technology and Materials, is composed by two chapters and describes emerging aspects of technology applied to biosensors. The subsequent section, entitled Biosensors for Health and including twenty chapters, is devoted to biosensor applications in the medical field. The last section, composed by two chapters, treats of the environmental and biosecurity applications of biosensors.

I want to express my appreciation and gratitude to all authors who contributed to this book with their research results and to InTech team, in particular to the Publishing Process Manager Ms. Mirna Cvijic that accomplished its mission with professionalism and dedication.

Editor
Pier Andrea Serra
University of Sassari
Italy

Part 1

Biosensor Technology and Materials

1

Fluorescent Biosensors for Protein Interactions and Drug Discovery

Alejandro Sosa-Peinado[1] and Martín González-Andrade[2]

[1]*Departamento de Bioquímica, Facultad de Medicina, Universidad Nacional Autónoma de México*

[2]*Facultad de Química, Universidad Nacional Autónoma de México*

México

1. Introduction

The powerful ability of proteins to bind selectively its ligand and interact specifically with other proteins during its functions, have been employed in the development of highly specific and robust biosensors (Medintz and Deschamps 2006; Vallee-Belisle and Plaxco 2010). To design protein biosensor is required to attach a transducer to the protein in order to monitor a specific interaction. The nature of this transducer is diverse, but fluorescent attachment has been used extensively by protein, in general are based in attachment in a the chemical groups and/or in the genetical fusion of green fluorescent proteins (GFP) or derived proteins (Deuschle, Okumoto et al. 2005; Campbell 2009; Wang, Nakata et al. 2009). In this review we are focus in the fluorescent biosensors based in site-specific fluorescent labeling, as a result of combining the chemical attachment by site-directed mutagenesis and/ or manipulation of genetic code. Given the enormous diversity in the nature of the fluorescent attachment to proteins, we are focused to the recent advances in monitoring protein-ligand and protein-protein, and their applications in different areas of research. Since the protein scaffold used as biosensor might be a pharmacological target (Cooper 2003), the design of robust biosensors, could be used for high-throughput screening in the search of new drugs (Cooper 2003).

2. General design of biosensor

A biosensor is a biological receptor able to monitor the concentration of a specific analyte or even more, could be selective to interact only with a particular conformation of a macromolecule, event typically associated to the allosteric proteins, that present changes in the protein conformation coupled to changes in the affinity for its ligand or another proteins (Wang, Nakata et al. 2009). In any case, for the biosensor design is required their appropriate transducer, and the nature of this could be diverse: optic, mechano-chemical, electro-chemical, acustic, etc. There is no a universal rationale for biosensor construction, therefore, should be taken in consideration several features for design: First, is the choice for the biological component, in general is a protein that provide the stereospecificity required for the wanted interaction, but in some cases nucleic acids are good sensors (aptamers). Enzymes are very specific, however in some cases the catalysis is not desirable, thus some enzymes have to be modified to impair the activity and conserve only the ligand binding property, or the ideal case is to use a protein that only bind the analyte to monitor. Accordingly, a family of proteins in the periplasmic space of bacteria fulfill the last requirement (Looger, Dwyer et al. 2003; de Lorimier, Tian et al. 2006). These proteins named periplasmic binding proteins (PBPs), present a conformational change upon ligand binding, as a first step to interact with a membrane transporters (ABC proteins), previous of the translocation of ligand to the interior to the cell (de Lorimier, Tian et al. 2006; Medintz and Deschamps 2006; Tsukiji, Miyagawa et al. 2009). The different members of these proteins are able to bind a large number of analytes, such a as: carbohydrates, amino acids, ions, hormones, heme-groups, etc. Thus several PBPs has been used to detect a specific ligand, the group of Hellinga has been able to construct constructed several fluorescent biosensors .

The Second consideration, is about the chemical nature of the fluorescent transducer, and the physicochemical property for which the signal is optimal. There are signals very sensitive to the polarity of the solvent, or to the electrochemical environment, pH, etc. In general several fluorescent groups have solvatochromic effects in which there is a low emission fluorescence in aqueous environment, but in low polar environment there is an increase of fluorescence emission associated to a blue-shifted emission spectrum. Since, when a protein interaction take place, this produce changes in solvent accessibility rearrangement of not covalent interaction, thus in many cases the fluorophore may sense the environment perturbation produced by the protein interaction. Also, there are fluorescents signals that are quenched when a ligand or another protein are in proximity of the label. When the protein present a notable conformational change, in some cases a pair donator-acceptor signals could be selected to generate Foster resonance energy transfer (FRET) biosensors, in which the fluorescence transference energy observed by fluorescence emission changed in a distance dependence when the conformational change take place.

Third consideration, is the selection of a position into the protein to introduce the signal, these position would generate low perturbation in the stability of the protein with full capacity to the specific interaction sought, and high sensitivity for detection, the advantage for label introduction by chemical methods, allow to introduce the label at any position of the protein. This may be the most difficult problem to predict the best place to introduce the signal to produce the high sensitive signal with a low perturbation of the ligand binding system. In many cases when the introduction of the signal is closer of the ligand binding site, allow the good signal. Now days, the structural information of proteins allow to evaluate *in silico* the effect of protein stability before the experimental work, from the protein data base (PDB), and the identification of structural binding motives or the ability to create a structural model from the homologues protein with know structure in combination with molecular modelling. A fourth factor to be considered is the robustness of the biosensor, to be reproducible, reversible, rapid for signal detection, and reagent free, altogether, these characteristics will determine if the designed biosensor could be able to monitor in real time in either cell environment or in a immobilized device (Looger, Dwyer et al. 2003; Vallee-Belisle and Plaxco 2010; Plaxco and Soh 2011). In general there are some advantage and limitations for these type of biosensors (Table 1).

	Advantage	Limitation
Fluorescent groups	The chemical nature is diverse, many are commercial available, is possible to select a broad range in light excitation in the UV, visible spectra. Are small and is possible to label at any position into the protein sequence.	The stability perturbation that may introduce the chemical group into the protein.
Position for labeling	Combined with the site directed mutagenesis is possible to introduce at any position wanted.	Stability perturbation, and undesired reaction, but this is overcome with incorporation of SH groups at specific positions.
Biological receptor	There are many ligand binding proteins, receptor, and enzymes for protein selection.	Modification of the ligand binding specificity for its ligand.

Table 1. Advantge and limitation for the inytroduction of fluorescent labels.

3. Biosensor based in chemical attachment of labels and genetic methods

The incorporation of fluorescent labels by combination of chemical-labeling methods simultaneously with molecular genetic methods are diverse, nonetheless, we can categorize in three major groups in terms of the method to label the chemical probe into the protein surface: i) incorporation of reactive free cysteine for thiol-fluorescent labeling by site directed labeling methods; ii) site specific incorporation of unnatural fluorescent amino acid based in a expansion of genetic code methods; and iii) incorporation by covalent chemical modification, some by post-photoaffinity labeling from the site directed labeling based in a thiol -fluorescent reactive, the signal incorporation could be at binding site (endosteric), outsite of the binding site (allosteric) or in the case of two fluorophores for fluorescence resonance energy transference (FRET) as described in Fig 1.

3.1 Biosensor based in site-directed mutagenesis and site-specific fluorescent labeling methodology

The addition of fluorescent signal to a protein by introduction of a reactive cysteine for a thiol-fluorescent group is consequence of both, the enormous chemical synthesis available to attach covalently fluorescent groups to the SH group present in the cysteine residue of proteins, and at the same time the well established molecular genetic methods to introduce a new residue by site directed mutagenesis. In particular the thiol groups of a cysteine is the most reactive nucleophile of protein residues, thus, is very effective to label only the SH residues without non-specific labeling. The large number of fluorescent probes could be excited in a broad range of light wavelength from the uv light to the visible range, and

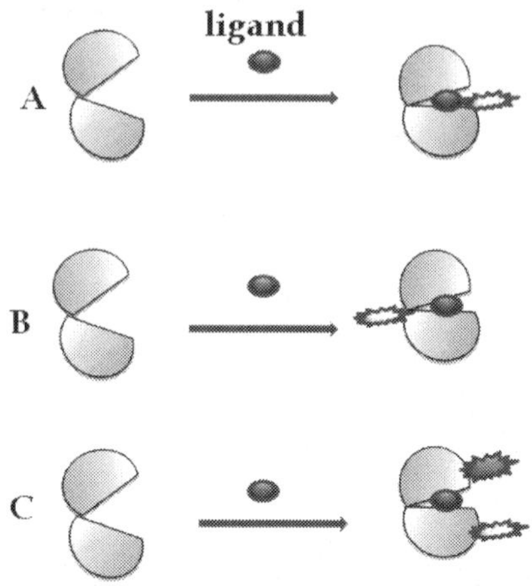

Fig. 1. Localization for fluorescent labeling. A, at the binding site, B, in allosteric site, and C, two fluorophore incoporation for FRET, when the distance between two signals changed by a conformational change..

several of these probes are commercially available (Toronto Chemical Research Inc., Invitrogen-Molecular Probes™, Sigma-Aldrich®). The cysteine residue are not frequently present in proteins, then, is possible eliminate cysteine residues by site directed mutagenesis to avoid unspecific labeling. Site specific labeling of proteins with fluorescent probes, requires careful choice of labeling chemistry, optimization of the labeling reaction, the complete characterization of labeled proteins for: labeling efficiency, retention of protein functionality and minimal structural perturbation (Altenbach, Klein-Seetharaman et al. 1999; Mansoor and Farrens 2004). Given that several of the labels are small chemical groups, the labeling at relatively exposed residues minimize the perturbation in the protein structure. This was demonstrated by Farrens and col by the specific incorporation of bromobimane in a helix-turn-helix motive after chemical modification of 21 consecutive single-cysteine mutants; the residues T115 to K135 of T4 lysozyme. The $\Delta\Delta G$ calculated from each 21 mutants and compared with the wild type enzyme indicated a minimal energy perturbation $\leq$ 1.5 kcal/mol, for those residues exposed $\geq$ 40 Å of solvent surface accessible, after chemical modifications. In this work was pointed out no energy destabilization of T4 lysozyme after fluorophore labeling unless the residue was buried into the protein structure. Thus having information about the protein topology, or the structure ligand binding domain, there is a good possibility to introduce a small fluorescent signal with low perturbation in the designed protein.

3.2 Biosensor based in the insertion of non-natural amino-acids

The use of amber stop codons has been allowed to acylate the tRNA with un-natural amino acids and enrich its chemical repertory into a protein. In addition to this method Honsaka and col has been developed the four base pare method to incorporate unnatural amino acids, among them have been synthesized *p*-aminophenylalanine derivatives bound to

BODIPY fluorophore. This approach was applied to incorporate two variants of fluorescent amino acids to calmodulin, an energy donor acceptor pair, to demonstrate the feasibility for FRET measurements when the distance between pairs change upon addition of calmodulin binding protein. This method allowed to study in solution the dynamics of the conformational change of calmodulin.

3.3 Biosensor based in post transcription modifications and chemical modification

Introducing a fluorescent signal without knowing about the sequence or the three dimensional structure, or binding domains for obtain a functional biosensor could be a very hard task, Hamachi and collaborators introduce the post-photoaffinity labeling modification (P-PALM) to introduce fluorescent molecule close of the active site of a enzyme without any genetic manipulation to introduce the signal into the protein (Nagase, Nakata et al. 2003; Nakata, Nagase et al. 2004). The main goal of this methodology to attach fluorescent labels in living cells or whole organisms, that is the reason to avoid genetic methods. Based in this approach this group developed a biosensor based in the scaffold of a lectin, a saccharide binding protein. To this end concavalin A (Con A) was used in presence of the P-PALM reagent. This reagent have three important characteristics (Fig. 2): 1) high affinity to the lectine, a saccharide moiety, to bind the Con A, 2) the photoactive moiety (diazirine) to label the protein by photoirradiation, and 3) a disulfide group to remove the original ligand to bind to the protein and allow at the same time a reactive site for chemical modification (the thiol group).

In other words the P-PALM is bounded to the protein by UV light irradiation when the ligand is anchored to the binding site of ConA by the saccharide moiety, then a reduction of the probe, generate a reactive SH for covalent modification with a thiol-reactive fluorophore, such as dansyl or fluorescein groups, then this lectin is transformed in fluorescent biosensor to saccharide (Fig 3).

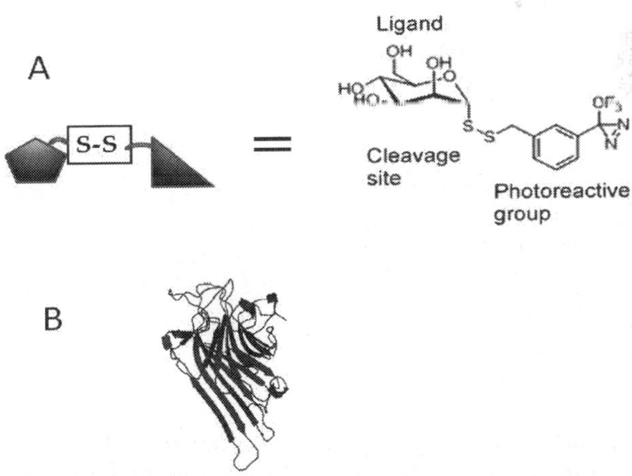

Fig. 2. P-PALM reactive and target. A is the molecular estructure of a post-photoaffinity labeling reagent P-PALM, and B is the structure of the target the concanalin A, the PDB Is is 1 VAM.

The advantage of this method is the introduction of several chemical labels without need to use genetic engineered methods (Fig. 3), with the additional property to attach several fluorescent moieties. For example the addition of the fluorescent pH indicator, SNARF, the biosensor was able to distinguish to differentiate several anomeric groups present in the saccharides (Nakata, Nagase et al. 2004; Ojida, Miyahara et al. 2004). The same group of Hamachi and collaborators has been developed a similar methodology, now based in the chemistry of tosyl group, named ligand directed tosyl (LDT) chemistry (Tsukiji, Miyagawa et al. 2009) that contained benzenesulfoamide as the specific moiety. This allow to synthesize tosyl derivatives that bind specifically to some proteins: carbonic anhydrase, FK506-binding protein, or congerin (beta-galactoside-binding lectin). This strategy was applied successfully to create biosensor *in vitro,* and inside the cells without genetic modification methodology. The applications around this methodologies are versatile, for example another development by the same group is the quenched ligand directed toysil (Q-LDT) chemistry (Tsukiji, Miyagawa et al. 2009; Tsukiji, Wang et al. 2009; Wang, Nakata et al. 2009), in this case after the photolabeling, the fluorescent signal is quenched, but when the ligand interact in the binding site, the quencher is released from the protein, and the increase of fluorescence signal is used to do a calibration of the ligand concentration in solution.

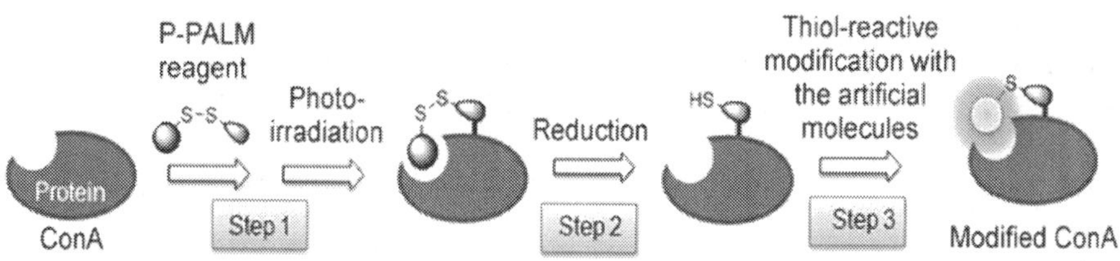

Fig. 3. Schema for the fluorescent labeling with a P-PALM reactive. In step 1 the P-PALM binds to the protein by photoirradiation, 2 reduction of the sample prepare a SH free and in 3, the fluorophores by specific chemical modification to SH group.

4. Biosensors for protein-ligand based in conformational changes

Several protein changed the conformation locally of globally when a ligand binds, this is in part explained by the conformational displacement or induced fit mechanisms present in proteins. Accordingly to recent view for the dynamical properties of proteins, from nuclear magnetic resonance (NMR) and molecular dynamics algorithms, it have been proposed that proteins are in dynamical equilibrium, and the presence of ligand should stabilize one of the extreme states. In this dynamics equilibrium point of view, several non-covalent interactions, such as hydrogen bound, hydrophobic interactions or van del Walls interactions are created at expenses to remove other interactions in different part of the protein, in a coupled process to the ligand binding event, in this sense if a suitable fluorescent signal is located into protein carring out the conformational change, should be an ideal for biosensor design when a fluorescent transducer is attached to the protein. The family of periplasmic binding proteins (PBPs) that presented a conformational change upon ligand binding has been used to create diverse biosensors based in the fluorescent incorporation by chemical modification with thiol-fluorescent reactive for cysteine. This work has been pioneered by Cass and col by introduction of fluorescent group into the maltoside binding protein (MBP) a PBP, and extensively developed by Hellinga and collaborators (de Lorimier, Smith et al. 2002). This family of proteins presented a bilobated structure with high similarity, that present at least two conformers: an open form in absence of ligand and a closed state bound to its ligand (Fig. 4). Given that the different member of this family are able to bind a diverse number of ligands, it have been developed a big number of biosensor for diverse ligands such as glucose, ribose, aminoacid, ions etc.

In the same line of research Hellinga and col. have been employed member of PBPs to developed approximately 300 different biosensor, by introduction of the signal in the binding site, or near of remote from the binding site, for example into the hinge that connect the structure of the two lobules in PBPs.

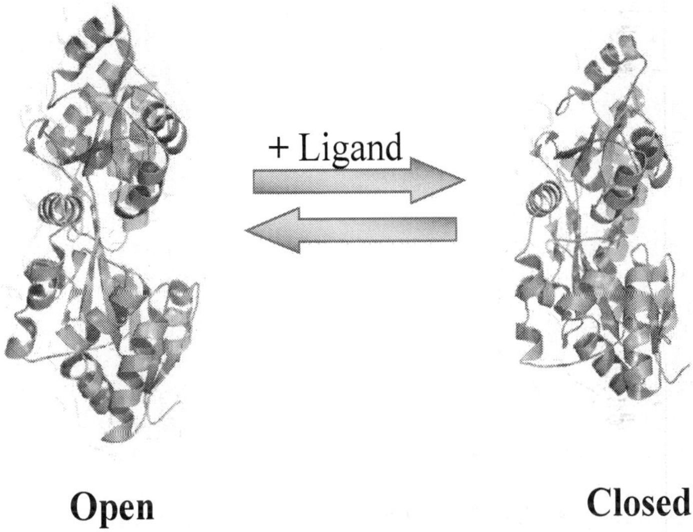

Fig. 4. Conformationa change present upon ligand binding in the maltoside binding protein, the PDD ID for open state is 1N3X and for the closed state is 1NL5.

The introduction of signal in the endosteric or allosteric sites allow to calibrate some of the signals to the concentration of ligand in solution, however only 4% of the 320 biosensor changed the fluorescence intensity to develop highly sensitive biosensor (Fig. 4). To improve the detection of the signal transduction, it was analyzed the molecular nature of fluorescence environment from a structural model for the maltose binding proteins and modified the fluorophore environment into the protein by site directed-mutagenesis, this study allow a increase in 400% of the signal intensity or signal, that point out the use of molecular modelling to improve the transduction signal to a high sensitive levels (Dattelbaum, Looger et al. 2005).

5. Biosensor to monitor protein-protein interactions

Specific protein–protein interactions are required for cellular communication processes, such as signal transduction cascades, transcription events, or transport process, etc. The determination of crystallographic structure of the protein complexes is not necessarily enough to explain the molecular basis of their specific interactions, therefore for a more dynamic study of protein-protein interactions in solution is combined with the introduction of labels in or near of interaction surface for the protein complex with structural models. For example, the use of fluorescent labels covalently attached for the proteins that participate of the primary events during the coagulation cascade were carried out; the interaction of the extracellular tissue factor (soluble TF) and the activated factor VII (Owenius, Osterlund et al. 2001). The results of this work indicated that the multi-probe methodology permits to obtain indirect binding constants between the two proteins in solution, and it was concluded that the tightness of the local interactions at the labeled positions was similar to the interactions detected inside of the interior of globular proteins.

The interface of actin myosin complex monitored by site-directed fluorescence and spin labeling techniques revealed a more complicated point of view for the interacting forces required for the active complex formation (LaConte, Voelz et al. 2002). The hypothesis of a simple transition of disordered weak interactions to strong-ordered interactions during the actin-myosin complex was not consistent with experimental. A strong-complex formation was indicated by a decrease in the mobility of the labels, but the labeled myosin indicated high mobility even after complex formation, also, solvent accessibility surface was decreased for actin-bound labels although was increased for myosin-bound probes.

The photoreceptor rhodopsin present a conformational change activated by light in order to form an active state (named MII). This state, interact and activated the G protein transducin for the initiation of the biochemical cascade during the vision process (Filipek, Stenkamp et al. 2003). Interactions of both proteins were monitored by the changes in the fluorescence of bimane specifically incorporated into the rhodopsin, with the carboxylic terminus of a G protein transducin (Janz and Farrens 2004), given that the tryptophan residue quenches the bimane fluorescence (Mansoor, McHaourab et al. 2002), this interaction is able to monitor protein-protein interactions or conformational changes in proteins. Mapping the interaction of tryptophan with bimane by fluorescence quenching in solution between rhodopsin and transducin, was detected the presence of a critical hydrophobic interaction that controls the affinity of this specific interaction (Janz and Farrens 2004). In a similar study for the binding and release of the arrestin to the photoreceptor rhodopsin were monitored in real time by the changes in the fluorescence spectra of arrestin labeled with bromobimane at the proposed surface-binding site of rhodopsin with the arrestin (Janz and Farrens 2004). These studies proposed that arrestin and retinal release from the rhodopsin receptor are a linked process (Sommer, Smith et al. 2005); thus, this innovative methodology has been used for study the dynamics of arrestin interactions on the mechanism of G-protein-coupled receptors (Sommer, Smith et al. 2006) which are the target of a big number of drugs designs.

6. Biosensor for robust detection of ligand interactions and drug design

Calmoduilin is a calcium binding proteins that interact with many cellular targets including soluble enzymes, ion-channels and primary pumps, resulting in a variety of essential downstream cellular effects (O'Neil and DeGrado 1990; Weinstein and Mehler 1994; Zhang and Yuan 1998; Zielinski 1998; Carafoli and Klee 1999; Berridge, et al. 2003), and the conformation of the protein which drastically change according to the calcium levels into the cell to regulate physiological processes (Fig. 5), therefore this protein represents an important drug target (Dagher, et al. 2006). Indeed, many CaM inhibitors are well known antipsychotic, smooth muscle relaxants, antitumoral and α-adrenergic blocking agents, among others. The interaction of CaM with its physiological targets depends on the exposure of two hydrophobic pockets (Fig. 5) following the conformational change elicited by Ca^{2+}-binding to the protein.

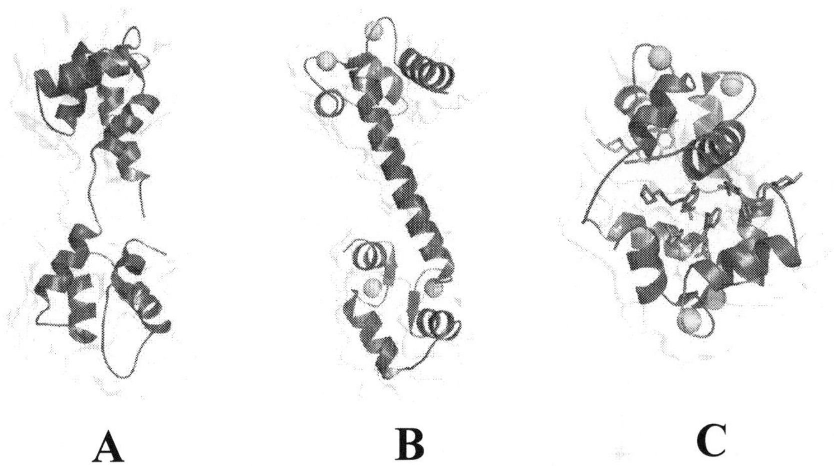

Fig. 5. Three-dimensional structures of the CaM in its different conformations: A) calcium-free (pdb code: 1CFD); B) with calcium (pdb code: 1CLL) and; C) with TFP (pdb code: 1LIN). The structures were drawn using the PyMOL program.

Many compounds including drugs, pesticides and research tools interact with CaM at the same hydrophobic sites provoking also conformational changes in the protein. Many of these substances behave as CaM antagonists, the best known structural examples of these interactions are the antipsychotic analogs of trifluoroperazine (Gangopadhyay, et al. 2004). In this sense several CaM has been used a protein target to interact with several protein by fluorescent attachment, for example: interaction between calmodulin (CaM) and a CaM-binding peptide of the ryanodine receptor (CaMBP) and its sub-fragments F1, has been measured by the mutant Thr31Cys with the fluorescent group badan attached (Sharma, Deo et al. 2005). A mutant of CaM coupled to three different environment-sensitive fluorophores (MDCC, acrylodan, and IANBD ester) was detected the CaM interaction with phenothiazines and related tryclic antidepressants (Douglass, Salins et al. 2002). Recently Gonález-Andrade and col, has been designed a alternative biosensing assay for CaM inhibitors by chemical modification of bromobimane at position 124 (Gonzalez-Andrade, et al. 2009; Figueroa, et al. 2010), that allowed to determine the IC_{50} and K_d of the CaM inhibitors in a same fluorescent assay Fig 6.

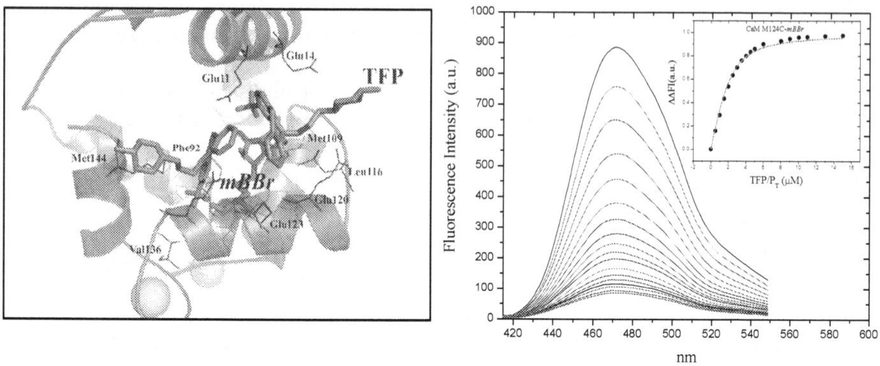

Fig. 6. Structural moeling of the trifluoroperazine into the binding site of calmodulin and fluoresence titration to compare with fluorescent changes.

7. Conclusions

The well established method to attach fluorescent labels into the structure of a protein mentioned above by chemical methods in combination in some cases with the molecular biology methodologies, is making available a broad number of proteins to monitor a diverse protein interactions. The selection of a protein receptor that should be a target form drug design for example the case of G protein coupled receptors (GPCR), that represent close of the 30 % of the drug market, or calmoduilin that participates in a large number of protein signals, provided a excellent protein receptor to be adapted in robust protein immobilization methods required in the development of new strategies in the drug research by high throughput screening.

8. Acknowledgments

This work was partially supported by grant 53633 from CONACYT, México. Martin González-Andrade acknowledges postdoctoral fellowship, awarded by DGAPA-UNAM.

9. References

Altenbach, C., J. Klein-Seetharaman, et al. (1999). Structural features and light-dependent changes in the sequence 59-75 connecting helices I and II in rhodopsin: a site-directed spin-labeling study. Biochemistry 38(25): 7945-7949.

Berridge, M. J., M. D. Bootman, et al. (2003). Calcium signalling: dynamics, homeostasis and remodelling. Nat Rev Mol Cell Biol 4(7): 517-529.

Campbell, R. E. (2009). Fluorescent-protein-based biosensors: modulation of energy transfer as a design principle. Anal Chem 81(15): 5972-5979.

Carafoli, E. and C. B. Klee (1999). Calcium as a cellular regulator. New York, Oxford University Press.

Cooper, M. A. (2003). Biosensor profiling of molecular interactions in pharmacology. Curr Opin Pharmacol 3(5): 557-562.

Dagher, R., C. Pigault, et al. (2006). Use of a fluorescent polarization based high throughput assay to identify new calmodulin ligands. Biochim Biophys Acta 1763(11): 1250-1255.

Dattelbaum, J. D., L. L. Looger, et al. (2005). Analysis of allosteric signal transduction mechanisms in an engineered fluorescent maltose biosensor. Protein Sci 14(2): 284-291.

de Lorimier, R. M., J. J. Smith, et al. (2002). Construction of a fluorescent biosensor family. Protein Sci 11(11): 2655-2675.

de Lorimier, R. M., Y. Tian, et al. (2006). Binding and signaling of surface-immobilized reagentless fluorescent biosensors derived from periplasmic binding proteins. Protein Sci 15(8): 1936-1944.

Deuschle, K., S. Okumoto, et al. (2005). Construction and optimization of a family of genetically encoded metabolite sensors by semirational protein engineering. Protein Sci 14(9): 2304-2314.

Douglass, P. M., L. L. Salins, et al. (2002). Class-selective drug detection: fluorescently-labeled calmodulin as the biorecognition element for phenothiazines and tricyclic antidepressants. Bioconjug Chem 13(6): 1186-1192.

Figueroa, et al. (2010). Fluorescence, circular dichroism, NMR, and docking studies of the interaction of the alkaloid malbrancheamide with calmodulin. J Enzyme Inhib Med Chem.

Filipek, S., R. E. Stenkamp, et al. (2003). G protein-coupled receptor rhodopsin: a prospectus. Annu Rev Physiol 65: 851-879.

Gangopadhyay, J. P., Z. Grabarek, et al. (2004). Fluorescence probe study of Ca2+-dependent interactions of calmodulin with calmodulin-binding peptides of the ryanodine receptor. Biochem Biophys Res Commun 323(3): 760-768.

Gonzalez-Andrade, M., M. Figueroa, et al. (2009). An alternative assay to discover potential calmodulin inhibitors using a human fluorophore-labeled CaM protein. Anal Biochem 387(1): 64-70.

Janz, J. M. and D. L. Farrens (2004). Rhodopsin activation exposes a key hydrophobic binding site for the transducin alpha-subunit C terminus. J Biol Chem 279(28): 29767-29773.

LaConte, L. E., V. Voelz, et al. (2002). Molecular dynamics simulation of site-directed spin labeling: experimental validation in muscle fibers. Biophys J 83(4): 1854-1866.

Looger, L. L., M. A. Dwyer, et al. (2003). Computational design of receptor and sensor proteins with novel functions. Nature 423(6936): 185-190.

Mansoor, S. E. and D. L. Farrens (2004). High-throughput protein structural analysis using site-directed fluorescence labeling and the bimane derivative (2-pyridyl)dithiobimane. Biochemistry 43(29): 9426-9438.

Mansoor, S. E., H. S. McHaourab, et al. (2002). Mapping proximity within proteins using fluorescence spectroscopy. A study of T4 lysozyme showing that tryptophan residues quench bimane fluorescence. Biochemistry 41(8): 2475-2484.

Medintz, I. L. and J. R. Deschamps (2006). Maltose-binding protein: a versatile platform for prototyping biosensing. Curr Opin Biotechnol 17(1): 17-27.

Nagase, T., E. Nakata, et al. (2003). Construction of artificial signal transducers on a lectin surface by post-photoaffinity-labeling modification for fluorescent saccharide biosensors. Chemistry 9(15): 3660-3669.

Nakata, E., T. Nagase, et al. (2004). Coupling a natural receptor protein with an artificial receptor to afford a semisynthetic fluorescent biosensor. J Am Chem Soc 126(2): 490-495.

O'Neil, K. T. and W. F. DeGrado (1990). How calmodulin binds its targets: sequence independent recognition of amphiphilic alpha-helices. Trends Biochem Sci 15(2): 59-64.

Ojida, A., Y. Miyahara, et al. (2004). Recognition and fluorescence sensing of specific amino acid residue on protein surface using designed molecules. Biopolymers 76(2): 177-184.

Owenius, R., M. Osterlund, et al. (2001). Spin and fluorescent probing of the binding interface between tissue factor and factor VIIa at multiple sites. Biophys J 81(4): 2357-2369.

Plaxco, K. W. and H. T. Soh (2011). Switch-based biosensors: a new approach towards real-time, in vivo molecular detection. Trends Biotechnol 29(1): 1-5.

Sharma, B., S. K. Deo, et al. (2005). Competitive binding assay using fluorescence resonance energy transfer for the identification of calmodulin antagonists. Bioconjug Chem 16(5): 1257-1263.

Sommer, M. E., W. C. Smith, et al. (2005). Dynamics of arrestin-rhodopsin interactions: arrestin and retinal release are directly linked events. J Biol Chem 280(8): 6861-6871.

Sommer, M. E., W. C. Smith, et al. (2006). Dynamics of arrestin-rhodopsin interactions: acidic phospholipids enable binding of arrestin to purified rhodopsin in detergent. J Biol Chem 281(14): 9407-9417.

Tsukiji, S., M. Miyagawa, et al. (2009). Ligand-directed tosyl chemistry for protein labeling in vivo. Nat Chem Biol 5(5): 341-343.

Tsukiji, S., H. Wang, et al. (2009). Quenched ligand-directed tosylate reagents for one-step construction of turn-on fluorescent biosensors. J Am Chem Soc 131(25): 9046-9054.

Vallee-Belisle, A. and K. W. Plaxco (2010). Structure-switching biosensors: inspired by Nature. Curr Opin Struct Biol 20(4): 518-526.

Wang, H., E. Nakata, et al. (2009). Recent progress in strategies for the creation of protein-based fluorescent biosensors. Chembiochem 10(16): 2560-2577.

Weinstein, H. and E. L. Mehler (1994). Ca(2+)-binding and structural dynamics in the functions of calmodulin. Annu Rev Physiol 56: 213-236.

Zhang, M. and T. Yuan (1998). Molecular mechanisms of calmodulin's functional versatility. Biochem Cell Biol 76(2-3): 313-323.

Zielinski, R. E. (1998). Calmodulin and Calmodulin-Binding Proteins in Plants. Annu Rev Plant Physiol Plant Mol Biol 49: 697-725.

2

AlGaN/GaN High Electron Mobility Transistor Based Sensors for Bio-Applications

Fan Ren[1], Stephen J. Pearton[2], Byoung Sam Kang[1] and Byung Hwan Chu[1]
[1]Department of Chemical Engineering, University Florida
[2]Department of Materials Science and Engineering, University of Florida
USA

1. Introduction

Chemical sensors have gained in importance in the past decade for applications that include homeland security, medical and environmental monitoring and also food safety. A desirable goal is the ability to simultaneously analyze a wide variety of environmental and biological gases and liquids in the field and to be able to selectively detect a target analyte with high specificity and sensitivity. In the area of detection of medical biomarkers, many different methods, including enzyme-linked immunsorbent assay (ELISA), particle-based flow cytometric assays, electrochemical measurements based on impedance and capacitance, electrical measurement of microcantilever resonant frequency change, and conductance measurement of semiconductor nanostructures. gas chromatography (GC), ion chromatography, high density peptide arrays, laser scanning quantitiative analysis, chemiluminescence, selected ion flow tube (SIFT), nanomechanical cantilevers, bead-based suspension microarrays, magnetic biosensors and mass spectrometry (MS) have been employed (Burlingame, Boyd and Gaskell 1996, Jackson and Chen 1996, Anderson, Bowden and Pickup 1996, Chen et al. 2003, Li et al. 2005, Zhang et al. 2006, Huber, Lang and Gerber 2008, Sandhu 2007, Zheng et al. 2005b). Depending on the sample condition, these methods may show variable results in terms of sensitivity for some applications and may not meet the requirements for a handheld biosensor.

For homeland security applications, reliable detection of biological agents in the field and in real time is challenging. During the anthrax attack on the World Bank in 2002, field tests showed 1200 workers to be positive, and all were sent home. 100 workers were provided antibiotics. However, confirmatory testing showed zero positives. False positives and false negatives can result due to very low volumes of samples available for testing and poor device sensitivities. Toxins such as ricin, botulinum toxin or enterotoxin B are environmentally stable, can be mass-produced and do not need advanced technologies for production and dispersal. The threat of these toxins is real. This is evident from the recent ricin detection from White House mail facilities and a US senator's office. Terrorists have already attempted to use botulinum toxin as a bio-weapon. Aerosols were dispersed at multiple sites in Tokyo, and at US military installations in Japan on at least 3 occasions between 1990 and 1995 by the Japanese cult Aum Shinrikyo (Greenfield et al. 2002). Four of the countries listed by the US government as "state sponsors of terrorism" (Iran, Iraq, North Korea, and Syria) (Greenfield et al. 2002) have developed, or are believed to be developing, botulinum toxin as a weapon (Cordesman 1998, Bermudez 2001). After the 1991 Persian Gulf War, Iraq admitted to the United Nations inspection team to having produced 19000 L of concentrated botulinum toxin, of which approximately 10000 L were loaded into military weapons. This toxin has not been fully accounted for and constitutes approximately 3 times the amount needed to kill the entire current human population by inhalation (Greenfield et al. 2002). A significant issue is the absence of a definite diagnostic method and the difficulty in differential diagnosis from other pathogens that would slow the response in case of a terror attack. This is a critical need that has to be met to have an effective response to terrorist attacks. Given the adverse consequences of a lack of reliable biological agent sensing on national security, there is a critical need to develop novel, more sensitive and reliable technologies for biological detection in the field (Arnon et al. 2001). Some specific toxins of interest include Enterotoxin type B (Category B, NIAID), Botulinum toxin (Category A NIAID) and ricin (Category B NIAID).

While the techniques mentioned above show excellent performance under lab conditions, there is also a need for small, handheld sensors with wireless connectivity that have the capability for fast responses. The chemical sensor market represents the largest segment for sales of sensors, including chemical detection in gases and liquids, flue gas and fire detection, liquid quality sensors, biosensors and medical sensors. Some of the major applications in the home include indoor air quality and natural gas detection. Attention is now being paid to more demanding applications where a high degree of chemical specificity and selectivity is required. For biological and medical sensing applications, disease diagnosis by detecting specific biomarkers (functional or structural abnormal enzymes, low molecular weight proteins, or antigen) in blood, urine, saliva, or tissue samples has been established. Most of the techniques mentioned earlier such as ELISA possesses a major limitation in that only one analyte is measured at a time. Particle-based assays allow for multiple detection by using multiple beads but the whole detection process is generally longer than 2 hours, which is not practical for in-office or bedside detection. Electrochemical devices have attracted attention due to their low cost and simplicity, but significant improvements in their sensitivities are still needed for use with clinical samples. Microcantilevers are capable of detecting concentrations as low as 10 pg/ml, but suffer from an undesirable resonant frequency change due to the viscosity of the medium and cantilever damping in the solution environment. Nano-material devices have provided an excellent option toward fast, label-free, sensitive, selective, and multiple detections for both preclinical and clinical applications. Examples of detection of biomarkers using electrical measurements with semiconductor devices include carbon nanotubes for lupus erythematosus antigen detection (Chen et al. 2003), compound semiconducting nanowires and In_2O_3 nanowires for prostate-specific antigen detection (Li et al. 2005), and silicon nanowire arrays for detecting prostate-specific antigen [(Zheng et al. 2005a)]. In clinical settings, biomarkers for a particular disease state can be used to determine the presence of disease as well as its progress.

Semiconductor-based sensors can be fabricated using mature techniques from the Si chip industry and/or novel nanotechnology approaches. Silicon based sensors are still the dominant component of the semiconductor segment due to their low cost, reproducible and controllable electronic response. However, these sensors are not suited for operation in harsh environments, for instance, high temperature, high pressure or corrosive ambients. Si will be etched by some of the acidic or basic aqueous solutions encountered in biological sensing. By sharp contrast, GaN is not etched by any acid or base at temperatures below a few hundred degrees. Therefore, wide band-gap group III nitride compound semiconductors (AlGaInN materials system) are alternative options to supplement silicon in these applications because of their chemical resistance, high temperature/high power capability, high electron saturation velocity and simple integration with existing GaN-based UV light-emitting diode, UV detectors and wireless communication chips.

A promising sensing technology utilizes AlGaN/GaN high electron mobility transistors (HEMTs). HEMT structures have been developed for use in microwave power amplifiers due to their high two dimensional electron gas (2DEG) mobility and saturation velocity. The conducting 2DEG channel of AlGaN/GaN HEMTs is very close to the surface and extremely sensitive to adsorption of analytes. HEMT sensors can be used for detecting gases, ions, pH values, proteins, and DNA.

The GaN materials system is attracting much interest for commercial applications of green, blue, and UV light emitting diodes (LEDs), laser diodes as well as high speed and high frequency power devices. Due to the wide-bandgap nature of the material, it is very thermally stable, and electronic devices can be operated at temperatures up to 500 °C. The GaN based materials are also chemically stable, and no known wet chemical etchant can etch these materials; this makes them very suitable for operation in chemically harsh environments. Due to the high electron mobility, GaN material based high electron mobility transistors (HEMTs) can operate at very high frequency with higher breakdown voltage, better thermal conductivity, and wider transmission bandwidths than Si or GaAs devices [(Makimoto, Yamauchi and Kumakura 2004, Zhang et al. 2003, Saito et al. 2006)].

An overlooked potential application of the GaN HEMT structure is sensors. The high electron sheet carrier concentration of nitride HEMTs is induced by piezoelectric polarization of the strained AlGaN layer in the hetero-junction structure of the AlGaN/GaN HEMT and the spontaneous polarization is very large in wurtzite III-nitrides. This provides an increased sensitivity relative to simple Schottky diodes fabricated on GaN layers or field effect transistors (FETs) fabricated on the AlGaN/GaN HEMT structure. The gate region of the HEMT can be used to modulate the drain current in the FET mode or use as the electrode for the Schottky diode. A variety of gas, chemical and health-related sensors based on HEMT technology have been demonstrated with proper surface functionalization on the gate area of the HEMTs, including the detection of hydrogen, mercury ion, prostate specific antigen (PSA), DNA, and glucose [(Jun et al. 2007, Yu et al. 2008, Wang et al. 2006a, Wang et al. 2007a, Anderson et al. 2008, Kim et al. 2003, Wang et al. 2005a, Schalwig et al. 2002, Luther, Wolter and Mohney 1999, Kang et al. 2005a, Wang et al. 2005b, Wright et al. 2009, Johnson et al. 2009, Lim et al. 2008, Tien et al. 2005a, Kryliouk et al. 2005, Tien et al. 2005b, Wang et al. 2005c, Eickhoff et al. 2003, Mehandru et al. 2004, Neuberger et al. 2001, Gangwani et al. 2007, Shen et al. 2004, Kang et al. 2007a, Kouche et al. 2005, Wang et al. 2007d, Kang et al. 2005d, Wang et al. 2007b, Chen et al. 2008, Pearton et al. 2007, Wang et al. 2007c, Kang et al. 2008, Kang et al. 2007d, Kang et al. 2004b, Lothian et al. 1992, Johnson et al. 2000, Kang et al. 2006, Kang et al. 2005c, Kang et al. 2007b, Kang et al. 2004a, Pearton et al. 2004)].

In this chapter, we discuss recent progress in the functionalization of these semiconductor sensors for applications in detection of pH measurement, biotoxins and other biologically important chemicals and the integration of these sensors into wireless packages for remote sensing capability.

2. Sensor functionalization

Specific and selective molecular functionalization of the semiconductor surface is necessary to achieve specificity in chemical and biological detection. Devices such as field effect transistors (FETs) can readily discriminate between adsorption of oxidizing and reducing gas molecules from the changes (increase or decrease) in the channel conductance. However, precise identification of a specific type of molecule requires functionalization of the surface with specific molecules or catalysts. Effective biosensing requires coupling of the unique functional properties of proteins, nucleic acids (DNA, RNA), and other biological molecules with the solid-state "chip" platforms. These devices take advantage of the specific, complementary interactions between biological molecules that are a fundamental aspect of biological function. Specific, complementary interactions are what permit antibodies to recognize antigens in the immune response, enzymes to recognize their target substrates, and the motor proteins of muscle to shorten during muscular contraction. The ability of biological molecules, such as proteins, to bind other molecules in a highly specific manner is the underlying principle of the "sensors" to detect the presence (or absence) of target molecules - just as it is in the biological senses of smell and taste.

One of the key technical challenges in fabricating hybrid biosensors is the junction between biological macromolecules and the inorganic scaffolding material (metals and semiconductors) of the chip. For actual device applications, it is often necessary to selectively modify a surface at micro- and even nano-scale, sometimes with different surface chemistry at different locations. In order to enhance detection speed, especially at very low analyte concentration, the analyte should be delivered directly to the active sensing areas of the sensors. A common theme for bio/chem sensors is that their operation often incorporates moving fluids. For example, sensors must sample a stream of air or water to interact with the specific molecules they are designed to detect.

The general approach to detecting biological species using a semiconductor sensor involves functionalizing the surface (e.g. the gate region of an ungated field effect transistor structure) with a layer or substance which will selectively bind the molecules of interest. In applications requiring less specific detection, the adsorption of reactive molecules will directly affect the surface charge and affect the near-surface conductivity. In their simplest form, the sensor consists of a semiconductor film patterned with surface electrodes and often heated to temperatures of a few hundred degrees Celsius to enhance dissociation of molecules on the exposed surface. Changes in resistance between the electrodes signal the adsorption of reactive molecules. It is desirable to be able to use the lowest possible operating temperature to maximize battery life in hand-held detection instruments. Electronic oxides such as ZnO as the sensing material are especially sensitive to reaction of target molecules with adsorbed oxygen or the oxygen in the lattice itself.

Biologically modified field effect transistors (bioFETs) have the potential to directly detect biochemical interactions in aqueous solutions. To enhance their practicality, the device must be sensitive to biochemical interactions on its surface, functionalized to probe specific biochemical interactions and must be stable in aqueous solutions for a range of pH and salt concentrations. Typically, the gate region of the device is covered with biological probes, which are used as receptor sites for the molecules of interest. The conductance of the device is changed as reaction occurs between these probes and appropriate species in solution.

Since GaN-based material systems are chemically stable, this should minimize degradation of adsorbed cells. The bond between Ga and N is ionic and proteins can easily attach to the

GaN surface. This is one of the key factors for making a sensitive biosensor with a useful lifetime. HEMT sensors have been used for detecting gases, ions, pH values, proteins, and DNA temperature with good selectivity by the modification of the surface in the gate region of the HEMT. The 2DEG channel is connected to an Ohmic-type source and drain contacts. The source-drain current is modulated by a third contact, a Schottky-type gate, on the top of the 2DEG channel. For sensing applications, the third contact is affected by the sensing environment, i.e. the sensing targets changes the charges on the gate region and behave as a gate. When charged analytes accumulate on the gate area, these charges form a bias and alter the 2DEG resistance. This electrical detection technique is simple, fast, and convenient. The detecting signal from the gate is amplified through the drain-source current and makes this sensor to be very sensitive for sensor applications. The electric signal also can be easily quantified, recorded and transmit, unlike fluorescence detection methods which need human inspection and are difficult to precisely quantify and transmit the data.

One drawback of HEMT sensors is a lack of selectivity to different analytes due to the chemical inertness of the HEMT surface. This can be solved by surface modification with detecting receptors. Sensor devices of the present disclosure can be used with a variety of fluids having environmental and bodily origins, including saliva, urine, blood, and breath. For use with exhaled breath, the device may include a HEMT bonded on a thermo-electric cooling device, which assists in condensing exhaled breath samples.

In our HEMT devices, the surface is generally functionalized with an antibody or enzyme layer. The success of the functionalization is monitored by a number of methods. Examples are shown in Figures 1 and 2. The first test is a change in surface tension when the functional layer is in place and the change in surface bonding can in some cases be seen by X-Ray Photoelectron Spectroscopy. Typically, a layer of Au is deposited on the gate region of the HEMT as a platform to attach a chemical such as thioglycolic acid, whose S-bonds readily attach to the Au. The antibody layer can then be attached to the thioglycolic acid. When the surface is completely covered by these functional layers, the HEMT will not be sensitive to buffer solutions or water that do not contain the antigen of interest, as shown in Figure 2. For detecting hydrogen, the gate region is functionalized with a catalyst metal such as Pt or Pd. In other cases, we immobilize an enzyme to catalyze reactions, as is used for the detection of glucose. In the presence of the enzyme glucose oxidase, glucose will react with oxygen to produce gluconic acid and hydrogen peroxide. Table I shows a summary of the surface functionalization layers we have employed for HEMT sensors to date. There are many additional options for detection of biotoxins and biological molecules of interest by use of different protein or antibody layers. The advantage of the biofet approach is that large arrays of HEMTs can be produced on a single chip and functionalized with different layers to allow for detection of a broad range of chemicals or gases.

3. pH Measurement

The measurement of pH is needed in many different applications, including medicine, biology, chemistry, food science, environmental science and oceanography. Solutions with a pH less than 7 are acidic and solutions with a pH greater than 7 are basic or alkaline. We have found that ZnO nanorod surfaces respond electrically to variations of the pH in electrolyte solutions introduced via an integrated microchannel [(Kang et al. 2005b)]. The ion-induced changes in surface potential are readily measured as a change in conductance of the single ZnO nanorods and suggest that these structures are very promising for a wide variety of sensor applications. An integrated microchannel was made from SYLGARD@ 184 polymer. Entry and exit holes in the ends of the channel were made with a small puncher (diameter less than 1mm) and the film immediately applied to the nanorod sensor. The pH solution was applied using a syringe autopipette (2-20ul).

Detection	Mechanism	Surface Functionalization
H_2	Catalytic dissociation	Pd, Pt
Pressure change	polarization	Polyvinylidene difluoride
Botulinum toxin	antibody	Thioglycolic acid/antibody
Proteins	Conjugation/hybridization	Aminopropylsilane/biotin
pH	Adsorption of polar molecules	Sc_2O_3, ZnO
Hg^{2+}	chelation	Thioglycolic acid/Au
KIM-1	antibody	KIM-1 antibody
Glucose	GO_X immobilization	ZnO nanorods
Prostate Specific Antigen	PSA antibody	Carboxylate succimdyl ester/PSA antibody
Lactic acid	LO_X immobilization	ZnO nanorods
Chloride ions	Anodization	Ag/AgCl electrodes; InN
Breast Cancer	antibody	Thyioglycolic acid/c-erbB antibody
CO_2	Absorption of water/charge	Polyethylenimine/starch
DNA	hybridization	3′-thiol-modified oligonucleotides
O_2	oxidation	InGaZnO

Table 1. Summary of surface functional layers used with HEMT sensors

Prior to the pH measurements, we used pH 4, 7, 10 buffer solutions to calibrate the electrode and the measurements at 25 °C were carried out in the dark or under ultra-violet(UV) illumination from 365 nm light using an Agilent 4156C parameter analyzer to avoid parasitic effects. The pH solution made by the titration method using HNO_3, NaOH and distilled water. The electrode was a conventional Acumet standard Ag/AgCl electrode. The nanorods showed a very strong photoresponse. The conductivity is greatly increased as a result of the illumination, as evidenced by the higher current. No effect was observed for illumination with below bandgap light. The photoconduction appears predominantly to originate in bulk conduction processes with only a minor surface trapping component. The adsorption of polar molecules on the surface of ZnO affects the surface potential and device characteristics. The current at a bias of 0.5V as a function of time from nanorods exposed for 60s to a series of solutions whose pH was varied from 2-12 was reduced upon exposure to these polar liquids as the pH is increased. The experiment was conducted starting at pH=7 and went to pH=2 or 12. The I-V measurement in air was slightly higher that in the

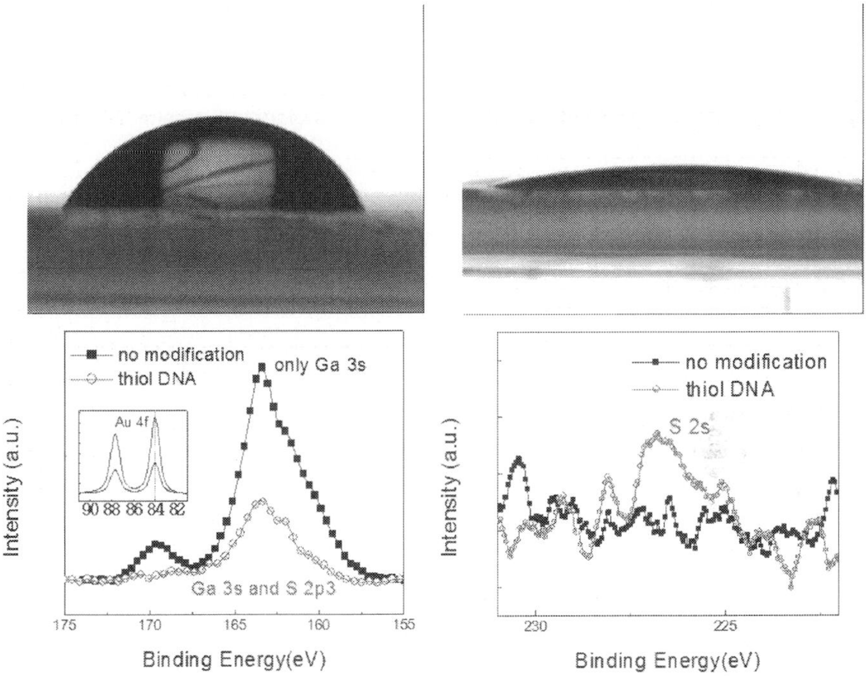

Fig. 1. Examples of a change in surface tension of the HEMT surface functionalization (top) and XPS measurement of formation of Au-S bonds after attachment of thioglycolic acid attachment to Au layer in gate region of HEMT.

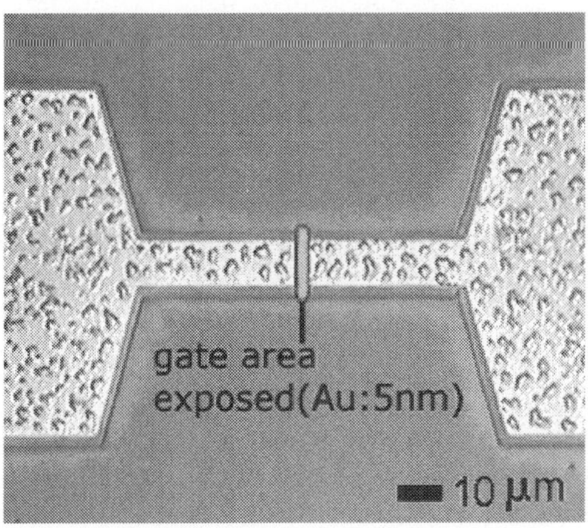

Fig. 2. Example of successful functionalization of HEMT surface-the device is no longer sensitive to water when the surface is completely covered with the functional layer.

pH=7(10-20%). The data in shows the sensor is sensitive to the concentration of the polar liquid and therefore could be used to differentiate between liquids into which a small amount of leakage of another substance has occurred. The conductance of the rods was higher under UV illumination but the percentage change in conductance is similar with and without illumination. The nanorods exhibited a linear change in conductance between pH 2-12 of 8.5nS/pH in the dark and 20nS/pH when illuminated with UV (365nm) light as shown at the bottom of Figure 16.The nanorods show stable operation with a resolution of ~0.1 pH over the entire pH range, showing the remarkable sensitivity to relatively small changes in concentration of the liquid.

Ungated AlGaN/ GaN HEMTs also exhibit large changes in current upon exposing the gate region to polar liquids. The polar nature of the electrolyte introduced led to a change of surface charges, producing a change in surface potential at the semiconductor /liquid interface. The use of Sc_2O_3 gate dielectric produced superior results to either a native oxide or UV ozone-induced oxide in the gate region. The ungated HEMTs with Sc_2O_3 in the gate region exhibited a linear change in current between pH 3-10 of 37μA/pH .The HEMT pH sensors show stable operation with a resolution of < 0.1 pH over the entire pH range. 100Å Sc_2O_3 was deposited as a gate dielectric through a contact window of SiN_x layer. Before oxide deposition, the wafer was exposed to ozone for 25 minutes. It was then heated in-situ at 300 °C cleaning for 10mins inside the growth chamber. The Sc_2O_3 was deposited by rf plasma-activated MBE at 100 °C using elemental Sc evaporated from a standard effusion at 1130 °C and O_2 derived from an Oxford RF plasma source. For comparison, we also fabricated devices with just the native oxide present in the gate region and also with the UV ozone -induced oxide. Figure 3 shows a scanning electron microscopy (SEM) image (top) and a cross-sectional schematic (bottom) of the completed device. The gate dimension of the device is $2 \times 50\ \mu m^2$. The pH solution was applied using a syringe autopipette (2-20ul).

Prior to the pH measurements, we used pH 4, 7, 10 buffer solutions from Fisher Scientific to calibrate the electrode and the measurements at 25 °C were carried out in the dark using an Agilent 4156C parameter analyzer to avoid parasitic effects. The pH solution made by the titration method using HCl, NaOH and distilled water. The electrode was a conventional Acumet standard Ag/AgCl electrode.

The adsorption of polar molecules on the surface of the HEMT affected the surface potential and device characteristics. Figure 4 shows the current at a bias of 0.25V as a function of time from HEMTs with Sc_2O_3 in the gate region exposed for 150s to a series of solutions whose pH was varied from 3-10. The current is significantly increased upon exposure to these polar liquids as the pH is decreased. The change in current was 37 μA/pH.

The HEMTs show stable operation with a resolution of ~0.1 pH over the entire pH range, showing the remarkable sensitivity of the HEMT to relatively small changes in concentration of the liquid. By comparison, devices with the native oxide in the gate region showed a higher sensitivity of ~70 μA/pA but a much poorer resolution of ~0.4 pH and evidence of delays in response of 10-15 secs. The latter may result from deep traps at the interface between the semiconductor and native oxide, whose density is much higher than at the Sc_2O_3-nitride interface. The devices with UV-ozone oxide in the gate region did not show these incubation times for detection of pH changes and showed similar sensitivities of gate source current as the Sc_2O_3 gate devices (~40 μA/pH) but with poorer resolution (~0.25 pH). Figure 9 shows that the HEMT sensor with Sc_2O_3 gate dielectric is sensitive to the concentration of the polar liquid and therefore could be used to differentiate between

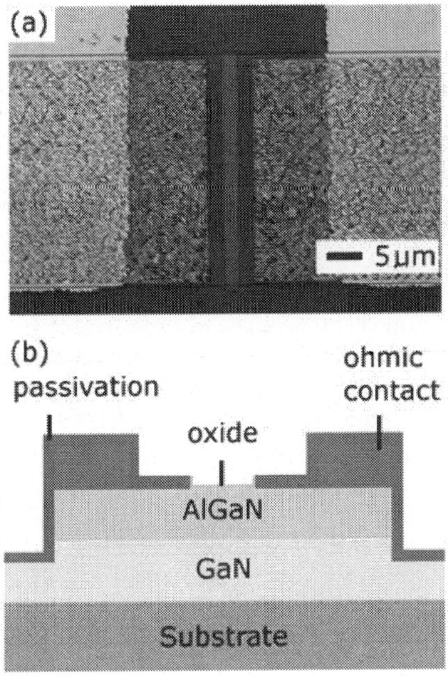

Fig. 3. (a) SEM and schematic of gateless HEMT. (b) Schematic of the pH sensor.

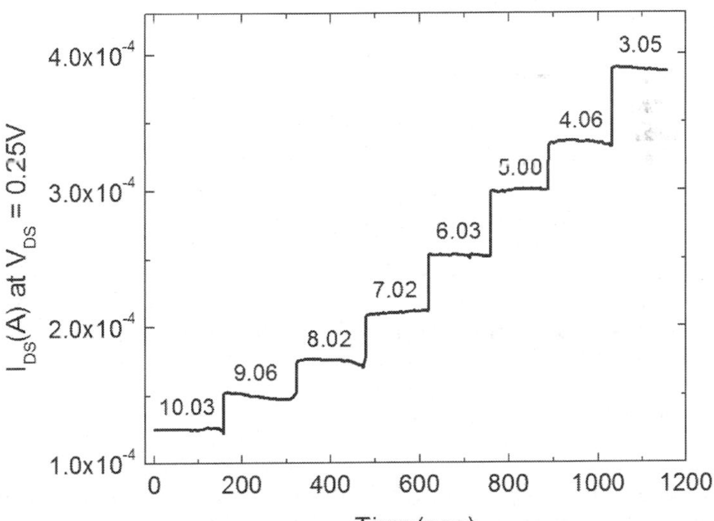

Fig. 4. Change in current in gateless HEMT at fixed source-drain bias of 0.25 V with pH from 3-10.

liquids into which a small amount of leakage of another substance has occurred. As mentioned earlier, the pH range of interest for human blood is 7-8. Figure 5 shows the current change in the HEMTs with Sc_2O_3 at a bias of 0.25V for different pH values in this range. Note that the resolution of the measurement is < 0.1 pH. There is still more to understand about the mechanism of the current reduction in relation to the adsorption of the polar liquid molecules on the HEMT surface. These molecules are bonded by van der-Waals type interactions and they screen surface change that is induced by polarization in the HEMT.

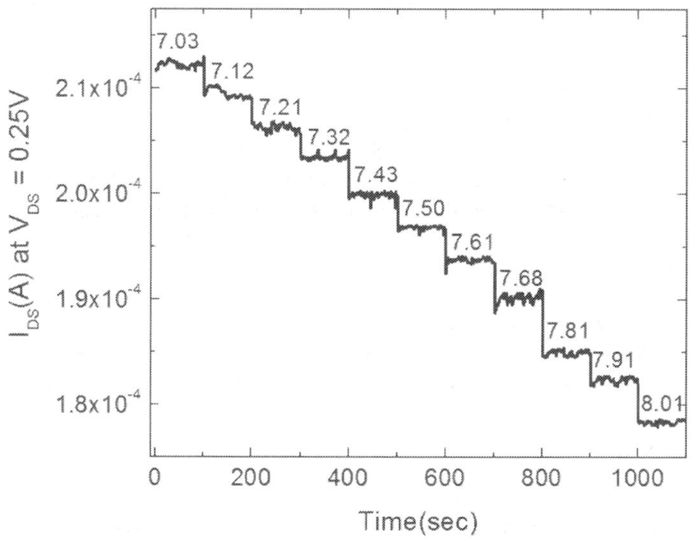

Fig. 5. Change in current in gateless HEMT at fixed source-drain bias of 0.25 V with pH from 7-8.

4. Sensing the pH value in the exhaled breath condensate

There is significant interest in developing rapid diagnostic approaches and improved sensors for determining early signs of medical problems in humans. Exhaled breath is a unique bodily fluid that can be utilized in this regard (Horvath et al. 2005, Namjou, Roller and McCann 2006, Machado et al. 2005, Kullmann et al. 2007, Vaughan et al. 2003, Hunt et al. 2000, Kostikas et al. 2002, Carpagnano et al. 2005, Gessner et al. 2003, Kullmann et al. 2008, Accordino et al. 2008, Czebe et al. 2008). Exhaled breath condensate pH is a robust and reproducible assay of airway acidity. For example, the blood pH range that is relevant for humans is 7-8. Humans, even when they are extremely ill, will not have a blood (or interstitial = space between cells in tissue) pH below 7. When they do drift below this value, it almost invariably equals mortality.

While most applications will detect substances or diseases in the breath as a gas or aerosol, breath can also be analyzed in the liquid phase as exhaled breath condensate (EBC). Analytes contained in the breath originating from deep within the lungs (alveolar gas) equilibrates with the blood, and therefore the concentration of molecules present in the breath is closely correlated with those found in the blood at any given time. EBC contains dozens of different biomarkers, such as adenosine, ammonia, hydrogen peroxide, isoprostanes, leukotrienes, peptide, cytokines and nitrogen oxide (Kullmann et al. 2008, Accordino et al. 2008, Czebe et al. 2008). Analysis of molecules in EBC is noninvasive and can provide a window on the metabolic state of the human body, including certain signs of cancer, respiratory diseases, liver and kidney functions.

As a diagnostic, exhaled breath offers advantages since samples can be collected and tested with results delivered in real time at the point of testing. Another advantage is that the sample can be collected non-invasively by asking a patient to blow into the disposable portion of a handheld testing device. Therefore, the sample collection method is hygienic for both the patient and the laboratory personnel. Exhaled breath can be used to detect various drugs, medications, their metabolites and markers, and this can be valuable in measuring both medication adherence and in determining the blood levels of these drugs and medications. Some of today's blood and urine-based tests might be replaced with simple breath-based testing. In consumer healthcare, diabetics would be able to test their glucose level, replacing painful and inconvenient finger-prick devices. For roadside screening of driving impairment, a point-of-care (POC) device similar in function to a handheld breath alcohol analyzer will detect drugs of abuse such as marijuana and cocaine. In workplace drug testing, a similar desktop device might eliminate the cost, embarrassment and inconvenience of workplace urine screening. In the setting of chronic oral drug therapy (e.g., treatment of schizophrenia with atypical antipsychotic medications), mortality/morbidity and the cost of health care will be markedly reduced by developing breath-based systems that document that drugs were orally ingested and entered the blood stream.

The glucose oxidase enzyme (GOx) is commonly used in biosensors to detect levels of glucose for diabetics. By keeping track of the number of electrons passed through the enzyme, the concentration of glucose can be measured. Due to the importance and difficulty of glucose immobilization, numerous studies have been focused on the techniques of immobilization of glucose with carbon nanotubes, ZnO nano-materials, and gold particles (Bloemen et al. 2007, Park, Boo and Chung 2006). ZnO-based nano-materials are especially interesting due to their non-toxic properties, low cost of fabrication and favorable electrostatic interaction between ZnO and the GOx lever. However, the activity of GOx is highly dependent on the pH value of the solution (Pandey et al. 2007). The pH value of a typical healthy person is between 7 and 8. This can vary significantly depending on the health condition of each individual, e.g. the pH value for patients with acute asthma was reported as low as 5.23 + 0.21 (n=22) as compared to 7.65 + 0.20 (n=19) for the control subjects (Kouassi, Irudayaraj and McCarty 2005). To achieve accurate glucose concentration measurement with immobilized GO_x, it is necessary to determine the pH value and glucose concentration with an integrated pH and glucose sensor.

AlGaN/GaN HEMTs can be used for measurements of pH in EBC and glucose, through integration of the pH and glucose sensor onto a single chip and with additional integration of the sensors into a portable, wireless package for remote monitoring applications. Figure 6 shows an optical microscopy image of an integrated pH and glucose sensor chip and cross-sectional schematics of the completed pH and glucose device. The gate dimension of the pH sensor device and glucose sensors was 20×50 μm^2.

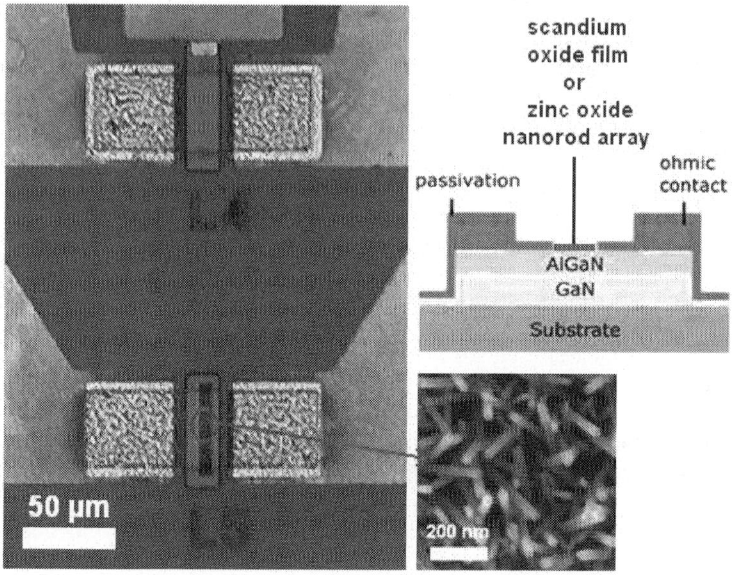

Fig. 6. SEM image of an integrated pH and glucose sensor. The insets show a schematic cross-section of the pH sensor and also an SEM of the ZnO nanorods grown in the gate region of the glucose sensor.

For the glucose detection, a highly dense array of 20-30 nm diameter and 2 µm tall ZnO nanorods were grown on the 20 × 50 μm^2 gate area. The lower right inset in Figure 6 shows closer view of the ZnO nanorod arrays grown on the gate area. The total area of the ZnO was increased significantly with the ZnO nanorods. The ZnO nanorod matrix provides a microenvironment for immobilizing negatively charged GO_x while retaining its bioactivity, and passes charges produced during the GO_x and glucose interaction to the AlGaN/GaN HEMT. The GOx solution was prepared with concentration of 10 mg/mL in 10 mM phosphate buffer saline (pH value of 7.4, Sigma Aldrich). After fabricating the device, 5 µl GO_x (~100 U/mg, Sigma Aldrich) solution was precisely introduced to the surface of the HEMT using a pico-liter plotter. The sensor chip was kept at 4 $^{\circ}C$ in the solution for 48 hours for GO_x immobilization on the ZnO nanorod arrays followed by an extensively washing to remove the un-immobilized GO_x.

To take the advantage of quick response (less than 1 sec) of the HEMT sensor, a real-time EBC collector is needed (Montuschi and Barnes 2002, Anh, Olthuis and Bergveld 2005). The amount of the EBC required to cover the HEMT sensing area is very small. Each tidal breath contains around 3 µl of the EBC. The contact angle of EBC on Sc_2O_3 has been measured to be less than 45°, and it is reasonable to assume a perfect half sphere of EBC droplet formed to cover the sensing area 4 × 50 μm^2 gate area. The volume of a half sphere with a diameter of 50 µm is around 3×10^{-11} liter. Therefore, 100,000 of 50 µm diameter droplets of EBC can be formed from each tidal breath. To condense entire 3 µl of water vapor, only ~ 7 J of energy need to be removed for each tidal breath, which can be easily achieved with a thermal electric module, a Peltier device, as shown in Figure 7. The schematic of the system for collecting the EBC is illustrated in Figure 8. The AlGaN/GaN HEMT sensor is directly mounted on the top of the Peltier unit (TB-8-0.45-1.3 HT 232, Kryotherm), as also shown in Figure 7, which can be cooled to precise temperatures by applying known voltages and currents to the unit. During our measurements, the hotter plate of the Peltier unit was kept at 21°C, and the colder plate was kept at 7 °C by applying bias of 0.7 V at 0.2 A. The sensor takes less than 2 sec to reach thermal equilibrium with the Peltier unit. This allows the exhaled breath to immediately condense on the gate region of the HEMT sensor.

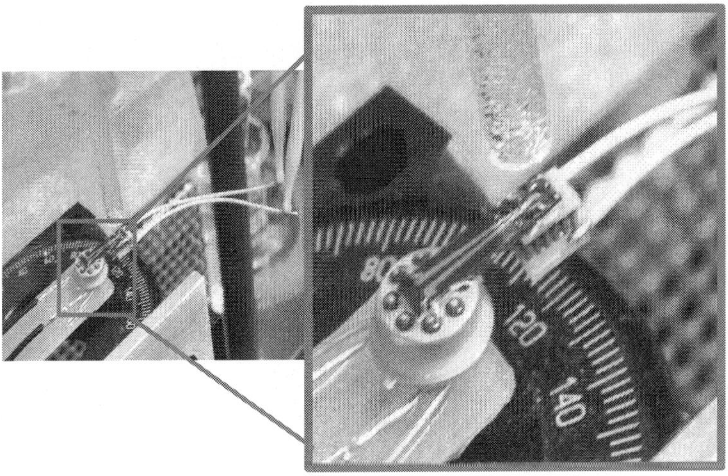

Fig. 7. Optical image of sensor mounted on Peltier cooler.

Prior to pH measurements of the EBC, a Hewlett Packard soap film flow meter and a mass flow controller were used to calibrate the flow rate of exhaled breath. The HEMT sensors were also calibrated and exhibited a linear change in current between pH 3-10 of 37μA/pH. Due to the difficulty to collect the EBC with different glucose concentration, the samples for glucose concentration detection were prepare from glucose diluted in PBS or DI water.

The HEMT sensors were not sensitive to switching of N_2 gas, but responded to applications of exhaled breath pulse inputs from a human test subject, as shown at the top of Figure 9 (top), which shows the current of a Sc_2O_3 capped HEMT sensor biased at 0.5V for exposure to different flow rates of exhaled breath (0.5-3.0 l/min). The flow rates are directly proportional to the intensity exhalation. Deep breath provides a higher flow rate. A similar study was conducted with pure N_2 to eliminate the flow rate effect on sensor sensitivity. The N_2 did not cause any change of drain current, but the increase of exhaled breath flow rate decreased the drain current proportionally from 0.5 L/min to a saturation value of 1 L/min. For every tidal breath, the beginning portion of the exhalation is from the physiologic dead space, and the gases in this space do not participate in CO_2 and O_2 exchange in the lungs. Therefore, the contents in the tidal breath are diluted by the gases from this dead space. For higher flow rate exhalation, this dilution effect is less effective. Once the exhaled breath flow rate is above 1L/min, the sensor current change reaches a limit. As a result, the test subject experiences hyper ventilation and the dilution becomes insignificant. Figure 9 (bottom) shows the time response of the sensors to much longer exhaled breaths.

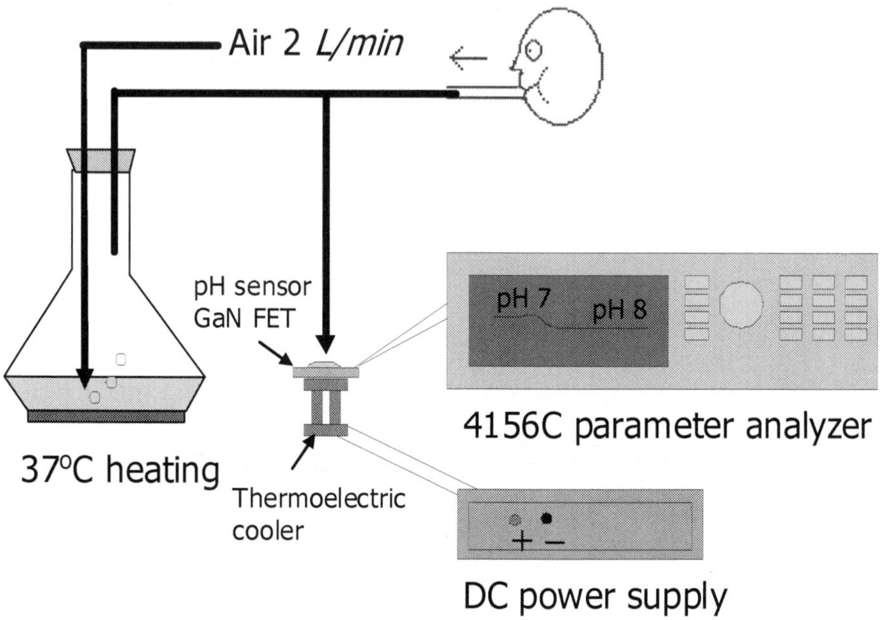

Fig. 8. Schematic of the system for collecting EBC.

The characteristic shape of the response curves is similar and is determined by the evaporation of the condensed EBC from the gate region of the HEMT sensor. The sensor is operated at 50 Hz and 10% duty cycle, which produces heat during operation. It only takes a few seconds for the EBC to vaporize from the sensing area and causes the spike-like response. The principal component of the EBC is water vapor, which represents nearly all of the volume (>99%) of the fluid collected in the EBC. The measured current change of the exhale breath condensate shows that the pH values are within the range between pH 7 and 8. This range is the typical pH range of human blood.

5. Glucose sensing

The glucose was sensed by ZnO nanorod functionalized HEMTs with glucose oxidase enzyme localized on the nanorods, shown in Figure 10. This catalyzes the reaction of glucose and oxygen to form gluconic acid and hydrogen peroxide. Figure 11 shows the real time glucose detection in PBS buffer solution using the drain current change in the HEMT sensor with constant bias of 250 mV. No current change can be seen with the addition of buffer solution at around 200 sec, showing the specificity and stability of the device. By sharp contrast, the current change showed a rapid response of less than 5 seconds when target glucose was added to the surface. So far, the glucose detection using Au nano-particle, ZnO nanorod and nanocomb, or carbon nanotube material with GOx immobilization is based on electrochemical measurement (Wang et al. 2006b, Wei et al. 2006, Yang et al. 2004, Hrapovic et al. 2004).

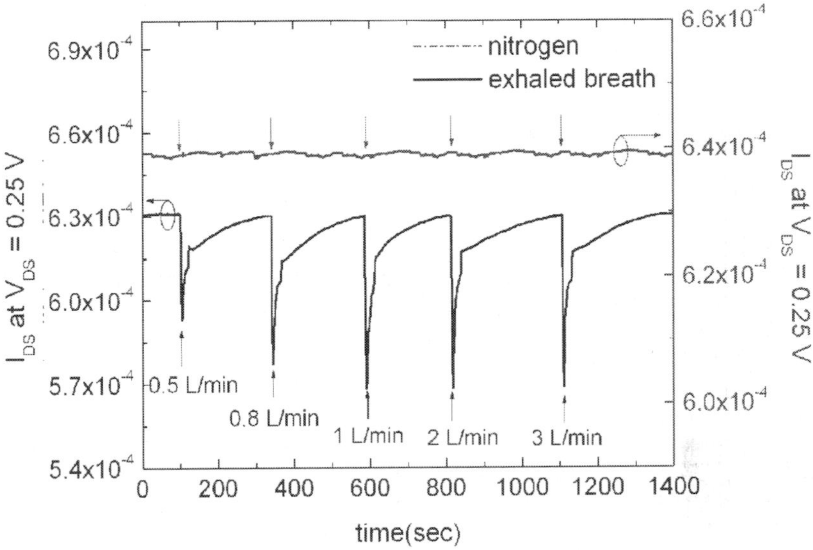

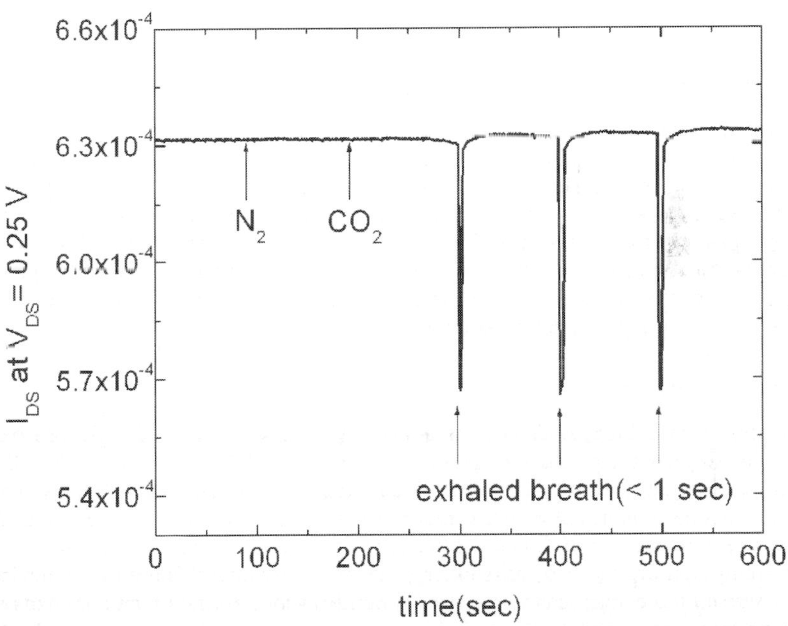

Fig. 9. Changes of drain current for HEMT sensor at fixed drain-source bias of 0.5 V with different flow rates or durations of exhaled breath from tidal breath to hyperventilation .The duration of the breath is 5 secs in the bottom figure.

Since there is a reference electrode required in the solution, the volume of sample can not be easily minimized. The current density is measured when a fixed potential applied between nano-materials and the reference electrode. This is a first order detection and the range of detection limit of these sensors is 0.5-70 μM. Even though the AlGaN/GaN HEMT based sensor used the same GOx immobilization, the ZnO nanorods were used as the gate of the HEMT. The glucose sensing was measured through the drain current of HEMT with a change of the charges on the ZnO nano-rods and the detection signal was amplified through the HEMT. Although the response of the HEMT based sensor is similar to that of an electrochemical based sensor, a much lower detection limit of 0.5 nM was achieved for the HEMT based sensor due to this amplification effect. Since there is no reference electrode required for the HEMT based sensor, the amount of sample only depends on the area of gate dimension and can be minimized. The sensors do not respond to glucose unless the enzyme is present, as shown in Figure 12.

Although measuring the glucose in the EBC is a noninvasive and convenient method for the diabetic application, the activity of the immobilized GO_x is highly dependent on the pH value of the solution. The GOx activity can be reduced to 80% for pH = 5 to 6. If the pH value of the glucose solution is larger than 8, the activity drops off very quickly (Kouassi et al. 2005). Figure 31 shows the time dependent source-drain current signals with constant drain bias of 500 mV for glucose detection in DI water and PBS buffer solution. 50 μl of PBS solution was introduced on the glucose sensor and no current change can be seen with the addition of buffer solution at 20 and 30 min. This stability is important to exclude possible noise from the mechanical change of the buffer solution. By sharp contrast, the current change showed a rapid response in less than 20 seconds when the sensor was dipped into the 100 ml of 10 mM glucose solution using DI water as the solvent. This sudden drain current increase indicated that GOx immediately reacted with glucose and oxygen was produced as a by-production of this reaction. However, the drain current gradually decreased. This was due to the oxygen produced in the GOx-glucose interaction reacting with water and changing the pH value adjacent the gate area. Since there was not agitation in the glucose solution, the solution around gate area became more basic and the activity of GOx decreased due to the high pH value environment from 60 to 85 min.

Because the lower activity of GOx in the high pH value condition, the amount of oxygen produced from GOx and glucose decreased as well during the period of 60-85 min. Once the OH^- ions produce from reaction between oxygen and water diffused away the gate area, the pH value decreased. Thus around 85 min, the pH value of the glucose solution around gate area decreased low enough to allow the activity of GOx to resume and the drain current of the glucose sensor showed another sudden increase. Then, the same process happened again and drain current of the glucose current gradually decreased for a second time.

On the contrary, when the glucose sensor was used in a pH controlled environment, the drain current stayed fairly constant, as shown in Figure 13. In this experiment, 50 μl of PBS solution was introduced on the glucose sensor to establish the base line of the sensor as in the previous experiment. Then, glucose of 10 nM concentration prepared in PBS solution was introduced to the gate area of the glucose sensor through a micro-injector. There was no glucose in the 50 μl PBS solution and the PBS solution was added at 20 and 30 min. It took time for the glucose solution to diffuse to the gate area of the sensor through the blank PBS and the drain current gradually increased corresponding to the glucose diffusion process. Since the fresh glucose was continuously provided to the sensor surface and the pH value of the glucose was controlled, once the concentration of the glucose reached equilibrium at the gate of the glucose sensor, the drain current of the glucose remained constant except in the presence of glucose solution, which was taken out from time to time using a micro-pipette. There were small oscillations of the drain current observed, which could be eliminated by using a microfluidic device for this experiment.

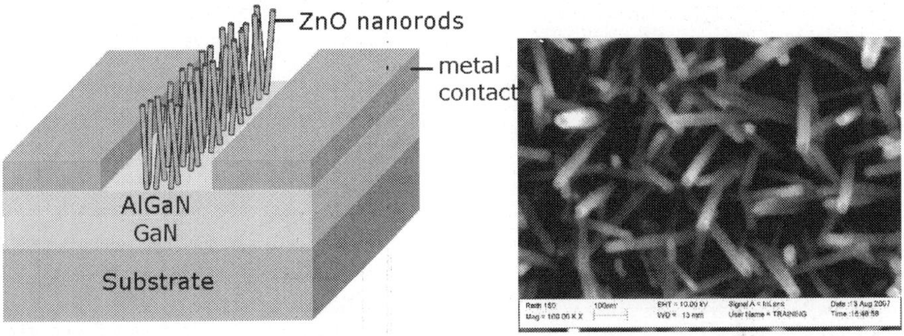

Fig. 10. (left) Schematic of ZnO nanorod functionalized HEMT and (right) SEM of nanorods on gate area.

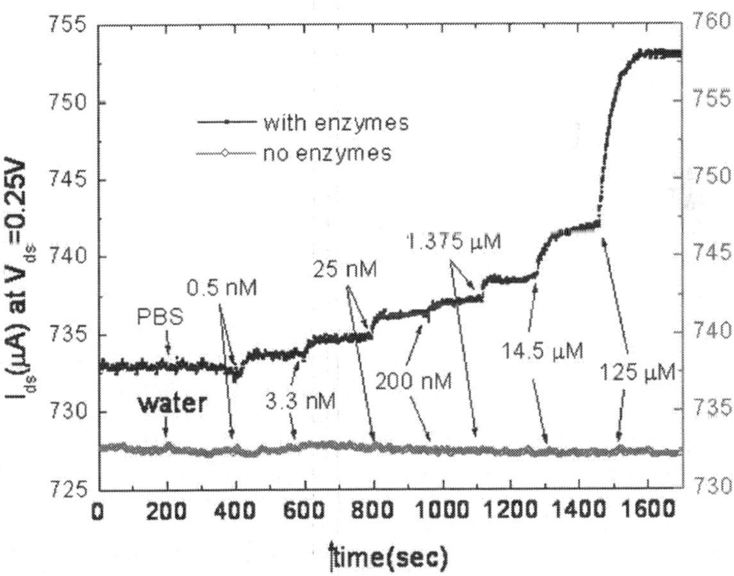

Fig. 11. Plot of drain current versus time with successive exposure of glucose from 500 pM to 125 μM in 10 mM phosphate buffer saline with a pH value of 7.4, both with and without the enzyme located on the nanorods.

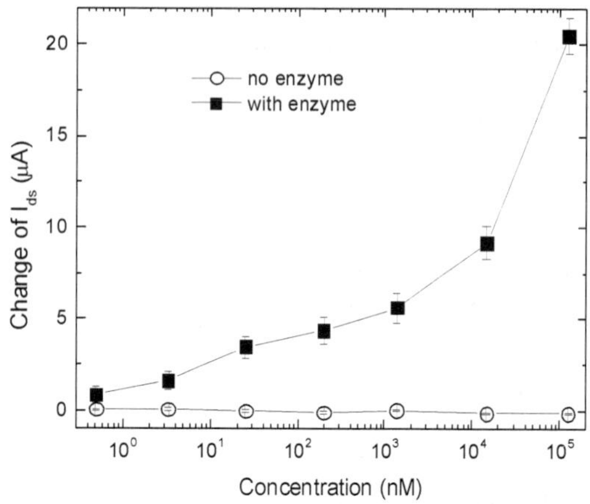

Fig. 12. Change in drain-source current in HEMT glucose sensors both with and without localized enzyme.

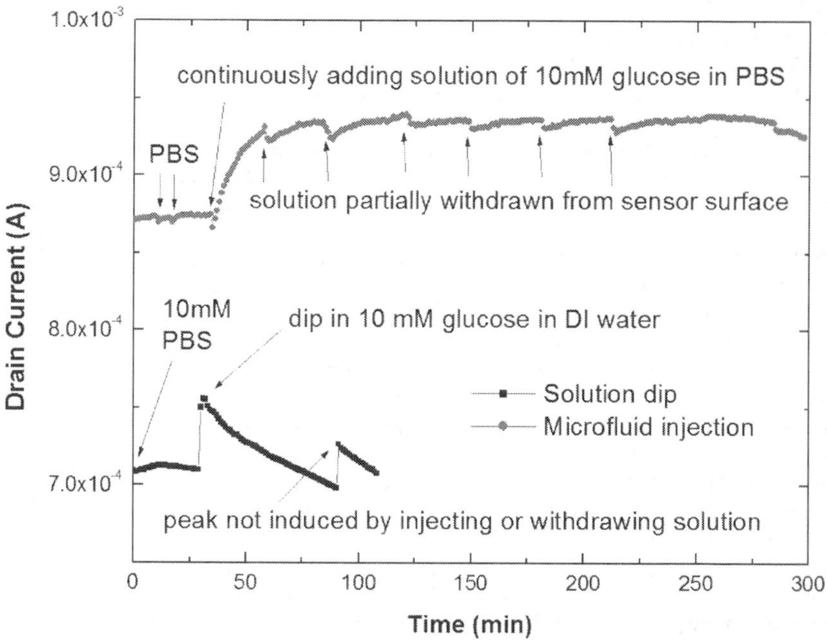

Fig. 13. Plot of drain current versus time by dipping the glucose sensor in 10 mM of glucose dissolved in DI water (black line) and exposing the sensor to continuously flow of 10 mM of glucose dissolved in phosphate buffer saline with a pH value of 7.4(red line).

The human pH value can vary significantly depending on the health condition. Since we cannot control the pH value of the EBC samples, we needed to measure the pH value while determine the glucose concentration in the EBC. With the fast response time and low volume of the EBC required for HEMT based sensor, a handheld and real-time glucose sensing technology can be realized.

6. Bio-toxin sensing

Reliable detection of biological agents in the field and in real time is challenging. Given the adverse consequences of a lack of reliable biological agent sensing on national security, there is a critical need to develop novel, more sensitive and reliable technologies for biological detection in the field (Arnon et al. 2001, Greenfield et al. 2002, Michaelson, Halpern and Kopans 1999, Harrison et al. 1998, McIntyre et al. 1999, Bigler et al. 2002, Paige and Streckfus 2007, Streckfus et al. 1999, Streckfus et al. 2000b, Streckfus et al. 2000a, Streckfus et al. 2001, Streckfus and Bigler 2005, Streckfus, Bigler and Zwick 2006, Chase 2000, Navarro et al. 1997, Bagramyan et al. 2008). The objective of this application is to develop and test a wireless sensing technology for detecting logicalb toxins. To achieve this objective, we have developed high electron mobility transistors (HEMTs) that have been demonstrated to exhibit some of the highest sensitivities for biological agents. Specific antibodies targeting Enterotoxin type B (Category B, NIAID), Botulinum toxin (Category A NIAID) and ricin (Category B NIAID), or peptide substrates for testing the toxin's enzymatic activity, have been conjugated to the HEMT surface. While testing still needs to be performed in the presence of cross-contaminants in biologically relevant samples, the initial results are very promising. A significant issue is the absence of a definite diagnostic method and the difficulty in differential diagnosis from other pathogens that would slow the response in case of a terror attack. Our aim is to develop reliable, inexpensive, highly sensitive, hand-held sensors with response times on the order of a few seconds, which can be used in the field for detecting biological toxins. This is significant because it would greatly improve our effectiveness in responding to terrorist attacks.

The current methods for toxin sensing in the field are generally not suited for field deployment and there is a need for new technologies. The current methods involve the use of HPLC, mass spectrometry and colorimetric ELISAs which are impractical because such tests can only be carried out at centralized locations, and are too slow to be of practical value in the field. These still tend to be the methods of choice in current detection of toxins, e.g. the standard test for botulinum toxin detection is the 'mouse assay', which relies on the death of mice as an indicator of toxin presence (Bagramyan et al. 2008). Clearly, such methods are slow and impractical in the field.

Antibody-functionalized Au-gated AlGaN/GaN high electron mobility transistors (HEMTs) show great sensitivity for detecting botulinum toxin. The botulinum toxin was specifically recognized through botulinum antibody, anchored to the gate area, as shown in Figure 14.

We investigated a range of concentrations from 0.1 ng/ml to 100 ng/ml. The source and drain current from the HEMT were measured before and after the sensor was exposed to 100 ng/ml of botulinum toxin at a constant drain bias voltage of 500 mV, as shown in Figure 16 (top). Any slight changes in the ambient of the HEMT affect the surface charges on the AlGaN/GaN. These changes in the surface charge are transduced into a change in the concentration of the 2DEG in the AlGaN/GaN HEMTs, leading to the decrease in the conductance for the device after exposure to botulinum toxin.

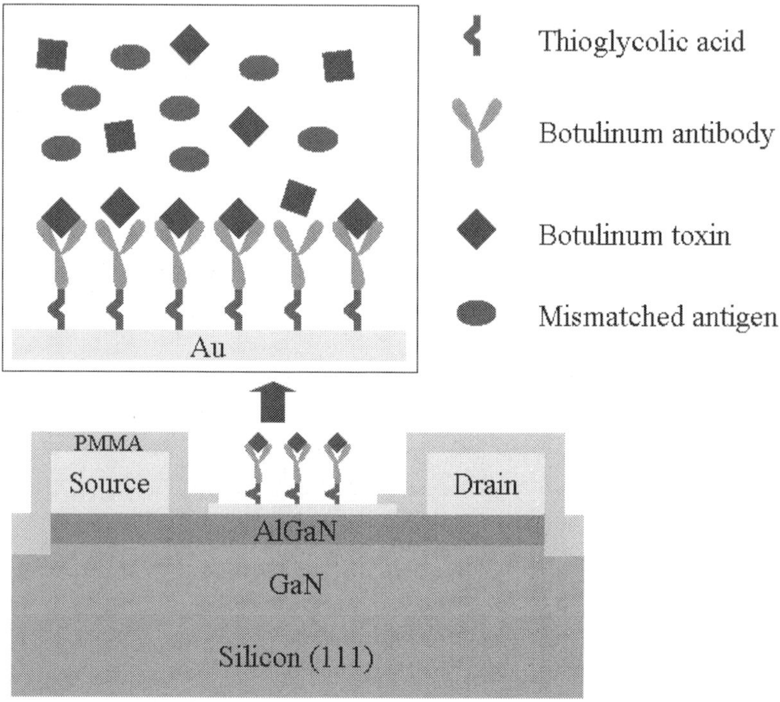

Fig. 14. Schematic of functionalized HEMT for botulinum detection.

Figure 16 (bottom) shows a real time botulinum toxin detection in PBS buffer solution using the source and drain current change with constant bias of 500 mV. No current change can be seen with the addition of buffer solution around 100 seconds, showing the specificity and stability of the device. In clear contrast, the current change showed a rapid response in less than 5 seconds when target 1 ng/ml botulinum toxin was added to the surface. The abrupt current change due to the exposure of botulinum toxin in a buffer solution was stabilized after the botulinum toxin thoroughly diffused into the buffer solution. Different concentrations (from 0.1 ng/ml to 100 ng/ml) of the exposed target botulinum toxin in a buffer solution were detected. The sensor saturates above 10ng/ml of the toxin. The experiment at each concentration was repeated four times to calculate the standard deviation of source-drain current response. The limit of detection of this device was below 1 ng/ml of botulinum toxin in PBS buffer solution. The source-drain current change was nonlinearly proportional to botulinum toxin concentration, as shown in Figure 15.
Figure 16 shows a real time test of botulinum toxin at different toxin concentrations with intervening washes to break antibody-antigen bonds. This result demonstrates the real-time capabilities and recyclability of the chip. Long term stability of the botulinum toxin sensor was also investigated with a package sensor. Figure 17 shows a photograph of the packaged sensor placed in a Petri dish for long term storage. PBS buffer solution was dropped on the active region of the sensor and the Petri dish as well. The Petri dish was then covered and sealed in order to keep the antibodies on the sensor in a PBS environment.

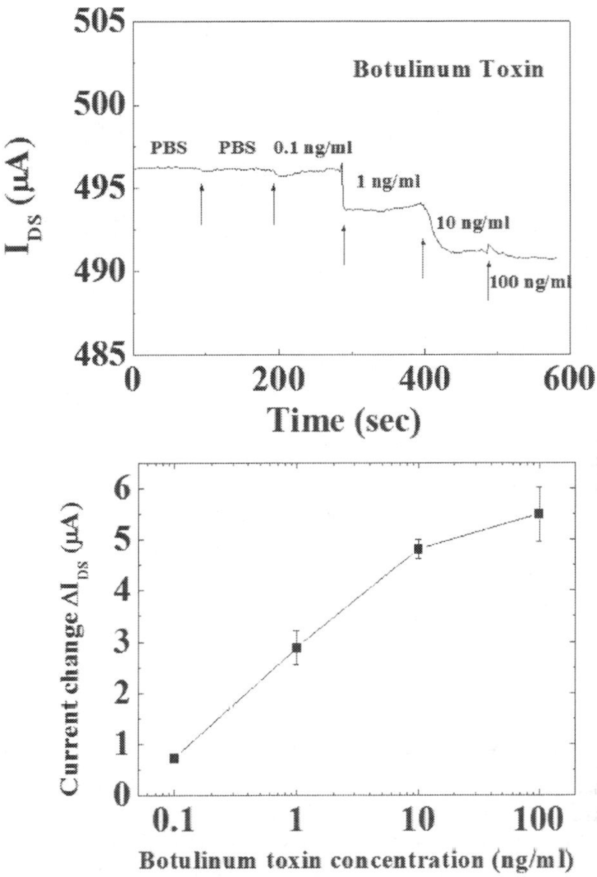

Fig. 15. Drain current of an AlGaN/GaN HEMT versus time for botulinum toxin from 0.1 ng/ml to 100 ng/ml(top) and change of drain current versus different concentrations from 0.1 ng/ml to 100 ng/ml of botulinum toxin (bottom).

Sensors were re-tested for the botulinum detection every three months. For those tests, the procedures of toxin detection and sensor surface reactivation were repeated for five times. This experiment demonstrated that after 9 month storage, the sensor still could detect the toxin and could be reactivated right after the test with PBS buffer solution rinse. This indicated that the toxin could be completely washed away from the antibodies. However, it was obvious that the detection sensitivity decreased after 9 months of storage. The decrease of the detection sensitivity drop after 9 month storage was not caused by the existence of the un-breakable toxin-antibody binding, but was rather due to the decrease of antibody activity. Another important finding was that the response time of the 9 month stored sensor increased from 5 seconds of the fresh sensor to around 10 seconds, when target toxins were exposed to the sensor. The longer response time may be also due to the decreased number of highly active sites on the antibodies after long term storage. This corresponds to the lower sensitivity of the sensor. The detailed mechanism needs further investigation.

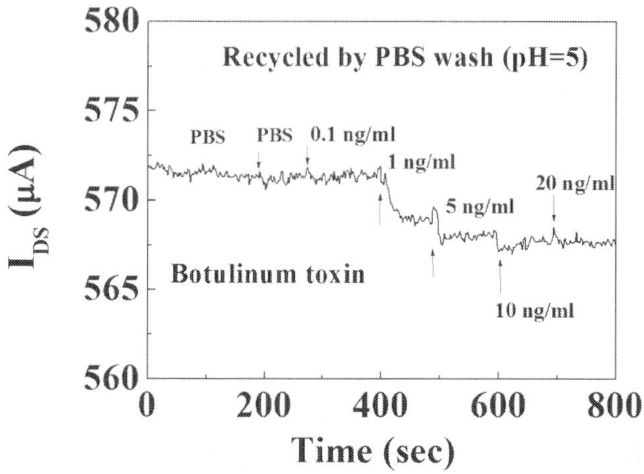

Fig. 16. Real-time test from a used botulinum sensor which was washed with PBS in pH 5 to refresh the sensor.

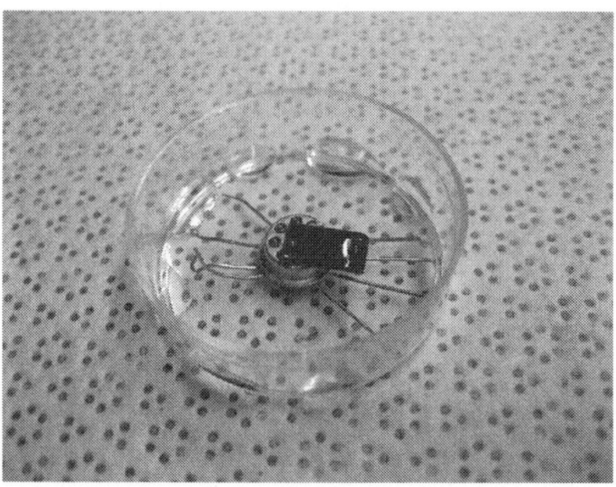

Fig. 17. Photograph of a packaged sensor placed in a Petri dish for long term storage.

Figure 18 shows the current changes of the sensors tested after different storage times at a fixed toxin concentration of 10 ng/ml against the first drain current measurement of the sensor. After 3, 6 and 9 months of storage, the current change drops 2%, 12% and 28%, respectively. Within 3 months of storage, this sensor showed almost the same sensitivity as when it was fresh. Although, after 6 and 9 months of storage, the sensor would need to be re-calibrated for toxin concentration determination usage, there is no need for recalibration for the use as the first responder of the detection for the presence or absence of the toxin.

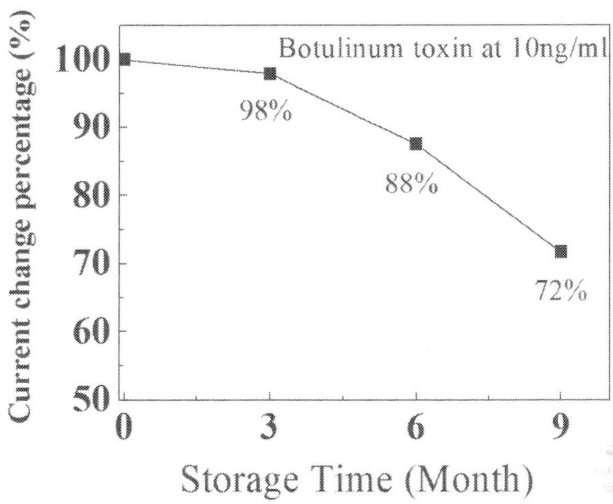

Fig. 18. The drain-source current change percentages of the initial, 3, 6 and 9 month stored sensors. The current change in the initial test is defined as 100%. The testing at the subsequent periods was defined relative to the initial test.

In summary, we have shown that through a chemical modification method, the Au-gated region of an AlGaN/GaN HEMT structure can be functionalized for the detection of botulinum toxin with a limit of detection less than 1 ng/ml. This electronic detection of biomolecules is a significant step towards a field-deployed sensor chip, which can be integrated with a commercial available wireless transmitter to realize a real-time, fast response and high sensitivity botulinum toxin detector.

7. Biomedical applications

7.1 Prostate cancer detection

Prostate cancer is the second most common cause of cancer death among men in the United States (Kelloff et al. 2004). The most commonly used serum marker for diagnosis of prostate cancer is prostate specific antigen (PSA) (Thompson and Ankerst 2007, Healy et al. 2007). The market size for prostate cancer testing is enormous. According to the American Cancer Society, prostate cancer is the most common form of cancer among men, other than skin cancer. It is estimated that during 2007, in the United States alone, 218,890 new cases of prostate cancer will be diagnosed and 1 in 6 men will be diagnosed with prostate cancer during his lifetime .

The American Cancer Society recommends health care professionals to offer the prostate-specific antigen (PSA) blood test and the digital rectal exam (DRE) yearly for men above the age of 50. Those men who have a higher risk, such as African Americans and men who have a first-degree relative diagnosed with prostate cancer should start testing at 45. Men who have several first-degree relatives diagnosed with prostate cancer should begin testing at 40. Since 1990, a recent awareness of cancers and the benefits of early detection have increased early detection tests for prostate cancer and they have grown to become fairly common. Prostate cancer can often be found early by testing the amount of prostate-specific antigen (PSA) in the patient's blood. It can also be detected on a digital rectal exam (DRE). If you have routine yearly exams and either one of these test results becomes abnormal, then any cancer you might have has likely been found at an early, more treatable stage.

The prostate cancer testing market is expected to grow over the upcoming years. As awareness of cancer and early detection increases, so too will the need for testing. Given the high demand for prostate cancer testing, one would think that there are many options for early detection. However, there are only two main ways for preliminary testing for prostate cancer: the prostate cancer antigen blood test and the digital rectal exam. Prostate-specific antigen (PSA) is made by cells in the prostate gland and although PSA is mostly found in semen, a certain amount is found in the blood as well. Most men have PSA levels under 4 nanograms per milliliter of blood. When prostate cancer develops, the PSA level usually goes up above 4 nanograms per milliliter; however, about 15% of men with a PSA below 4 will have prostate cancer on biopsy. If the patient's PSA level is between 4 and 10, their chance of having prostate cancer is about 25%. If the patient's PSA level is above 10, there is more than a 50% chance they have prostate cancer, which increases as the PSA level goes up. If the patient's PSA level is high, the doctor may advise a prostate biopsy to find out if they have cancer.

Generally PSA testing approaches are costly, time-consuming and need sample transportation. A number of different electrical measurements have been used for rapid detection of PSA(Wang 2006, Fernández-Sánchez et al. 2004, Hwang et al. 2004, Wee et al. 2005, Wang et al. 2009, Anderson et al. 2009). For example, electrochemical measurements based on impedance and capacitance are simple and inexpensive but need improved sensitivities for use with clinical samples (Wang 2006, Fernández-Sánchez et al. 2004). Resonant frequency changes of an anti-PSA antibody coated microcantilever enable a detection sensitivity of ~ 10 pg/ml but this micro-balance approach has issues with the effect of the solution on resonant frequency and cantilever damping (Fernández-Sánchez et al. 2004, Hwang et al. 2004). Antibody-functionalized nanowire FETs coated with antibody provide for low detection levels of PSA (Wang et al. 2009, Anderson et al. 2009), but the scale-up potential is limited by the expensive e-beam lithography requirements. Antibody functionalized Au-gated AlGaN/GaN HEMTs shown schematically in Figure 19 were found to be effective for detecting PSA at low concentration levels.

The PSA antibody was anchored to the gate area through the formation of carboxylate succinimdyl ester bonds with immobilized thioglycolic acid. The HEMT drain-source current showed a response time of less than 5 seconds when target PSA in a buffer at clinical concentrations was added to the antibody-immobilized surface. The devices could detect a range of concentrations from 1 μg/ml to 10 pg/ml. The lowest detectable concentration was two orders of magnitude lower than the cut-off value of PSA measurements for clinical detection of prostate cancer. Figure 20 shows the real time PSA detection in PBS buffer solution using the source and drain current change with constant bias of 0.5V(Kang et al. 2007c). No current change can be seen with the addition of buffer solution or nonspecific bovine serum albumin (BSA), but there was a rapid change when10 ng/ml PSA was added to the surface. The abrupt current change due to the exposure of PSA in a buffer solution could be stabilized after the PSA diffused into the buffer solution. The ultimate detection limit appears to be a few pg/ml (Kang et al. 2007c).

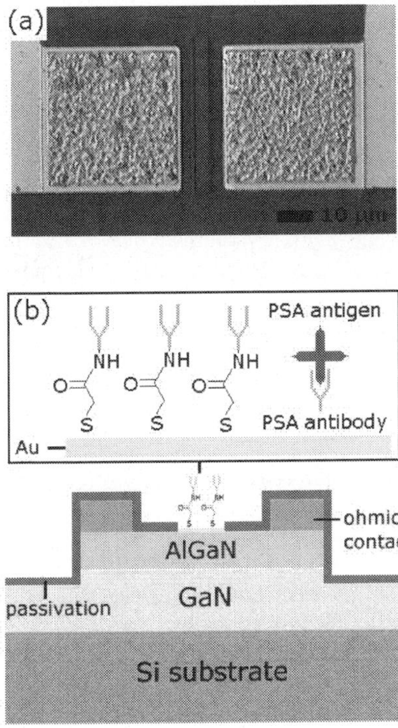

Fig. 19. Schematic of HEMT sensor functionalized for PSA detection.

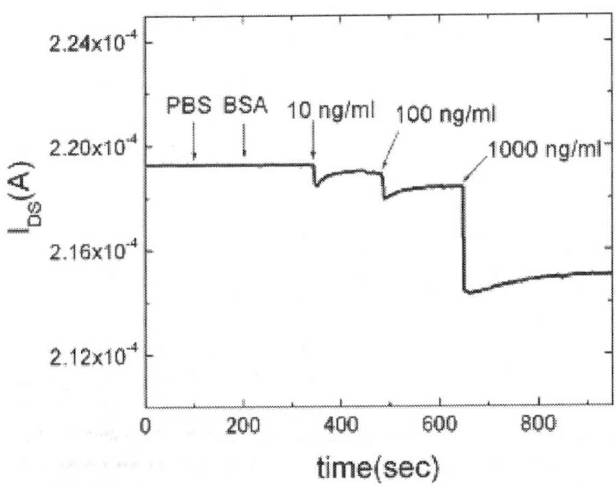

Fig. 20. Drain current versus time for PSA detection when sequentially exposed to PBS, BSA, and PSA

7.2 Kidney injury molecule detection

Problems such as Acute Kidney Injury (AKI) or Acute Renal Failure (ARF) are unfortunately still associated with a high mortality rate (Thadhani, Pascual and Bonventre 1996, Chertow et al. 1998, Bonventre and Weinberg 2003). An important biomarker for early detection of AKI is the urinary antigen known as kidney injury molecule-1 or KIM-1(Ichimura et al. 1998) and this is generally carried out with the ELISA technique discussed earlier (Vaidya and Bonventre 2006, Vaidya et al. 2006, Lequin 2005). The biomarker can also be detected with particle-based flow cytometric assay, but the cycle time is several hours (Vignali 2000). Electrical measurement approaches based on carbon nanotubes (Chen et al. 2003), nanowires of In_2O_3 (Li et al. 2005) or Si (Zheng et al. 2005b, Patolsky, Zheng and Lieber 2006a, Patolsky, Zheng and Lieber 2006b, Patolsky et al. 2007, Han et al. 2005), or Si or GaN FETs look promising for fast and sensitive detection of anibodies and potentially for molecules such as KIM-1(Thadhani et al. 1996, Chertow et al. 1998, Bonventre and Weinberg 2003, Ichimura et al. 1998, Vaidya and Bonventre 2006, Vaidya et al. 2006, Lequin 2005, Vignali 2000, Chen et al. 2003, Li et al. 2005, Zheng et al. 2005b, Patolsky et al. 2006a, Patolsky et al. 2006b, Patolsky et al. 2007, Han et al. 2005).
The functionalization scheme in the gate region began with thioglycolic acid followed by KIM-1 antibody coating (Wang et al. 2007d). The gate region was deposited with a 5 nm thick Au film. Then the Au was conjugated to specific KIM-1 antibodies with a self-assembled monolayer of thioglycolic acid. The HEMT source-drain current showed a clear dependence on the KIM-1 concentration in phosphate-buffered saline (PBS) buffer solution, as shown in Figure 21 where the time dependent source-drain current at a bias of 0.5 V is plotted for KIM-1 detection in PBS buffer solution. The limit of detection (LOD) was 1ng/ml using a 20 μm ×50 μm gate sensing area (Wang et al. 2007d).

7.3 Breast cancer detection

The market size for breast cancer testing is vast - nearly 200,000 women and 1,700 men were diagnosed in 2006 alone. Although lucrative, competition in this industry is strong. Growth potential is possible, however, as the most effective and widely used diagnostic exam for breast cancer, the mammogram, is potentially harmful due to radiation exposure. Other, less popular, exams that do not involve radiation tend to be both invasive and expensive. Currently, the overwhelming majority of patients are screened for breast cancer by mammography . This procedure involves a high cost to the patient and is invasive (radiation) which limits the frequency of screening. Breast cancer is currently the most common female malignancy in the world, representing 7% of the more than 7.6 million cancer-related deaths worldwide. Breast cancer accounts for over 30% of all new diagnoses in women aged 20-49 and 50-69, and 20% among older women. As a result, more than one million mammograms are performed each year. According to the National Breast Cancer Foundation, it is estimated that nearly 200,000 women and 1,700 men will be diagnosed with breast cancer this year.
When breast cancer is discovered early on, there is a much better chance of successful treatment. Therefore it is highly recommended that women check their breasts monthly from the age of 20. Clinical breast examinations should be conducted every three years from ages 20-39 and an annual mammogram for women 50 and older. Work by Michaelson et al. (Michaelson et al. 1999) indicates a 96% survival rate if patients could be screened every three months. Thus, mortality in breast cancer patients could be reduced by increasing the frequency of screening. However this is not feasible presently due to the lack of cheap and reliable technologies that can screen breast cancer non-invasively.

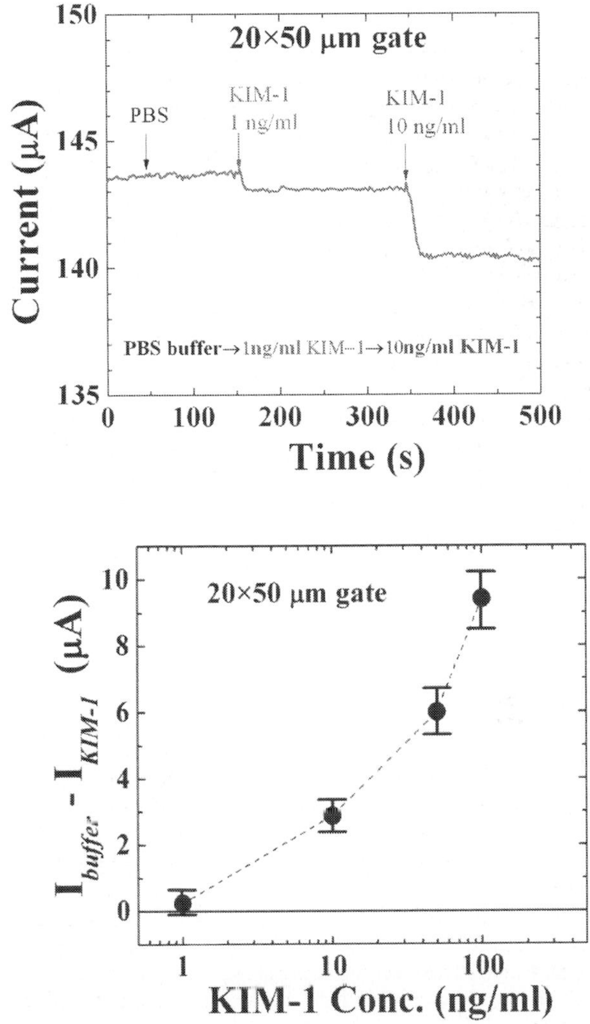

Fig. 21. Time dependent current signal when exposing the HEMT to 1ng/ml and 10ng/ml KIM-1 in PBS buffer.

There is recent evidence to suggest that salivary testing for makers of breast cancer may be used in conjunction with mammography (Bigler et al. 2002, Harrison et al. 1998, McIntyre et al. 1999, Streckfus et al. 1999, Streckfus et al. 2000b, Streckfus et al. 2000a, Streckfus et al. 2001, Streckfus and Bigler 2005, Streckfus et al. 2006, Chase 2000). Saliva-based diagnostics for the protein c-erbB-2, have tremendous prognostic potential (Streckfus and Bigler 2005,

Paige and Streckfus 2007). Soluble fragments of the c-erbB-2 oncoprotein and the cancer antigen 15-3 were found to be significantly higher in the saliva of women who had breast cancer than in those patients with benign tumors (Streckfus et al. 2006). Other studies have shown that epidermal growth factor (EGF) is a promising marker in saliva for breast cancer detection (Paige and Streckfus 2007, Navarro et al. 1997). These initial studies indicate that the saliva test is both sensitive and reliable and can be potentially useful in initial detection and follow-up screening for breast cancer. However, to fully realize the potential of salivary biomarkers, technologies are needed that will enable facile, sensitive, specific detection of breast cancer.

Antibody-functionalized Au-gated AlGaN/GaN high electron mobility transistors (HEMTs) show promise for detecting c-erbB-2 antigen. The c-erbB-2 antigen was specifically recognized through c-erbB antibody, anchored to the gate area. We investigated a range of clinically relevant concentrations from 16.7 μg/ml to 0.25 μg/ml.

The Au surface was functionalized with a specific bi-functional molecule, thioglycolic acid. We anchored a self-assembled monolayer of thioglycolic acid, $HSCH_2COOH$, an organic compound and containing both a thiol (mercaptan) and a carboxylic acid functional group, on the Au surface in the gate area through strong interaction between gold and the thiol-group of the thioglycolic acid. The devices were first placed in the ozone/UV chamber and then submerged in 1 mM aqueous solution of thioglycolic acid at room temperature. This resulted in binding of the thioglycolic acid to the Au surface in the gate area with the COOH groups available for further chemical linking of other functional groups. The device was incubated in a phosphate buffered saline (PBS) solution of 500 μg/ml c-erbB-2 monoclonal antibody for 18 hours before real time measurement of c-erbB-2 antigen.

After incubation with a PBS buffered solution containing c-erbB-2 antibody at a concentration of 1 μg/ml, the device surface was thoroughly rinsed off with deionized water and dried by a nitrogen blower. The source and drain current from the HEMT were measured before and after the sensor was exposed to 0.25 μg/ml of c-erbB-2 antigen at a constant drain bias voltage of 500 mV. Any slight changes in the ambient of the HEMT affect the surface charges on the AlGaN/GaN. These changes in the surface charge are transduced into a change in the concentration of the 2DEG in the AlGaN/GaN HEMTs, leading to the slight decrease in the conductance for the device after exposure to c-erbB-2 antigen.

Figure 22 shows real time c-erbB-2 antigen detection in PBS buffer solution using the source and drain current change with constant bias of 500 mV. No current change can be seen with the addition of buffer solution around 50 seconds, showing the specificity and stability of the device. In clear contrast, the current change showed a rapid response in less than 5 seconds when target 0.25 μg/ml c-erbB-2 antigen was added to the surface. The abrupt current change due to the exposure of c-erbB-2 antigen in a buffer solution was stabilized after the c-erbB-2 antigen thoroughly diffused into the buffer solution. Three different concentrations (from 0.25 μg/ml to 16.7 μg/ml) of the exposed target c-erbB-2 antigen in a buffer solution were detected. The experiment at each concentration was repeated five times to calculate the standard deviation of source-drain current response.

The limit of detection of this device was 0.25 μg/ml c-erbB-2 antigen in PBS buffer solution. The source-drain current change was nonlinearly proportional to c-erbB-2 antigen concentration, as shown in Figure 23. Between each test, the device was rinsed with a wash buffer of 10 mM, pH 6.0 phosphate buffer solution containing 10 mM KCl to strip the antibody from the antigen.

Clinically relevant concentrations of the c-erbB-2 antigen in the saliva and serum of normal patients are 4-6 μg/ml and 60-90 μg/ml respectively. For breast cancer patients, the c-erbB-2 antigen concentrations in the saliva and serum are 9-13 μg/ml and 140-210 μg/ml, respectively. Our detection limit suggests that HEMTs can be easily used for detection of clinically relevant concentrations of biomarkers. Similar methods can be used for detecting other important disease biomarkers and a compact disease diagnosis array can be realized for multiplex disease analysis.

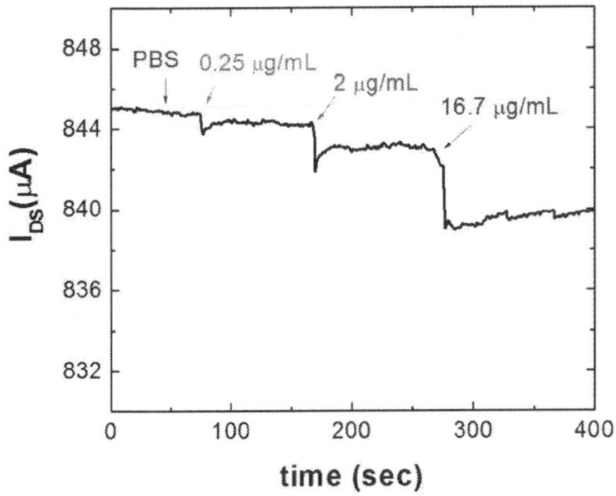

Fig. 22. Drain current of an AlGaN/GaN HEMT over time for c-erbB-2 antigen from 0.25 μg/ml to 17 μg/ml.

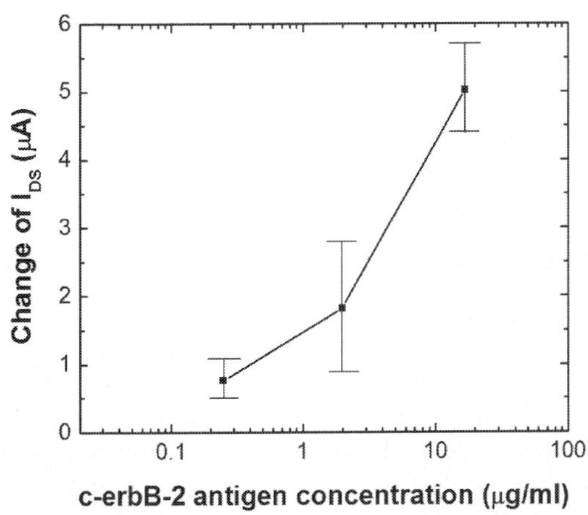

Fig. 23. Drain current as a function of c-erbB-2 antigen concentrations from 0.25 μg/ml to 17 μg/ml.

7.4 Lactic acid detection

Lactic acid can also be detected with ZnO nanorod-gated AlGaN/GaN HEMTs. Interest in developing improved methods for detecting lactate acid has been increasing due to its importance in areas such as clinical diagnostics, sports medicine, and food analysis. An accurate measurement of the concentration of lactate acid in blood is critical to patients that are in intensive care or undergoing surgical operations as abnormal concentrations may lead to shock, metabolic disorder, respiratory insufficiency, and heart failure. Lactate acid concentration can also be used to monitor the physical condition of athletes or of patients with chronic diseases such as diabetes and chronic renal failure. In the food industry, lactate level can serve as an indicator of the freshness, stability and storage quality. For the reasons above, it is desirable to develop a sensor capable of simple and direct measurements, rapid response, high specificity, and low cost. Recent researches on lactate acid detection mainly focus on amperometric sensors with lactate acid specific enzymes attached to an electrode with a mediator (Parra et al. 2006, Phypers and Pierce 2006, Lin, Shih and Chau 2007, Spohn et al. 1996, Pohanka and Zboril 2008, Suman et al. 2005, Haccoun et al. 2006, Di et al. 2007). Examples of materials used as mediators include carbon paste, conducting copolymer, nanostructured Si_3N_4 and silica materials. Other methods of detecting lactate acid include utilizing semiconductors (Lupu et al. 2007) and electro-chemiluminescent materials (Marquette, Degiuli and Blum 2000).

A ZnO nanorod array, which was used to immobilize lactate oxidase oxidase (LOx), was selectively grown on the gate area using low temperature hydrothermal decomposition as illustrated in Figure 24. The array of one-dimensional ZnO nanorods provided a large effective surface area with high surface-to-volume ratio and a favorable environment for the immobilization of LOx.

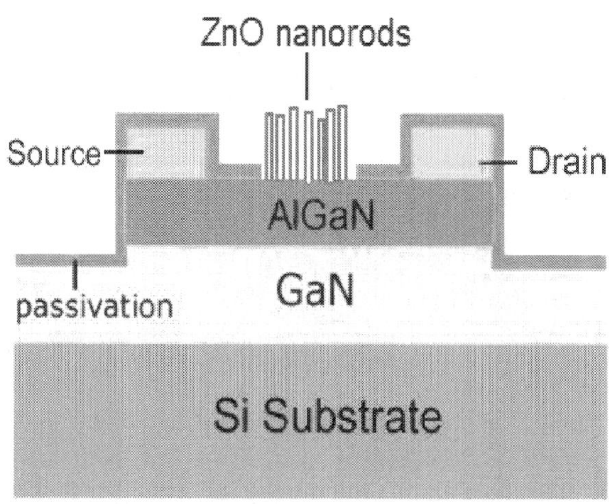

Fig. 24. Schematic cross sectional view of the ZnO nanorod gated HEMT for lactic acid detection.

The AlGaN/GaN HEMT drain-source current showed a rapid response when various concentrations of lactate acid solutions were introduced to the gate area of the HEMT sensor. The HEMT could detect lactate acid concentrations from 167 nM to 139 μM. Figure 25 shows a real time detection of lactate acid by measuring the HEMT drain current at a constant drain-source bias voltage of 500 mV during exposure of HEMT sensor to solutions with different concentrations of lactate acid. The sensor was first exposed to 20 μl of 10 mM PBS and no current change could be detected with the addition of 10 μl of PBS at approximately 40 seconds, showing the specificity and stability of the device. By contrast, a rapid increase in the drain current was observed when target lactate acid was introduced to the device surface. The sensor was continuously exposed to lactate acid concentrations from 167 nM to 139 μM.

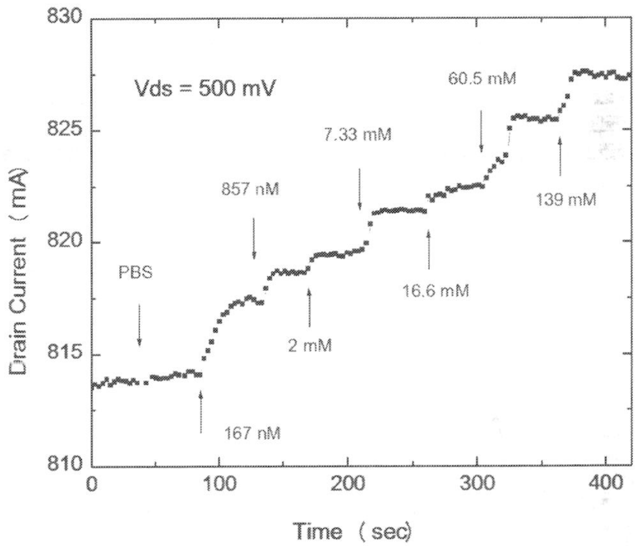

Fig. 25. Drain current as a function of the time with successive exposure to lactate acid from 167 nM to 139 μM.

As compared with the amperometric measurement based lactate acid sensors, our HEMT sensors do not require a fixed reference electrode in the solution to measure the potential applied between the nano-materials and the reference electrode. The lactate acid sensing with the HEMT sensor was measured through the drain current of HEMT with a change of the charges on the ZnO nanorods and the detection signal was amplified through the HEMT. Although the time response of the HEMT sensors is similar to that of electrochemical based sensors, a significant change of drain current was observed for exposing the HEMT to the lactate acid at a low concentration of 167 nM due to this amplification effect. In addition, the amount of sample, which is dependent on the area of gate dimension, can be minimized for the HEMT sensor due to fact no reference electrode is required. Thus, measuring lactate acid in the exhaled breath condensate (EBC) can be achieved as a noninvasive method.

7.5 Chloride ion detection

Chlorine is widely used in the manufacture of many products and items directly or indirectly, i.e. in paper product production, antiseptic, dye-stuffs, food, insecticides, paints, petroleum products, plastics, medicines, textiles, solvents, and many other consumer products. It is used to kill bacteria and other microbes in drinking water supplies and waste water treatment. Excess chlorine also reacts with organics and forms disinfection by-products such as carcinogenic chloroform, which is harmful to human health. Thus, to ensure the safety of public health, it is very important to accurately and effectively monitor chlorine residues, typically in the form of chloride ion concentration, during the treatment and transport of drinking water (Taylor and Hong 2000, Walker, Hall and Hurst 1990, Cook and Miles 1980, Elsheimer 1987, Verma and Parthasarathy 1996, Graule et al. 1989, Kumar, Venkatesh and Maiti 2004, Blackwell et al. 1997). In addition, the chloride ion is an essential mineral for humans, and is maintained to a total body chloride balance in body fluids such as serum, blood, urine, exhaled breath condensate etc., by the kidneys. Variations in the chloride ion concentration in serum may serve as an index of renal diseases, adrenalism, pneumonia and, thus, the measurement of this parameter is clinically important (Walker et al. 1990, Davidsson et al. 2005, Davidsson et al. 2007, Niimi et al. 2004, Effros et al. 2002).

7.5.1 HEMT Functionalized with Ag/AgCl

(HEMTs) with a Ag/AgCl gate are found to exhibit significant changes in channel conductance upon exposing the gate region to various concentrations of chorine ion solutions, as shown in Figure 26. The Ag/AgCl gate electrode, prepared by potentiostatic anodization, changes electrical potential when it encounters chorine ions. This gate potential changes lead to a change of surface charge in the gate region of the HEMT, inducing a higher positive charge on the AlGaN surface, and increasing the pizeo-induced charge density in the HEMT channel. These anions create an image positive charge on the Ag gate metal for the required neutrality, thus increasing the drain current of the HEMT. The HEMT source-drain current showed a clear dependence on the chorine concentration (Walker et al. 1990).

Figure 27 shows the time dependence of Ag/AgCl HEMT drain current at a constant drain bias voltage of 500mV during exposure to solutions with different chlorine ion concentrations. The HEMT sensor was first exposed to DI water and no change of the drain current was detected with the addition of DI water at 100 seconds. This stability was important to exclude possible noise from the mechanical change of the NaCl solution. By sharp contrast, there was a rapid response of HEMT drain current observed in less than 30 seconds when target of 1×10^{-8} M NaCl solution was switched to the surface at 175 sec. The abrupt current change due to the exposure of chlorine in NaCl solution stabilized after the chlorine thoroughly diffused into the water to reach a steady state. When Ag/AgCl gate metal encountered chorine ions, the electrical potential of the gate was changed, inducing a higher positive charge on the AlGaN surface, and increased the pizeo-induced charge density in the HEMT channel. 1×10^{-7} M of NaCl solution was then applied at 382 second and it was accompanied with a larger signal corresponding to the higher chlorine concentration. Further real time tests were carried out to explore the detection of higher Cl^- ion concentrations. The sensors was exposed to 10^{-8} M, 10^{-7} M, 10^{-6} M, 10^{-5} M and 10^{-4} M solutions continuously and repeated five times to obtain the standard deviation of source-drain current response for each concentration. The limit of detection of this device was $1\times10^{-}$

[8] M chlorine in DI-water. Between each test, the device was rinsed with DI water. These results suggest that our HEMT sensors are recyclable with simple DI water rinse. The presence of the Ag/AgCl gate leads to a logarithmic dependence of current on the concentration of NaCl.

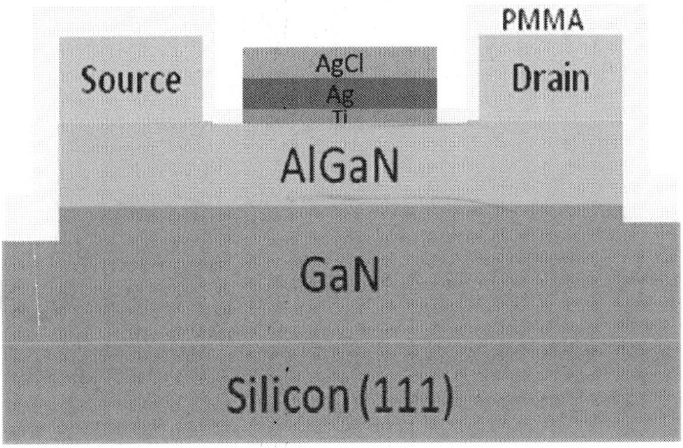

Fig. 26. Schematic cross sectional view of a Ag/AgCl gated HEMT.

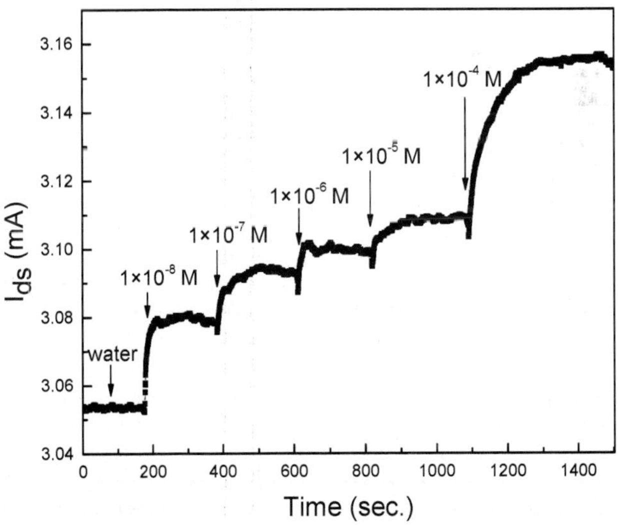

Fig. 27. Time dependent drain current of a Ag/AgCl gated AlGaN/GaN HEMT exposed to different concentrations of NaCl solutions (bottom).

7.5.2 HEMT Functionalized with InN

Real time detection of chloride ion detection with AlGaN/GaN high electron mobility transistors (HEMTs) with an InN thin film in the gate region has also been demonstrated. The sensor, shown schematically in Figure 28, exhibited significant changes in channel conductance upon exposure to various concentrations of NaCl solutions. The InN thin film, deposited by Molecular Beam Epitaxy, provided fixed surface sites for reversible anion coordination. The potential change in the gate area induced a change of the piezo-induced charge density in the electron channel in the HEMT. The sensor was tested over the range of 100nM to 100μM NaCl solutions.

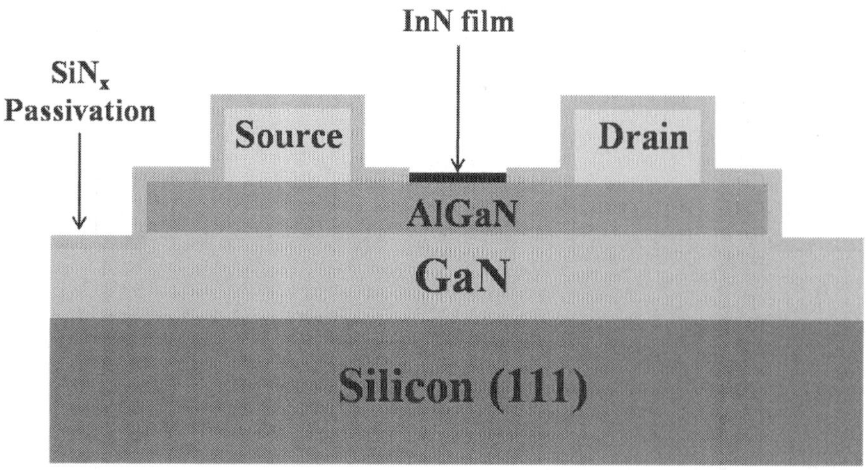

Fig. 28. Cross section schematic of the InN-gated HEMT.

Figure 29 also shows the results of real time detection of Cl^- ions by measuring the HEMT drain current at a constant drain bias voltage of 500mV during exposure to solutions of different chloride ion concentrations. The HEMT sensor was first exposed to DI water and no change of the drain current was detected with the addition of DI water at 100 seconds. The small spike in the current is due to mechanical disturbance of the HEMT surface when the water was added. By sharp contrast, a rapid response of HEMT drain current was observed in less than 20 seconds when target of 100 nM NaCl solution was exposed to the surface at 200 seconds. The abrupt current change stabilized after the sodium chloride solution thoroughly diffused into water and reached a steady state. When the InN gate metal encountered chloride ion, the electrical potential of the gate was changed and resulted in the increase the pizeo-induced charge density in the HEMT channel. A larger signal change was observed when 1μM of NaCl solution was applied at 300 seconds. The sensor was exposed to higher Cl^- ion concentrations of 10μM and 100μM sequentially for a further real time test. The test was repeated with the same sensor for five times to obtain the standard deviation of source-drain current response for each concentration. The sensor can be reusable by washing it with DI water and drying with nitrogen gas. The limit of detection of this device was 100nM chloride ions in DI water. The presence of the InN gate leads to a logarithmic dependence of current on the concentration for NaCl.

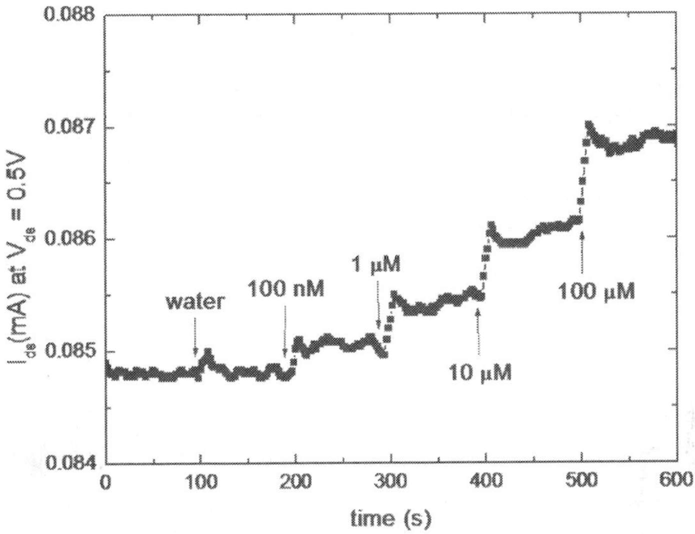

Fig. 29. Real time source-drain current at a constant bias of 500mV as different concentrations of Cl- ions were added.

7.6 Traumatic Brain Injury

TBI is one of the most frequent causes of morbidity and mortality on the modern battlefield. U.S. casualties in Iraq are suffering a greater percentage of brain injuries than in previous wars. One of the contributing factors is the proliferation of the use of Improvised Explosive Device (IED) against US warfighters (Warden , Langlois, Rutland-Brown and Thomas 2004). Recent assessments have indicated that about 65 % of casualties are correlated with brain injuries. Traumatic brain injury, including concussion are also growing medical problem among civilians, with almost 2 million cases in the US each year (Langlois et al. 2004). The development of a fast response and portable TBI sensor can have tremendous impact in early diagnosis, and proper management of TBI. Accurate and early diagnosis of a soldier's health in acute care environments can significantly simplify decisions about situation management. For example, decisions need to be made about whether to admit or discharge injured soldiers or to transfer other facility with advanced diagonal system, such as computer tomography (CT) and magnetic resonance imaging (MRI) scans. The capability to detect, in real time, markers in body fluids of soldiers can result in better patient outcomes especially in the battlefield or remote areas, where complicated and expensive CT and MRI scans are not available. For example, traumatic brain injury (TBI) is one of the most frequent causes of morbidity and mortality on the modern battlefield (Warden , Langlois et al. 2004). U.S. casualties in Iraq are suffering a greater percentage of brain injuries than in previous wars. Recent assessments have indicated that about 65 % of casualties are correlated with brain injuries, and concussion is a growing medical problem. The development of a fast response and portable TBI sensor can have tremendous impact in early diagnosis, and proper management of TBI

Preliminary results show the TBI antibody can be functionalized on the HEMT surface and fast response of TBI antigen was achieved. The detection of limit of detection (LOD) was in the 10th of μg/ml range, however this is not low enough for practical use. The typical TBI antigen concentration in the TBI patient's serum is in the range of ng/ml. We have used HEMT sensors to detect the kidney injury molecules and prostate specific antigen and achieved the LOD in the range of 1-10 pg/ml range. The reason for higher LOD for the TBI antigen detection was due to the much smaller size of the TBI antigen. Smaller antigens carry less charges, thus provide less effect on the drain current of the HEMT sensor. Based on the promising biomarker and device data, we have recently used HEMTs for detecting a biomarker UCH-L1 (BA0127) antigen involved in Traumatic Injury Molecule. The gate region was functionalized with a specific antibody to traumatic brain injury antigen. The HEMT current showed a decrease as a function of TBI antigen concentration in PBS buffer (Figure 30). This shows the time dependent current change in BA0127 (UCH-L1) antibody modified HEMTs upon exposure to 2 μg/ml, and then to 16.9, 80, and 188 μg/ml of BA0127 (UCH-L1) in PBS buffer. The response time is around 6 seconds. The preliminary limit of detection (LOD) was found to be 20 μg/ml, demonstrating the potential for TBI detection with accurate, rapid, noninvasive, and high throughput capabilities.

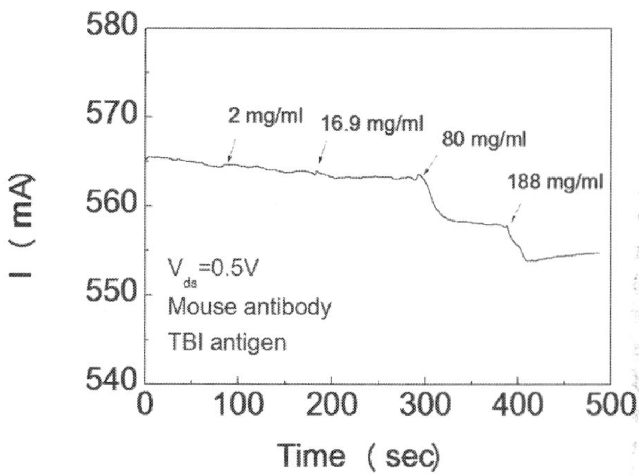

Fig. 30. Time dependent current signal when exposing the HEMT to 2 μg/ml to 188 μg/ml BA0127 TBI antigen in PBS buffer.

8. Endocrine disrupter exposure level meassurement

There have been many reports evaluating the adverse effects of endocrine disrupters (ED) on reproduction in wild animals, especially in aquatic environments (Mosconi et al. 2002, Sumpter and Jobling 1995, Matozzo et al. 2008a, Watson et al. 2007, Garcia-Reyero et al. 2006, Porte et al. 2006, Hinck et al. 2008). A wide range of chemicals are considered EDs, including naturally occurring or improperly disposed estrogens and anthropogenic chemicals that were heavily used in the past. These chemicals promote feminization in wild life and also pose a threat to public health. Some reports suggest that ED can influence fetal development (Bern 1998) or act as a carcinogen (Davis et al. 1993, Yager and Liehr 1996,

Liehlr 2001). Therefore, it is beneficial to develop tools that could accurately monitor the level of ED exposure.

Vitellogenin (Vtg) is a major egg yolk precursor protein that can be used as a biomarker to indicate an organism's exposure to ED (Heppell et al. 1995). The gene for this protein is expressed in the liver of oviparous animals under the control of estrogen (Matozzo et al. 2008b, Heppell et al. 1995, Carmon, Baltus and Luck 2005b, Hahn et al. 2006, Eidem et al. 2006, Sabo-Attwood et al. 2007, Denslow et al. 1999, Garcia-Reyero et al. 2009, Chertow et al. 1998). Male fish, under natural conditions, should have very low doses of Vtg since they do not produce eggs. However, if male fish are exposed to estrogen or to estrogen mimics in the environment, the Vtg gene is turned on. The dynamic range of this protein in normal male fish is 10-50 ng/ml in plasma and ~20 mg/ml in females producing eggs (Denslow et al. 1999). There have been reports of finding as much as 100 mg/ml in some fish that were induced with estrogen (Garcia-Reyero et al. 2009). While the dynamic range is over 6 orders of magnitude, one normally finds 1~100 μg/ml in plasma in exposed males (Denslow et al. 1999). Although Vtg from one species is limited in its application as a probe for another, some segments of Vtg are highly conserved among species, suggesting the possibility of developing antibodies with wide cross-reactivity (Denslow et al. 1999). Enzyme-linked-immunosorbent-assay (ELISA) (Heppell et al. 1995, Eidem et al. 2006, Sabo-Attwood et al. 2007, Denslow et al. 1999, Garcia-Reyero et al. 2009), quartz crystal microbalance (Carmon, Baltus and Luck 2005a), and yeast cell-based assay (Hahn et al. 2006) are typically used as the Vtg detection methods, however, these methods are not suitable for on-field, real-time measurements.

Figure 31 shows the results of real time detection of Vtg by measuring the HEMT at constant drain bias voltage of 500 mV with an Agilent 4156C parameter analyzer at 25°C. Purified Vtg solutions were prepared in 10mM PBS and introduced to the sensor surface by a syringe autopipette (0.5-2μL). The drain current measurement began with 10 μL of PBS placing on the HEMT surface. Before introducing the Vtg solutions, an additional 1μL drop of PBS was added to the sensor. Other than the small disturbance at 50 seconds, no change of the drain current was detected. The disturbance in the current was due to mechanical disturbance of the HEMT surface and the level went back to its original state. In comparison, a rapid response of HEMT drain current was observed in less than 10 seconds when the sensor was exposed to 5μg/mL of Vtg at 100 seconds. The abrupt current change stabilized after the VTG thoroughly diffused into the solution and reached a steady state. When the antigen encountered the antibody, the electrical potential of the gate was changed and resulted in the increase of the pizeo-induced charge density in the HEMT channel.

A larger signal change was observed when 10μg/mL of Vtg was added at 200 seconds. There was PBS solution on the sensor already. In order to achieve the 10μg/mL of Vtg on the sensor, higher concentration than 10μg/mL was needed to be used to add on the sensor. Thus, an abrupt spike of the drain current change was observed due to the exposure of higher Vtg concentration solution to the sensing area, which was stabilized after the Vtg thoroughly diffused into the solution on the top of the sensing area. The sensor was exposed to higher Vtg concentrations of 50μg/mL and 100μg/mL sequentially for further real time test. The test was repeated with the same sensor for three times. The sensors were rinsed with 10mM PBS at pH=6 because antibodies have optimal reactivity at pH=7.4 and will release the antigen at a lower pH.

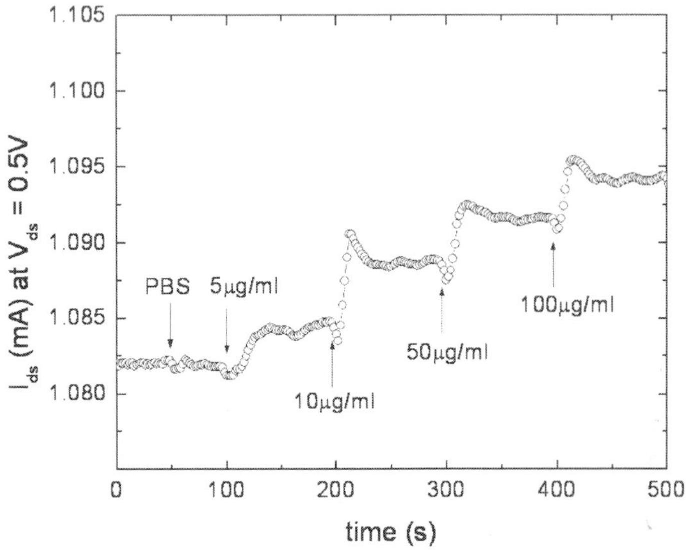

Fig. 31. Real time source-drain current of sensors when introduced to 5, 10, 50, and 100 μg/mL of vitellogenin

Figure 32 (top) shows Vtg detection results with actual male and female largemouth bass serum samples. The male serum contained no vitellogenin whereas the female serum contained 8mg/mL of Vtg. In contrast to PBS solutions, serum has many proteins that can interfere with the correct sensor reading. Therefore, it was necessary to block the unreacted carboxylic groups on the sensor. 1mg/mL bovine serum albumin (BSA) solution was applied to the sensor for 3 hours and washed thoroughly with PBS to remove the excess BSA. An important factor that influences the sensor performance is the Debye length of the solution (Curreli et al. 2008). Electrolytes that are present in the solution can screen the field effect from the antigen-antibody interaction. In solutions such as serum, the Debye length is greatly reduced and causes lower sensitivity of the device. Therefore, dilution of largemouth bass serum was needed to detect Vtg in the solution. The serum was diluted to 1% in 10mM PBS. The measurement started with 1% male serum containing no Vtg on the sensor. At 100 seconds, additional diluted male serum was added to confirm that there was no current change due to the serum background. By contrast, the current increased when drops of 1% female serum containing Vtg were added every 100 seconds.

Figure 32 (bottom) shows the drain current changes as a function of the Vtg concentration. Each concentration was repeated five times to obtain the standard deviation of source-drain current response for each concentration. The source-drain current change is nonlinearly proportional to Vtg concentration. Between each test, the device was rinsed with a wash buffer of 10 μM phosphate buffer solution containing 10 μM KCl with pH 6 to strip the antigen from the antibody. Successful detection in serum samples shows that HEMTs have potential as biological sensors in real-world applications.

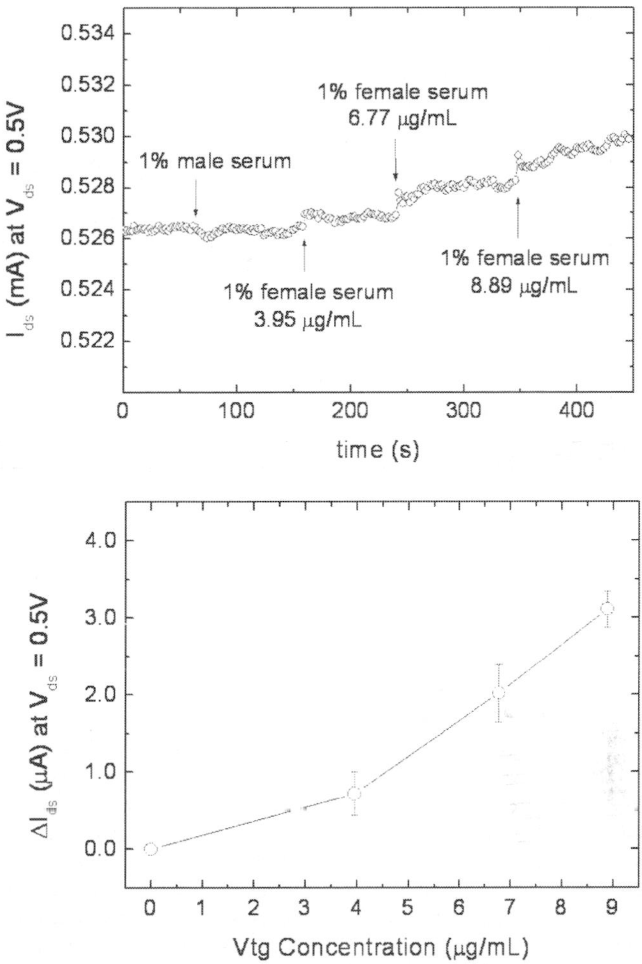

Fig. 32. (top) Real time detection of vitellogenin in largemouth bass serum. (bottom) Drain current change in HEMT as a function of vitellogenin concentration

9. Wireless sensors

With many of the sensor applications, it is desirable to have the detected signal transmitted wirelessly to a central location. This could be part of an unmanned system for biotoxin detection or part of a personal medical monitoring system in which a patient could breathe into a hand-held device that then transmits the encrypted signal to a doctor's office. This would allow for less numerous visits to doctor's offices and less problems with false positive tests because data could be accumulated over an extended period and a more reliable baseline established.

A prototype of a remote hydrogen sensing system was installed in a Ford dealership in Orlando (Greenway Ford), which is a test site for a hydrogen-fueled vehicle program supported by Florida State Government, since August 2006. The hydrogen-fueled buses and cars are stored and have maintenance performed on them in a large work area at the Ford dealership. Our hydrogen sensing system includes four on-site sensors, power management subsystem, wireless transmitter and receiver connect to a computer. An intelligent monitoring software developed by our team is used to control data logging and tracking of each individual sensor as well as defining and implementing the monitoring states, transitions, and actions of the hydrogen sensor network. It can trigger an alarm and/or send messages to computers, cell phones or PDAs, when a preset hydrogen threshold level is detected. Also, the software is able to warn the users of potential sensor failure, power outages and network failures through cell phone network and Internet. Currently, the cost of electronic parts including wireless transceiver and detection circuits is less than $20 in small quantity. In large quantity, it can be lower than $10. If the complete wireless transceiver and detection circuit are designed and integrated on a custom IC for mass production, the cost should be in the range of $5-8, similar to Bluetooth wireless chips. The sensors themselves can be mass-produced for 5-10 cents each according to Nitronex, Inc. A schematic block diagram of sensor module and wireless network server is shown in Figure 33.

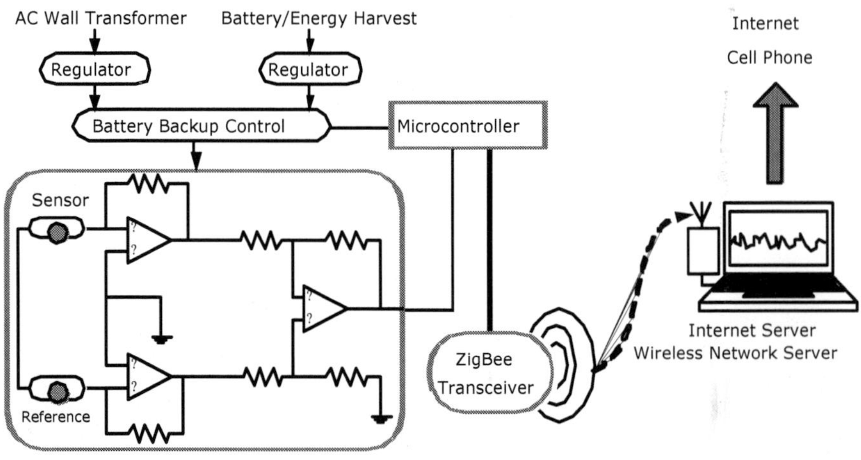

Fig. 33. Schematic of remote data transmission system for sensors.

As shown in the Figure 34, we have also developed a pen-sized portable, re-configurable wireless transceiver integrated with pH sensor has been designed and fabricated. The wireless transmitter and receiver pair was designed to acquire EBC data and transmit it wirelessly. This system is able to interface multiple different sensors and consists of a transmitter and receiver pair. The transmitter was designed such that it is the size of a marker-pen so that it could be used as an ultra-portable lightweight handheld device. The transmitter is designed to be operated on an ultra-low-power mode. The transmitter is also equipped with an on-board recharging circuit, which can be powered by using a standard mini-USB cable. The transmitter consumes on average 80μA. The transmitter and receiver pair is designed to operate at 2.4GHz with range of up to 20ft line-of-sight. The receiver has USB 2.0 connectivity, which relays EBC data from the transmitter to a PC while powering the receiver. The transmitter is designed to integrate with various different sensors through a connector. The transmitter can be reset for the required input signal range to trigger the alarm through the bi-directional wireless communication for a different sensing application. Thus this system is reconfigurable over-the-air. The wireless circuits only consume a power level around 1 μW. If the sensor consumes a similar power level, the battery installed on the transmitter package can last more than one month. This EBC sensing pair of devices can be mass-produced cost effectively well below $100 each pair. The sensor occupies the tip of the pen-shaped layout in Figure 34 and runs off a 75mA Li ion polymer rechargeable battery. Figure 34 illustrated the package sensors mounted on a circuit board containing the detection circuit and microcontroller and the wireless transmitter for data collection. The sensor module is fully integrated on an FR4 PC board and is packaged with battery. The dimension of the sensor module package is: 4.5" × 2.9" × 2". The maximum line of sight range between the sensor module and the base station is 150m. The base station of the wireless sensor network server is also integrated in a single module (3.0" × 2.7" × 1.1") and is ready to be connected to a laptop by a USB cable. The base station draws its power from the laptop's USB interface, thus do not require any battery or wall AC transformer, which reduces its form factor. The PC is used to record the sensing data, send the data to internet, and take actions when the hydrogen is detected.

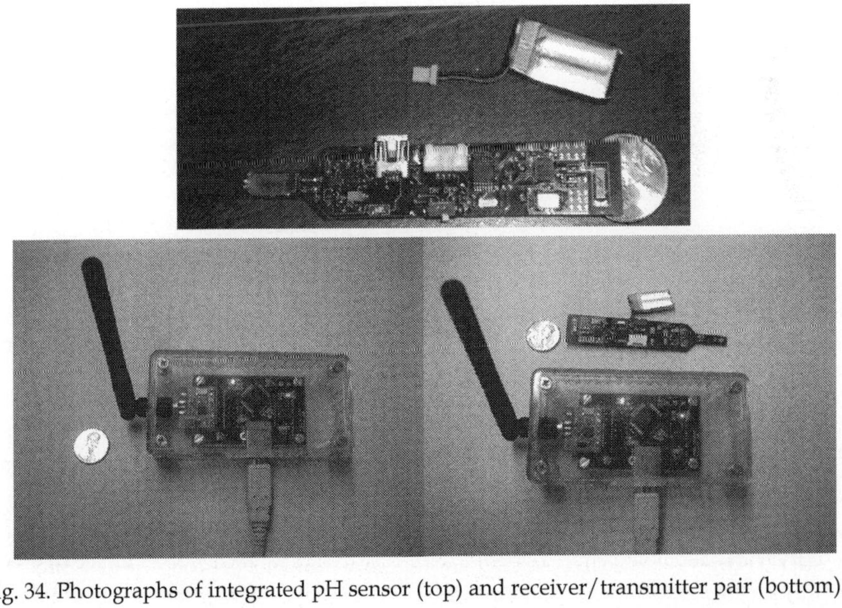

Fig. 34. Photographs of integrated pH sensor (top) and receiver/transmitter pair (bottom).

A client program has also been developed to receive the sensor data remotely. The remote client can get a real-time log of the system for 10 minutes via the client program. In addition, a full data log will be obtained via accessing the server using a ftp client as the server program incorporates a full data logging functionality. When the current of any of the sensors exceeds a preset level, the server program will automatically execute the phone-dialing program, reporting the emergency to relevant personnel. A web server was developed using MATLAB (Mathworks Inc) to share the collected sensor data via the Internet. The data display time range can be chosen real-time, 85 minutes, 15 hours and 6 day.

10. Summary

We have summarized recent progress in AlGaN/GaN HEMT sensors. These devices can take advantage of the advantages of microelectronics, including high sensitivity, possibility of high-density integration, and mass manufacturability. The goal is to realize real-time, portable and inexpensive chemical and biological sensors and to use these as handheld exhaled breath, saliva, urine, or blood monitors with wireless capability. Frequent screening can catch the early development of diseases, reduce the suffering of the patients due to late diagnoses, and lower the medical cost. For example, a 96 % survival rate has been predicted in breast cancer patients if the frequency of screening is every three months. This frequency cannot be achieved with current methods of mammography due to high cost to the patient and invasiveness (radiation).

There are many possible applications, including:

Diabetes/Glucose Testing -The population of diabetics is large and growing. There are in excess of 150 million diabetics in the world and some believe this number will double by 2010. Although the frequent monitoring of glucose levels is strongly encouraged by health professionals most of the glucose testing products currently on the market are uncomfortable for the user and dissatisfaction is high. Less invasive products are also less effective and have been unable to gain market share. Conditions are favorable for the introduction of an effective, non-invasive product.

Breast Cancer Testing - The market size for breast cancer testing is vast – nearly 200,000 women and 1,700 men were diagnosed in 2006 alone. Although lucrative, competition in this industry is strong. Growth potential is possible, however, as the most effective and widely used diagnostic exam for breast cancer, the mammogram, is potentially harmful due to radiation exposure. Other, less popular, exams that do not involve radiation tend to be both invasive and expensive.

Asthma Testing - Asthma testing products are increasingly in demand. 1 in 20 Americans suffers from asthma and this number stands to increase in the near future. Despite this, the market for pre-attack testing materials is undersaturated. Only one product has reached the marketplace and although inexpensive this product is also relatively inaccurate. Other potential competition may be more accurate but has yet to reach the market.

Prostate Testing - Because 1 in 6 men will be diagnosed with prostate cancer during his lifetime, the market for testing products is also quite large. While two tests currently possess the bulk of the market, they either inaccurate or invasive or both. Because of this relatively weak competitive market new entry possibilities are strong.

Narcotics Testing - Toxicology screens are the most common narcotics testing products currently on the market. Used regularly by law enforcement agencies, medical facilities, and

corporate businesses tests are inexpensive and effective. More advanced technology has also been developed to in an effort to monitor discrete drug levels in an individual's system.
HEMT sensors show promising results for protein, DNA, prostate cancer, kidney injury molecules, pH values of solutions, mercury ions as well glucose in the exhaled breath condensate. The method relies on an amplification of small changes in antibody-structure due to binding to antigens. The characteristics of these sensors include fast response (liquid phase-5 to 10 seconds and gas phase- milli-second), digital output signal, small device size (less than $100 \times 100\ \mu m^2$) and chemical and thermal stability.
Given the ever increasing incidence of diabetes in both the United States and abroad the market for diabetes testing and supplies is large and growing. Moreover, prevalent market-wide dissatisfaction with current testing alternatives - due to discomfort, inaccuracy, and/or cost - leads us to believe that the diabetes testing market is by far the most promising one for this technology. Although possible concerns include a difficult government certification process and insurance coverage, a survey of possible competition shows similar products to be either nonexistent or in an embryonic stage of development, meaning possible market entry can be made carefully and strategically.
Like the market for diabetes testing, the market for breast cancer testing is also highly promising. Although numerous testing alternatives exist the market size is huge and growing - in 2005 the testing market in the United States alone was worth well in excess of $1 billion - and the most common diagnostic methods involve some level of discomfort and/or exposure to radiation giving it the same kind of patient dissatisfaction found among diabetes. Because testing is performed less frequently, however, its larger market may prove less lucrative and market entry is highly dependent upon government regulations and insurance coverage. Barring these difficulties market entry (if made carefully) should be relatively easy.
There are still some critical issues. First, the sensitivity for certain antigens (such as prostate or breast cancer) needs to be improved further to allow sensing in body fluids other than blood (urine, saliva). Second, a sandwich assay allowing the detection of the same antigen using two different antibodies (similar to ELISA) needs to be tested. Third, integrating multiple sensors on a single chip with automated fluid handling and algorithms to analyze multiple detection signals, and fourth, a package that will result in a cheap final product is needed. Fourth, the stability of surface functionalization layers in some cases is not conducive to long-term storage and this will limit the applicability of those sensors outside of clinics. There is certainly a need for detection of multiple analytes simultaneously. However, there are many such approaches and acceptance from the clinical community is generally slow for many reasons, including regulatory concerns.

11. Acknowledgments

The work at UF is partially supported by the Office of Naval Research (ONR) under Contract number 00075094 monitored by Dr. Chagaan Baatar, NSF under contract number ECCS 0901711 monitored by Dr. Yogesh B. Gianchandani, NASA Kennedy Space Center Grant NAG 10-316 monitored by Mr. Daniel E. Fitch, and by Superfund Basic Research Program Grant RO1ES015449.

12. References

Learn About Cancer. American Cancer Society.
What is Breast Cancer? United States Department of Health and Human Services.

Accordino, R., A. Visentin, A. Bordin, S. Ferrazzoni, E. Marian, F. Rizzato, C. Canova, R. Venturini & P. Maestrelli (2008) Long-term repeatability of exhaled breath condensate pH in asthma. *Respiratory Medicine,* 102, 377-381.

Anderson, J. L., E. F. Bowden & P. G. Pickup (1996) Dynamic electrochemistry: Methodology and application. *Analytical Chemistry,* 68, R379-R444.

Anderson, T., F. Ren, S. Pearton, B. Kang, H. Wang, C. Chang & J. Lin (2009) Advances in Hydrogen, Carbon Dioxide, and Hydrocarbon Gas Sensor Technology Using GaN and ZnO-Based Devices. *Sensors,* 9, 4669-4694.

Anderson, T., H. Wang, B. Kang, F. Ren, S. Pearton, A. Osinsky, A. Dabiran & P. Chow (2008) Effect of bias voltage polarity on hydrogen sensing with AlGaN/GaN Schottky diodes. *Applied Surface Science,* 255, 2524-2526.

Anh, D. T. V., W. Olthuis & P. Bergveld (2005) A hydrogen peroxide sensor for exhaled breath measurement. *Sensors and Actuators B-Chemical,* 111, 494-499.

Arnon, S. S., R. Schechter, T. V. Inglesby, D. A. Henderson, J. G. Bartlett, M. S. Ascher, E. Eitzen, A. D. Fine, J. Hauer, M. Layton, S. Lillibridge, M. T. Osterholm, T. O'Toole, G. Parker, T. M. Perl, P. K. Russell, D. L. Swerdlow, K. Tonat & B. Working Grp Civilian (2001) Botulinum toxin as a biological weapon - Medical and public health management. *Jama-Journal of the American Medical Association,* 285, 1059-1070.

Bagramyan, K., J. R. Barash, S. S. Arnon & M. Kalkum (2008) Attomolar Detection of Botulinum Toxin Type A in Complex Biological Matrices. *Plos One,* 3.

Bermudez, J. 2001. *The armed forces of North Korea.* IB Tauris.

Bern, H. A. (1998) The fragile fetus. *Journal of Clean Technology Environmental Toxicology and Occupational Medicine,* 7, 25-32.

Bigler, L. R., C. F. Streckfus, L. Copeland, R. Burns, X. L. Dai, M. Kuhn, P. Martin & S. A. Bigler (2002) The potential use of saliva to detect recurrence of disease in women with breast carcinoma. *Journal of Oral Pathology & Medicine,* 31, 421-431.

Blackwell, P. A., M. R. Cave, A. E. Davis & S. A. Malik (1997) Determination of chlorine and bromine in rocks by alkaline fusion with ion chromatography detection. *Journal of Chromatography A,* 770, 93-98.

Bloemen, K., G. Lissens, K. Desager & G. Schoeters (2007) Determinants of variability of protein content, volume and pH of exhaled breath condensate. *Respiratory Medicine,* 101, 1331-1337.

Bonventre, J. V. & J. M. Weinberg (2003) Recent advances in the pathophysiology of ischemic acute renal failure. *Journal of the American Society of Nephrology,* 14, 2199-2210.

Burlingame, A., R. Boyd & S. Gaskell (1996) Mass Spectrometry. *Anal. Chem,* 68, 599-652.

Carmon, K., R. Baltus & L. Luck (2005a) A biosensor for estrogenic substances using the quartz crystal microbalance. *Analytical Biochemistry,* 345, 277-283.

Carmon, K. S., R. E. Baltus & L. A. Luck (2005b) A biosensor for estrogenic substances using the quartz crystal microbalance. *Analytical Biochemistry,* 345, 277-283.

Carpagnano, G. E., M. P. F. Barbaro, O. Resta, E. Gramiccioni, N. V. Valerio, P. Bracciale & G. Valerio (2005) Exhaled markers in the monitoring of airways inflammation and its response to steroid's treatment in mild persistent asthma. *European Journal of Pharmacology,* 519, 175-181.

Chase, W. R. (2000) Salivary markers: their role in breast cancer detection. *J Mich Dent Assoc,* 82, 12.

Chen, K., H. Wang, B. Kang, C. Chang, Y. Wang, T. Lele, F. Ren, S. Pearton, A. Dabiran, A. Osinsky & P. Chow (2008) Low Hg(II) ion concentration electrical detection with AlGaN/GaN high electron mobility transistors. *Sensors And Actuators B-Chemical,* 134, 386-389.

Chen, R. J., S. Bangsaruntip, K. A. Drouvalakis, N. W. S. Kam, M. Shim, Y. M. Li, W. Kim, P. J. Utz & H. J. Dai (2003) Noncovalent functionalization of carbon nanotubes for highly specific electronic biosensors. *Proceedings of the National Academy of Sciences of the United States of America,* 100, 4984-4989.

Chertow, G. M., E. M. Levy, K. E. Hammermeister, F. Grover & J. Daley (1998) Independent association between acute renal failure and mortality following cardiac surgery. *American Journal of Medicine,* 104, 343-348.

Cook, J. M. & D. L. Miles. 1980. Methods for the chemical analysis of groundwater, *Report, 80/5*. Institute of Geological. Sciences.

Cordesman, A. (1998) Weapons of mass destruction in the Gulf and greater Middle East: force trends, strategy, tactics and damage effects. *Washington DC: Center for Strategic and International Studies*, 18–52.

Curreli, M., R. Zhang, F. N. Ishikawa, H. K. Chang, R. J. Cote, C. Zhou & M. E. Thompson (2008) Real-Time, Label-Free Detection of Biological Entities Using Nanowire-Based FETs. *Ieee Transactions on Nanotechnology,* 7, 651-667.

Czebe, K., I. Barta, B. Antus, M. Valyon, I. Horvath & T. Kullmann (2008) Influence of condensing equipment and temperature on exhaled breath condensate pH, total protein and leukotriene concentrations. *Respiratory Medicine,* 102, 720-725.

Davidsson, A., K. N. Sjosward, L. Lundman & B. Schmekel (2005) Quantitative assessment and repeatability of chlorine in exhaled breath condensate - Comparison of two types of condensators. *Respiration,* 72, 529-536.

Davidsson, A., M. Soderstrom, K. N. Sjosward & B. Schmekel (2007) Chlorine in breath condensate - A measure of airway affection in pollinosis? *Respiration,* 74, 184-191.

Davis, D. L., H. L. Bradlow, M. Wolff, T. Woodruff, D. G. Hoel & H. Antonculver (1993) Medical Hypothesis - Xenoestrogens As Preventable Causes Of Breast-Cancer. *Environmental Health Perspectives,* 101, 372-377.

Denslow, N. D., M. C. Chow, K. J. Kroll & L. Green (1999) Vitellogenin as a biomarker of exposure for estrogen or estrogen mimics. *Ecotoxicology,* 8, 385-398.

Di, J. W., J. J. Cheng, Q. A. Xu, H. I. Zheng, J. Y. Zhuang, Y. B. Sun, K. Y. Wang, X. Y. Mo & S. P. Bi (2007) Direct electrochemistry of lactate dehydrogenase immobilized on silica sol-gel modified gold electrode and its application. *Biosensors & Bioelectronics,* 23, 682-687.

Effros, R. M., K. W. Hoagland, M. Bosbous, D. Castillo, B. Foss, M. Dunning, M. Gare, W. Lin & F. Sun (2002) Dilution of respiratory solutes in exhaled condensates. *American Journal of Respiratory and Critical Care Medicine,* 165, 663-669.

Eickhoff, M., J. Schalwig, G. Steinhoff, O. Weidemann, L. Görgens, R. Neuberger, M. Hermann, B. Baur, G. Müller & O. Ambacher (2003) Electronics and sensors based on pyroelectric AlGaN/GaN heterostructures–Part B: Sensor applications. *physica status solidi (c)*, 1908-1918.

Eidem, J. K., H. Kleivdal, K. Kroll, N. Denslow, R. van Aerle, C. Tyler, G. Panter, T. Hutchinson & A. Goksoyr (2006) Development and validation of a direct homologous quantitative sandwich ELISA for fathead minnow (Pimephales promelas) vitellogenin. *Aquatic Toxicology,* 78, 202-206.

Elsheimer, H. N. (1987) Application Of An Ion-Selective Electrode Method To The Determination Of Chloride In 41 International Geochemical Reference Materials. *Geostandards Newsletter,* 11, 115-122.

Fernández-Sánchez, C., C. McNeil, K. Rawson & O. Nilsson (2004) Disposable noncompetitive immunosensor for free and total prostate-specific antigen based on capacitance measurement. *Anal. Chem,* 76, 5649-5656.

Gangwani, P., S. Pandey, S. Haldar, M. Gupta & R. S. Gupta (2007) Polarization dependent analysis of AlGaN/GaN HEMT for high power applications. *Solid-State Electronics,* 51, 130-135.

Garcia-Reyero, N., D. S. Barber, T. S. Gross, K. G. Johnson, M. S. Sepulveda, N. J. Szabo & N. D. Denslow (2006) Dietary exposure of largemouth bass to OCPs changes expression of genes important for reproduction. *Aquatic Toxicology,* 78, 358-369.

Garcia-Reyero, N., K. J. Kroll, L. Liu, E. F. Orlando, K. H. Watanabe, M. S. Sepulveda, D. L. Villeneuve, E. J. Perkins, G. T. Ankley & N. D. Denslow (2009) Gene expression responses in male fathead minnows exposed to binary mixtures of an estrogen and antiestrogen. *Bmc Genomics,* 10.

Gessner, C., S. Hammerschmidt, H. Kuhn, H. A. Seyfarth, U. Sack, L. Engelmann, J. Schauer & H. Wirtz (2003) Exhaled breath condensate acidification in acute lung injury. *Respiratory Medicine,* 97, 1188-1194.

Graule, T., A. Vonbohlen, J. A. C. Broekaert, E. Grallath, R. Klockenkamper, P. Tschopel & G. Tolg (1989) Atomic Emission And Atomic-Absorption Spectrometric Analysis Of High-Purity Powders For The Production Of Ceramics. *Fresenius Zeitschrift Fur Analytische Chemie,* 335, 637-642.

Greenfield, R. A., B. R. Brown, J. B. Hutchins, J. J. Iandolo, R. Jackson, L. N. Slater & M. S. Bronze (2002) Microbiological, biological, and chemical weapons of warfare and terrorism. *American Journal of the Medical Sciences,* 323, 326-340.

Haccoun, J., B. Piro, V. Noel & M. C. Pham (2006) The development of reagentless lactate biosensor based on a novel conducting polymer. *Bioelectrochemistry,* 68, 218-226.

Hahn, T., K. Tag, K. Riedel, S. Uhlig, K. Baronian, G. Gellissen & G. Kunze (2006) A novel estrogen sensor based on recombinant Arxula adeninivorans cells. *Biosensors & Bioelectronics,* 21, 2078-2085.

Han, D. I., D. S. Kim, J. E. Park, J. K. Shin, S. H. Kong, P. Choi, J. H. Lee & G. Lim (2005) Detection of streptavidin-biotin protein complexes using three-dimensional MOSFET in the Si micro-fluidic channel. *Japanese Journal of Applied Physics Part 1-Regular Papers Brief Communications & Review Papers,* 44, 5496-5499.

Harrison, T., L. Bigler, M. Tucci, L. Pratt, F. Malamud, J. T. Thigpen, C. Streckfus & H. Younger (1998) Salivary sIgA concentrations and stimulated whole saliva flow rates among women undergoing chemotherapy for breast cancer: an exploratory study. *Spec Care Dentist,* 18, 109-12.

Healy, D. A., C. J. Hayes, P. Leonard, L. McKenna & R. O'Kennedy (2007) Biosensor developments: application to prostate-specific antigen detection. *Trends in Biotechnology,* 25, 125-131.

Heppell, S. A., N. D. Denslow, L. C. Folmar & C. V. Sullivan (1995) Universal Assay Of Vitellogenin As A Biomarker For Environmental Estrogens. *Environmental Health Perspectives,* 103, 9-15.

Hinck, J. E., V. S. Blazer, N. D. Denslow, K. R. Echols, R. W. Gale, C. Wieser, T. W. Maya, M. Ellersiecke, J. J. Coyle & D. E. Tillitt (2008) Chemical contaminants, health indicators, and reproductive biomarker responses in fish from rivers in the Southeastern United States. *Science of the Total Environment,* 390, 538-557.

Horvath, I., J. Hunt, P. J. Barnes & A. E. T. F. E. Breath (2005) Exhaled breath condensate: methodological recommendations and unresolved questions. *European Respiratory Journal,* 26, 523-548.

Hrapovic, S., Y. L. Liu, K. B. Male & J. H. T. Luong (2004) Electrochemical biosensing platforms using platinum nanoparticles and carbon nanotubes. *Analytical Chemistry,* 76, 1083-1088.

Huber, F., H. P. Lang & C. Gerber (2008) BIOSENSORS New leverage against superbugs. *Nature Nanotechnology,* 3, 645-646.

Hunt, J. F., K. Z. Fang, R. Malik, A. Snyder, N. Malhotra, T. A. E. Platts-Mills & B. Gaston (2000) Endogenous airway acidification - Implications for asthma pathophysiology. *American Journal of Respiratory and Critical Care Medicine,* 161, 694-699.

Hwang, K. S., J. H. Lee, J. Park, D. S. Yoon, J. H. Park & T. S. Kim (2004) In-situ quantitative analysis of a prostate-specific antigen (PSA) using a nanomechanical PZT cantilever. *Lab on a Chip,* 4, 547-552.

Ichimura, T., J. V. Bonventre, V. Bailly, H. Wei, C. A. Hession, R. L. Cate & M. Sanicola (1998) Kidney injury molecule-1 (KIM-1), a putative epithelial cell adhesion molecule containing a novel immunoglobulin domain, is up-regulated in renal cells after injury. *Journal of Biological Chemistry,* 273, 4135-4142.

Jackson, K. W. & G. R. Chen (1996) Atomic absorption, atomic emission, and flame emission spectrometry. *Analytical Chemistry,* 68, R231-R256.

Johnson, J., Y. H. Choi, A. Ural, W. Lim, J. S. Wright, B. P. Gila, F. Ren & S. J. Pearton (2009) Growth and Characterization of GaN Nanowires for Hydrogen Sensors. *Journal of Electronic Materials,* 38, 490-494.

Johnson, J. W., B. Luo, F. Ren, B. P. Gila, W. Krishnamoorthy, C. R. Abernathy, S. J. Pearton, J. I. Chyi, T. E. Nee, C. M. Lee & C. C. Chuo (2000) Gd2O3/GaN metal-oxide-semiconductor field-effect transistor. *Applied Physics Letters,* 77, 3230-3232.

Jun, J., B. Chou, J. Lin, A. Phipps, X. Shengwen, K. Ngo, D. Johnson, A. Kasyap, T. Nishida, H. T. Wang, B. S. Kang, F. Ren, L. C. Tien, P. W. Sadik, D. P. Norton, L. F. Voss & S. J. Pearton (2007) A hydrogen leakage detection system using self-powered wireless hydrogen sensor nodes. *Solid-State Electronics,* 51, 1018-1022.

Kang, B., S. Kim, F. Ren, J. Johnson, R. Therrien, P. Rajagopal, J. Roberts, E. Piner, K. Linthicum, S. Chu, K. Baik, B. Gila, C. Abernathy & S. Pearton (2004a) Pressure-induced changes in the conductivity of AlGaN/GaN high-electron mobility-transistor membranes. *Applied Physics Letters,* 85, 2962-2964.

Kang, B., G. Louche, R. Duran, Y. Gnanou, S. Pearton & F. Ren (2004b) Gateless AlGaN/GaN HEMT response to block co-polymers. *Solid-State Electronics,* 48, 851-854.

Kang, B., R. Mehandru, S. Kim, F. Ren, R. Fitch, J. Gillespie, N. Moser, G. Jessen, T. Jenkins & R. Dettmer (2005a) Hydrogen sensors based on Sc2O3/AlGaN/GaN high electron mobility transistors. *physica status solidi (c),* 2, 2672-2675.

Kang, B., S. Pearton, J. Chen, F. Ren, J. Johnson, R. Therrien, P. Rajagopal, J. Roberts, E. Piner & K. Linthicum (2006) Electrical detection of deoxyribonucleic acid hybridization with AlGaN/GaN high electron mobility transistors. *Applied Physics Letters,* 89, -.

Kang, B., F. Ren, Y. Heo, L. Tien, D. Norton & S. Pearton (2005b) pH measurements with single ZnO nanorods integrated with a microchannel. *Applied Physics Letters,* 86, -.

Kang, B., F. Ren, L. Wang, C. Lofton, W. Tan, S. Pearton, A. Dabiran, A. Osinsky & P. Chow (2005c) Electrical detection of immobilized proteins with ungated AlGaN/GaN high-electron-mobility transistors. *Applied Physics Letters,* 87, -.

Kang, B., H. Wang, T. Lele, Y. Tseng, F. Ren, S. Pearton, J. Johnson, P. Rajagopal, J. Roberts, E. Piner & K. Linthicum (2007a) Prostate specific antigen detection using AlGaN/GaN high electron mobility transistors. *Applied Physics Letters,* 91, -.

Kang, B., H. Wang, F. Ren, B. Gila, C. Abernathy, S. Pearton, D. Dennis, J. Johnson, P. Rajagopal, J. Roberts, E. Piner & K. Linthicum (2008) Exhaled-breath detection using AlGaN/GaN high electron mobility transistors integrated with a Peltier element. *Electrochemical And Solid State Letters,* 11, J19-J21.

Kang, B., H. Wang, F. Ren, S. Pearton, T. Morey, D. Dennis, J. Johnson, P. Rajagopal, J. Roberts, E. Piner & K. Linthicum (2007b) Enzymatic glucose detection using ZnO nanorods on the gate region of AlGaN/GaN high electron mobility transistors. *Applied Physics Letters,* 91, -.

Kang, B. S., S. Kim, F. Ren, B. P. Gila, C. R. Abernathy & S. J. Pearton (2005d) Comparison of MOS and Schottky W/Pt-GaN diodes for hydrogen detection. *Sensors and Actuators B-Chemical,* 104, 232-236.

Kang, B. S., H. T. Wang, T. P. Lele, Y. Tseng, F. Ren, S. J. Pearton, J. W. Johnson, P. Rajagopal, J. C. Roberts, E. L. Piner & K. J. Linthicum (2007c) Prostate specific antigen detection using AlGaN/GaN high electron mobility transistors. *Applied Physics Letters,* 91.

Kang, B. S., H. T. Wang, F. Ren, B. P. Gila, C. R. Abernathy, S. J. Pearton, J. W. Johnson, P. Rajagopal, J. C. Roberts, E. L. Piner & K. J. Linthicum (2007d) pH sensor using AlGaN/GaN high electron mobility transistors with Sc2O3 in the gate region. *Applied Physics Letters,* 91.

Kelloff, G. J., D. S. Coffey, B. A. Chabner, A. P. Dicker, K. Z. Guyton, P. D. Nisen, H. R. Soule & A. V. D'Amico (2004) Prostate-specific antigen doubling time as a surrogate marker for evaluation of oncologic drugs to treat prostate cancer. *Clinical Cancer Research,* 10, 3927-3933.

Kim, J., B. P. Gila, C. R. Abernathy, G. Y. Chung, F. Ren & S. J. Pearton (2003) Comparison of Pt/GaN and Pt/4H-SiC gas sensors. *Solid-State Electronics,* 47, 1487-1490.

Kostikas, K., G. Papatheodorou, K. Ganas, K. Psathakis, P. Panagou & S. Loukides (2002) pH in expired breath condensate of patients with inflammatory airway diseases. *American Journal of Respiratory and Critical Care Medicine,* 165, 1364-1370.

Kouassi, G., J. Irudayaraj & G. McCarty (2005) Activity of glucose oxidase functionalized onto magnetic nanoparticles. *Biomagnetic research and technology,* 3, 1.

Kouche, A. E. L., J. Lin, M. E. Law, S. Kim, B. S. Kim, F. Ren & S. T. Pearton (2005) Remote sensing system for hydrogen using GaN Schottky diodes. *Sensors and Actuators B-Chemical,* 105, 329-333.

Krylriouk, O., H. Park, H. Wang, B. Kang, T. Anderson, F. Ren & S. Pearton (2005) Pt-coated InN nanorods for selective detection of hydrogen at room temperature. *Journal Of Vacuum Science & Technology B,* 23, 1891-1894.

Kullmann, T., I. Barta, E. Csiszer, B. Antus & I. Horvath (2008) Differential Cytokine Pattern in the Exhaled Breath of Patients with Lung Cancer. *Pathology & Oncology Research,* 14, 481-483.

Kullmann, T., I. Barta, Z. Lazar, B. Szili, E. Barat, M. Valyon, M. Kollai & I. Horvath (2007) Exhaled breath condensate pH stanclardised for CO2 partial pressure. *European Respiratory Journal,* 29, 496-501.

Kumar, S. D., K. Venkatesh & B. Maiti (2004) Determination of chloride in nuclear-grade boron carbide by ion chromatography. *Chromatographia,* 59, 243-245.

Langlois, J., W. Rutland-Brown & K. Thomas. 2004. *Traumatic brain injury in the United States: emergency department visits, hospitalizations, and deaths*. Dept. of Health and Human Services, Centers for Disease Control and Prevention, Division of Acute Care, Rehabilitation Research and Disability Prevention, National Center for Injury Prevention and Control.

Lequin, R. M. (2005) Enzyme Immunoassay (EIA)/Enzyme-Linked Immunosorbent Assay (ELISA). *Clinical Chemistry,* 51, 2415-2418.

Li, C., M. Curreli, H. Lin, B. Lei, F. N. Ishikawa, R. Datar, R. J. Cote, M. E. Thompson & C. W. Zhou (2005) Complementary detection of prostate-specific antigen using ln(2)O(3) nanowires and carbon nanotubes. *Journal of the American Chemical Society,* 127, 12484-12485.

Liehlr, J. G. (2001) Genotoxicity of the steroidal oestrogens oestrone and oestradiol: possible mechanism of uterine and mammary cancer development. *Human Reproduction Update,* 7, 273-281.

Lim, W., J. S. Wright, B. P. Gila, J. L. Johnson, A. Ural, T. Anderson, F. Ren & S. J. Pearton (2008) Room temperature hydrogen detection using Pd-coated GaN nanowires. *Applied Physics Letters,* 93.

Lin, C. L., C. L. Shih & L. K. Chau (2007) Amperometric L-Lactate sensor based on sol-gel processing of an enzyme-linked silicon alkoxide. *Analytical Chemistry,* 79, 3757-3763.

Lothian, J. R., J. M. Kuo, F. Ren & S. J. Pearton (1992) Plasma and Wet Chemical Etching of IN0.5GA0.5P. *Journal of Electronic Materials,* 21, 441-445.

Lupu, A., A. Valsesia, F. Bretagnol, P. Colpo & F. Rossi (2007) Development of a potentiometric biosensor based on nanostructured surface for lactate determination. *Sensors and Actuators B-Chemical,* 127, 606-612.

Luther, B. P., S. D. Wolter & S. E. Mohney (1999) High temperature Pt Schottky diode gas sensors on n-type GaN. *Sensors and Actuators B-Chemical,* 56, 164-168.

Machado, R. F., D. Laskowski, O. Deffenderfer, T. Burch, S. Zheng, P. J. Mazzone, T. Mekhail, C. Jennings, J. K. Stoller, J. Pyle, J. Duncan, R. A. Dweik & S. C. Erzurum (2005) Detection of lung cancer by sensor array analyses of exhaled breath. *American Journal of Respiratory and Critical Care Medicine,* 171, 1286-1291.

Makimoto, T., Y. Yamauchi & K. Kumakura (2004) High-power characteristics of GaN/InGaN double heterojunction bipolar transistors. *Applied Physics Letters,* 84, 1964-1966.

Marquette, C. A., A. Degiuli & L. J. Blum (2000) Fiberoptic biosensors based on chemiluminescent reactions. *Applied Biochemistry and Biotechnology,* 89, 107-115.

Matozzo, V., F. Gagne, M. Marin, F. Ricciardi & C. Blaise (2008a) Vitellogenin as a biomarker of exposure to estrogenic compounds in aquatic invertebrates: A review. *Environment International,* 34, 531-545.

Matozzo, V., F. Gagne, M. G. Marin, F. Ricciardi & C. Blaise (2008b) Vitellogenin as a biomarker of exposure to estrogenic compounds in aquatic invertebrates: A review. *Environment International,* 34, 531-545.

McIntyre, R., L. Bigler, T. Dellinger, M. Pfeifer, T. Mannery & C. Streckfus (1999) Oral contraceptive usage and the expression of CA 15-3 and c-erbB-2 in the saliva of healthy women. *Oral Surgery Oral Medicine Oral Pathology Oral Radiology and Endodontics,* 88, 687-690.

Mehandru, R., B. Luo, B. Kang, J. Kim, F. Ren, S. Pearton, C. Pan, G. Chen & J. Chyi (2004) AlGaN/GaN HEMT based liquid sensors. *Solid-State Electronics,* 48, 351-353.

Michaelson, J. S., E. Halpern & D. B. Kopans (1999) Breast cancer: Computer simulation method for estimating optimal intervals for screening. *Radiology,* 212, 551-560.

Montuschi, P. & P. J. Barnes (2002) Analysis of exhaled breath condensate for monitoring airway inflammation. *Trends in Pharmacological Sciences,* 23, 232-237.

Mosconi, G., O. Carnevali, M. F. Franzoni, E. Cottone, I. Lutz, W. Kloas, K. Yamamoto, S. Kikuyama & A. M. Polzonetti-Magni (2002) Environmental Estrogens and reproductive biology in amphibians. *General and Comparative Endocrinology,* 126, 125-129.

Namjou, K., C. B. Roller & P. J. McCann (2006) The breathmeter - A new laser device to analyze your health. *Ieee Circuits & Devices,* 22, 22-28.

Navarro, M. A., R. Mesia, O. DiezGibert, A. Rueda, B. Ojeda & M. C. Alonso (1997) Epidermal growth factor in plasma and saliva of patients with active breast cancer and breast cancer patients in follow-up compared with healthy women. *Breast Cancer Research and Treatment,* 42, 83-86.

Neuberger, R., G. Müller, O. Ambacher & M. Stutzmann (2001) Ion-induced modulation of channel currents in AlGaN/GaN high-electron-mobility transistors. *physica status solidi (a),* 183, R10-R12.

Niimi, A., L. T. Nguyen, O. Usmani, B. Mann & K. F. Chung (2004) Reduced pH and chloride levels in exhaled breath condensate of patients with chronic cough. *Thorax,* 59, 608-612.

Paige, S. Z. & C. F. Streckfus (2007) Salivary analysis in the diagnosis and treatment of breast cancer: a role for the general dentist. *Gen Dent,* 55, 156-7; quiz 158, 167-8.

Pandey, P., S. P. Singh, S. K. Arya, V. Gupta, M. Datta, S. Singh & B. D. Malhotra (2007) Application of thiolated gold nanoparticles for the enhancement of glucose oxidase activity. *Langmuir,* 23, 3333-3337.

Park, S., H. Boo & T. D. Chung (2006) Electrochemical non-enzymatic glucose sensors. *Analytica Chimica Acta,* 556, 46-57.

Parra, A., E. Casero, L. Vazquez, F. Pariente & E. Lorenzo (2006) Design and characterization of a lactate biosensor based on immobilized lactate oxidase onto gold surfaces. *Analytica Chimica Acta,* 555, 308-315.

Patolsky, F., B. Timko, G. Zheng & C. Lieber (2007) Nanowire-based nanoelectronic devices in the life sciences. *Mrs Bulletin,* 32, 142-149.

Patolsky, F., G. Zheng & C. Lieber (2006a) Fabrication of silicon nanowire devices for ultrasensitive, label-free, real-time detection of biological and chemical species. *Nature Protocols,* 1, 1711-1724. (2006b) Nanowire sensors for medicine and the life sciences. *Nanomedicine,* 1, 51-65.

Pearton, S. J., B. S. Kang, S. K. Kim, F. Ren, B. P. Gila, C. R. Abernathy, J. S. Lin & S. N. G. Chu (2004) GaN-based diodes and transistors for chemical, gas, biological and pressure sensing. *Journal of Physics-Condensed Matter,* 16, R961-R994.

Pearton, S. J., T. Lele, Y. Tseng & F. Ren (2007) Penetrating living cells using semiconductor nanowires. *Trends in Biotechnology,* 25, 481-482.

Phypers, B. & J. Pierce (2006) Lactate physiology in health and disease. *Continuing Education in Anaesthesia, Critical Care & Pain,* 6, 128.

Pohanka, M. & P. Zboril (2008) Amperometric biosensor for D-lactate assay. *Food Technology and Biotechnology,* 46, 107-110.

Porte, C., G. Janer, L. Lorusso, M. Ortiz-Zarragoitia, M. Cajaraville, M. Fossi & L. Canesi (2006) Endocrine disruptors in marine organisms: Approaches and perspectives. *Comparative Biochemistry And Physiology C-Toxicology & Pharmacology,* 143, 303-315.

Sabo-Attwood, T., J. L. Blum, K. J. Kroll, V. Patel, D. Birkhoiz, N. J. Szabo, S. Z. Fisher, R. McKenna, M. Campbell-Thompson & N. D. Denslow (2007) Distinct expression and activity profiles of largemouth bass (Micropterus salmoides) estrogen receptors in response to estradiol and nonylphenol. *Journal of Molecular Endocrinology,* 39, 223-237.

Saito, W., T. Domon, I. Omura, M. Kuraguchi, Y. Takada, K. Tsuda & M. Yamaguchi (2006) Demonstration of 13.56-MHz class-E amplifier using a high-voltage GaN power-HEMT. *Ieee Electron Device Letters,* 27, 326-328.

Sandhu, A. (2007) Biosensing - New probes offer much faster results. *Nature Nanotechnology,* 2, 746-748.

Schalwig, J., G. Muller, U. Karrer, M. Eickhoff, O. Ambacher, M. Stutzmann, L. Gorgens & G. Dollinger (2002) Hydrogen response mechanism of Pt-GaN Schottky diodes. *Applied Physics Letters,* 80, 1222-1224.

Shen, L., R. Coffie, D. Buttari, S. Heikman, A. Chakraborty, A. Chini, S. Keller, S. P. DenBaars & U. K. Mishra (2004) High-power polarization-engineered GaN/AlGaN/GaN HEMTs without surface passivation. *Ieee Electron Device Letters,* 25, 7-9.

Spohn, U., D. Narasaiah, L. Gorton & D. Pfeiffer (1996) A bienzyme modified carbon paste electrode for the amperometric detection of L-lactate at low potentials. *Analytica Chimica Acta,* 319, 79-90.

Streckfus, C. & L. Bigler (2005) The use of soluble, salivary c-erbB-2 for the detection and post-operative follow-up of breast cancer in women: the results of a five-year translational research study. *Adv Dent Res,* 18, 17-24.

Streckfus, C., L. Bigler, T. Dellinger, X. L. Dai, W. J. Cox, A. McArthur, A. Kingman & J. T. Thigpen (2001) Reliability assessment of soluble c-erbB-2 concentrations in the saliva of healthy women and men. *Oral Surgery Oral Medicine Oral Pathology Oral Radiology and Endodontics,* 91, 174-179.

Streckfus, C., L. Bigler, T. Dellinger, X. L. Dai, A. Kingman & J. T. Thigpen (2000a) The presence of soluble c-erbB-2 in saliva and serum among women with breast carcinoma: A preliminary study. *Clinical Cancer Research,* 6, 2363-2370.

Streckfus, C., L. Bigler, T. Dellinger, M. Pfeifer, A. Rose & J. T. Thigpen (1999) CA 15-3 and c-erbB-2 presence in the saliva of women. *Clin Oral Investig,* 3, 138-43.

Streckfus, C., L. Bigler, M. Tucci & J. T. Thigpen (2000b) A preliminary study of CA15-3, c-erbB-2, epidermal growth factor receptor, cathepsin-D, and p53 in saliva among women with breast carcinoma. *Cancer Investigation,* 18, 101-109.

Streckfus, C. F., L. R. Bigler & M. Zwick (2006) The use of surface-enhanced laser desorption/ionization time-of-flight mass spectrometry to detect putative breast cancer markers in saliva: a feasibility study. *Journal of Oral Pathology & Medicine,* 35, 292-300.

Suman, S., R. Singhal, A. L. Sharma, B. D. Malthotra & C. S. Pundir (2005) Development of a lactate biosensor based on conducting copolymer bound lactate oxidase. *Sensors and Actuators B-Chemical,* 107, 768-772.

Sumpter, J. P. & S. Jobling (1995) Vitellogenesis as a Biomarker for Estrogenic Contamination of the Aquatic Environment. *Environmental Health Perspectives,* 103, 173-178.

Taylor, J. S. & S. K. Hong (2000) Potable water quality and membrane technology. *Laboratory Medicine,* 31, 563-568.

Thadhani, R., M. Pascual & J. V. Bonventre (1996) Medical progress - Acute renal failure. *New England Journal of Medicine,* 334, 1448-1460.

Thompson, I. M. & D. P. Ankerst (2007) Prostate-specific antigen in the early detection of prostate cancer. *Canadian Medical Association Journal,* 176, 1853-1858.

Tien, L., P. Sadik, D. Norton, L. Voss, S. Pearton, H. Wang, B. Kang, F. Ren, J. Jun & J. Lin (2005a) Hydrogen sensing at room temperature with Pt-coated ZnO thin films and nanorods. *Applied Physics Letters,* 87, -.

Tien, L., H. Wang, B. Kang, F. Ren, P. Sadik, D. Norton, S. Pearton & J. Lin (2005b) Room-temperature hydrogen-selective sensing using single Pt-coated ZnO nanowires at microwatt power levels. *Electrochemical and Solid State Letters,* 8, G230-G232.

Vaidya, V. S. & J. V. Bonventre (2006) Mechanistic biomarkers for cytotoxic acute kidney injury. *Expert Opinion on Drug Metabolism & Toxicology,* 2, 697-713.

Vaidya, V. S., V. Ramirez, T. Ichimura, N. A. Bobadilla & J. V. Bonventre (2006) Urinary kidney injury molecule-1: a sensitive quantitative biomarker for early detection of kidney tubular injury. *American Journal of Physiology-Renal Physiology,* 290, F517-F529.

Vaughan, J., L. Ngamtrakulpanit, T. N. Pajewski, R. Turner, T. Nguyen, A. Smith, P. Urban, S. Hom, B. Gaston & J. Hunt (2003) Exhaled breath condensate pH is a robust and reproducible assay of airway acidity. *European Respiratory Journal,* 22, 889-894.

Verma, R. & R. Parthasarathy (1996) Neutron activation analysis for chlorine in Zr-2.5 wt% Nb coolant tube material. *Journal of Radioanalytical and Nuclear Chemistry,* 214, 391-397.

Vignali, D. A. A. (2000) Multiplexed particle-based flow cytometric assays. *Journal of Immunological Methods,* 243, 243-255.

Walker, H., W. Hall & J. Hurst. 1990. *Clinical methods: the history, physical and laboratory examinations*. Butterworths Stoneham, MA.

Wang, H., T. Anderson, B. Kang, F. Ren, C. Li, Z. Low, J. Lin, B. Gila, S. Pearton, A. Osinsky & A. Dabiran (2007a) Stable hydrogen sensors from AlGaN/GaN heterostructure diodes with TiB2-based Ohmic contacts. *Applied Physics Letters*, 90, 252109.

Wang, H., T. Anderson, F. Ren, C. Li, Z. Low, J. Lin, B. Gila, S. Pearton, A. Osinsky & A. Dabiran (2006a) Robust detection of hydrogen using differential AlGaN/GaN high electron mobility transistor sensing diodes. *Applied Physics Letters*, 89, -.

Wang, H., B. Kang, T. Chancellor, T. Lele, Y. Tseng, F. Ren, S. Pearton, A. Dabiran, A. Osinsky & P. Chow (2007b) Selective detection of Hg (II) ions from Cu(II) and Pb(II) using AlGaN/GaN high electron mobility transistors. *Electrochemical and Solid State Letters*, 10, J150-J153.

Wang, H., B. Kang, F. Ren, R. Fitch, J. Gillespie, N. Moser, G. Jessen, T. Jenkins, R. Dettmer, D. Via, A. Crespo, B. Gila, C. Abernathy & S. Pearton (2005a) Comparison of gate and drain current detection of hydrogen at room temperature with AlGaN/GaN high electron mobility transistors. *Applied Physics Letters*, 87, 172105.

Wang, H., B. Kang, F. Ren, L. Tien, P. Sadik, D. Norton, S. Pearton & J. Lin (2005b) Detection of hydrogen at room temperature with catalyst-coated multiple ZnO nanorods. *Applied Physics A-Materials Science & Processing*, 81, 1117-1119.

(2005c) Hydrogen-selective sensing at room temperature with ZnO nanorods. *Applied Physics Letters*, 86, 243503.

Wang, H. T., B. S. Kang, T. F. Chancellor, T. P. Lele, Y. Tseng, F. Ren, S. J. Pearton, W. J. Johnson, P. Rajagopal, J. C. Roberts, E. L. Piner & K. J. Linthicum (2007c) Fast electrical detection of Hg(II) ions with AlGaN/GaN high electron mobility transistors. *Applied Physics Letters*, 91.

Wang, H. T., B. S. Kang, F. Ren, S. J. Pearton, J. W. Johnson, P. Rajagopal, J. C. Roberts, E. L. Piner & K. J. Linthicum (2007d) Electrical detection of kidney injury molecule-1 with AlGaN/GaN high electron mobility transistors. *Applied Physics Letters*, 91.

Wang, J. (2006) Electrochemical biosensors: Towards point-of-care cancer diagnostics. *Biosensors & Bioelectronics*, 21, 1887-1892.

Wang, J. X., X. W. Sun, A. Wei, Y. Lei, X. P. Cai, C. M. Li & Z. L. Dong (2006b) Zinc oxide nanocomb biosensor for glucose detection. *Applied Physics Letters*, 88.

Wang, Y., B. Chu, K. Chen, C. Chang, T. Lele, G. Papadi, J. Coleman, B. Sheppard, C. Dungen, S. Pearton, J. Johnson, P. Rajagopal, J. Roberts, E. Piner, K. Linthicum & F. Ren (2009) Fast detection of a protozoan pathogen, Perkinsus marinus, using AlGaN/GaN high electron mobility transistors. *Applied Physics Letters*, 94, -.

Warden, D. Blast Injury. In *Defense and Veterans Brain Injury center*.

Watson, C. S., N. N. Bulayeva, A. L. Wozniak & R. A. Alyea (2007) Xenoestrogens are potent activators of nongenomic estrogenic responses. *Steroids*, 72, 124-134.

Wee, K. W., G. Y. Kang, J. Park, J. Y. Kang, D. S. Yoon, J. H. Park & T. S. Kim (2005) Novel electrical detection of label-free disease marker proteins using piezoresistive self-sensing micro-cantilevers. *Biosensors & Bioelectronics*, 20, 1932-1938.

Wei, A., X. W. Sun, J. X. Wang, Y. Lei, X. P. Cai, C. M. Li, Z. L. Dong & W. Huang (2006) Enzymatic glucose biosensor based on ZnO nanorod array grown by hydrothermal decomposition. *Applied Physics Letters*, 89.

Wright, J. S., W. Lim, B. P. Gila, S. J. Pearton, F. Ren, W. T. Lai, L. C. Chen, M. S. Hu & K. H. Chen (2009) Pd-catalyzed hydrogen sensing with InN nanobelts. *Journal of Vacuum Science & Technology B,* 27, L8-L10.

Yager, J. D. & J. G. Liehr (1996) Molecular mechanisms of estrogen carcinogenesis. *Annual Review of Pharmacology and Toxicology,* 36, 203-232.

Yang, Y. H., H. F. Yang, M. H. Yang, Y. L. Liu, G. L. Shen & R. Q. Yu (2004) Amperometric glucose biosensor based on a surface treated nanoporous ZrO2/chitosan composite film as immobilization matrix. *Analytica Chimica Acta,* 525, 213-220.

Yu, X., C. Li, Z. N. Low, J. Lin, T. J. Anderson, H. T. Wang, F. Ren, Y. L. Wang, C. Y. Chang, S. J. Pearton, C. H. Hsu, A. Osinsky, A. Dabiran, P. Chow, C. Balaban & J. Painter (2008) Wireless hydrogen sensor network using AlGaN/GaN high electron mobility transistor differential diode sensors. *Sensors and Actuators B-Chemical,* 135, 188-194.

Zhang, A. P., L. B. Rowland, E. B. Kaminsky, J. W. Kretchmer, R. A. Beaupre, J. L. Garrett, J. B. Tucker, B. J. Edward, J. Foppes & A. F. Allen (2003) Microwave power SiC MESFETs and GaNHEMTs. *Solid-State Electronics,* 47, 821-826.

Zhang, J., H. P. Lang, F. Huber, A. Bietsch, W. Grange, U. Certa, R. McKendry, H. J. Guntgerodt, M. Hegner & C. Gerber (2006) Rapid and label-free nanomechanical detection of biomarker transcripts in human RNA. *Nature Nanotechnology,* 1, 214-220.

Zheng, G., F. Patolsky, Y. Cui, W. Wang & C. Lieber (2005a) Multiplexed electrical detection of cancer markers with nanowire sensor arrays. *Nature Biotechnology,* 23, 1294-1301.

Zheng, G. F., F. Patolsky, Y. Cui, W. U. Wang & C. M. Lieber (2005b) Multiplexed electrical detection of cancer markers with nanowire sensor arrays. *Nature Biotechnology,* 23, 1294-1301.

Part 2

Biosensors for Health

3

Biosensors for Health Applications

Cibele Marli Cação Paiva Gouvêa
Universidade Federal de Alfenas
Brazil

1. Introduction

The ability to assess health status, disease onset and progression, and monitor treatment outcome through a non-invasive method is the main aim to be achieved in health care promotion and delivery and research. There are three prerequisites to reach this goal: specific biomarkers that indicates a healthy or diseased state; a non-invasive approach to detect and monitor the biomarkers; and the technologies to discriminate the biomarkers.

The early disease diagnosis is crucial for patient survival and successful prognosis of the disease, so that sensitive and specific methods are required for that. Among the numerous mankind diseases, three of them are relevant because of their worldwide incidence, prevalence, morbidity and mortality, namely diabetes, cardiovascular disease and cancer.

In recent years, the demand has grown in the field of medical diagnostics for simple and disposable devices that also demonstrate fast response times, are user-friendly, cost-efficient, and are suitable for mass production. Biosensor technologies offer the potential to fulfill these criteria through an interdisciplinary combination of approaches from nanotechnology, chemistry and medical science.

The emphasis of this chapter is on the recent advances on the biosensors for diabetes, cardiovascular disease and cancer detection and monitoring. An overview at biorecognition elements and transduction technology will be presented as well as the biomarkers and biosensing systems currently used to detect the onset and monitor the progression of the selected diseases. The last part will discuss some challenges and future directions on this field.

2. Biorecognition elements and transduction technology

2.1 Biorecognition elements

Clinical analyses are no longer carried out exclusively in the clinical chemistry laboratory. Measurements of analytes in biological fluids are routinely performed in various locations, including hospital, by caregivers in non-hospital settings and by patients at home. Biosensors (bioanalytical sensors) for the measurement of analytes of interest in clinical chemistry are ideally suited for these new applications. These factors make biosensors very attractive compared to contemporary chromatographic and spectroscopic techniques.

A biosensor can be generally defined as a device that consists of a biological recognition system and a transducer, for signal processing, to deduce and quantity a particular analyte (Hall, 1990). Biosensors provide advanced platforms for biomarker analysis with the advantages of being easy to use, rapid and robust as well as offering multianalyte testing capability; however a specific biomarker is necessary. Biomarkers are molecules that can be objectively measured and evaluated as indicators of normal or disease processes and pharmacologic responses to therapeutic intervention (Rusling et al., 2010).

The first biosensor was reported by Clark and Lyons (1962) for glucose in blood measurement. They coupled the enzyme glucose oxidase to an amperometric electrode for PO_2. The enzyme-catalyzed oxidation of glucose consumed O_2 and lowered PO_2 that was sensed, proportionally to the glucose concentration in the sample. The enzyme-based sensor was the first generation of biosensors and in the subsequent years a variety of biosensors for other clinically important substances were developed. Therefore, biosensors can be categorized according to the biological recognition element (enzymatic, immuno, DNA and whole-cell biosensors; Spichiger-Keller, 1998) or the signal transduction method (electrochemical, optical, thermal and mass-based biosensors; Wanekaya et al., 2008) (Fig 1).

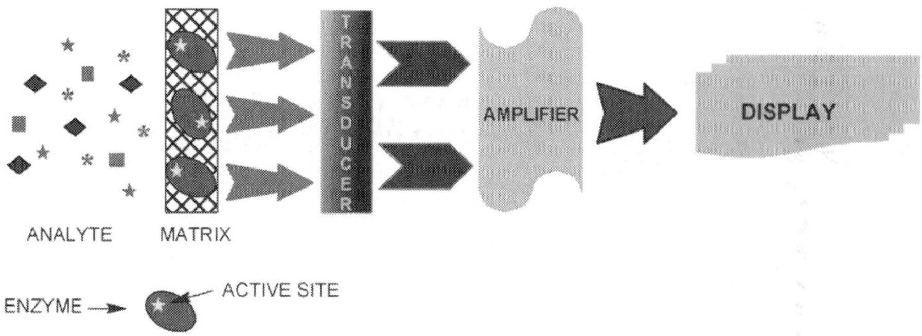

Fig. 1. Schematic of a biosensor (Arya et al., 2008).

Substantial amounts of published work on the enzyme-based biosensors are found in the literature due to their medical applicability, commercial availability or ease of enzyme isolation and purification from different sources and also enzymes can be used in combination for detection of a target analyte (D'Orazio, 2003). By acting as biocatalytic elements, the enzymatic reaction is accompanied by the consumption or production of species such as CO_2, NH_3, H_2O_2, H^+, O_2 or by the activation/inhibition activity that can be detected easily by various transducers and correlate this species to the substrates. Amongst various enzymes, glucose oxidase, horseradish peroxidase, and alkaline phosphatase have been employed in most biosensor studies (Laschi et al., 2000; Wang, 2000). The detection limit is satisfactory or exceeded but the enzyme stability is still a problem, especially considering a long period of time. A major advantage of enzyme-based biosensors is the ability, in some cases, to modify catalytic properties or substrate specificity by genetic engineering. The major limitation is the lack of specificity in differentiating among compounds of similar classes (Buerk, 1993; 2001; D'Orazio, 2003).

Affinity biosensors have received considerable attention in the last years, since they provide information about binding of antibodies to antigens, cell receptors to their ligands, DNA/RNA to complementary sequences of nucleic acids and functioning enzymatic pathways that allow the screening of gene products for metabolic functions.

Immunosensors are based on the high selectivity of the antibody-antigen reaction. The specific interaction is sensed by a transducer and measurements can be obtained directly, in minutes, rather than the hours required for visualizing results of an ELISA test

(Spangler et al., 2001). Either an antigen or antibody can be immobilized onto a surface of support in an array format (Huang et al., 2004) and participates in a biospecific interaction with the other component, allowing detection and quantification of an analyte of interest (Stefan et al., 2000). The sensors may operate either as direct or as indirect sensors often referred to homogeneous and heterogeneous immunosensors, respectively. Antibodies are the critical part of an immunosensor to provide sensitivity and specificity. As the antibody-antigen complex is almost irreversible, only a single immunoassay can be performed (Buerk, 1993) although intensive research effort has been directed toward the regeneration of renewable antibody surfaces. Reproducibility is another concern, partly due to the antibody orientation and immobilization onto the sensor surface. Immunosensors are inherently more versatile than enzyme-based biosensors because antibodies are more selective and specific. Immunosensors are currently been used for infectious diseases diagnosis (Huang et al., 2004).

DNA analysis is the most recent and most promising application of biosensors to clinical chemistry. DNA is well suited for biosensing because the base pairing interactions between complementary sequences are both specific and robust. DNA biosensors employ immobilized relatively short synthetic single-stranded oligodeoxynucleotides that hybridizes to a complementary target DNA in the sample (Palecek, 2002). Hybridization can be performed either in solution or on solid supports. The system can be used for repeated analysis since the nucleic acid ligands can be denatured to reverse binding and then regenerated (Ivnitski et al., 1999). However, considerable research is still needed to develop methods for directly targeting natural DNA present in organisms and in human blood with high detection sensitivity (Palecek, 2002). Accurate tests for recognizing DNA sequences, usually, need to multiply small amounts of DNA into readable quantities using the polymerase chain reaction (PCR). Some of the new gene chips are sensitive enough to eliminate the need for target amplification, a time-consuming process. This improvement has stimulated the development of DNA biosensors with a view toward rapid analysis for point-of-care diagnostics for infectious disease, testing cancer and genetic disease diagnosis and measurement of drug resistance or susceptibility, and even a whole cancer circulating cell can be identified (Liu et al., 2009).

Whole-cell biosensors are based in the general metabolic status of bacteria, fungi, yeasts, animal or plant cells that are the recognition elements. Whole cells can easily be manipulated and adapted to consume and degrade new substrates. Many enzymes and co-factors that co-exist in the cells give them the ability to consume and hence detect a large number of chemicals. However, this may compromise their selectivity (Ding et al., 2008).

The sensing molecule, in general, is hold on a solid support, the matrix. Chemical properties of a desired support decide the method of immobilization and the operational stability of a biosensor. In particular, it should be resistant to a wide range of physiological pHs, temperature, ionic strength and chemical composition. The ability to co-immobilize more than one biologically active component is desirable in some cases. Conducting polymers, carbon nanotubes, nanoparticles, sol-gel/hydro-gels and self-assembled monolayer are common used to immobilize a variety of sensing molecules (Arya et al., 2008).

2.2 Transduction technology

The interaction of the analyte with the bioreceptor is designed to produce an effect measured by the transducer, which converts the information into a measurable signal. A variety of transducer methods have been feasible toward the development of biosensor technology; however the most common methods are electrochemical, optical and piezoelectric (Buerk, 1993; Collings & Caruso 1997; Wang, 2000).

Electrochemical sensors measure the electrochemical changes that occur when analytes interact with a sensing surface of the detecting electrode. The electrochemical assay is simple, reliable, has a low detection limit and a wide dynamic range due to the fact that the electrochemical reactions occur at the electrode–solution interfaces. Based on that and cost competitiveness, more than half of the biosensors, reported in the literature, are based on electrochemical transducers (Meadows, 1996). The electrical changes can be potentiometric (a change in the measured voltage between the indicator and reference electrodes), amperometric (a change in the measured current at a given applied voltage), or conductometric (a change in the ability of the sensing material to transport charge). Amperometry is the electrochemical technique usually applied in commercially available biosensors for clinical analyses that detect redox reactions. The electrochemical platform is suited for enzyme-based and DNA/RNA sensors, field monitoring applications (e.g. hand-held) and miniaturization toward the fabrication of an implantable biosensor.

Optical transducers can be used to monitor affinity reactions and have been applied to quantitate antigenic species of interest in clinical chemistry and to study the kinetics and affinity of antigen–antibody and DNA interactions. Of particular interest have been direct optical transducers based on methods such as internal reflectance spectroscopy, surface plasmon resonance and evanescent wave sensing. Light entering an optical device is directed through optical fibers or planar waveguides toward a sensing surface and reflected back out again. The reflected light is monitored, using a detector such as a photodiode, revealing information about the physical events occurring at the sensing surface. The measured optical signals often include absorbance, fluorescence, chemiluminescence, surface plasmon resonance (to probe refractive index), or changes in light reflectivity. Optical biosensors are preferable for screening a large number of samples simultaneously; however, they cannot be easily miniaturized for insertion into the bloodstream. Most optical methods of transduction require a spectrophotometer to detect signal changes.

Mass sensors can produce a signal based on the mass of chemicals that interact with the sensing film, usually a vibrating piezoelectric quartz crystal. Acoustic wave devices, made of piezoelectric materials, are the most common sensors, which bend when a voltage is applied to the crystal. Acoustic wave sensors are operated by applying an oscillating voltage at the resonant frequency of the crystal, and measuring the change in resonant frequency when the target analyte interacts with the sensing surface. Because a significant amount of nonspecific adsorption occurs in solutions, piezoelectric sensors have received their widest use in gas phase analyses. Extremely high sensitivities are possible with these devices detecting femtogram levels of drug vapors. Similarly to optical detection, piezoelectric detection requires large sophisticated instruments to monitor the signal.

Generation of heat during a reaction can be used in a calorimetric based biosensor. Changes in solution temperature caused by the reaction are measured and compared to a sensor with no reaction to determine the analyte concentration. This approach is well suited for enzyme/substrate reactions that cause changes in solution temperature but not for receptor-ligand reactions because there is no temperature change at steady-state and transient measurements are very difficult to make. Calorimetric microsensors have been manufactured for detection of cholesterol in blood serum based on the enzymatically produced heat of oxidation and decomposition reactions (Caygill et al., 2010).

3. Biosensors for diabetes applications

3.1 Glucose as diabetes biomarker

About 3% of the population worldwide suffers from diabetes, a leading cause of death, and its incidence is growing fast. Diabetes is a syndrome of disordered metabolism resulting in abnormally high blood sugar levels. Diabetic individuals are at a greater heart disease, stroke, high blood pressure, blindness, kidney failure, neurological disorders risk and other health related complications without diligent monitoring blood glucose concentrations. Through patient education, regular examinations and tighter blood glucose monitoring, many of these complications can be reduced significantly (Turner & Pickup, 1985; Lasker, 1993). Optimal management of diabetes involves patients measuring and recording their own blood glucose levels. Under normal physiological condition, the concentration of fasting plasma glucose is in the range 6.1–6.9 $mmolL^{-1}$, so the variation of the blood glucose level can indicate diabetes mellitus, besides other conditions. Consequently, quantitation of the glucose content is of extreme importance, as it is the main diabetes biomarker. The American Diabetes Association recommends that insulin-dependent type 1 diabetics self-monitor blood glucose 3–4 times daily, while insulin-dependent type 2 diabetics monitor once-daily (American, 1997). However, frequent self-monitoring of glucose concentrations is difficult, given the time, the inconvenience and the discomfort involved with the traditional measurement technique. Several methods for glucose analysis have been reported. However, most of these methods involve complex procedures or are expensive in terms of costs. Therefore it is necessary to develop a simple, sensitive, accurate, micro-volume and low-cost approach for glucose analysis which is appropriate for rapid field tests and is also effective as an alternative to the existing methods.

3.2 Biosensors for glucose measuring

Glucose can be monitored by invasive and non-invasive technologies. Glucose biosensor was the first reported biosensor (Clark & Lyons, 1962) and after that a great number of different glucose biosensors were developed, including implantable sensors for measuring glucose in blood or tissue. Glucose sensors are now widely available as small, minimally invasive devices that measure interstitial glucose levels in subcutaneous fat (Cengiz & Tamborlane, 2009). Requirements of a sensor for *in vivo* glucose monitoring include miniaturization of the device, long-term stability, elimination of oxygen dependency, convenience to the user and biocompatibility. Long-term biocompatibility has been the main requirement and has limited the use of *in vivo* glucose sensors, both subcutaneously and intravascular, to short periods of time. Diffusion of low-molecular-weight substances from the sample across the polyurethane sensor outer membrane results in loss of sensor sensitivity. In order to address the problem, microdialysis or ultrafiltration technology has been coupled with glucose biosensors. The current invasive glucose monitors commercially available use glucose oxidase-based electrochemical methods and the electrochemical sensors are inserted into the interstitial fluid space. Most sensors are reasonably accurate although sensor error including drift, calibration error, and delay of the interstitial sensor value behind the blood value are still present (Castle & Ward, 2010). The glucose biosensor is the most widely used example of an electrochemical biosensor which is based on a screen-printed amperometric disposable electrode. This type of biosensor has been used widely throughout the world for glucose testing in the home bringing diagnosis to on site analysis.

Non-invasive glucose sensing is the ultimate goal of glucose monitoring and the main approaches being pursued for glucose sensor development are: near infrared spectroscopy, excreted physiological fluid (tears, sweat, urine, saliva) analysis, microcalorimetry, enzyme electrodes, optical sensors, sonophoresis and iontophoresis, both of which extract glucose from the skin (Koschwanez & Reichert, 2007; Beauharnois et al., 2006; Chu et al., 2011). Despite the relative ease of use, speed and minimal risk of infection involved with infrared spectroscopy, this technique is hindered by the low sensitivity, poor selectivity, frequently required calibrations, and difficulties with miniaturization. Problems surrounding direct glucose analysis through excreted physiological fluids include a weak correlation between excreted fluids and blood glucose concentrations. Exercise and diet that alter glucose concentrations in the fluids also produce inaccurate results (Pickup et al., 2005). The desire to create an artificial pancreas drives for continued research efforts in the biosensor area. Nevertheless, the drawbacks of *in vivo* biosensors must be solved before such an insulin modulating system can be achieved.

4. Biosensors for cardiovascular diseases applications

4.1 Cardiovascular disease biomarkers

Cardiovascular diseases are highly preventable, yet they are major cause of death of humans over the world. One of the most important reasons of the increasing incidences of cardiovascular diseases and cardiac arrest is hypercholesterolemia, i.e. increased concentration of cholesterol in blood (Franco et al., 2011). Hence estimation of cholesterol level in blood is important in clinical applications. The early evaluation of patients with symptoms that indicates an acute coronary syndrome is of great clinical relevance. Biomarkers have become increasingly important in this setting to supplement electrocardiographic findings and patient history because one or both can be misleading. Cardiac troponin is the only marker used routinely nowadays in this setting because it is specific from the myocardial tissue, easily detected, and useful for therapeutic decision making. Determination of the level of other non-myocardial tissue-specific markers might also be helpful, such as myeloperoxidase, copeptin, growth differentiation factor 15 and C-reactive protein (CRP). CRP, which reflects different aspects of the development of atherosclerosis or acute ischemia, is one of the plasma proteins known as acute-phase proteins and its levels rise dramatically during inflammatory processes occurring in the body. This increment is due to a rise in the plasma concentration of IL-6, which is produced predominantly by macrophages as well as adipocytes. CRP can rise as high as 1000-fold with inflammation. CRP was found to be the only marker of inflammation that independently predicts the risk of a heart attack.

4.2 Biosensors in cardiovascular disease

Biosensors for cholesterol measurement comprise the majority of the published articles in the field of cardiovascular diseases. In the fabrication of cholesterol biosensor for the estimation of free cholesterol and total cholesterol, mainly cholesterol oxidase (ChOx) and cholesterol esterase (ChEt) have been employed as the sensing elements (Arya et al., 2008) (Fig. 2). Electrochemical transducers have been effectively utilized for the estimation of cholesterol in the system (Charpentier & Murr, 1995; Singh et al., 2006; Zhou et al., 2006; Arya et al., 2007). Based on number and reliability of optical methods, a variety of optical transducers have been employed for cholesterol sensing, namely monitoring: luminescence, change in color of dye, fluorescence and others (Arya et al., 2008). Other cardiovascular disease biomarkers are also quantified. CRP measurement rely mainly on immunosensing technologies with optical, electrochemical and acoustic transducers besides approaches to simultaneous analytes measurement (Albrecht et al., 2008; Heyduk et al., 2008; McBride & Cooper, 2008; Niotis et al., 2010; Qureshi et al., 2010a,b; Sheu et al., 2010; Zhou et al., 2010). Silva et al. (2010) incorporated streptavidin polystyrene microspheres to the electrode surface of SPEs in order to increase the analytical response of the cardiac troponin T and Park et al. (2009) used an assay based on virus nanoparticles for troponin I highly sensitive and selective diagnostic, a protein marker for a higher risk of acute myocardial infarction.

Early and accurate diagnosis of cardiovascular disease is crucial to save many lives, especially for the patients suffering the heart attack. Accurate and fast quantification of cardiac muscle specific biomarkers in the blood enables accurate diagnosis and prognosis and timely treatment of the patients. It is apparent that increasing incidences of cardiovascular diseases and cardiac arrest in contemporary society denote the necessity of the availability of cholesterol and other biomarkers biosensors. However, only a few have been successfully launched in the market. One of the reasons lays in the optimization of critical parameters, such as enzyme stabilization, quality control and instrumentation design. The efforts directed toward the development of cardiovascular disease biosensors have resulted in the commercialization of a few cholesterol biosensors. A better comprehension of the bioreagents immobilization and technological advances in the microelectronics are likely to speed up commercialization of the much needed biosensors for cardiovascular diseases.

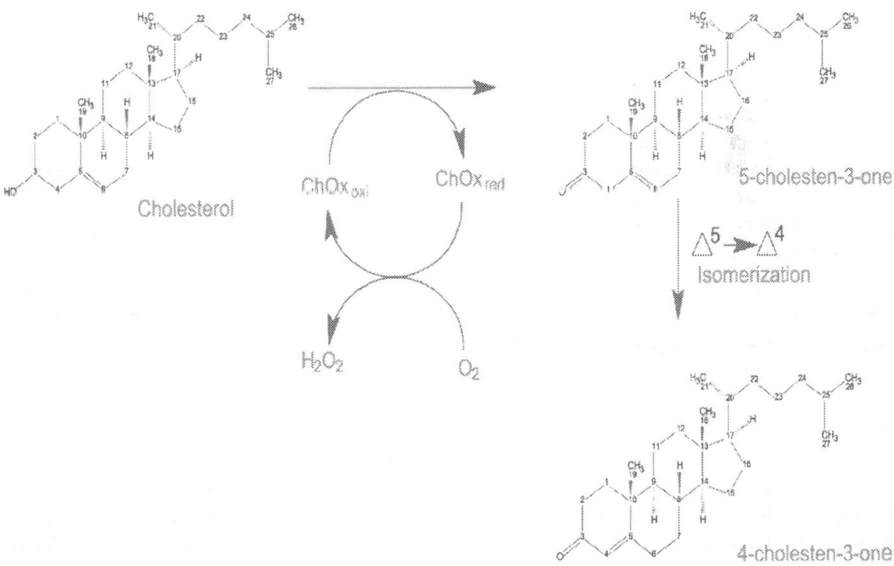

Fig. 2. Pathway of cholesterol oxidase enzyme reaction (Arya et al., 2008).

5. Biosensors for cancer applications

5.1 Cancer biomarkers

Cancer is the leading cause of death in economically developed countries and the second leading cause of death in developing countries. This disease continues to increase globally largely because of the aging and growth of the world population alongside an increasing adoption of cancer-causing behaviors, particularly smoking. Breast cancer is the most frequently diagnosed cancer and the leading cause of cancer death among females and lung cancer is the leading cancer site in males. Breast cancer is now also the leading cause of cancer death among females in economically developing countries, a shift from the previous decade during which the most common cause of cancer death was cervical cancer (Jemal et al., 2011). Solid cancers are a leading cause of morbidity and mortality worldwide, primarily due to the failure of effective clinical detection and treatment of metastatic disease in distant sites (Chambers et al., 2002; Pantel & Brakenhoff, 2004). Cancer can be caused by a range of factors, both genetic and environmental. Chemical, physical and biological factors such as the exposure to carcinogenic chemicals, radiation, bacterial (e.g. stomach cancer), viral infections (e.g. cervical cancer) and toxins (aflatoxin; e.g. liver cancer) can lead to cancer development (Vineis et al., 2010). As the causes of cancer are so diverse, clinical testing is also very complex. The multi-factorial changes (genetic and epigenetic) can cause the onset of the disease and the formation of cancer cells. However, no single gene is universally altered during this process, but a set of them that brings difficulties to the correct disease diagnosis. All the changes which take place, in the tumors from different locations (organ), as well within tumors from the same location, can be so variable and overlapping that it is difficult to select a specific change or marker for the diagnosis of specific cancers. Therefore, a range of biomarkers can potentially be analyzed for disease diagnosis. These biomarkers or molecular signatures can be produced either by the tumor itself or by the body in response to the presence of cancer (Robert, 2010). Several cancer biomarkers are listed in Table 1.

The analysis of biomarkers in body fluids such as blood, urine and others is one of the methods applied in the detection of the disease. Multi-marker profiles, both presence and concentration level, can be essential for the diagnosis of early disease onset. These methods should provide information to assist clinicians in making successful treatment decisions and increasing patient survival rate (Tothill, 2009). A range of biomarkers have been identified with different types of cancers. These include DNA modifications, RNA, proteins (enzymes and glycoproteins), hormones and related molecules, molecules of the immune system, oncogenes and other modified molecules. Several biomarkers are current being studied, including genes and proteins; however few of them have routine cancer clinical testing importance because of their complexity. The development of protein based biomarkers for biosensors use in cancer diagnosis is more attractive than genetic markers due to protein abundance, recovery and cost effective technique for the development of point-of-care devices (Li et al., 2010).

5.2 Biosensors in cancer disease

Existing methods of screening for cancer are heavily based on cell morphology using staining and microscopy which are invasive techniques. Furthermore, tissue removal can miss cancer cells at the early onset of the disease. Biosensor-based detection becomes practical and advantageous for cancer clinical testing, since it is faster, more user-friendly, less expensive and less technically demanding than microarray or proteomic analyses. However, significant technical development is still needed, particularly for protein based biosensors. For cancer diagnosis multi-array sensors would be beneficial for multi-marker analysis. A range of molecular recognition molecules have been used for biomarker detection, being antibodies the most widely used. More recently, synthetic (artificial) molecular recognition elements such as nanomaterials, aptamers, phage display peptides, binding proteins and synthetic peptides as well as metal oxides materials have been fabricated as affinity materials and used for analyte detection and analysis (Sadik et al., 2009; Khati, 2010). Antibodies (monoclonal and polyclonal) have been applied in cancer diagnostics tests targeting cancer cells and biomarkers. Polyclonal antibodies can be raised against any biomarker or cells and with the introduction of high throughput techniques, applying these molecules in sensors has been successful. The use of monoclonal antibodies however, results in more specific tests. The drawbacks include that monoclonal antibodies are more difficult to maintain and can be more expensive than polyclonal antibodies (Huang et al., 2010). Replacing natural biomolecules with artificial receptors or biomimics has therefore become an attractive area of research in recent years. The advantages of using these molecules are that they are robust, more stable, less expensive to produce and can be modified easily to aid immobilization on the sensor surface as well as adding labels as the maker for detection (Liu et al., 2007). Those molecules can be synthesized after a selection from combinatorial libraries with higher specificity and sensitivity when compared to the antibody molecule.

Breast	ER,PR, HER2, CA15-3, CA125, CA27.29, CEA BRCA1, BRCA2, MUC-1, CEA, NY-BR-1, ING-1
Bladder	BAT, FDP, NMP22, HA-Hase, BLCA-4, CYFRA 21-1
Cervix	P53, Bcl-2, Brn-3a, MCM, SCC-Ag, TPA, CYFRA 21-1, VEGF, M-CSF
Colon	HNPCC, FAP, CEA, CA19-9, CA24-2, p53
Esophagus	SCC
Leukemia	Chromosomal aberrations
Liver	AFP, CEA
Lung	NY-ESO-1, CEA, CA19-9, SCC, CYFRA21-1, NSE
Melanoma	Tyrosinase, NY-ESO-1
Ovarian	CA125, AFP, hCG, p53, CEA
Pancreas	CA19-9, CEA, MIC-1
Prostate	PSA, PAP
Solid tumors	Circulating tumour cells in biological fluids, expression of targeted growth factor receptors
Stomach	CA72-4, CEA, CA19-9

Table 1. Cancer biomaker

For cancer biomarkers analysis, bioaffinity based electrochemical biosensors are usually applied to detect gene mutations of biomarkers and protein biomarkers. Electrochemical affinity sensors based on antibodies offer great selectivity and sensitivity for early cancer diagnosis and these include amperometric, potentiometric and impedimetric/conductivity devices. Amperometric and potentiometric transducers have been the most commonly used, but much attention in recent years has been devoted to impedance based transducers since they are classified as label-free detection sensors. However, much of the technology is still at the research stage (Lin & Ju, 2005; Wang, 2006). Besides based on antibodies, electrochemical devices have been developed based on DNA hybridization and used for cancer gene mutation detection. In this type of device a single stranded DNA sequence is immobilized on the electrode surface where DNA hybridization takes place (Ahmed, 2008). ELISA based assays conducted on the electrode surface are the most frequently used techniques for cancer protein markers analysis, such as CEA. In this method the antibody (or antigen) is labeled with an enzyme such as horseradish peroxidase (HRP), or alkaline phosphatase (AP) and these will then catalyze an added substrate to produce an electroactive species which can then be detected on an electrochemical transducer. Electrochemical detection of rare circulating tumor cells has the potential to provide clinicians with a standalone system to detect and monitor changes in cell numbers throughout therapy, conveniently and frequently for efficient cancer treatment (Chung et al., 2011).

Many commercially available platforms use fluorescence labels as the detection system. However, the instruments used for signal readout are usually expensive and are more suitable for laboratory settings. As an example the Affymetrix gene chip (Affymetrix Inc., Santa Clara, USA) can be used for screening cancer and cancer gene identification. Other biosensor platforms such as grating couplers, resonant mirrors and surface plasmon based systems have also been used for cancer biomarkers diagnosis. These are classified as label-free and real-time affinity reaction detection systems. Different SPR based biosensors have been developed for cancer markers detection based on the above optical systems (Tothill, 2009). Recently, microcantilever based sensors have also been applied for early-stage diagnosis of hepatocellular carcinoma (Liu et al., 2009b).

In spite of the achieved development in cancer biosensing, the point-of-care testing is not yet available. In order to achieve this goal challenges must be overcome such as: development of reproducible biomarker assays; improvement in recognition ligands; development of multi-channel biosensors; advances in sample preparation; device miniaturization and integration; development of more sensitive transducers; microfluidics integration; advanced manufacturing techniques and cost reduction (Rasooly & Jacobson, 2006).

6. Conclusion

A precise diagnostic for a disease is essential for a successful treatment and recovery of patients suffering from it. Diagnostics methods must be simple, sensitive and able to detect multiple biomarkers that exist at low concentrations in biological fluids. Biosensors can fulfill these requirements. However, biosensor devices need to be further developed and improved to face these new challenges to allow, for example, multiplex analysis of several biomarkers where arrays of sensors need to be developed on the same chip.

Biosensors are firmly established for application in clinical chemical analysis. Biosensors for measurement of blood metabolites such as glucose, lactate, urea and creatinine, using both electrochemical and optical modes of transduction, are commercially developed and used routinely in the laboratory, in point-of-care settings and, in the case of glucose, for self-testing. While immunosensors have difficulty competing with traditional immunoassay based mainly on sensitivity requirements, they hold promise for testing where some sensitivity can be sacrificed for improved ease of use and faster time to result, such as in near-patient testing for cardiac and cancer markers. Although biosensors are used for several clinical applications, few biosensors have been developed for cardiovascular and cancer-related clinical testing. Development of molecular tools, both genomic and proteomic, to profile tumors and produce molecular signatures, based on genetic and epigenetic signatures, changes in gene expression and protein profiles and protein posttranslational modifications has opened new opportunities for utilizing biosensors in cancer testing. Harnessing the potential of biosensors is challenging because of cancer's complexity and diversity. Successful development of biosensor-based cancer testing will require continued development and validation of biomarkers and development of ligands for those biomarkers, as well as continued development of sample preparation methods and multi-channel biosensors able to analyze many cancer markers simultaneously. The use of biosensors for cancer clinical testing may increase assay speed and flexibility, enable multi-target analyses and automation and reduced costs of diagnostic testing. Biosensors have the potential to deliver molecular testing to the community health care setting and to underserved populations. Cancer biomarkers identified from basic and clinical research, and from genomic and proteomic analyses must be validated. Ligands and probes for these markers can then be combined with detectors to produce biosensors for cancer-related clinical testing. Point-of-care cancer testing requires integration and automation of the technology as well as development of appropriate sample preparation methods (Rasooly & Jacobson, 2006).

A clear direction for future work in biosensor research is in molecular diagnostics. Improving the sensitivity of DNA biosensors for a single-molecule detection in an unamplified sample is an important goal to achieve. This goal will require enhancing the signal-to-noise rate, improving the signal produced by the biochemical reaction or increasing the sensitivity of the transducer while reducing background noise. Ultrasensitive transducer technologies will be required. Some recent examples of transduction modes with enhanced sensitivity include microcantilevers for the detection of mass changes upon detection of a binding event and quartz crystal microbalances capable of monitoring formation and rupturing of chemical bonds by sensing acoustic emissions. The latter has demonstrated sensitivity to detect a single virus particle. Increasing the arrays amplitude for more complete and rapid DNA sequencing information is another area of focus, and improvements in this area may ultimately be limited by resolution of the detection transducer. DNA chips are being incorporated into total analysis systems, including microfluidics and the biosensor on a single structure. These systems should include, in the future, no need for sample preparation, a user-friendly handling system, chemical analysis and signal acquisition capabilities. Central to development of lab-on-a-chip analysis system will be the homogeneous sensing formats and microfabrication technologies for DNA analysis. One recent step towards a homogeneous assay has been the development of synthetic polymeric probes that emit fluorescence only after the hybridization to native DNA targets, allowing monitoring of hybridization in real time without the need for separation steps. Further development and improvement of nanotechnologies will be needed to produce nanoscale devices, with expanded sizes of arrays using reduced sample volume. The future of such devices for rapid determination of a disease could be especially used for point-of-care application. However, cost and quality control of these devices must be strictly adjusted for the accurate devices to gain popular acceptance. Homogeneous assay formats, removing the need for sample preparation and amplification steps and mass fabrication will be important to lowering cost.

Molecular biology will play a central role in the future of biosensor development, for example, to improve biocomponent stability, and for the development of aptamers. The highly reproducible synthetic approach and ease of immobilization of aptamers hold great promise for the custom design of future biosensors for molecular diagnostics (D'Orazio, 2003). Future innovation in biosensor technology to include biomarkers patterns, software and microfluidics can make these devices of high potential for health applications. The concept of using nanomaterials in the development of sensors for biomarkers diagnosis will make these devices highly sensitive and more applicable for point-of-care early diagnosis. Early diagnosis will aid in the increase in the survival rate of patients and successful development of biosensors for disease diagnosis and monitoring will require appropriate funding to move the technology from research through to the realization of commercial products.

Biosensor research and development over the past decades have demonstrated that it is still a relatively young technology. The rationale behind the slow and limited technology transfer could be attributed to cost considerations and some key technical barriers. Many of the more recent major advances had to await miniaturization technologies that are just becoming available through research in the electronic and optical solid state circuit industries. Analytical chemistry has changed considerably, driven by automation, miniaturization, and system integration with high throughput for multiple tasks. Such requirements pose a great challenge in biosensor technology which is often designed to detect one single or a few target analytes. Successful biosensors must be versatile to support interchangeable biorecognition elements, and in addition miniaturization must be feasible to allow automation for parallel sensing with ease of operation at a competitive cost. The future is very bright for biosensors. These advancements will, however, require a concerted multi-disciplinary approach for the sensor systems to successfully make the very big jump from the research and development laboratory to the market place. Combination of several new techniques, derived from physical chemistry, molecular biology, biochemistry, thick and thin film physics, materials science and electronics with the necessary expertise has revealed the promise for development of viable clinical useful biosensor.

7. References

Ahmed, FE. (2008). Mining the oncoproteome and studying molecular interactions for biomarker development by 2DE, ChIP and SPR technologies. *Expert Review of Proteomics*, Vol.5, No.3, pp. 469-496.

Albrecht, C.; Kaeppel, N. & Gauglitz, G. (2008). Two immunoassay formats for fully automated CRP detection in human serum. *Analytical and Bioanalytical Chemistry*, Vol.391, No.5, pp. 1845-1852.

American diabetes association. (1997). Clinical practice recommendations 1997 - Introduction. *Diabetes Care*, Vol.20, No. Suppl 1, pp. S1–S70.

Arya, SK.; Datta, M. & Malhotra, BD. (2008). Recent advances in cholesterol biosensor. *Biosensors and Bioelectronics*, Vol.23, No.7, pp. 1083-1100.

Arya, SK.; Prusty, AK.; Singh, SP.; Solanki, PR.; Pandey, MK.; Datta, M. & Malhotra, BD. (2007). Cholesterol biosensor based on N-(2-aminoethyl)-3-aminopropyl-trimethoxysilane self-assembled monolayer. *Analytical Biochemistry*, Vol.363, No.2, pp. 210-218.

Beauharnois, ME.; Neelamegham, S. & Matta, KL. (2006). Quantitative measurement of selectin-ligand interactions: assays to identify a sweet pill in a library of carbohydrates. *Methods in Molecular Biology*, Vol.347, pp. 343-358.

Buerk, DG. (1993). *Biosensors: Theory and Applications*. Technomic Publishing Company, ISBN 0-87762-975-7, Lancaster, UK.

Castle, JR. & Ward, WK. (2010). Amperometric glucose sensors: sources of error and potential benefit of redundancy. *Journal of Diabetes Science and Technology*, Vol.4, No. 1, pp. 221-225.

Caygill, RL.; Blair, GE. & Millner, PA. (2010). A review on viral biosensors to detect human pathogens. *Analytica Chimica Acta*, Vol.681, No. 12, pp. 8-15.

Cengiz, E. & Tamborlane, WV. (2009). A tale of two compartments: interstitial versus blood glucose monitoring. *Diabetes Technology and Therapeutics*, Vol.11, No. Suppl 1, pp. S11-S16.

Chambers, AF.; Groom, AC. & MacDonald, IC. (2002). Dissemination and growth of cancer cells in metastatic sites. *Nature Reviews Cancer*, Vol.2, No. 8, pp. 563–572.

Charpentier, L. & Murr, NE. (1995). Amperometric determination of cholesterol in serum with use of a renewable surface peroxidase electrode. *Analytica Chimica Acta*, Vol.318, No1, pp. 89–93.

Chu, MX.; Miyajima, K.; Takahashi, D.; Arakawa, T.; Sano, K.; Sawada, S.; Kudo, H.; Iwasaki, Y.; Akiyoshi, K.; Mochizuki, M. & Mitsubayashi, K. (2011). Soft contact lens biosensor for in situ monitoring of tear glucose as non-invasive blood sugar assessment. *Talanta*, Vol.83, No.3, pp. 960-965.

Chung, YK.; Reboud, J.; Lee, KC.; Lim, HM.; Lim, PY.; Wang, KY.; Tang, KC.; Ji, H. & Chen, Y. (2011). An electrical biosensor for the detection of circulating tumor cells. *Biosensors and Bioelectronics*, Vol.26, No. 5, pp. 2520-2526.

Clark Jr., LC. & Lyons, C. (1962). Electrode systems for continuous monitoring in cardiovascular surgery. *Annals of the New York Academy of Sciences*, Vol.102, No.1, pp. 29-45.

Collings, AF. & Caruso, F. (1997). Biosensors: recent advances. *Reports on Progress in Physics*, Vol.60, No.11, 1397-1445.

Ding, L.; Du, D.; Zhang, X. & Ju, H. (2008). Trends in cell-based electrochemical biosensors. *Current Medicinal Chemistry*, Vol.15, No.30, pp. 3160-3170.

D'Orazio, P. (2003). Biosensors in clinical chemistry. *Clinica Chimica Acta*, Vol.334, No. 1-2, pp. 41-69.

Franco, M.; Cooper, RS.; Bilal, U. & Fuster, V. (2011). Challenges and opportunities for cardiovascular disease prevention. *American Journal of Medicine*, Vol.24, No.2, pp. 95-102.

Hall, EAH. (1990). *Biosensors*. Open University Press, ISBN-10: 0335151612, Cambridge, UK.

Heyduk, E.; Dummit, B.; Chang, YH. & Heyduk, T. (2008). Molecular pincers: antibody-based homogeneous protein sensors. *Analytical Chemistry*, Vol.80, No. (13):5152-9.

Huang, L.; Muyldermans, S. & Saerens, D. (2010). Nanobodies®: proficient tools in diagnostics. *Expert Review of Molecular Diagnostics*, Vol.10, No. 6, pp. 777-785.

Huang, R.; Lin, Y.; Shi, Q.; Flowers, L.; Ramachandran, S.; Horowitz, IR.; et al. (2004). Enhanced protein profiling arrays with ELISA-based amplification for high-throughput molecular changes of tumor patients' plasma. *Clinical Cancer Research*, Vol.10, No.2, pp. 598-609.

Ivnitski, D.; Abdel-Hamid, I.; Atanasov, P. & Wilkins, E. (1999). Biosensors for detection of pathogenic bacteria. *Biosensors and Bioelectronics*, Vol.14, No.7, pp. 599-624.

Jemal, A.; Bray, F.; Center, MM.; Ferlay, J.; Ward, E. & Forman, D. (2011). Global cancer statistics. *CA: A Cancer Journal for Clinicians*, Vol. 61, doi:10.3322/caac.20107.

Khati, M. The future of aptamers in medicine. (2010). *Journal of Clinical Pathology*, Vol.63, No.6, pp. 480-487.

Koschwanez, HE. & Reichert, WM. (2007). In vitro, in vivo and post explantation testing of glucose-detecting biosensors: current methods and recommendations. *Biomaterials*, Vol.28, No. 25, pp. 3687-3703.

Laschi, S.; Franek, M. & Mascini, M. (2000). Screen-printed electrochemical immunosensors for PCB detection. *Electroanalysis*, Vol.12, No.16, pp. 1293-1298.

Lasker, RD. (1993). The Diabetes Control and Complications Trial - Implications for Policy and Practice. *New England Journal of Medicine*, Vol.329, No. 14, pp. 1035-1036.

Li, Z.; Wang, Y.; Wang, J.; Tang, Z.; Pounds, JG. & Lin, Y. (2010). Rapid and sensitive detection of protein biomarker using a portable fluorescence biosensor based on quantum dots and a lateral flow test strip. *Analytical Chemistry*, Vol.15;82, No.16, pp. 7008-7014.

Lin, J. & Ju, H. (2005). Electrochemical and chemiluminescent immunosensors for tumor markers. *Biosensors and Bioelectronics*, Vol.20, No.8, pp. 1461-1470.

Liu, G.; Mao, X.; Phillips, JA.; Xu, H.; Tan, W.& Zeng, L. (2009a). Aptamer-nanoparticle strip biosensor for sensitive detection of cancer cells. *Analytical Chemistry*, Vol.81, No. 24, pp. 10013-10018.

Liu, GL.; Rosa-Bauza, YT.; Salisbury, CM.; Craik, C.; Ellman, JA.; Chen, FF. & Lee, LP. (2007). Peptide-nanoparticle hybrid SERS probes for optical detection of protease activity. *Journal of Nanoscience and Nanotechnology*, Vol.7, No.7, pp. 2323-2330.

Liu, Y.; Li, X.; Zhang, Z.; Zuo, G.; Cheng, Z. & Yu, H. (2009b). Nanogram per milliliter-level immunologic detection of alpha-fetoprotein with integrated rotating-resonance microcantilevers for early-stage diagnosis of heptocellular carcinoma. *Biomedical Microdevices*, Vol.11, No.1, pp. 183-191.

McBride, JD. & Cooper, MA. (2008). A high sensitivity assay for the inflammatory marker C-Reactive protein employing acoustic biosensing. *Journal of Nanobiotechnology*, Vol.6, pp. 5, 6:5doi:10.1186/1477-3155-6-5.

Meadows, D. (1996). Recent developments with biosensing technology and applications in the pharmaceutical industry. *Advanced Drug Delivery Reviews*, Vol.21, No.3, pp. 179-189.

Niotis, AE.; Mastichiadis, C.; Petrou, PS.; Christofidis, I.; Kakabakos, SE.; Siafaka-Kapadai, A.; & Misiakos, K. (2010). Dual-cardiac marker capillary waveguide fluoroimmunosensor based on tyramide signal amplification. *Analytical and Bioanalytical Chemistry*, Vol.396, No. 3, pp. 1187-1196.

Palecek, E. (2002). Past, present and future of nucleic acids electrochemistry. *Talanta*, Vol. 56, No.5, pp. 809-819.

Pantel, K. & Brakenhoff, RH. (2004). Dissecting the metastatic cascade. *Nature Reviews Cancer*, Vol.4, No. 6, pp. 448-456.

Park, JS.; Cho, MK.; Lee, EJ.; Ahn, KY.; Lee, KE.; Jung, JH.; Cho, Y.; Han, SS.; Kim, YK. & Lee, J. (2009). A highly sensitive and selective diagnostic assay based on virus nanoparticles. *Nature Nanotechnology*, Vol.4, No. 4, pp. 259-264.

Pickup, JC.; Hussain, F.; Evans, ND. & Sachedina, N. (2005). In vivo glucose monitoring: the clinical reality and the promise. *Biosensors and Bioelectronics*, Vol.20, No. 10, pp. 1897-902.

Qureshi, A.; Gurbuz, Y.; Kallempudi, S. & Niazi, JH. (2010a). Label-free RNA aptamer-based capacitive biosensor for the detection of C-reactive protein. *Physical Chemistry Chemical Physics*, Vol.12, No.32, pp. 9176-982.

Qureshi, A.; Niazi, JH.; Kallempudi, S. & Gurbuz, Y. (2010b). Label-free capacitive biosensor for sensitive detection of multiple biomarkers using gold interdigitated capacitor arrays. *Biosensors and Bioelectronics*, Vol.25, No. 10, pp. 2318-2323.

Rasooly, A, Jacobson J. (2006). Development of biosensors for cancer clinical testing. *Biosensors and Bioelectronics*, Vol.21, No. 10, pp. 1851-1858.

Robert, J. (2010). Polymorphismes génétiques. *Bulletin du Cancer*, Vol.97, No. 11, pp. 1253-1264.

Rusling, JF.; Kumar, CV.; Gutkind, JS. & Patel, V. (2010). Measurement of biomarker proteins for point-of-care early detection and monitoring of cancer. *Analyst*, Vol.135, No. 10, pp. 2496-2511.

Sadik, OA.; Aluoch, AO. & Zhou, A. (2009). Status of biomolecular recognition using electrochemical techniques. *Biosensors and Bioelectronics*, 24, No.9, pp. 2749-2765.

Sheu, BC.; Lin, YH.; Lin, CC.; Lee, AS.; Chang, WC.; Wu, JH.; Tsai, JC. & Lin, S. (2010). Significance of the pH-induced conformational changes in the structure of C-reactive protein measured by dual polarization interferometry. *Biosensors and Bioelectronics*, Vol.26, No. 2, pp. 822-827.

Silva, BV.; Cavalcanti, IT.; Mattos, AB.; Moura, P.; Sotomayor, MP. & Dutra, RF. (2010). Disposable immunosensor for human cardiac troponin T based on streptavidin-microsphere modified screen-printed electrode. *Biosensors and Bioelectronics*, Vol.26, No. 3, pp. 1062-1067.

Singh, S.; Solanki, PR.; Pandey, MK. & Malhotra, BD. (2006). Covalent immobilization of cholesterol esterase and cholesterol oxidase on polyaniline films for application to cholesterol biosensor. *Analytica Chimica Acta*, Vol.568, No.1-2, pp. 126–132.

Spangler, BD.; Wilkinson, EA.; Murphy, JT. & Tyler, BJ. (2001). Comparison of the Spreeta® surface plasmon resonance sensor and a quartz crystal microbalance for detection of Escherichia coli heat-labile enterotoxin. *Analytica Chimica Acta*, Vol.444, No.1, pp. 149-161.

Spichiger-Keller, UE. (1998). *Chemical sensors and biosensors for medical and biological applications*. Weinheim: Wiley-VCH, ISBN 978-352-7612-28-4, Verlag, GmbH.

Stefan, RI.; van Staden, JF. & Aboul-Enein, HY. (2000). Immunosensors in clinical analysis. *Fresenius' Journal of Analytical Chemistry*, Vol.366, No.6-7, pp. 659-668.

Tothill, IE. (2009). Biosensors for cancer markers diagnosis. *Seminars in Cell and Developmental Biology*, Vol.20, No.1, pp. 55-62.

Turner, APF. & Pickup, JC. (1985). Diabetes-mellitus - biosensors for research and management. *Biosensors*, Vol.1, No. 1, pp. 85–115.

Vineis, P.; Schatzkin, A. & Potter, JD. (2010). Models of carcinogenesis: an overview. *Carcinogenesis*, Vol.31, No. 10, pp. 1703-1709

Wanekaya, AK., Chen, W. & Mulchandani, A. (2008). Recent biosensing developments in environmental security. *Journal of Environmental Monitoring*, Vol. 10, No. 6, pp. 703-712.

Wang, J. (2000). Analytical Electrochemistry. 2nd ed. Wiley-VCH, ISBN 0471-28272-3, New York, USA.

Wang, J. (2006). Electrochemical biosensors: towards point of care cancer diagnostics. *Biosensors and Bioelectronics*, Vol.21, No.10, pp. 1887-1892.

Zhou, F.; Lu, M.; Wang, W.; Bian, ZP.; Zhang, JR. & Zhu, JJ. (2010). Electrochemical immunosensor for simultaneous detection of dual cardiac markers based on a poly(dimethylsiloxane)-gold nanoparticles composite microfluidic chip: a proof of principle. *Clinical Chemistry*, Vol. 56, No. 11. pp. 1701-1707.

Zhou, N.; Wang, J.; Chen, T.; Yu, Z. & Li, G. (2006.) Enlargement of gold nanoparticles on the surface of a self-assembled monolayer modified electrode: a mode in biosensor design. *Analytical Chemistry*, Vol.78, No. 14, pp. 5227–5230.

4

Nanobiosensor for Health Care

Nada F. Atta, Ahmed Galal and Shimaa M. Ali
Department of Chemistry, Faculty of Science, Cairo University, Giza
Egypt

1. Introduction

A chemical sensor: is a device that transforms chemical information, ranging from the concentration of a specific sample component to total composition analysis, into an analytically useful signal (IUPAC).
Biosensors: are analytical tools for the analysis of bio-material samples to gain an understanding of their bio-composition, structure and function by converting a biological response into an electrical signal (Figure 1). The analytical devices composed of a biological recognition element directly interfaced to a signal transducer which together relate the concentration of an analyte (or group of related analytes) to a measurable response. The term 'biosensor' is often used to cover sensor devices used in order to determine the concentration of substances and other parameters of biological interest even where they do not utilise a biological system directly.

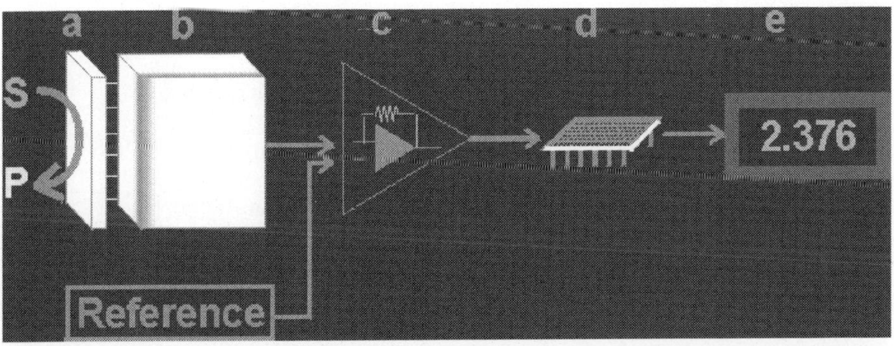

Fig. 1. Schematic diagram showing the main components of a biosensor. The biocatalyst (a) converts the substrate to product. This reaction is determined by the transducer (b) which converts it to an electrical signal. The output from the transducer is amplified (c), processed (d) and displayed (e). *(http://www.lsbu.ac.uk/biology/enztech/biosensors.html)*

The key part of a biosensor is the transducer (shown as the 'black box' in Figure 1) which makes use of a physical change accompanying the reaction. This may be:
1. the heat output (or absorbed) by the reaction (calorimetric biosensors),
2. changes in the distribution of charges causing an electrical potential to be produced (potentiometric biosensors),

3. movement of electrons produced in a redox reaction (amperometric biosensors),
4. light output during the reaction or a light absorbance difference between the reactants and products (optical biosensors), or
5. effects due to the mass of the reactants or products (piezo-electric biosensors).

There are three so-called 'generations' of biosensors; First generation biosensors where the normal product of the reaction diffuses to the transducer and causes the electrical response, second generation biosensors which involve specific 'mediators' between the reaction and the transducer in order to generate improved response, and third generation biosensors where the reaction itself causes the response and no product or mediator diffusion is directly involved.

The electrical signal from the transducer is often low and superimposed upon a relatively high and noisy (i.e. containing a high frequency signal component of an apparently random nature, due to electrical interference or generated within the electronic components of the transducer) baseline. The signal processing normally involves subtracting a 'reference' baseline signal, derived from a similar transducer without any biocatalytic membrane, from the sample signal, amplifying the resultant signal difference and electronically filtering (smoothing) out the unwanted signal noise. The relatively slow nature of the biosensor response considerably eases the problem of electrical noise filtration. The analogue signal produced at this stage may be output directly but is usually converted to a digital signal and passed to a microprocessor stage where the data is processed, converted to concentration units and output to a display device or data store.

Biosensors represent a rapidly expanding field, at the present time, with an estimated 60% annual growth rate; the major impetus coming from the health-care industry (e.g. 6% of the western world are diabetic and would benefit from the availability of a rapid, accurate and simple biosensor for glucose) but with some pressure from other areas, such as food quality appraisal and environmental monitoring. The estimated world analytical market is about 12,000,000,000 year^{-1} of which 30% is in the health care area. There is clearly a vast market expansion potential as less than 0.1% of this market is currently using biosensors.

2. The history of biosensor development

1916	First report on the immobilisation of proteins: adsorption of invertase on activated charcoal
1922	First glass pH electrode
1956	Invention of the oxygen electrode (Clark)
1962	First description of a biosensor: an amperometric enzyme electrode for glucose (Clark)
1969	First potentiometric biosensor: urease immobilised on an ammonia electrode to detect urea
1970	Invention of the Ion-Selective Field-Effect Transistor (ISFET) (Bergveld)
1972/5	First commercial biosensor: Yellow Springs Instruments glucose biosensor
1975	First microbe-based biosensor First immunosensor: ovalbumin on a platinum wire Invention of the pO_2 / pCO_2 optode

1976	First bedside artificial pancreas (Miles)
1980	First fibre optic pH sensor for *in vivo* blood gases (Peterson)
1982	First fibre optic-based biosensor for glucose
1983	First surface plasmon resonance (SPR) immunosensor
1984	First mediated amperometric biosensor: ferrocene used with glucose oxidase for the detection of glucose
1987	Launch of the MediSense ExacTech™ blood glucose biosensor
1990	Launch of the Pharmacia BIACore SPR-based biosensor System
1992	i-STAT launches hand-held blood analyser
1996	Glucocard launched
1996	Abbott acquires MediSense for $867 million
1998	Launch of LifeScan FastTake blood glucose biosensor
1998	Merger of Roche and Boehringer Mannheim to form Roche Diagnostics
2001	LifeScan purchases Inverness Medical's glucose testing business for $1.3billion
1999-Current	BioNMES, Quantum dots, Nanoparticles, Nanocantilever, Nanowire and Nanotube

Table 1. Defining events in the history of biosensor development

3. Basic characteristics of a biosensor

A successful biosensor must possess at least some of the following beneficial features:

1. The biocatalyst must be highly specific for the purpose of the analyses, be stable under normal storage conditions and, except in the case of colorimetric enzyme strips and dipsticks (see later), show good stability over a large number of assays (i.e. much greater than 100).
2. The reaction should be as independent of such physical parameters as stirring, pH and temperature as is manageable. This would allow the analysis of samples with minimal pre-treatment. If the reaction involves cofactors or coenzymes these should, preferably, also be co-immobilised with the enzyme.
3. The response should be accurate, precise, reproducible and linear over the useful analytical range, without dilution or concentration. It should also be free from electrical noise.
   a. **Linearity:** Maximum linear value of the sensor calibration curve. Linearity of the sensor must be high for the detection of high substrate concentration.
   b. **Sensitivity:** The value of the electrode response per substrate concentration.
   c. **Selectivity:** Interference of chemicals must be minimised for obtaining the correct result.
   d. **Response time:** The necessary time for having 95% of the response.
4. If the biosensor is to be used for invasive monitoring in clinical situations, the probe must be tiny and biocompatible, having no toxic or antigenic effects. If it is to be used in fermenters it should be sterilisable. This is preferably performed by autoclaving but no

biosensor enzymes can presently withstand such drastic wet-heat treatment. In either case, the biosensor should not be prone to fouling or proteolysis.

5. The complete biosensor should be cheap, small, portable and capable of being used by semi-skilled operators.
6. There should be a market for the biosensor. There is clearly little purpose developing a biosensor if other factors (e.g. government subsidies, the continued employment of skilled analysts, or poor customer perception) encourage the use of traditional methods and discourage the decentralisation of laboratory testing.

4. Types of biosensors

1. **Resonant Biosensors:** in this type of biosensor, an acoustic wave transducer is coupled with an antibody (bio-element). When the analyte molecule (or antigen) gets attached to the membane, the mass of the membrane changes. The resulting change in the mass subsequently changes the resonant frequency of the transducer. This frequency change is then measured.
2. **Optical-detection Biosensors:** the output transduced signal that is measured is light for this type of biosensor. The biosensor can be made based on optical diffraction or electrochemiluminescence. In optical diffraction based devices, a silicon wafer is coated with a protein via covalent bonds. The wafer is exposed to UV light through a photo-mask and the antibodies become inactive in the exposed regions. When the diced wafer chips are incubated in an analyte, antigen-antibody bindings are formed in the active regions, thus creating a diffraction grating. This grating produces a diffraction signal when illuminated with a light source such as laser. The resulting signal can be measured or can be further amplified before measuring for improved sensitivity.
3. **Thermal-detection Biosensors:** this type of biosensor is exploiting one of the fundamental properties of biological reactions, namely absorption or production of heat, which in turn changes the temperature of the medium in which the reaction takes place. They are constructed by combining immobilized enzyme molecules with temperature sensors. When the analyte comes in contact with the enzyme, the heat reaction of the enzyme is measured and is calibrated against the analyte concentration. The total heat produced or absorbed is proportional to the molar enthalpy and the total number of molecules in the reaction. The measurement of the temperature is typically accomplished via a thermistor, and such devices are known as enzyme thermistors. Their high sensitivity to thermal changes makes thermistors ideal for such applications. Unlike other transducers, thermal biosensors do not need frequent recalibration and are insensitive to the optical and electrochemical properties of the sample. Common applications of this type of biosensor include the detection of pesticides and pathogenic bacteria.
4. **Ion-Sensitive Biosensors:** these are semiconductor FETs having an ion-sensitive surface. The surface electrical potential changes when the ions and the semiconductor interact. This change in the potential can be subsequently measured. The Ion Sensitive Field Effect Transistor (ISFET) can be constructed by covering the sensor electrode with a polymer layer. This polymer layer is selectively permeable to 4 analyte ions. The ions diffuse through the polymer layer and in turn cause a change in the FET surface potential. This type of biosensor is also called an ENFET (Enzyme Field Effect Transistor) and is primarily used for pH detection.

5. **Electrochemical Biosensors:** electrochemical biosensors are mainly used for the detection of hybridized DNA, DNA-binding drugs, glucose concentration, etc. The underlying principle for this class of biosensors is that many chemical reactions produce or consume ions or electrons which in turn cause some change in the electrical properties of the solution which can be sensed out and used as measuring parameter. Electrochemical biosensors can be classified based on the measuring electrical parameters as: (1) conductimetric, (2) amperometric and (3) potentiometric.
   a. *Conductimetric*: the measured parameter is the electrical conductance / resistance of the solution. When electrochemical reactions produce ions or electrons, the overall conductivity or resistivity of the solution changes. This change is measured and calibrated to a proper scale. Conductance measurements have relatively low sensitivity. The electric field is generated using a sinusoidal voltage (AC) which helps in minimizing undesirable effects such as Faradaic processes, double layer charging and concentration polarization.
   b. *Amperometric*: this high sensitivity biosensor can detect electroactive species present in biological test samples. Since the biological test samples may not be intrinsically electro-active, enzymes are needed to catalyze the production of radio-active species. In this case, the measured parameter is current.
   c. *Potentiometric*: in this type of sensor the measured parameter is oxidation or reduction potential of an electrochemical reaction. The working principle relies on the fact that when a ramp voltage is applied to an electrode in solution, a current flow occurs because of electrochemical reactions. The voltage at which these reactions occur indicates a particular reaction and particular species.

5. Biosensors applications

Biosensors can have a variety of biomedical, industry, and military applications as shown in Figure 2. The major application so far is in blood glucose sensing because of its abundant market potential. However, biosensors have tremendous potential for commercialization in other fields of application as well. In spite of this potential, however, commercial adoption has been slow because of several technological difficulties. For example, due to the presence of biomolecules along with semiconductor materials, biosensor contamination is a major issue.

6. Nanobiosensors based on gold nanoparticles (GNPs)

Many interests have been directed to the biosensing of drugs and biological molecules . The nanotechnology of sol-gel based on molecular recognition and nanoparticles play a very important role in scientific researches (Atta et al., 2009a, 2009b, 2009c, 2010a, 2010b, 2010c, 2010d, 2011a, 2011b, 2011c). Due to extremely small size of nanomaterials they are more readily taken up by the human body. Nanomaterials are able to cross biological membranes and access cells, tissues and organs that larger-sized particles normally cannot. Nanoparticles are stable, solid colloidal particles and range in size from 10 to 1,000 nm. Drugs can be absorbed onto the particle surface, entrapped inside the particle, or dissolved within the particle matrix. Nanoparticles have benefits because of its size. Because of their size they can easily enter small places. Nanoparticles have attracted the attention of scientists because of their multifunctional character. Nanoparticles have large surface area to volume ratio, that helps in diffusion also leading to special properties such as increased heat and chemical resistance.

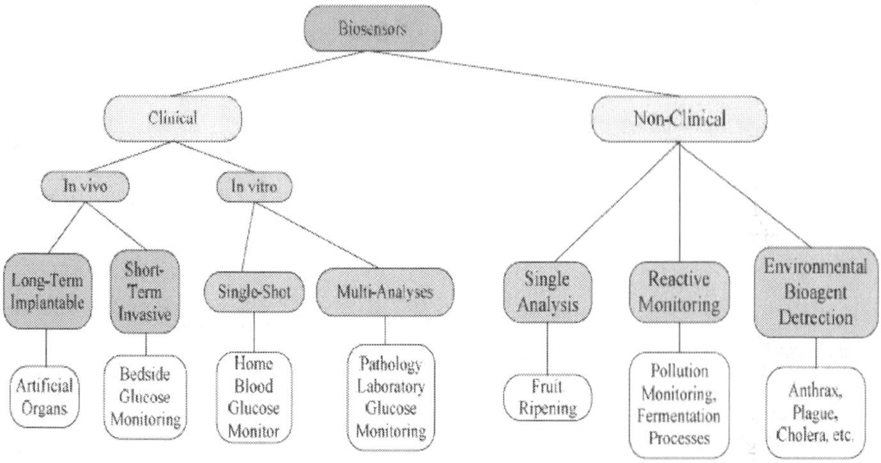

Fig. 2. Biosensors applications

The development of active nanostructures, capable of performing a function or executing a specific task, is currently a major focus of research efforts in bio-/nanotechnology. One already highly successful nanodevice paradigm is the nanosensor: a designed nanostructure, which can provide information about its local environment through its response. Nanomaterials are exquisitely sensitive chemical and biological sensors. Each sensor should be sensitive for one chemical or biological component of a substance. Thus, by having sensor arrays it is possible to tell the composition of an unknown substance. The application area will be wide, encompassing food industry, detection of pollution, medical sector, brewery etc. A nanobiosensor also referred to a nanosensor, is a biosensor with dimensions on the nanometer scale (1 nm = 10^{-9} m). So, Nanosensors are any biological, chemical, or physical sensory points used to convey information about nanoparticles to the macroscopic world. Though humans have not yet been able to synthesize nanosensors, predictions for their use mainly include various medicinal purposes and as gateways to building other nanoproducts, such as computer chips that work at the nanoscale and nanorobots. Presently, there are several ways proposed to make nanosensors, including top-down lithography, bottom-up assembly, and molecular self-assembly.Various kinds of nanomaterials have been being actively investigated for their applications in biosensors, such as gold nanoparticles (GNPs), carbon nanotubes (CNTs), magnetic nanoparticles and quantum dots which have been applied for the detection of DNA, RNA, proteins, glucose, pesticides and other small molecules from clinical samples, food industrial samples, as well as environmental monitoring.

Metal nanoparticles, such as silver (Ag), gold (Au), platinum (Pt) and palladium (Pd) nanoparticles have attracted much interest in the construction of biosensors due to their unique chemical and physical properties. Nanoparticles can offer many advantages, such as large surface-to-volume ratio, high surface reaction activity and strong adsorption ability to immobilize the desired biomolecules. Gold nanoparticles, in particular, have been widely used to construct biosensors because of their excellent ability to immobilize biomolecules. Many kinds of biosensors, such as enzyme sensor, immunosensor and DNA sensor, with improved analytical performances have been prepared based on the application of gold nanoparticles. gold nanoparticles (GNPs) are not only better conductor but also offer good microenvironment for retaining the activity of enzyme. They can bind directly with enzymes without disrupting its biological recognition properties. Nowadays, it is revealed that GNPs also exhibit excellent catalytic effects on many important chemical reactions. In addition, GNPs are able to reduce the insulating effect of the protein shell and thus enhance electron transfer in the reaction processes. So far, the oxidation of carbon monoxide, electrochemical oxidation of methanol and hydrogenation of unsaturated substrates and many others are all based on the catalytic effect of GNPs. The most interesting point of GNPs is that their catalytic effect is highly size-dependent. The unique active sites and electronic states of GNPs can lead to their anomalous catalytic activity although the mechanism is still not fully understood.

6.1 Glucose biosensors

The maintenance of glucose level in human or animal blood is very important and any deviance from the normal glucose level may arouse sickness and disease. Thus, fast and accurate detection of the glucose level in blood is of significance to human health. The glucose biosensor has been also widely used as a clinical indicator of diabetes and in the food industry for quality control. Among the various detection methods, enzyme-based electrodes have been extensively studied because of their high selectivity and sensitivity. In1962, Clark and Lyons developed the first enzyme electrode (Clark & & Lyons, 1962). Clark used platinum (Pt) electrodes to detect oxygen. The enzyme glucose oxidase(GOx) was placed very close to the surface of platinum by physically trapping it against the electrodes with a piece of dialysis membrane. The enzyme activity changes depending on the surrounding oxygen concentration. Glucose reacts with glucose oxidase (GOx) to form gluconic acid while producing two electrons and two protons, thus reducing GOx. The reduced GOx, surrounding oxygen, electrons and protons (produced above) react to form hydrogen peroxide and oxidized GOx (the original form). This GOx can again react with more glucose. The higher the glucose content, more oxygen is consumed. On the other hand, lower glucose content results in more hydrogen peroxide. Hence, either the consumption of oxygen or the production of hydrogen peroxide can be detected by the help of platinum electrodes and this can serve as a measure for glucose concentration. Since then, a lot of interests have been put on enzyme-based biosensors. Various techniques such as spectrophotometric, electrochemical, chemiluminescence, fluorescence, and oxygen(O_2) sensor methods have been reported. Most of these methods are based on the immobilization of the enzyme glucose oxidase (GOx) on a solid substrate. Usually the immobilized enzyme can be reused for certain times. The performance of an enzyme-based biosensor relies heavily on the properties of the supporting materials. They should provide a good environment for enzyme immobilization and should be able to maintain their biological activity. Lots of materials have been used for enzyme immobilization including inorganic materials, organic materials and biomaterials. Biomaterials are considered to be more ideal enzyme immobilization platform since they are more biocompatible with enzymes. Among these biomaterials, eggshell membrane (ESM) has been proved to be an effective and stable enzyme immobilization bio-platform because it not only maintains the enzyme activity but also extends the shelf-life of the immobilized enzyme. GNPs were in situ synthesized and deposited on an ESM and the GNPs-coated ESM was subsequently immobilized with GOx to form a GOx-GNPs/ESM which was positioned on the surface of an O_2 electrode to accomplish a glucose biosensor (Zhenga et al., 2010). GNPs are proposed to speed up the enzymatic reactions with the following reaction schemes:

$$\text{Glucose} + \text{GOx-FAD} \rightarrow \text{Gluconolatone} + \text{GOx-FADH}_2 \quad (1)$$

$$\text{GOx-FADH}_2 + O_2 \xrightarrow{\text{GNPs}} \text{GOx-FAD} + H_2O_2 \quad (2)$$

GOx catalyzes the oxidation of β-d-glucose to gluconolactone and finally hydrolyzes to gluconic acid with a concomitant consumption of dissolved O_2. The depletion of dissolved O_2 can be simply monitored by an O_2 electrode. GOx can be easily immobilized with high loading and activity because of the large surface area of the membrane and the attachment of enzyme to the GNPs. Moreover, GNPs can facilitate the electron transfer of enzyme to oxygen acceptor and enhance the mediated bioelectrocatalytic oxidation of glucose, thus improving the sensitivity of detection. As a result, the GOx-GNPs/ESM biosensor should display higher sensitivity and possesses potential for clinical determination of glucose in human serum. GNPs on GOx/ESM can improve the calibration sensitivity (30 % higher than GOx/ESM without GNPs), stability (87.3% of its initial response to glucose after 10-week storage) and shortens the response time (<30 s) of the glucose biosensor. The linear working range for the GOx-GNPs/ESM glucose biosensor is 8.33 μM to 0.966 mM glucose with a detection limit of 3.50 μM (S/N=3). The biosensor has been successfully applied to determine the glucose in human blood serum samples and the results compared well to a standard spectrophotometric method commonly used in hospitals.

Blood serum sample	Concentration of glucose[a] (mM)	Concentration of glucose[b] (mM)	RSD[c] (%)	Glucose added (mM)	Glucose found (mM)	Recovery (%)	RSD[c] (%)
1	3.10	3.09	0.78	0.400	0.390	97.5	1.59
2	2.60	2.89	3.29	0.400	0.393	98.3	0.86
3	3.13	3.01	2.97	0.400	0.389	97.3	0.99
4	3.55	3.65	3.76	0.400	0.378	94.5	2.92
5	3.19	3.18	3.06	0.400	0.368	92.0	4.04
6	3.72	3.91	3.94	0.400	0.417	104	1.86
7	3.56	3.76	4.06	0.400	0.421	105	1.67

[a] Determined by the spectrophotometric method in hospital.
[b] Determined by the GOx-GNPs/ESM glucose biosensor.
[c] Three replicates were performed.

Table 2. Determination and recovery of glucose in blood serum samples using the GOx-GNPs/ESM glucose biosensor (Zhenga et al., 2010).

Biopolymer chitosan is a polysaccharide derived by deacetylation of chitin. It has primary amino groups that have pKa values of about 6.3. At pH below the pKa, most of the amino groups are protonated, making chitosan a water-soluble polyelectrolyte. When the pH is raised above the pKa, the amino groups are deprotonated, and chitosan becomes insoluble. Chitosan is inexpensive and displays an excellent film-forming ability, biocompatibility, nontoxicity, high mechanical strength, and a susceptibility to chemical modifications. The stabilization of gold nanoparticles with chitosan has been extensively reported (Santos et al., 2004, Esumi et al., 2003) . As chitosan in solution is protonated and positively charged, it can be adsorbed onto the surfaces of gold nanoparticles, stabilizing and protecting the nanoparticles, and further construct. Examples of biosensors based on the excellent properties of chitosan and gold nanoparticles were next described (Luo et al., 2005). Gold nanoparticles, which were prepared in advance through the reduction of $HAuCl_4$ with citrate, can be self-assembly onto electrodeposited chitosan films and then immobilize enzymes effectively. And also they can be mixed with chitosan and enzymes to construct biosensors through simple one-step electrodeposition. However, in both of these systems, gold nanoparticles need to be prepared previously, which prolongs the whole time of biosensor preparation and makes the procedure a bit complicated. Recently, several methods for the formation of gold nanoparticles on the surface of electrodes directly through the electrochemical reduction of $HAuCl_4$ have been reported. Mena et al. compared different strategies for the construction of amperometric enzyme biosensors using gold nanoparticle-modified electrodes (Mena et al., 2005). Compton et al. investigated electrochemical detection of As(III) at a gold nanoparticle-modified glassy carbon (GC) electrode which was fabricated by the electrochemical deposition of Au nanoparticles onto GC (Dai et al., 2004). By this means, one can synthesize gold nanoparticles on the surface of electrode directly in a short of time, and the sizes of the nanoparticles can be controlled by different conditions of electrochemical deposition with the advantageous properties being kept. Thus, a simple method for fabricating a chitosan film containing gold nanoparticles have been reported (Du et al., 2007b) in which $HAuCl_4$ solution is mixed with chitosan and electrochemically reduced to gold nanoparticles directly, and the produced gold nanoparticles were stabilized by chitosan and electrochemically deposited onto the glass carbon electrode under a certain voltage along with chitosan. The whole procedure cost only about 10 min. Then a model enzyme, glucose oxidase (GOx), was assembled on the chitosan gold nanoparticles modified electrode. The linear range of the glucose biosensor is from 5.0×10^{-5} to 1.30×10^{-3} M with a Michaelis-Menten constant of 3.5 mM and a detection limit of about 13 μM.

During the last years, numerous works have been published concerning the use of the silica sol-gel technology as a strategy to preserve the catalytic activity of enzymes after the immobilization step. In this sense, the polymeric network generated by sol-gel technology can be used as an adequate matrix in which several compounds, including biological material, can be encapsulated through physical entrapment rather than by covalent bonding leading to a non aggressive approach. Particularly, the sol-gel network provides a biocompatible environment for enzyme protection exhibiting additional advantages such as simplicity of preparation, chemical inertness, high stability, physical rigidity, renewable surface and tuneable properties. The final properties of the sol-gel matrix play a key role in the biosensor performance and can be easily controlled by varying some parameters such as the precursor or the preparation conditions (pH, ratio of compounds, etc). Various precursors have been reported in the literature for the preparation of the sol-gel network, but among them the most used for enzyme encapsulation are oxysilanes such as methyltrimethoxy-silane (MTMOS), tetramethoxysilane (TMOS), 3-aminopropyltriethoxysilane (APTOS) and tetraethoxysilane (TEOS) (Wang et al., 1998, Walcarius, 2001, Salimi et al., 2004, Kumar et al., 2006, Pauliukaite et al., 2006, Singh et al., 2007). The preparation and characterization of a new organic-inorganic hybrid composite material from a three-dimensional silica polymer network, obtained by means of the sol-gel technology using tetraethoxysilane as precursor was reported (Barbadilloa et al., 2009). This matrix provides an excellent network allowing the encapsulation of gold nanoparticles, conductive material (graphite powder, C) and a biosensing molecule such as glucose oxidase (GOx), chosen as amodel since it is a stable, inexpensive and well-studied enzyme. This composite material combines the advantages induced from both the silica matrix, which enables the incorporation of the other elements while keeping the enzymatic activity of the assembly, and the presence of nanostructures, which enhances the electroactive area. As a consequence, the resulting biosensor TEOS/GNPs/GOx/C exhibits a wider linear range concentration, higher sensitivity and higher accuracy, when compared with a similar composite containing GOx but free of GNPs (TEOS/GOx/C). Taking into account the good performance of the resulting biosensor, this approach is a promising route for designing a wide range of biosensors.

Biosensor	Sensitivity (μAmM^{-1})	Linear range (mM)	Applied potential (V)	Accuracy (R.S.D.)
TEOS/GOx/C (Barbadilloa et al., 2009)	1.73	1-20	+0.25	1.1% (n=8)
TEOS/AuNPs/GOx/C (Barbadilloa et al., 2009)	2.43	0.5-55	+0.25	0.5% (n=8)
Sol-gel/chitosan/GOx (Chen et al.2003)	0.27	Up to 14	+0.35	2% (n=7)
Fc/Ormosil/GOx/GP (Pandey et al., 2003)	1.76	Up to 35	+0.35	-
Sol-gel/CNT/GOx/Bppg (Salimi et al., 2004)	0.20	0.2-20	+0.3	1.8% (n=10)
Sol-gel/GOx/chitosan/PB/GC (Tan et al., 2005)	0.42	0.05-26	-0.05	3.8% (n=8)
Sol-gel/PNR/GOx (Pauliukaite et al.2006)	0.06	0.05-0.6	-0.25	-
Sol-gel/GOx/PtNPs-CNT (Yang et al., 2006)	0.28	1-25	+0.1	5.1% (n=10)
Sol-gel/PVA/GOx/SPE (Zuo et al., 2008)	0.44	0-4.1	-0.5	-
Sol-gel/GOx/PB/GC (Liang et al., 2008)	0.84	0.01-5.8	0	1.8% (n=8)
Solgel/GOx/CNT/chitosan/PtNP/GC (Kang et al., 2008)	2.08	0.001-6.0	+0.1	-

Table 3. A comparison between various biosensors based on sol-gel technology (Barbadilloa et al., 2009).

The oxidase-based amperometric biosensors previously relied on the immobilization of oxidase enzymes on the surface of various electrodes. However, electron transfer efficiency of redox enzymes is poor in the absence of mediator, because enzyme active sites are deeply embedded inside the protein. The sensitivity of resulted biosensors can be significantly improved by the immobilization of mediators in the matrices. Among the different mediators described in the literature, ferrocene (Fc) and its derivatives, first reported by Cass et al. (Cass et al., 1984), have proved to be the most efficient electron transfers for the GOx enzymatic reaction. There are a lot of cases about ferrocene (Fc) and its derivatives introduced to enzyme biosensor as the mediator. However, leakage has been a main problem for the entrapment of mediators due to their low molecular weight in polymer matrices. In order to prevent the leakage of mediator, mediator can be linked covalently with polymer or with high molecular weight compounds before immobilization on the surface of electrode. Gorton et al. (Gorton et al., 1990) studied ferrocene-containing siloxane polymer modified electrode surface with a poly (ester-sulfuric acid) cation-exchanger to improve the stability of the mediator. Another alternative method is to synthesize a few Fc derivatives with specific functional groups (Jönsson et al., 1989, Foulds & Lowe, 1988), but the preparation methods are complicated. For instance, Jönsson et al. (Jönsson et al., 1989) used hydroxymethyl Fc and anthracene carboxylic acid to synthesize anthracene substituted ferrocene. The other alternative method to increase the stability of Fc and its derivatives is the formation of inclusion complex with cyclodextrin (CD), a class of torpidly shaped cycloamyloses with a hydrophilic outer surface and a hydrophobic inner cavity, which makes the dissolubility of Fc decrease. Several investigations have been made to study the characterization of interacting Fc–CD system and their roles. Liu et al. (Liu et al., 1998) developed the sensitive biosensor for glucose by immobilizing glucose oxidase in β-cyclodextrin via cross-linking and by including ferrocene in the cavities of dextrin polymer via host–guest reaction. Zhang et al. (Zhang et al., 2000) successfully used ferrocene with β-cyclodextrin to prepare β-CD/Fc inclusion complex modified carbon paste electrode. The water-soluble inclusion complex of 1,1-dimethylferrocene with (2- hydroxypropyl)-β-CD has been used in bioelectrocatalysis (Bersier et al., 1991). Gold nanoparticles were capped by inclusion complex between mono- 6-thio-β-cyclodextrin and ferrocene through -SH, which resulted into stable fixation of ferrocene on the surface of gold nanoparticles (Chen & Diao, 2009). Then, the glucose biosensors were constructed by using GNPs/CD–Fc as the building block. The composite nanoparticles showed excellent efficiency of electron transfer between the GOx and the electrode for the electrocatalysis of glucose. The sensor (GNPs/CD–Fc/GOD) showed a relatively fast response time (5 s), low detection limit (15 μM, S/N = 3), and high sensitivity (ca. 18.2 $mA.M^{-1}.cm^{-2}$) with a linear range of 0.08–11.5 mM of glucose. The excellent sensitivity was possibly attributed to the presence of the GNPs/CD-Fc film that can provide a convenient electron tunneling between the protein and the electrode. In addition, the biosensor demonstrated high anti-interference ability, stability and natural life. The good stability and natural life can be attributed to the following two aspects: on the one hand, the fabrication process was mild and no damage was made on the enzyme molecule, on the other hand, the GNPs possessed good biocompatibility that could retain the bioactivity of the enzyme molecules immobilized on the electrode.

In comparison with spherical nanoparticles, one-dimensional (1-D) nanomaterials, especially nanowires, possess a number of unique physical and electronic properties that endow them with new and important activities. The excellent properties of nanowires are due to several beneficial features arising from their shape anisotropy on the electrochemical reaction at electrodes: (i) facile pathways for the electron transfer by reducing the number of interfaces between the nanoparticle catalysts and (ii) effective surface exposure to work as active catalytic sites in the electrode–electrolyte interface. It has been reported that enzymes can be adsorbed onto these nanostructures, because these materials provide large surface area for enzyme loading and friendly microenvironment to stabilize the immobilized enzymes. Recent results suggest the possibility of incorporating large numbers of nanowires into large-scale arrays and complex hierarchical structures for high-density biosensors, electronics, and optoelectronics. Biosensors based on nanowires showed improved signal-to-noise ratios, high faradaic current density, fast electron-transfer rate, enhanced sensitivities, better detection limit. Recently, increasing research interest in biosensor filed has been focused on composite materials based on 1-D materials and noble metal nanoparticles with a synergistic effect. Materials for such purposes include carbon nanotubes, carbon nanofibers, redox mediators and metal nanoparticles.

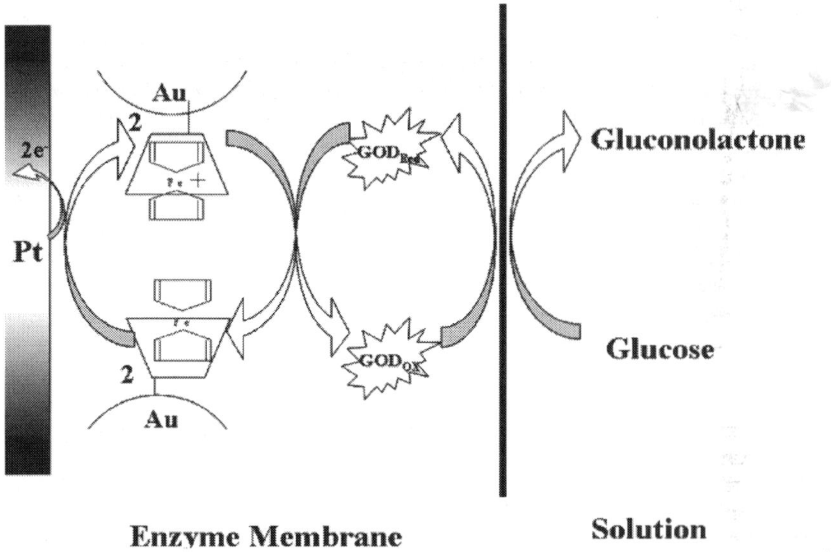

Fig. 3. Schematic illustration of sensing mechanism for electrocatalytic glucose on the GNPs/CD-Fc/GOD modified platinum electrode surface (Chen & Diao, 2009).

For example, coupling carbon nanofibers with palladium nanoparticles resulted in a remarkable improvement of the electroactivity of the composite materials towards reduction of H_2O_2 and oxidation of β-nicotinamide adenine dinucleotide in reduced form (NADH) (Huang et al., 2008). Zou et al. reported a glucose biosensor based on electrodeposition of platinum nanoparticles onto multiwalled carbon nanotubes (Zou et al., 2008). Wu et al. constructed a glucose biosensor based on multi-walled carbon nanotubes and GNPs by layer-by-layer self-assembly technique (Wu et al., 2007). Taking advantage of the nanowires and GNPs, a novel glucose biosensor was developed, based on the immobilization of glucose oxidase (GOx) with cross-linking in the matrix of bovine serum albumin (BSA) on a Pt electrode, which was modified with gold nanoparticles decorated Pb nanowires (GNPs-

PbNWs) (Wanga et al., 2009). Pb nanowires (PbNWs) were synthesized by an l-cysteine-assisted self-assembly route, and then gold nanoparticles (GNPs) were attached onto the nanowire surface through -SH-Au specific interaction. The synergistic effect of PbNWs and GNPs made the biosensor exhibit excellent electrocatalytic activity and good response performance to glucose. In pH 7.0, the biosensor showed the sensitivity of 135.5μA.mM^{-1}.cm^{-2}, the detection limit of 2 μM (S/N = 3), and the response time <5 s with a linear range of 5-2200 μM. Furthermore, the biosensor exhibits good reproducibility, long-term stability and relative good anti-interference.

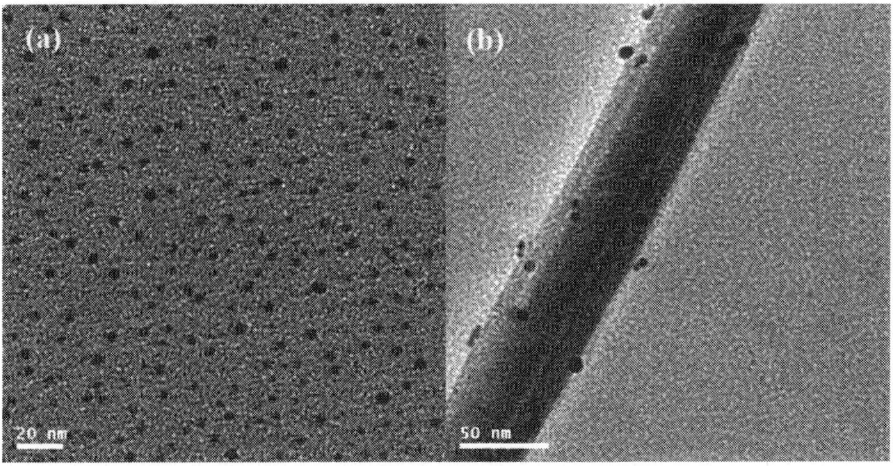

Fig. 4. TEM images of (a) GNPs, (b) GNPs-PbNWs (Wanga et al., 2009).

6.2 Cholesterol biosensors

Cholesterol is a fundamental parameter in the diagnosis of coronary heart disease, arteriosclerosis, and other clinical (lipid) disorders and in the assessment of the risks of thrombosis and myocardial infarction. The clinical analysis of cholesterol in serum samples is important in the diagnosis and prevention of a large number of clinical disorders such as hypertension, cerebral thrombosis and heart attack. Hence, it is important to develop a reliable and sensitive biosensor which can permit a suitable and rapid determination of cholesterol. Ideally, the total cholesterol concentration in a healthy person's blood should be less than 200 mg/dL (<5.17 mM). The borderline high is defined as 200–239 mg/dL (5.17–6.18 mM), and the high value is defined as above 240 mg/dL (≥6.21 mM) (Shen & Liu, 2007). Different analytical methods have been used for the determination of cholesterol for instance colorimetric, spectrometric and electrochemical methods. Among these methods, electrochemical detection of cholesterol has achieved significant attention due to the rapid determination, simplicity, and low cost. Thus, amperometric biosensors are more attractive due to their low detection limit and enzyme stabilization can be easily achieved. Especially, the enzyme based cholesterol sensors have gained special focus taking the advantages of good stability, high sensitivity and wide linear range they hold a leading position among the presently available biosensor systems. Recently, many scientists and biologists focused on the preparation of newer nanocomposite with good biocompatibility that could be the promising matrices for enzyme immobilization which can enhance the selectivity and sensitivity of the biosensors. Among the natural biocompatible macromolecules, chitosan (CS) is the biodegradable polymer obtained from marine versatile biopolymer-chitin. CS fibers situate apart from all other biodegradable natural fibers in several inherent properties such as outstanding biocompatibility, non-toxicity, biodegradability, high mechanical strength, fast metal complexation and hydrophilicity for enzyme immobilization. CS nanofibers (NFs) have remarkable characteristic such as exceptionally minute pore size with very outsized surface area-to-volume proportion, high porosity and diameters of the fiber was in nanometer scale. These properties of CSNFs hold fine enzyme immobilization scaffold and it was exploited for biosensor applications. These interesting matrices provide high surface area for high enzyme loading and compatible micro-environment helping enzyme stability. Besides, CS provides direct contact between enzyme active site and electrode. Enzyme immobilization is currently the gigantic increasing subject of considerable interest because the use of enzyme is frequently inadequate due to their availability in tiny quantity, instability, high cost and the limited possibility of economic recoveries of these bio-catalysts from an effective response unify. For a good enzyme immobilization, biocompatibility is the one of the most important key requisite that benefits the enzymatic bio-transformations to construct the biosensors. So, increase the biocompatibility of the support, various surface modification protocol have often been used such as adsorption, coating, self-assembly and graft polymerization. Among these techniques, it is relatively graceful and efficient to directly bind natural bio-macromolecules on the support surface to form a bio-mimetic compatible layer for enzyme immobilization. In the recent years, there is a trend to use nanostructured materials as supports for enzyme immobilization, since the large surface area to volume ratio of nanosize materials can effectively improve to the loading enzyme per unit to volume ratio of support and the excellent catalytic efficiency of the immobilized enzyme. Both nanofibers and nanoparticles were explored for this purpose. Recent developments in the field of nanobiotechnology, metal nanoparticles (MNPs) find numerous applications. Among the MNPs, GNPs be widely used for the catalytic and biological application. GNPS provides adequate micro-environment to enhance DET between biomolecule and electrode. In the fabrication of a cholesterol biosensor, cholesterol oxidase (ChOx) is most commonly used as the biosensing element. Cholesterol oxidase catalyzes the oxidation of cholesterol to H_2O_2 and cholest-4-en-3-one in the presence of oxygen. The enzymatic reaction in the use of cholesterol oxidase (ChOx) as a receptor can be described as follows:

ChOx

$$\text{Cholesterol} + O_2 \rightarrow \text{Cholest-4-en-3-one} + H_2O_2$$

The electro-oxidation current of hydrogen peroxide is detected after application of a suitable potential to the system. The major problem for amperometric detection is the overestimation of the response current due to interferences such as ascorbic acid. This problem can be overcome by using a combination of two or three enzymes, which are more selective for the analyte of interest (Bongiovanni et al., 2001) or by devising techniques to eliminate or reduce the interference. A novel amperometric cholesterol biosensor was fabricated by the immobilization of ChOx (cholesterol oxidase) onto the chitosan nanofibers/gold nanoparticles (designated as CSNFs/AuNPs) composite network (NW) (Gomathia et al., 2010). The fabrication involves preparation of chitosan nanofibers (CSNFs) and subsequent electrochemical loading of gold nanoparticles. Field emission scanning electron microscopy

(FE-SEM) was used to investigate the morphology of CSNFs (sizes in the range of 50–100 nm) and spherical GNPs. The CSNF-GNPs/ChOx biosensor exhibited a wide linear response tocholesterol (concentration range of 1-45 μM), good sensitivity (1.02 μA/μM), low response time (5 s) and excellent long term stability. The combined existence of GNPs within CSNFs NW provides the excellent performance of the biosensor towards the electrochemical detection of cholesterol.

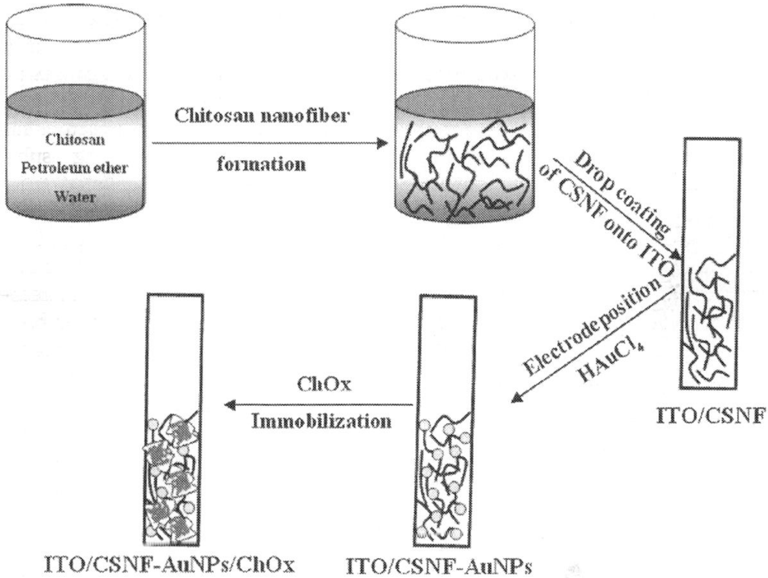

Fig. 5. Fabrication of CSNF-GNPs/ChOx biosensor electrode (Gomathia et al., 2010).

Many researchers have reported the inclusion of metal nanoparticles with a catalytic effect in polymer modified electrodes to decrease the overpotential applied to the amperometric biosensors (Safavi et al., 2009, Hrapovic et al., 2004, Ren et al., 2005, Huang et al., 2004). Amperometric cholesterol biosensors based on carbon nanotube-chitosan-platinum-cholesterol oxidase nanobiocomposite was fabricated for cholesterol determination at an applied potential of 0.4 V (Tsai et al., 2008). To improvethe selectivity of the biosensor, Gopalana et al. reported the construction of a cholesterol biosensor by monitoring the reduction current of H_2O_2 at −0.05 V (Gopalana et al., 2009). Bimetallic alloys are widely used in catalysis and sensing fields. Owing to the interaction between two components in bimetallic alloys, they generally show many favorable properties in comparison with the corresponding monometallic counterparts, which include high catalytic activity, catalytic selectivity, and better resistance to deactivation. Among various bimetallic alloys, gold-platinum (AuPt) alloy is very attractive. It has excellent catalysis and resistance to deactivation due to the high synergistic action between gold and platinum (Xiao et al., 2009). Owing to these advantages of bimetallic nanoparticles, it becomes significant to develop AuPt nanoparticles for application in electrochemical sensors with appropriate characteristics such as high sensitivity, fast response time, wide linear range, better selectivity, and reproducibility. An electrodeposition method was applied to form gold-platinum (AuPt) alloy nanoparticles on the glassy carbon electrode (GCE) modified with a mixture of an ionic liquid (IL) and chitosan (Ch) (AuPt-Ch-IL/GCE). AuPt-Ch-IL/GCE electrocatalyzed the reduction of H_2O_2 and thus was suitable for the preparation of biosensors. Cholesterol oxidase (ChOx) was then, immobilized on the surface of the electrode by cross-linking ChOx and chitosan through addition of glutaraldehyde (ChOx/AuPt-Ch-IL/GCE) (Safavia & Farjamia, 2011). The fabricated biosensor exhibited two wide linear ranges of responses to cholesterol in the concentration ranges of 0.05–6.2 mM and 6.2–11.2 mM. The sensitivity of the biosensor was 90.7 $\mu A.mM^{-1}.cm^{-2}$ and the limit of detection was 10 μM of cholesterol. The response time was less than 7 s. The Michaelis-Menten constant (Km) was found as 0.24 mM. The effect of the addition of 1 mM ascorbic acid and glucose was tested on the amperometric response of 0.5 mM cholesterol and no change in response current of cholesterol was observed.

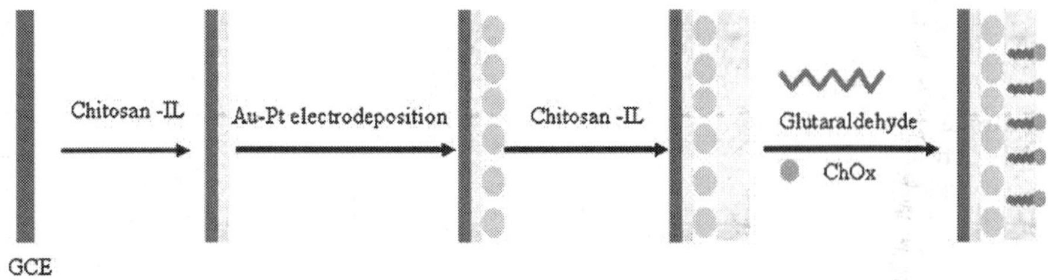

Fig. 6. Schematic illustration of preparation procedures of ChOx/AuPt-Ch-IL/GCE (Safavia & Farjamia, 2011).

6.3 Tyrosinase biosensors

Phenolic compounds often exist in the wastewaters of many industries, causing problems for our living environment. Many of them are very toxic, showing adverse effects on animal and plants. Therefore, the identification and quantification of such compounds are very important for environment monitoring. Some methods are available for the phenolic compound assay, including gas or liquid chromatography and spectrophotometry (Chriswell et al. 1975, Poerschmann et al., 1997). However, demanding sample pretreatments, low sensitivities, and time-consuming manipulations limit their practical applications. A great amount of effort has been devoted to the development of simple and effective analytical methods for the determination of phenolic compounds. Among them, amperometric biosensor based on tyrosinase has been shown to be a very simple and convenient tool for phenol assay due to its high sensitivity, effectiveness, and simplicity (Wang et al., 2002, Dempsey et al., 2004, Rajesh et al., 2004, Xue & Shen, 2002, Zhang et al., 2003, Wang et al., 2000a, Yu et al. 2003, Campuzano et al., 2003, Tatsuma & Sato, 2004). The immobilization of tyrosinase is a crucial step in the fabrication of phenol biosensor. The earlier reports on the immobilization methods included polymer entrapment (Wang et al., 2002, Dempsey et al., 2004), electropolymerization (Dempsey et al., 2004, Rajesh et al., 2004), sol-gels (Rajesh et al., 2004, Yu et al. 2003), self-assembled monolayers (SAMs)1 (Campuzano et al., 2003, Tatsuma et al., 2004), and covalent linking (Anh et al., 2002, Rajesh et al., 2004a). However, some of these immobilizations are relatively complex, requiring the use of solvents that are unattractive to the environment and result in relatively poor stability and bioactivity of tyrosinase. Recent years have seen increased interest in searching for simple and reliable schemes to immobilize enzymes. The biocompatible nanomaterials have their unique advantages in enzyme immobilization. They could retain the activity of enzyme well due to the desirable microenvironment, and they could enhance the direct electron transfer between the enzyme's active sites and the electrode (Gorton et al., 1999, Jia et al., 2002). In spite of the big amount of literature on tyrosinase electrochemical biosensors, two general limitations need to be solved yet in order to improve their practical usefulness. One of them concerns the stability of the biosensors. Although many efforts have been made to improve the useful lifetime and reusability of tyrosinase electrodes, searching for appropriate microenvironments for retaining the biological activity of the enzyme, its inherent instability provokes that this useful lifetime is too short for practical applications in many cases. On the other hand, the low concentration levels of phenolic compounds that should be detected due to their classification as priority pollutants, requires that the tyrosinase biosensors are capable to achieve a high sensitivity. The aim of this work is the design of a new tyrosinase bioelectrode able to improve significantly these important analytical characteristics with respect to previous designs. The new bioelectrode design is based on the combination of the advantageous properties of a graphite–Teflon composite electrode matrix for the immobilization of enzymes, and the use of colloidal gold nanoparticles. In this new design, both the enzyme tyrosinase and gold nanoparticles are incorporated into the composite electrode matrix by simple physical inclusion. The use of graphite–Teflon composite pellets for the construction of enzyme electrodes has been extensively reported (Serra et al., 2002, GuzmanVazquez de Pradaet al., 2003, Pena et al., 2001). The resulting bioelectrodes are easily renewable by polishing and allow incorporation of biomolecules and other modifiers with no covalent attachments, thus making the electrode fabrication procedure easy, fast and cheap. On the other hand, electrochemical biosensors created by coupling biological recognition elements with electrochemical transducers based on or modified with gold nanoparticles are playing an increasingly important role in biosensor research over the last few years (Yanez-Sedeno & Pingarron, 2005). So, colloidal gold allows proteins to retain their biological activity upon adsorption (Doron et al., 1995, Brown et al., 1996, Mena et al., 2005) and modification of electrodes with this type of nanoparticles provides a microenvironment similar to that of the redox proteins in native systems, reducing the insulating effect of the protein shell for the direct electron transfer through the conducting tunnels of gold nanocrystals (Liu et al., 2003a). Surface morphology of gold nanoparticles, and the interaction between the nanoparticles and the electrode surface, are significant factors which contribute to improve the electrical contact between the redox protein and the electrode material (Shipway et al., 2000). In this context, biosensors based on the immobilization of enzymes on gold nanoparticles for the determination of hydrogen peroxide, nitrite, glucose and phenols (Tang & Jiang, 1998, Xiao et al., 2000, Gu et al., 2001, Liu & Ju, 2002, Jia et al., 2002, Liu & Ju, 2003, Liu et al., 2003b, Xiao et al., 2003, Carralero-Sanz et al., 2005) have been recently reported.

The preparation of a tyrosinase biosensor based on the immobilization of the enzyme onto a glassy carbon electrode modified with electrodeposited gold nanoparticles (Tyr-nAu-GCE) was reported (Carralero-Sanz et al., 2005). The enzyme immobilized by cross-linking with glutaraldehyde retains a high bioactivity on this electrode material. Under the optimized working variables (a Au electrodeposition potential of −200mV for 60 s, an enzyme loading of 457 U, a detection potential of −0.10V and a 0.1 mol. L^{-1} phosphate buffer solution of pH 7.4 as working medium) the biosensor exhibited a rapid response to the changes in the substrate concentration for all the phenolic compounds tested: phenol, catechol, caffeic acid, chlorogenic acid, gallic acid and protocatechualdehyde. A R.S.D. of 3.6% (n = 6) was obtained from the slope values of successive calibration plots for catechol with the same Tyr-nAu-GCE with no need to apply a cleaning procedure to the biosensor. The useful lifetime of one single biosensor was of at least 18 days, and a R.S.D. of 4.8% was obtained for the slope values of catechol calibration plots obtained with five different biosensors. The Tyr-nAu-GCE was applied for the estimation of the phenolic compounds content in red and white wines. A good correlation of the results (r = 0.990) was found when they were plotted versus those obtained by using the spectrophotometric method involving the Folin-Ciocalteau reagent.

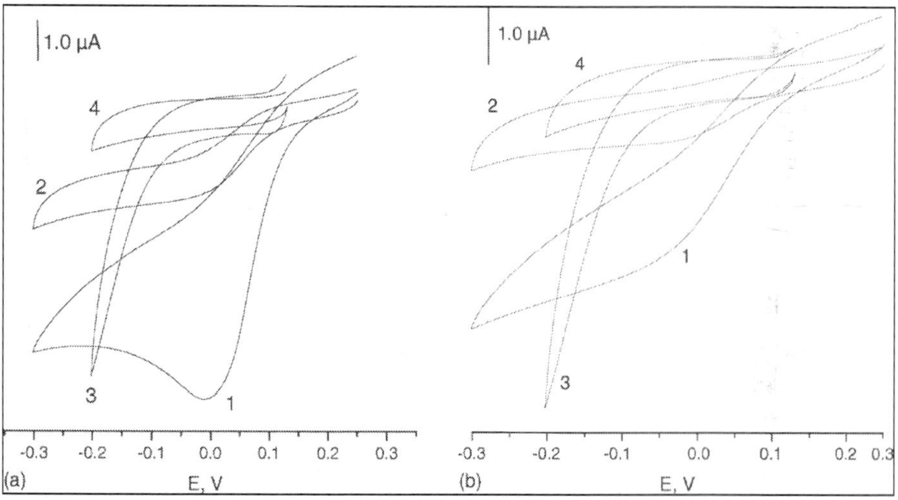

Fig. 7. Cyclic voltammograms for 2.0×10^{-4} mol.L^{-1} solutions of catechol (a) and caffeic acid (b), at: (1) Tyr-nAu-GCE; (2) Tyr-GCE; (3) Au-GCE; (4) GCE; v = 25mVs−1. Supporting electrolyte: 0.05 mol.L^{-1} phosphate buffer (pH 7.4) (Carralero-Sanz et al., 2005).

The design of a new tyrosinase biosensor with improved stability and sensitivity was reported (Carralero-Sanz et al., 2006). The biosensor design is based on the construction of a graphite–Teflon composite electrode matrix in which the enzyme and colloidal gold nanoparticles are incorporated by simple physical inclusion. The Tyr–Au_{coll}–graphite–Teflon biosensor exhibited suitable amperometric responses at −0.10 V for the different phenolic compounds tested (catechol; phenol; 3,4-dimethylphenol; 4-chloro-3-methylphenol; 4-chlorophenol; 4- chloro-2-methylphenol; 3-methylphenol and 4-methylphenol). The limits of detection obtained were 3 nM for catechol, 3.3 μM for 4- chloro- 2-methylphenol, and approximately 20 nM for the rest of phenolic compounds. The presence of colloidal gold into the composite matrix gives rise to enhanced kinetics of both the enzyme reaction and the electrochemical reduction of the corresponding *o*-quinones at the electrode surface, thus allowing the achievement of a high sensitivity. The biosensor exhibited an excellent renewability by simple polishing, with a lifetime of at least 39 days without apparent loss of the immobilized enzyme activity. The usefulness of the biosensor for the analysis of real samples was evaluated by performing the estimation of the content of phenolic compounds in water samples of different characteristics.

A highly efficient enzyme-based screen printed electrode (SPE) was obtained by using covalent attachment between 1-pyrenebutanoic acid, succinimidyl ester (PASE) adsorbing on the graphene oxide (GO) sheets and amines of tyrosinase-protected gold nanoparticles (Tyr-Au) (Song et al., 2010). Herein, the bi-functional molecule PASE was assembled onto GO sheets. Subsequently, the Tyr-Au was immobilized on the PASE-GO sheets forming a biocompatible nanocomposite, which was further coated onto the working electrode surface of the SPE. Attributing to the synergistic effect of GO-Au integration and the good biocompatibility of the hybrid-material, the fabricated disposable biosensor (Tyr-Au/PASE-GO/SPE) exhibited a rapid amperometric response (less than 6 s) with a high sensitivity and good storage stability for monitoring catechol. This method shows a good linearity in the range from 8.3×10^{-8} to 2.3×10^{-5} M for catechol with a squared correlation coefficient of 0.9980, a quantitation limit of 8.2×10^{-8} M (S/N = 10) and a detection limit of 2.4×10^{-8} M (S/N = 3). The Michaelis-Menten constant was measured to be 0.027 mM. This disposable tyrosinase biosensor could offer a great potential for rapid, cost-effective and on-field analysis of phenolic compounds.

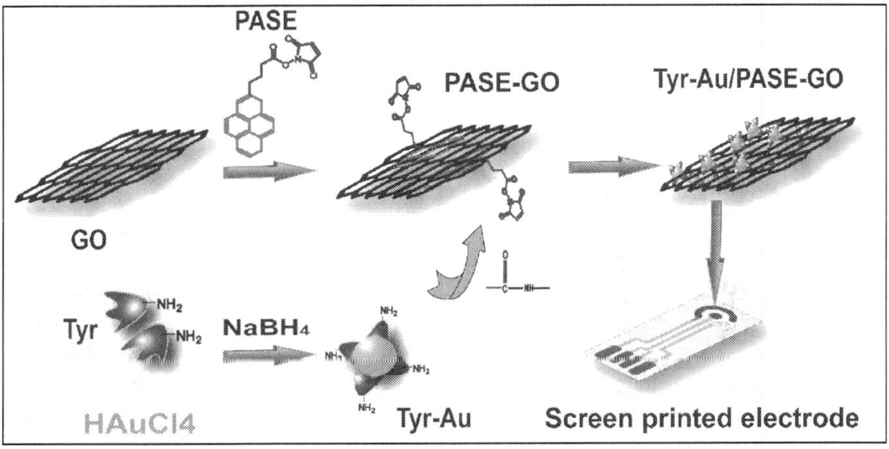

Fig. 8. Assembling process of Tyr-Au/PASE-GO on SPE (Song et al., 2010).

6.4 Urease biosensors

Kidneys perform key roles in various body functions, including excreting metabolic waste products such as urea from the bloodstream, regulating the hydrolytic balance of the body, and maintaining the pH of body fluids. The level of urea in blood serum is the best measurement of kidney function and staging of kidney diseases. The normal urea level in serum ranges from 15 to 40 mg/dL (i.e., 2.5–7.5 mM). An increase in urea concentration causes renal failure such as acute or chronic urinary tract obstruction with shock, burns, dehydration, and gastrointestinal bleeding, whereas a decrease in urea concentration causes hepatic failure, nephritic syndrome, and cachexia. Therefore, there is an urgent need to develop a device that rapidly monitors urea concentration in the body. Most existing urea biosensors utilize urease (Urs) as the sensing element. The available Urs on the electrode surface hydrolyzes urea into NH_4^+ and HCO_3^-ions. The concentration of urea is measured by monitoring the librated ions using a transducer such as amperometric, potentiometric, optical, thermal, or piezoelectric. Although various urea biosensors that use a range of transducers have been studied extensively, the Urs-based amperometric urea biosensor is considered one of the most promising approaches because it offers fast, simple, and low-cost detection. The response time of such a biosensor is directly associated with the hydrolysis rate of urea on the electrode surface; therefore, rapid production of NH_4^+ ions on the electrode will lead to a highly sensitive biosensor. It is well established that the performance of biosensors greatly depends on the physicochemical properties of the electrode materials, enzyme immobilization procedure, and enzyme concentration on the electrode surface. Many electrode materials have been used to fabricate urea biosensors. However, there is an ongoing demand for new types of electrode materials that can provide the Urs enzyme with better stability and performance for *in vitro* urea measurement. In this context, the use of nanomaterials to fabricate biosensors is one of the most exciting approaches because nanomaterials have a unique structure and high surface-to-volume ratio. The surfaces of nanomaterials can also be tailored in the molecular scale in order to achieve various desirable properties. Many attempts have been made to fabricate a third-generation biosensor with self-assembly technology; however, these approaches were based on planar self-assembly that may only offer limited available surface area on the electrode, which can compromise the performance of the biosensor. Meanwhile, gold nanoparticles have played an increasingly important role for biosensor applications over the last decade.

Gold nanoparticles can (1) provide a stable surface for the immobilization of biomolecules without compromising their biological activities and (2) permit direct electron transfer from the redox biomolecules to the bulk electrode materials, thereby enhancing the electrochemical sensing ability. For example, Shipway et al. systematically studied the new electronic, photoelectronic, and sensoring systems that used gold nanoparticle superstructures on the electrode surface (Shipway et al., 2000). In addition, previous studies indicated that biological macromolecules such as enzymes can generally retain their enzymatic and electrochemical activity after being immobilized onto the gold nanoparticles (Brown et al., 1996, Xiao et al., 1999). Anamperometric biosensor was fabricated for the quantitative determination of urea in aqueous medium using hematein, a pH-sensitive natural dye (Tiwari et al., 2009). The urease (Urs) covalently immobilized onto an electrode made of gold nanoparticles functionalized with hyperbranched polyester-BoltronR H40 (H40–Au) coated onto an indium–tin oxide (ITO) covered glass substrate. The covalent linkage between the Urs enzyme and H40–Au nanoparticles provided the resulting enzyme electrode (Urs/H40–Au/ITO) with a high level of enzyme immobilization and excellent lifetime stability. The biosensor based on Urs/H40–Au/ITO as the working electrode showed a linear current response to the urea concentration ranging from 0.01 to 35 mM. The urea biosensor exhibited a sensitivity of 7.48nA/mMwith a response time of 3 s. The Michaelis–Menten constant for the Urs/H40–Au/ITO biosensor was calculated to be 0.96mM, indicating the Urs enzyme immobilized on the electrode surface had a high affinity to urea.

A renewable potentiometric urease inhibition biosensor based on self-assembled gold nanoparticles has been developed for the determination of mercury ions (Yang et al., 2006a).

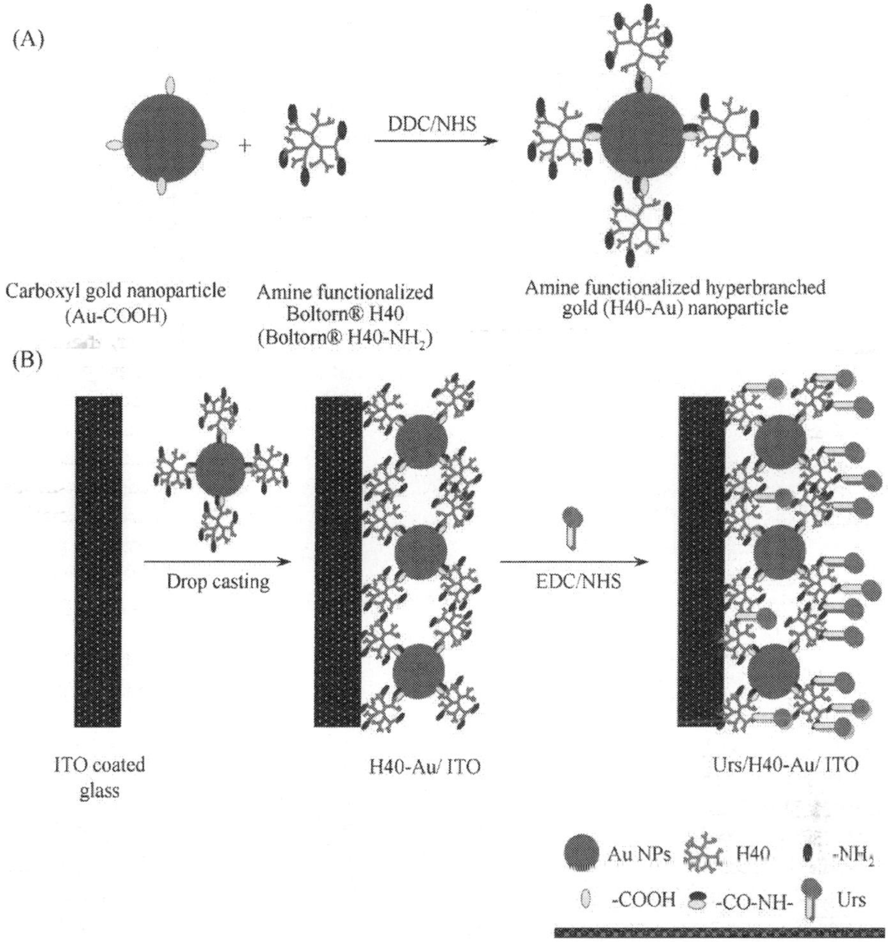

Fig. 9. Schematic presentation of the [A] preparation of hyperbranched gold (H40–Au) nanoparticles and [B] fabrication of H40–Au/ITO and Urs/H40–Au/ITO electrodes(Tiwari et al., 2009).

Gold nanoparticles were chemically adsorbed on the PVC-NH2 matrix membrane pH electrode surface containing *N,N*didecylaminomethylbenzene (DAMAB) as a neutral carrier and urease was then immobilized on the gold nanoparticles. The linear range of determination of Hg^{2+} was 0.09–1.99 μmol.L^{-1} with a detection limit of 0.05 μmol.L^{-1}. The advantages of self-assembled immobilization are low detection limit, fast response and ease regeneration. The assembled gold nanoparticles and inactive enzyme layers denatured by Hg^{2+} can be rinsed out via a saline solution with acid and alkali successively. This sensor is generally of great significance for inhibitor determination, especially in comparison with expensive base transducers.

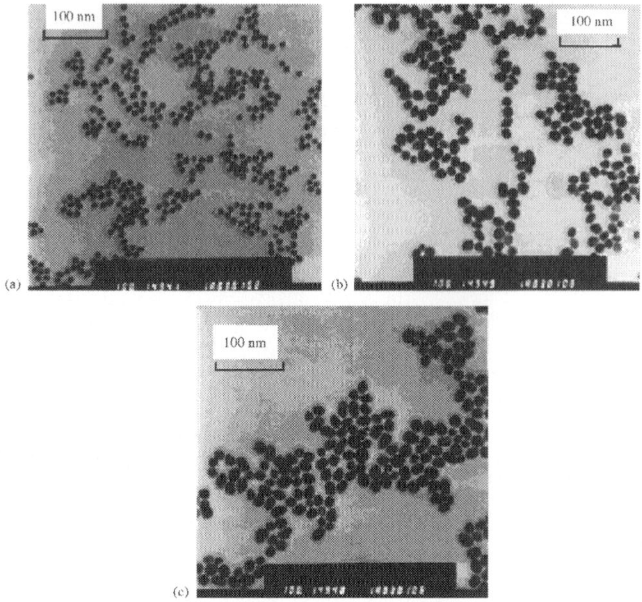

Fig. 10. TEM of gold nanoparticles with different size: 12 nm (a), 20 nm (b) and 35 nm (c) (Yang et al., 2006a).

6.5 Acetylcholinesterase biosensors

Carbamate and organophosphate pesticides have come into widespread use in agriculture because of their high insecticidal activity and relatively low environmental persistence. However, overuse of these pesticides results in pesticide residues in food, water and environment, and leads to a severe threat to human health due to their high toxicity to acetylcholinesterase (AChE), which is essential for the functioning of the central nervous system in humans. For these reasons, it has great significance to develop a fast, reliable and inexpensive analytical method for determination of trace amounts of these pesticides. Common analytical techniques for determination of these compounds, such as gas and liquid chromatography are sensitive, reliable and precise. However, these methods require expensive instrumentation, complicated pretreatment procedure and professional operators, which limit their application for real-time detection of these compounds. In order to simplify procedure and decrease cost, enzyme based biosensors could be a reliable and promising alternative to classical methods because of their simple fabrication, easy operation, high sensitivity and selectivity. It is well known that acetylthiocholine chloride (ATCl) can be catalytically hydrolyzed by AChE to thiocholine (TCh), which could be electrochemically oxidized at special potential. The hydrolysis reaction of ATCl would be inhibited by carbamate and organophosphorous pesticides, because AChE could irreversibly combine with these pesticides, which results in AChE inactivation to give low TCh concentration and low oxidation current. Therefore, based on the inhibition of carbamate and organophosphate pesticides on the AChE activity, the concentrations of pesticides would be monitored by measuring the electrochemical oxidation peak current of TCh. The key aspect in construction of this kind of biosensor is the immobilization of AChE on the solid electrode surface with high electron transfer rate and bioactivity. In order to settle it, a variety of matrix materials have been employed, among them, GNPs have attracted enormous interest in the fabrication of electrochemical biosensors for possessing conductive sensing interface, catalytic properties and conductivity properties. Moreover, GNPs can provide an environment similar to that of proteins in a native system and allow protein molecules more freedom in orientation, which will reduce the insulating property of protein shell and facilitate the electron transfer through the conducting tunnel of GNPs. Gold nanoparticles were synthesized *in situ* and electrodeposited onto Au substrate (Dua et al., 2008). The GNPs modified interface facilitates electron transfer across self-assembled monolayers of 11-mercaptoundecanoic acid (MUA). After activation of surface carboxyl groups with 1-ethyl-3-(3-dimethylaminopropyl) carbodiimide and *N*-hydroxysuccinimide, the interface displayed good stability for immobilization of biomolecules. The immobilized acetylcholinesterase (AChE) showed excellent activity to its substrate, leading to a stable AChE biosensor. Under the optimal experimental conditions, the inhibition of malathion on AChE biosensor was proportional to its concentration in two ranges, from 0.001 to 0.1 $\mu g.mL^{-1}$ and from 0.1 to 25 $\mu g.mL^{-1}$, with detection limit of 0.001 $\mu g.mL^{-1}$. The simple method showed good reproducibility and acceptable stability, which had potential application in biosensor design.

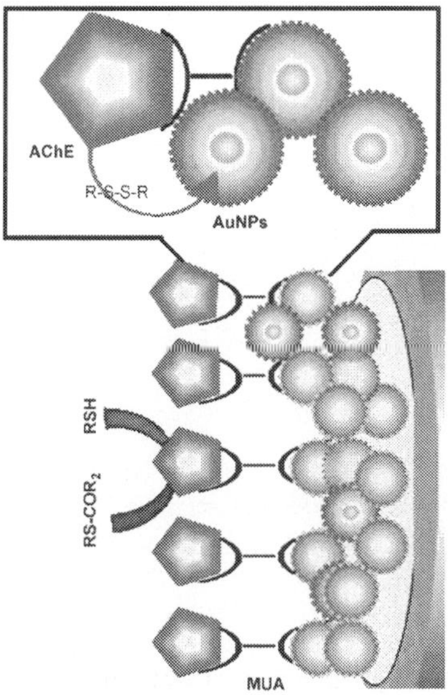

Fig. 11. Principle of GNPs served as mediator for electron transfer across SAMs for AChE biosensor design (Dua et al., 2008).

GNPs are particularly attractive for fabricating electrochemical sensors and biosensor. However, GNPs are inherently instable and apt to agglomerate. In order to settle this problem, it is necessary to use protective agents. SF is a natural protein, which can be extracted from silkworm cocoon. Due to the unique properties of SF with thermal stability, nontoxicity, low cost and biocompatibility, it is widely used as a substrate for enzyme immobilization. Furthermore, GNPs could be in situ produced by the reduction of SF at room temperature, in which SF acts as both reducing agent and protector. It has been demonstrated that GNPs and SF could interact to form a bioconjugate, and this kind of GNPs–SF colloid possessed a stable and highly dispersed nature. A sensitive and stable amperometric biosensor for the detection of methyl paraoxon, carbofuran and phoxim had been developed based on immobilization of acetylcholinasterase (AChE) on gold nanoparticles and silk fibroin (SF) modified platinum electrode (Yin et al., 2009). The SF provided a biocompatible microenvironment around the enzyme molecule to stabilize its biological activity and effectively prevented it from leaking out of platinum electrode surface. In the presence of acetylthiocholine chloride (ATCl) as a substrate, GNPs promoted electron transfer reaction at a lower potential and catalyzed the electrochemical oxidation of thiocholine (TCh), thus increasing detection sensitivity. Under optimum conditions, the inhibition percentages of methyl paraoxon, carbofuran and phoxim were proportional to their concentrations in the range of $6x10^{-11}$–$5x10^{-8}$ M, $2x10^{-10}$–$1x10^{-7}$ M and $5x10^{-9}$–$2x10^{-7}$ M, respectively. The detection limits were found to be $2x10^{-11}$ M for methyl paraoxon, $1x10^{-10}$ M for carbofuran and $2x10^{-9}$ M for phoxim. Moreover, the fabricated biosensor had good reproducibility and acceptable stability. The biosensor is a promising new tool for pesticide analysis.

A novel interface embedded in situ gold nanoparticles (GNPs) in chitosan hydrogel was constructed by one-step electrochemical deposition in solution containing tetrachloroauric (III) acid and chitosan (Du et al., 2007a). This deposited interface possessed excellent biocompatibility and good stability. The immobilized AChE, as a model, showed excellent activity to its substrate and provided a quantitative measurement of organophosphate pesticides involved in the inhibition action. Operational parameters, including the deposition time, tetrachloroauric (III) acid concentration have been optimized. Under the optimal electrodeposition, an amperometric sensor for the fast determination of malathion and monocrotophos, respectively was developed with detection limit of 0.001 $\mu g.mL^{-1}$. The simple method showed good fabrication reproducibility and acceptable stability, which provided a new avenue for electrochemical biosensor design.

6.6 Horseradish peroxidase

Over the last years, considerable efforts have been devoted to the development of horseradish peroxidase (HRP, EC 1.11.1.7, H_2O_2 oxidoreductase)-based mediatorless electrochemical biosensors for the fast, simple, selective and accurate quantification of H_2O_2. This interest is justified by the industrial, chemical and biomedical applications of this oxidant compound. In addition, H_2O_2 constitutes a relevant biochemical mediator in many cellular processes, as well as a by-product of several oxidases with analytical applications. Different strategies has been described for connecting the catalytic active site of HRP with electrode surfaces, in order to construct such kind of third generation H_2O_2 biosensors in which the direct electron transfer between the enzyme and the electrode is allowed without the use of any natural or artificial redox mediator. Among these methods, it should be highlighted the use of electroconductive polymers (Zhaoyang et al., 2006, Luo et al., 2006, Mala Ekanayake et al., 2009), metal nanoparticles (Zhaoyang et al., 2006, Luo et al., 2006,

Mala Ekanayake et al., 2009, Jeykumari et al., 2008, Schumb et al., 1995, Ferreira et al., 2004, Alonso Lomillo et al., 2005, Pingarron et al., 2008), redox polymers and sol–gel materials (Wang et al., 2000, Jia et al., 2005, Garca et al., 2007), DNA (Song et al., 2006) and carbon nanotubes (Jeykumari et al., 2008) as wiring materials for HRP. On the other hand, the immobilization strategy to be employed is another key factor to consider in the design of an enzyme biosensor. This approach should favor the maintenance of the active enzyme conformation as well as provide a favorable hydrophilic microenvironment around the biocatalyst in order to contribute to the best catalytic performance of the enzyme (Song et al., 2006, Villalonga et al., 2007). In this regard, it has been previously reported the preparation of highly active and stable biocatalysts by the polyelectrostatic immobilization of enzymes in polysaccharide-coated supports (Gomez et al., 2006). In addition, several ionic polysaccharides such as sodium alginate (Camacho et al., 2007, Ionescu et al., 2006, Cosnier et al., 2004) and chitosan and its derivatives (Qin et al., 2006, Li et al., 2008), have been successfully used as coating materials for preparing robust enzyme biosensors. Horseradish peroxidase was cross-linked with cysteamine-capped Au nanoparticles and further immobilized on sodium alginate-coated Au electrode through polyelectrostatic interactions (Chico et al., 2009). The electrode was employed for constructing a reagentless amperometric biosensor for H_2O_2. The electrode showed linear response (poised at -400 mV vs. Ag/AgCl) toward H_2O_2 concentration between 20 μM and 13.7 mM at pH 7.0. The biosensor reached 95% of steady-state current in about 15 s, and its sensitivity was 40.1 mA/M.cm^2. The detection limit of the enzyme-based electrode was determined as 3 μM, at a signal-to-noise ratio of three. The electrode retained 97% of its initial analytical response after 1 month of storage at 4 °C in 50 mM sodium phosphate buffer, pH 7.0. The stability of the biosensor was significantly reduced when it was incubated in high ionic strength solutions, retaining only 44% of its initial response after 1 month of storage at 4 °C in 1 M NaCl ionic strength in 50 mM sodium phosphate buffer, pH 7.0.

The preparation of horseradish peroxidase (HRP)-GNPs-silk fibroin (SF) modified glassy carbon electrode (GCE) by one step procedure was reported (Yina et al., 2009). The enzyme electrode showed a quasi-reversible electrochemical redox behavior with a formal potential of −210mV (vs. SCE) in 0.1M phosphate buffer solution at pH 7.1. The response of the biosensor showed a surface-controlled electrochemical process with one electron transfer accompanying with one proton. The cathodic transfer coefficient was 0.42, the electron transfer rate constant was 1.84 s^{-1} and the surface coverage of HRP was 1.8×10^{-9} mol.cm^{-2}. The experimental results indicated that GNPs–SF composite matrix could not only steadily immobilize HRP, but also efficiently retain its bioactivity. The biosensor displayed an excellent and quick electrocatalytic response to the reduction of H_2O_2.

A novel method for fabrication of horseradish peroxidase (HRP) biosensor has been developed by self-assembling gold nanoparticles on thiol-functionalized poly(styrene-*co*-acrylic acid) (St-*co*-AA) nanospheres (Xu et al., 2004). At first, a cleaned gold electrode was immersed in thiol-functionalized poly(St-*co*-AA) nanosphere latex prepared by emulsifier-free emulsion polymerization of St with AA and function with dithioglycol to assemble the nanospheres, then gold nanoparticles were chemisorbed onto the thiol groups. Finally, horseradish peroxidase was immobilized on the surface of the gold nanoparticles. The sensor displayed an excellent electrocatalytical response to reduction of H_2O_2 without the aid of an electron mediator. The sensor was highly sensitive to hydrogen peroxide with a detection limit of 4.0 μmol.L^{-1}, and the linear range was from 10.0 μmol.L^{-1} to 7.0 mmol.L^{-1}.

The biosensor retained more than 97.8% of its original activity after 60 days of use. Moreover, the studied biosensor exhibited good current repeatability and good fabrication reproducibility.

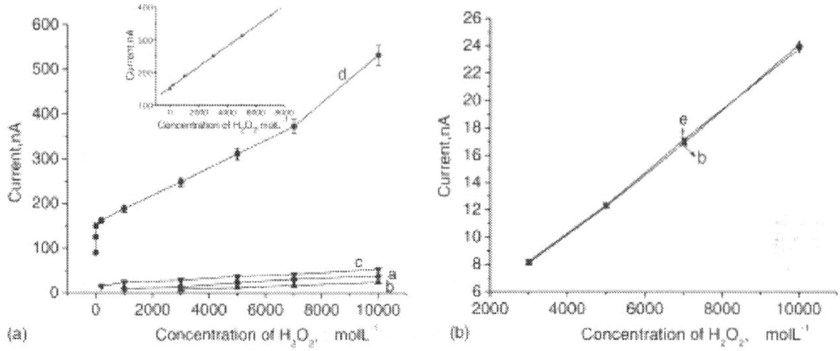

Fig. 12. Steady-state amperometric responses of electrodes to the reduction of H_2O_2 in the stirring PB under elimination of oxygen: (a) the non-modified gold electrode; (b) the latex modified electrode; (c) the gold nanoparticle modified electrode before HRP addition; (d) the gold nanoparticle modified electrode after HRP addition; (e) the latex modified electrode after HRP addition; Applied potential, −200mV; supporting electrolyte, 100 mmol.L^{-1} pH 7 (Xu et al., 2004).

A one-step method for fabrication of horseradish peroxidase (HRP) biosensor has been developed (Di et al., 2005). The gold nanoparticles and HRP were simultaneously embedded in silica sol-gel network on gold electrode surface in the presence of cysteine. The immobilized HRP exhibited direct electrochemical behavior toward the reduction of hydrogen peroxide. The heterogeneous electron transfer rate constant was evaluated to be 7.8 s^{-1}. The biosensor displayed an excellent elctrocatalytic response to the reduction of H_2O_2 without any mediator. The calibration range of H_2O_2 was from 1.6 μmol.L^{-1} to 3.2 mmol.L^{-1} and a detection limit of 0.5 μmol.L^{-1} at a signal-to- noise ratio of 3. The biosensor exhibited high sensitivity, rapid response and long-term stability.

The design and development of a screen printed carbon electrode (SPCE) on a polyvinyl chloride substrate as a disposable sensor is described (Tangkuaram et al., 2007). Six configurations were designed on silk screen frames. The SPCEs were printed with four inks: silver ink as the conducting track, carbon ink as the working and counter electrodes, silver/silver chloride ink as the reference electrode and insulating ink as the insulator layer. Selection of the best configuration was done by comparing slopes from the calibration plots generated by the cyclic voltammograms at 10, 20 and 30mM $K_3Fe(CN)_6$ for each configuration. The electrodes with similar configurations gave similar slopes. The 5th configuration was the best electrode that gave the highest slope. Modifying the best SPCE configuration for use as a biosensor, horseradish peroxidase (HRP) was selected as a biomaterial bound with gold nanoparticles in the matrix of chitosan (HRP/GNP/CHIT). Biosensors of HRP/SPCE, HRP/CHIT/SPCE and HRP/GNP/CHIT/SPCE were used in the amperometric detection of H_2O_2 in a solution of 0.1M citrate buffer, pH 6.5, by applying a potential of −0.4 V at the working electrode. All the biosensors showed an immediate response to H_2O_2. The effect of HRP/GNP incorporated with CHIT (HRP/GNP/CHIT/SPCE) yielded the highest performance. The amperometric response of HRP/GNP/CHIT/SPCE retained over 95% of the initial current of the 1st day up to 30 days of storage at 4 °C. The biosensor showed a linear range of 0.01–11.3 mM H_2O_2, with a detection limit of 0.65 μM H_2O_2 (S/N = 3). The low detection limit, long storage life and wide linear range of this biosensor make it advantageous in many applications, including bioreactors and biosensors.

6.7 DNA biosensors

DNA biosensors for the detection of nucleic acid sequences have attracted ever increasing interests in connection with highly demanding research efforts directed to gene analysis, clinical disease diagnosis, or even forensic applications (Service, 1998, Butler, 2006, Staudt, 2001, Farace et al., 2002, Reisberga et al., 2006). Various techniques including optical, electrochemistry, surface plasmon resonance spectroscopy, and quartz crystal microbalance, etc have been well developed for DNA detection (Rosi & Mirkin, 2005, Gerion et al., 2003, Drummond et al., 2003, He et al., 2000). Among them, electrochemistry offer great advantages such as simple, rapid, low-cost and high sensitivity (Lao et al., 2005). A key issue faced with any DNA hybridization biosensor is the immobilization amount and accessibility of probe DNA for hybridization recognition (Moses et al., 2004, Lowe et al., 2003, Ding et al., 2008, Ostatná et al., 2005). Increasing the immobilization amount and controlling over the molecular orientation of probe DNA would markedly improve the performance properties of DNA biosensor. It has been well elaborated that the immobilization amount and the molecular orientation of probe single-stranded DNA could remarkably influence the operational performance of DNA electrochemical biosensor (Liu et al., 2008, Basuray et al., 2009). Therefore, numerous different immobilization strategies have been proposed and employed aimed at improving the link stability between DNA and transducer surface (Cederquist et al., 2008), or increasing the amountof immobilized DNA (Liu et al., 2005), and sometimes simplifying the immobilization procedure (Kjllman et al., 2008). In order to achieve this goal, nanomaterials could be used as an elegant solution for the control of DNA immobilization and hybridization. For a decade, metal nanoparticles have shown huge potential in the fields of biosensing, diagnostics and molecular therapeutics because of its excellent optical and electrical properties (Brown et al., 1996, Bao et al., 2003, Ma et al., 2004, Kidambi et al., 2004). Owing to the large surface area and biocompatibility with biosystem, gold nanoparticles have been shown as a good candidate for enhancement of DNA immobilization and hybridization and they have been directly linked onto the biosensor surface via various strategies such as covalent linking, electrodeposition, electroless deposition, sol–gel, etc (Li et al., 2007, Yamada et al., 2003, Zhao et al., 2007, Jena& Raj, 2007). The self-assembly of GNPs on the electrode surface could be easily achieved via the use of a bi-functional chemical linking agent such as 1,6-hexanedithiol, cysteamine. Although these self-assembly methods are very simple and rapid, the formed monolayer on the electrode surface are usually insulated or could not offer a good electrical conductivity between GNPs and electrode surface, which is not especially favorable for the fabrication of electrochemical sensor or biosensor.

A novel protocol for development of DNA electrochemical biosensor based on GNPs modified glassy carbon electrode (GCE) was proposed (Li et al., 2011), which was carried out by the self-assembly of GNPs on the mercaptophenyl film (MPF) via simple electrografting of in situ generated mercaptophenyl diazonium cations. The resulting MPF was covalently immobilized on GCE surface via C–C bond with high stability, which was desirable in fabrication of excellent performance biosensors. Probe DNA was self-assembled on GNPs through the well-known Au–thiol binding. The recognition of fabricated DNA electrochemical biosensor toward complementary single-stranded DNA was determined by differential pulse voltammetry with the use of $Co(phen)_3^{3+}$ as the electrochemical indicator. Taking advantage of amplification effects of GNPs and stability of MPF, the developed biosensor could detect target DNA with the detection limit of 7.2×10^{-11} M, which also exhibits good selectivity, stability and regeneration ability for DNA detection. DNA biosensor which was based on the self-assembly of GNPs on the mercapto-diazoaminobenzene monolayer modified electrode was also reported (Liet al., 2010a). The mercapto-diazoaminobenzene monolayer was obtained by covalent immobilization of 4-aminothiophenol (4-ATP) molecules onto another 4-ATP monolayer functionalized gold electrode bydiazotization-coupling reaction. The DNA immobilization and hybridization on the GNPs modified electrode was further investigated. The prepared GNPs–ATP–diazo-ATP film demonstrated efficient electron transfer ability for the electroactive species toward the electrode surface due to a large conjugated structure of the mercapto-diazoaminobenzene monolayer. The recognition of fabricated electrochemical DNA biosensor toward complementary single-stranded DNA was determined by differential pulse voltammetry with the use of $Co(phen)_3^{3+}$ as an electrochemical indicator. A linear detection range for the complementary target DNA was obtained from 3.01×10^{-10} to 1.32×10^{-8} M with a detection limit of 9.10×10^{-11} M. The fabricated biosensor also possessed good selectivity and could be regenerated easily.

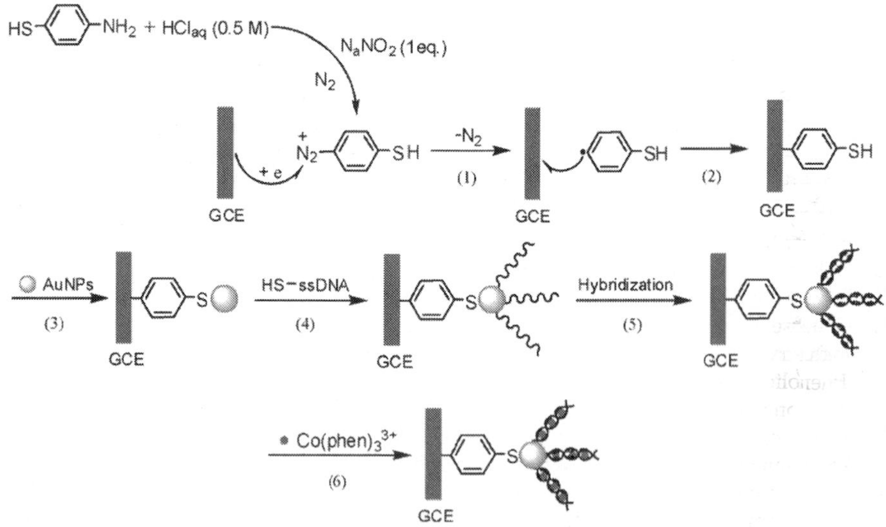

Fig. 13. Schematic representation of the fabrication of DNA biosensor (Li et al., 2011).

Colloidal gold nanoparticles and carboxyl group-functionalized CdS Nanoparticles (CdS NPs) were immobilized on the Au electrode surface to fabricate a novel electrochemical

DNA biosensor (Du et al., 2009). Both GNPs and CdS NPs, well known to be good biocompatible and conductive materials, could provide larger surface area and sufficient amount of binding points for DNA immobilization. DNA immobilization and hybridization were characterized with differential pulse voltammetry (DPV) by using $[Co(phen)_2(Cl)(H_2O)]Cl\cdot 2H_2O$ as an electrochemical hybridization indicator. With this approach, the target DNA could be quantified at a linear range from 2.0×10^{-10} to 1.0×10^{-8} M, with a detection limit of 2.0×10^{-11} M by 3σ. In addition, the biosensor exhibited a good repeatability and stability for the determination of DNA sequences.

Layers for DNA immobilization	Detection limit ($mol.L^{-1}$)
Au and CdS NPs (Du et al., 2009)	2.0×10^{-11}
LBL Au NPs and MWCNTs (Ma et al., 2008)	7.5×10^{-12}
CNTs (Niu et al., 2011)	1.4×10^{-10}
Pt NPs and CNTs (Zhu et al., 2005)	1.0×10^{-11}
ZrO_2/SWNTs/PDC/GCE (Yang et al., 2007)	1.38×10^{-12}
Multilayer gold nanoparticles (Tsai et al., 2005)	1×10^{-11}
Conducting polyaniline nanotube (Chang et al., 2007)	3.759×10^{-14}
CdS nanoparticles and polypyrrole (Peng et al., 2006)	1×10^{-9}

Table 4. The performance comparison of various fabricated DNA biosensors (Du et al., 2009).

7. Conclusion

Nanotechnology has been widely and successively applied in the field of sensing of drugs and biological molecules. The most important example of nanosensors are gold nanoparticles (GNPs) which offer many advantages, such as large surface-to-volume ratio, high surface reaction activity and strong adsorption ability to immobilize the desired biomolecules, good microenvironment for retaining the activity of enzyme, excellent catalytic effects on many important chemical reactions, their catalytic effect is highly size-dependent thus, the unique active sites and electronic states of GNPs can lead to their anomalous catalytic activity.

The biomaterials to be sensed include a large variety of materials such as:

1. Glucose and cholesterol which are largely attributed to the human health and the food industry.
2. Phenolic compounds whose identification and quantification are very important for environment monitoring.
3. Some carbamate and organophosphate pesticides which affect food, water and environment, and leads to a severe threat to human health.
4. H_2O_2 whose quantification is justified by the industrial, chemical and biomedical applications of this oxidant compound. In addition, H_2O_2 constitutes a relevant biochemical mediator in many cellular processes, as well as a by-product of several oxidases with analytical applications.
5. DNA and nucleic acids sequences detection which are directed to gene analysis, clinical disease diagnosis, or even forensic applications.

8. Copyright permissions

Final version after cut& edit	Licence no. according to "Copyright Clearance Center"
Fig1	(http://www.lsbu.ac.uk/biology/enztech/biosensors.html)
Table1	Not published
Fig2	Not published
Table2	2634100245226
Table3	2634101412860
Fig3	2633701365374
Fig4	2633701475869
Fig5	2634161086239
Fig6	2633710689524
Fig7	2633710837251
Fig8	2634150357126
Fig9	2633710969058
Fig10	2633711095490
Fig11	2633711408445
Fig12	2633720091311
Fig13	2633720380564
Table4	2634110691438

9. References

Alonso Lomillo, M.A.A.; Ruiz, J.G. & Pascual, F.J.M. (2005). Biosensor based on platinum chips for glucose determination. Analytical Chimica Acta, Vol.547, No.2, pp.209–214.

Anh, T.M.; Dzyadevych, S.V.; Soldatkin, A.P.; Chien, N.D.; Renault, N.J. & Chovelon, J.M. (2002). Development of tyrosinase biosensor based on pH-sensitive field-effect transistors for phenols determination in water solutions. Talanta, Vol.56, No.4, pp.627–634.

Atta, N.F. & Abdel-Mageed, A.M. (2009). Smart electrochemical sensor for some neurotransmitters using imprinted sol-gel films. Talanta, Vol.80, pp.511-518.

Atta, N.F. & El-Kady, M.F. (2009a). Poly(3-methylthiophene)/palladium sub-micro-modified sensor electrode. Part II: Voltammetric and EIS studies, and analysis of catecholamine neurotransmitters, ascorbic acid and acetaminophen. Talanta, Vol.79, pp.639-647.

Atta, N.F. & El-Kady, M.F. (2010a). Novel poly(3-methylthiophene)/Pd nanoparticles sensor: Synthesis, characterization and its application to the simultaneous analysis of dopamine and ascorbic acid in biological fluid. Sensors & Actuators B: Chemical, Vol.145, pp.299-310.

Atta, N.F.; Galal, A. & Ahmed, R.A. (2011a). Direct and simple electrochemical determination of morphine at PEDOT modified Pt electrode. Electroanalysis, Vol.23, pp,1-10.

Atta, N.F.; Galal, A. & Ahmed, R.A. (2011b). Poly(3,4-ethylene-dioxythiophene) electrode for the selective determination of dopamine in presence of sodium dodecyl sulfate. Bioelectrochemistry, Vol.80, pp.132-141.

Atta, N.F.; Galal, A. & El-Kady, M.F. (2009b). Palladium nanoclusters-coated poly(furan) as a novel sensor for catecholamine neurotransmitters and paracetamol. Sensors & Actuators B: Chemical, Vol.141, pp.566-574.

Atta, N.F.; Galal, A. & El-Kady, M.F. (2010b). Simultaneous determination of catecholamines, uric acid and ascorbic acid at physiological levels using poly(N-methylpyrrole)/Pd-nanoclusters sensor. Analytical Biochemistry, Vol.400, pp.78-88.

Atta, N.F.; Galal, A.; Abu-Attia, F.M. & Azab, S.M. (2010c). Carbon paste gold nanopatricles sensor for the selective determination of dopamine in buffered solutions. Journal of Electrochemical Society, Vol.157, pp.F116-F123.

Atta, N.F.; Galal, A.; Abu-Attia, F.M. & Azab, S.M. (2011c). Characterization and electrochemical investigations of micellar/drug interactions. Electrochimica Acta, Vol.56, pp.2510-2517.

Atta, N.F.; Hamed, M.M. & Abdel-Mageed, A.M. (2010d). Computational investigation and synthesis of a sol-gel imprinted materials for sensing application of some biologically active molecules. Analytical Chimica Acta, Vol.667, pp.63-70.

Bao, L.L.; Mahurin, S.M.; Haire, R.G. & Dai, S. (2003). Silver-Doped Sol−Gel Film as a Surface-Enhanced Raman Scattering Substrate for Detection of Uranyl and Neptunyl Ions. Analytical Chemistry, Vol.75, No.23, pp.6614–6620.

Barbadilloa, M.; Caseroa, E.; Petit-Domíngueza, M.D.; Vázquezb, L.; Parientea, F. & Lorenzoa, E. (2009). Gold nanoparticles-induced enhancement of the analytical response of an electrochemical biosensor based on an organic–inorganic hybrid composite material. Talanta, Vol.80, No.2, pp.797–802.

Basuray, S.; Senapati, S.; Aijian, A.; Mahon, A.R. & Chang, H. (2009). Shear and AC Field Enhanced Carbon Nanotube Impedance Assay for Rapid, Sensitive, and Mismatch-Discriminating DNA Hybridization. ACS Nano, Vol.3, pp.1823–1830.

Bersier, P.M.; Bersier, J. & Klingert, B. (1991). Electrochemistry of cyclodextrins and cyclodextrin inclusion complexes. Electroanalysis, Vol.3, No.6, pp.443-455.

Bongiovanni, C.; Ferri, T.; Poscia, A.; Varalli, M.; Santucci, R. & Desideri, A. (2001). An electrochemical multienzymatic biosensor for determination of cholesterol. Bioelectrochemistry, Vol.54, No.1, pp.17–22.

Brown, K.R.; Fox, A.P. & Natan, M.J. (1996). Stereoselective Total Synthesis of Natural (+)-Streptazolin via a Palladium-Catalyzed Enyne Bicyclization Approach. Journal of the American Chemical Society, Vol.118, No.5, pp.1154–1157.

Butler, J.M. (2006). Genetics and genomics of core short tandem repeat loci used in human identity testing. Journal of Forensic Science, Vol.51, pp.253–265.

Camacho, C.; Matas, J.C.; Garca, D.; Simpson, B.K. & Villalonga R. (2007). Amperometric enzyme biosensor for hydrogen peroxide via Ugi multicomponent reaction. Electrochemistry Communications, Vol.9, No.7, pp.1655–1660.

Campuzano, S.; Serra, B.; Pedrero, M.; Javier, Manuel de Villena, F. & Pingarron, J.M. (2003). Amperometric flow-injection determination of phenolic compounds at self-assembled monolayer-based tyrosinase biosensors. Analytical Chimica Acta , Vol.494, pp.187–197.

Carralero-Sanz, V.; Mena, M.L.; Gonzalez-Cortes, A.; Yanez-Sedeno, P. & Pingarron, J.M. (2006). Development of a high analytical performance-tyrosinase biosensor based on a composite graphite–Teflon electrode modified with gold nanoparticles. Biosensors and Bioelectronics, Vol.22, No.5, pp.730–736.

Carralero-Sanz, V.; Mena, M.L.; Gonzalez-Cortes, A.; Yanez-Sedeno, P. & Pingarron, J.M. (2005). Development of a tyrosinase biosensor based on gold nanoparticles-modified glassy carbon electrodes: Application to the measurement of a bioelectrochemical polyphenols index in wines. Analytical Chimica Acta, Vol.528, No.1, pp.1–8.

Cass A.E.G.; Davis G.; Francis G.D.; Hill H.A.O.; Aston W.J.; Higgins I.J.; Plotkin E.V.; Scott, L.D.L. & Turner, A.P.F. (1984). Ferrocene-mediated enzyme electrode for amperometric determination of glucose. Analytical Chemistry, Vol.56, No.4, pp.667-671.

Cederquist, K.B.; Golightly, R.S. & Keating, C.D. (2008). Molecular Beacon−Metal Nanowire Interface: Effect of Probe Sequence and Surface Coverage on Sensor Performance. Langmuir, Vol.24, No.16, pp.9162–9171.

Chang, H.X.; Yuan, Y.; Shi, N.L. & Guan, Y.F. (2007). Electrochemical DNA Biosensor Based on Conducting Polyaniline Nanotube Array. Analytical Chemistry, Vol.79, No.13, pp.5111–5115.

Chen, M. & Diao, G. (2009). Electrochemical study of mono-6-thio-β-cyclodextrin/ferrocene capped on gold nanoparticles: Characterization and application to the design of glucose amperometric biosensor. Talanta, Vol.80, No.2, pp.815–820.

Chen, X.; Jia, J. & Dong, S. (2003). Organically Modified Sol-Gel/Chitosan Composite Based Glucose Biosensor. Electroanalysis, Vol.15, No.7, pp.S608–612.

Chico, B.; Camacho, C.; Pérez, M.; Longo, M.A.; Sanromán, M.A.; Pingarrón, J.M. & Villalonga, R. (2009). Polyelectrostatic immobilization of gold nanoparticles-modified peroxidase on alginate-coated gold electrode for mediatorless biosensor construction. Journal of Electroanalytical Chemistry, Vol.629, No.1-2, pp.126–132.

Chriswell, C.D.; Chang, R.C. & Fritz, J.S. (1975). Chromatographic determination of phenols in water. Analytical Chemistry, Vol.47, No.8, pp.1325–1329.

Clark, L.C. & Lyons, C. (1962). Electrode systems for continuous monitoring in cardiovascular surgery. Annals of the New York Academy of Sciences, Vol.102, No. 1, pp. 29–45.

Cosnier, S.; Mousty, C.; de Melo, J.; Lepellec, A.; Novoa, A.; Polyak, B. & Marks, R.S. (2004). Organic Phase PPO Biosensors Prepared by Multilayer Deposition of Enzyme and Alginate Through Avidin-Biotin Interactions. Electroanalysis, Vol.16, No.24, pp.2022–2029.

Dai, X.; Nekrassova, O.; Hyde, M.E. & Compton, R.G. (2004). Anodic Stripping Voltammetry of Arsenic(III) Using Gold Nanoparticle-Modified Electrodes. Analytical Chemistry, Vol.76, No.19, pp.5924-5929.

Dempsey, E.; Diamond, D. & Collier, A. (2004). Development of a biosensor for endocrine disrupting compounds based on tyrosinase entrapped within a poly(thionine) film. Biosensors and Bioelectronics, Vol.20, No.2, pp.367– 377.

Di, J.; Shen, C.; Peng, S.; Tu, Y. & Li, S. (2005). A one-step method to construct a third-generation biosensor based on horseradish peroxidase and gold nanoparticles embedded in silica sol–gel network on gold modified electrode. Analytical Chimica Acta, Vol.553, No.1-2, pp.196–200.

Ding, C.F.; Zhao, F.; Zhang, M.L. & Zhang, S.S. (2008). Hybridization biosensor using 2,9-dimethyl-1,10-phenantroline cobalt as electrochemical indicator for detection of hepatitis B virus DNA. Bioelectrochemistry, Vol.72, No.1, pp.28–33.

Doron, A.; Katz, E. & Willner, I. (1995). Organization of Au-colloids as monolayer films onto ITO-glass surfaces: Application of the metal-colloid films as base interfaces to construct redox-active and photoactive self-assembled monolayers. Langmuir, Vol.11, pp.1313–1317.

Drummond, T.G.; Hill, M.G. & Barton, J.K. (2003). Electrochemical DNA sensors. Nature Biotechnology, Vol.21, pp.1192–1199.

Du, D.; Ding, J.; Cai, J. & Zhang, A. (2007a). One-step electrochemically deposited interface of chitosan-gold nanoparticles for acetylcholinesterase biosensor design. Journal of Electroanalytical Chemistry, Vol.605, No.1, pp.53–60.

Du, P.; Li, H.; Mei, Z. & Liu, S. (2009). Electrochemical DNA biosensor for the detection of DNA hybridization with the amplification of Au nanoparticles and CdS nanoparticles. Bioelectrochemistry, Vol.75, No.1, pp.37–43.

Du, Y.; Luo, X.; Xu, J. & Chen, H. (2007b). A simple method to fabricate a chitosan-gold nanoparticles film and its application in glucose biosensor. Bioelectrochemistry, Vol.70, No.2, pp.342–347.

Dua, D.; Ding, J.; Cai, J.; Zhang, J. & Liua, L. (2008). In situ electrodeposited nanoparticles for facilitating electron transfer across self-assembled monolayers in biosensor design. Talanta, Vol.74, No.5, pp.1337–1343.

Esumi, K.; Takei, N. & Yoshimura, T. (2003). Antioxidant-potentiality of gold–chitosan nanocomposites. Colloids and Surfaces B: Biointerfaces, Vol.32, No.2, pp.117–125.

Farace, G.; Lillie, G.; Hianik, T.; Payne, P. & Vadgama, P. (2002). Reagentless biosensing using electrochemical impedance spectroscopy. Bioelectrochemistry, Vol.55, No.1-2, pp.1–3.

Ferreira, S.M.; Lerner, S.F.; Brunzini, R.; Evelson, P.A. & Llesuy, S.F. (2004). Oxidative stress markers in aqueous humor of glaucoma patients. American Journal of Ophthalmology, Vol.137, No.1, pp.62–69.

Foulds, N.C. & Lowe, C.R. (1988). Immobilization of glucose oxidase in ferrocene-modified pyrrole polymers. Analytical Chemistry, Vol.60, No.22, pp.2473-2478.

Garca, A.; Peniche-Covas, C.; Chico, B.; Simpson, B.K. & Villalonga, R. (2007). Ferrocene Branched Chitosan for the Construction of a Reagentless Amperometric Hydrogen Peroxide Biosensor. Macromolecular Bioscience, Vol.7, No.4, pp.435–439.

Gerion, D.; Chen, F.; Kannan, B.; Fu, A.; Parak, W.J.; Chen, D.J.; Majumdar, A. & Alivisatos, A.P. (2003). Room-Temperature Single-Nucleotide Polymorphism and Multiallele DNA Detection Using Fluorescent Nanocrystals and Microarrays. Analytical Chemistry, Vol.75, No.18, pp.4766–4772.

Gomathia, P.; Ragupathy, D.; Choic, J.H.; Yeumc, J.H.; Leeb, S.C.; Kimb, J.C.; Leed, S.H. & Ghima, H.D. (2010). Fabrication of novel chitosan nanofiber/gold nanoparticles composite towards improved performance for a cholesterol sensor. Sensors and Actuators B: Chemical, In press.

Gomez, L.; Ramrez, H.L.; Villalonga, M.L.; Hernndez, J. & Villalonga, R. (2006). Immobilization of chitosan-modified invertase on alginate-coated chitin support via polyelectrolyte complex formation. Enzyme and Microbial Technology, Vol.38, No.1-2, pp.22–27.

Gopalana, A.I.; Leea, K.P. & Ragupathya, D. (2009). Development of a stable cholesterol biosensor based on multi-walled carbon nanotubes–gold nanoparticles composite covered with a layer of chitosan-room-temperature ionic liquid network. Biosensors and Bioelectronics, Vol.24, No.7, pp.2211-2217.

Gorton, L.; Karan, H.I.; Hale, P.D.; Inagaki, T.; Okamoto, Y. & Skotheim, T.A. (1990). A glucose electrode based on carbon paste chemically modified with a ferrocene-containing siloxane polymer and glucose oxidase, coated with a poly(ester-sulfonic acid) cation-exchanger. Analytical Chimica Acta, Vol.228, pp.23-30.

Gorton, L.; Lindgren, A.; Larsson, T.; Munteanu, F.D.; Ruzgas, T. & Gazaryan, I. (1999). Direct electron transfer between heme-containing enzymes and electrodes as basis for third generation biosensors. Analytical Chimica Acta , Vol.400, pp.91-108.

Gu, H.; Yu, A. & Chen, H. (2001). Direct electron transfer and characterization of hemoglobin immobilized on a Au colloid-cysteamine-modified gold electrode. Journal of Electroanalytical Chemistry, Vol.516, No.1-2, pp.119-126.

GuzmanVazquez de Prada, A.; Pena, N.; Mena, M.L.; Reviejo, A.J. & Pingarron, J.M. (2003). Graphite-Teflon composite bienzyme amperometric biosensors for monitoring of alcohols. Biosensors and Bioelectronics, Vol.18, No.10, pp.1279-1288.

He, L.; Musick, M.D.; Nicewarner, S.R.; Salinas, F.G.; Benkovic, S.J.; Natan, M.J. & Keating, C.D. (2000). Colloidal Au-Enhanced Surface Plasmon Resonance for Ultrasensitive Detection of DNA Hybridization. Journal of the American Chemical Society, Vol.122, No. 32, pp.9071-9077.

Hrapovic, S.; Liu, Y.; Male, K.B. & Luong J.H.T. (2004). Electrochemical Biosensing Platforms Using Platinum Nanoparticles and Carbon Nanotubes. Analytical Chemistry, Vol.76, No.4, pp.1083-1088.

Huang, H.; Yuan, Q. & Yang, X. (2004). Preparation and characterization of metal-chitosan nanocomposites. Colloids & Surfaces B: Biointerfaces, Vol.39, No.1-2, pp.31-37.

Huang, J.S.;Wang, D.W.; Hou, H.Q. & You, T.Y. (2008). Electrospun Palladium Nanoparticle-Loaded Carbon Nanofibers and Their Electrocatalytic Activities towards Hydrogen Peroxide and NADH. Advanced Functional Materials, Vol.18, No.3, pp.441-448.

Ionescu, R.E.; Abu-Rabeah, K.; Cosnier, S.; Durrieu, C.; Chovelon, J.M. & Marks, R.S. (2006). Amperometric Algal Chlorella vulgaris Cell Biosensors Based on Alginate and Polypyrrole-Alginate Gels. Electroanalysis, Vol.18, No.11, pp.1041-1046.

Jena, B.K. & Raj, C.R. (2007). Ultrasensitive nanostructured platform for the electrochemicalsensing of hydrazine. Journal of Physical Chemistry: C, Vol.111, pp.6228-6232.

Jeykumari, D.R.S. & Narayanan, S.S. (2008). Fabrication of bienzyme nanobiocomposite electrode using functionalized carbon nanotubes for biosensing applications. Biosensors and Bioelectronics, Vol.23, No.11, pp.1686-1693.

Jia, J.; Wang, B.; Wu, A.; Cheng, G.; Li, Z. & Dong, S. (2002). A Method to Construct a Third-Generation Horseradish Peroxidase Biosensor: Self-Assembling Gold Nanoparticles to Three-Dimensional Sol-Gel Network. Analytical Chemistry, Vol.74, No.9, pp. 2217-2223.

Jia, N.; Zhou, Q.; Liu, L.; Yan, M. & Jiang, Z. (2005). Direct electrochemistry and electrocatalysis of horseradish peroxidase immobilized in sol-gel-derived tin oxide/gelatin composite films. Journal of Electroanalytical Chemistry, Vol.580, No.2, pp.213-221.

Jönsson, G.; Gorton, L. & Pettersson, L. (1989). Mediated electron transfer from glucose oxidase at a ferrocene-modified graphite electrode. Electroanalysis, Vol.1, No.1, pp.49-54.

Kang, X.; Mai, Z.; Zou, X.; Cai P. & Mo, J. (2008). Glucose biosensors based on platinum nanoparticles-deposited carbon nanotubes in sol-gel chitosan/silica hybrid. Talanta, Vol.74, No.4, pp.879–886.

Kidambi, S.; Dai, J.H.; Li, J. & Bruening, L.M. (2004). Selective Hydrogenation by Pd Nanoparticles Embedded in Polyelectrolyte Multilayers. Journal of the American Chemical Society, Vol.126, No.9, pp.2658–2659.

Kjllman, T.H.M.; Peng, H.; Soeller, C. & Travas-Sejdic, J. (2008). Effect of Probe Density and Hybridization Temperature on the Response of an Electrochemical Hairpin-DNA Sensor. Analytical Chemistry, Vol.80, No.24, pp.9460–9466.

Kumar, A.; Pandey, R.R. & Brantley, B. (2006). Tetraethylorthosilicate film modified with protein to fabricate cholesterol biosensor. Talanta, Vol.69, No.3, pp.700–705.

Lao, R.J.; Song, S.P.; Wu, H.P.; Wang, L.H.; Zhang, Z.Z.; He, L. & Fan, C.H. (2005). Electrochemical Interrogation of DNA Monolayers on Gold Surfaces. Analytical Chemistry, Vol.77, No.19, pp.6475–6480.

Li, D.; Yan, Y.; Wieckowska, A. & Willner, I. (2007). Amplified electrochemical detection of DNA through the aggregation of Au nanoparticles on electrodes and the incorporation of methylene blue into the DNA-crosslinked structure. Chemical Communications, No.34, pp.3544–3546.

Li, F.; Fengb, Y.; Dongb, P.; Yangb, L. & Tang, B. (2011). Gold nanoparticles modified electrode via simple electrografting of in situ generated mercaptophenyl diazonium cations for development of DNA electrochemical biosensor. Biosensors and Bioelectronics, Vol.26, No.5, pp.1947–1952.

Li, W.; Yuan, R.; Chai, Y.; Zhou, L.; Chen, S. & Li, N. (2008). Immobilization of horseradish peroxidase on chitosan/silica sol–gel hybrid membranes for the preparation of hydrogen peroxide biosensor. Journal of Biochemical & Biophysical Methods, Vol.70, No.6, pp.830–837.

Liang, R.; Jiang, J. & Quiu, J. (2008). Preparation of GOD/Sol-Gel Silica Film on Prussian Blue Modified Electrode for Glucose Biosensor Application. Electroanalysis, Vol.20, No.24, pp.2642–2648.

Liu, G.; Wan, Y.; Gau, V.; Zhang, J.; Wang, L.; Song, S. & Fan, C. (2008). An Enzyme-Based E-DNA Sensor for Sequence-Specific Detection of Femtomolar DNA Targets. Journal of the American Chemical Society, Vol.130, No.21, pp.6820–6825.

Liu, H.Y.; Li, H.B.; Ying, T.L.; Sun, K.; Qin, Y.Q. & Qi, D.Y. (1998). Amperometric biosensor sensitive to glucose and lactose based on co-immobilization of ferrocene, glucose oxidase, β-galactosidase and mutarotase in β-cyclodextrin polymer. Analytical Chimica Acta , Vol.358, No.2, pp.137-144.

Liu, S. & Ju, H. (2002). Renewable reagentless hydrogen peroxide sensor based on direct electron transfer of horseradish peroxidase immobilized on colloidal gold-modified electrode. Analytical Biochemistry, Vol.307, No.1, pp.110–116.

Liu, S. & Ju, H. (2003). Reagentless glucose biosensor based on direct electron transfer of glucose oxidase immobilized on colloidal gold modified carbon paste electrode. Biosensors and Bioelectronics, Vol.19, No.3, pp.177–183.

Liu, S.; Leech, D. & Ju, H. (2003a). Application of Colloidal Gold in Protein Immobilization, Electron Transfer, and Biosensing. Analytical Letters, Vol.36, pp.1–19.

Liu, S.; Yu, J. & Ju, H. (2003b). Renewable phenol biosensor based on a tyrosinase-colloidal gold modified carbon paste electrode. Journal of Electroanalytical Chemistry, Vol.540, pp.61–67.

Liu, S.F.; Li, Y.F.; Li, J.R. & Jiang, L. (2005). Enhancement of DNA immobilization and hybridization on gold electrode modified by nanogold aggregates. Biosensors and Bioelectronics, Vol.21, No.5, pp.789–795.

Lowe, L.B.; Brewer, S.H.; Kramer, S.; Fuierer, R.R.; Qian, G.G.; Agbasi-Porter, C.O.; Moses, S.; Franzebm, S. & Feldheim, D.L. (2003). Laser-Induced Temperature Jump Electrochemistry on Gold Nanoparticle-Coated Electrodes. Journal of the American Chemical Society, Vol.125, No.47, pp.14258–14259.

Luo, X.; Killard, A.J.; Morrin, A. & Smyth, M.R. (2006). Enhancement of a conducting polymer-based biosensor using carbon nanotube-doped polyaniline. Analytical Chimica Acta, Vol.575, No.1, pp.39–44.

Luo, X.L.; Xu, J.J.; Zhang, Q.; Yang, G.J. & Chen, H.Y. (2005). Electrochemically deposited chitosan hydrogel for horseradish peroxidase immobilization through gold nanoparticles self-assembly. Biosensors and Bioelectronics, Vol.21, No.1, pp.190-196.

Ma, H.Y.; Zhang, L.P.; Pan, Y. & Zhang, K.Y. (2008). A Novel Electrochemical DNA Biosensor Fabricated with Layer-by-Layer Covalent Attachment of Multiwalled Carbon Nanotubes and Gold Nanoparticles. Electroanalysis, Vol.20, No.11, pp.1220–1226.

Ma, R.; Sasaki, T. & Bando, Y. (2004). Layer-by-Layer Assembled Multilayer Films of Titanate Nanotubes, Ag- or Au-Loaded Nanotubes, and Nanotubes/Nanosheets with Polycations. Journal of the American Chemical Society, Vol.126, No.33, pp.10382–10388.

Mala Ekanayake, E.M.I.; Preethichandra, D.M.G. & Kaneto, K. (2008). Bi-functional amperometric biosensor for low concentration hydrogen peroxide measurements using polypyrrole immobilizing matrix. Sensors and Actuators B: Chemical, Vol.132, No.1, pp.166–171.

Mena, M.L.; Yanez-Sedeno, P. & Pingarron, J.M. (2005). A comparison of different strategies for the construction of amperometric enzyme biosensors using gold nanoparticle-modified electrodes. Analytical Biochemistry, Vol.336, No.1, pp.20-27.

Moses, S.; Brewer, S.H.; Lowe, L.B.; Lappi, S.E.; Gilvey, L.B.G.; Sauthier, M.; Tenent, R.C.; Feldheim, D.L. & Franzen, S. (2004). Characterization of single- and double-stranded DNA on gold surfaces. Langmuir, Vol.20, pp.11134–11140.

Niu, S.Y.; Zhao, M.; Ren, R. & Zhang, S.S. (2011). Carbon nanotube-enhanced DNA biosensor for DNA hybridization detection using Manganese(II)-schiff base complex as hybridization indicator. Journal of Inorganic Biochemistry, In press.

Ostatná, V.; Dolinnaya, N.; Andreev, S.; Oretskaya, T.; Wang, J. & Hianik, T. (2005).The detection of DNA deamination by electrocatalysis at DNA-modified electrodes. Bioelectrochemistry, Vol. 67, No., pp.205–210.

Pandey, P.C.; Upadhyay, S.; Shukla, N.K. & Sharma, S. (2003). Studies on the electrochemical performance of glucose biosensor based on ferrocene encapsulated ORMOSIL and glucose oxidase modified graphite paste electrode. Biosensors and Bioelectronics, Vol.18, No.10, pp.1257–1268.

Pauliukaite, R.; Paquim, A.M.C.; Oliveira-Brett, A.M. & Brett, C.M.A. (2006). Electrochemical, EIS and AFM characterisation of biosensors: Trioxysilane sol–gel encapsulated glucose oxidase with two different redox mediators. Electrochimica Acta, Vol.52, No.1, pp.1–8.

Pena, N.; Ruiz, G.; Reviejo, A.J. & Pingarron, J.M. (2001). Graphite−Teflon Composite Bienzyme Electrodes for the Determination of Cholesterol in Reversed Micelles. Application to Food Samples. Analytical Chemistry, Vol.73, No.6, pp.1190–1195.

Peng, H.; Soeller, C.; Cannell, M.B.; Bowmaker, G.A.; Cooney, R.P. & Sejdic, J.T. (2006). Electrochemical detection of DNA hybridization amplified by nanoparticles. Biosensors and Bioelectronics, Vol.21, No.9, pp.1727–1736.

Pingarron, J.M.; Yoez-Sedeo, P. & Gonzlez-Cortés, A. (2008). Gold nanoparticle-based electrochemical biosensors. Electrochimica Acta, Vol.53, No.19, pp.5848–5866.

Poerschmann, J.; Zhang, Z.Y.; Kopinke, F.D. & Pawliszyn, J. (1997). Solid Phase Microextraction for Determining the Distribution of Chemicals in Aqueous Matrices. Analytical Chemistry, Vol.69, No.4, pp.597–600.

Qin, X.; Chun, M.; Ni-Na, L.; Jun-Jie, Z. & Jian, S. (2006). Immobilization of horseradish peroxidase on O-carboxymethylated chitosan/sol-gel matrix. Reactive & Functional Polymers, Vol.66, No.8, pp.863–870.

Rajesh; Takashima, W. & Kaneto K. (2004a). Amperometric phenol biosensor based on covalent immobilization of tyrosinase onto an electrochemically prepared novel copolymer poly (N-3-aminopropyl pyrrole-co-pyrrole) film. Sensors and Actuators B: Chemical, Vol.102, No.2, pp.271–277.

Rajesh; Takashima, W. & Kaneto, K. (2004). Amperometric tyrosinase based biosensor using an electropolymerized PTS-doped polypyrrole film as an entrapment support. Reactive & Functional Polymers, Vol.59, pp.163– 169.

Reisberga, S.; Piroa, B.; Noela, V. & Pham, M.C. (2006). Selectivity and sensitivity of a reagentless electrochemical DNA sensor studied by square wave voltammetry and fluorescence. Bioelectrochemistry, Vol.69, No.2, pp.172–179.

Ren, X.; Meng, X. & Tang, F. (2005). Preparation of Ag–Au nanoparticle and its application to glucose biosensor. Sensors and Actuators B: Chemical, Vol.110, No.2, pp.358-363.

Rosi, N.L. & Mirkin, C.A. (2005). Nanostructures in biodiagnostics. Chemical Reviews, Vol.105, pp.1547–1562.

Safavi, A.; Maleki, N. & Farjami, E. (2009). Electrodeposited Silver Nanoparticles on Carbon Ionic Liquid Electrode for Electrocatalytic Sensing of Hydrogen Peroxide. Electroanalalysis, Vol.21, No.13, pp.1533–1538.

Safavia, A. & Farjamia, F. (2011). Electrodeposition of gold–platinum alloy nanoparticles on ionic liquid–chitosan composite film and its application in fabricating an amperometric cholesterol biosensor. Biosensors and Bioelectronics, Vol.26, No.5, pp.2547–2552.

Salimi, A.; Compton, R.G. & Hallaj, R. (2004). Glucose biosensor prepared by glucose oxidase encapsulated sol-gel and carbon-nanotube-modified basal plane pyrolytic graphite electrode. Analytical Biochemistry, Vol.333, No.1, pp.49–56.

Santos, D.S.; Goulet, P.J.G.; Pieczonka, N.P.W.; Oliveira, O.N. & Aroca, R.F. (2004). Gold nanoparticle embedded, self-sustained chitosan films as substrates for surface-enhanced raman scattering. Langmuir, Vol.20, pp.10273–10277.

Schumb, W.C.; Satterfield, C.N. & Wentworth, R.L. (1995). Hydrogen Peroxide, Reinhold, New York.

Serra, B.; Jimenez, S.; Mena, M.L.; Reviejo, A.J. & Pingarron, J.M. (2002). Composite electrochemical biosensors: a comparison of three different electrode matrices for the construction of amperometric tyrosinase biosensors. Biosensors and Bioelectronics, Vol.17, No.3, pp.217–226.

Service, R.F. (1998). Coming soon: the pocket DNA sequencer. Science, Vol.282, pp.399–401.

Shen, J. & Liu, C.C. (2007). Development of a screen-printed cholesterol biosensor: Comparing the performance of gold and platinum as the working electrode material and fabrication using a self-assembly approach. Sensors and Actuators B: Chemical, Vol.120, No. 2, pp.417–425.

Shipway, A.N.; Lahav, M. & Willner, I. (2000). Nanostructured Gold Colloid Electrodes. Advanced Materials, Vol.12, No.13, pp.993–998.

Singh, S.; Singhal, R. & Malhotra, B.D. (2007). Immobilization of cholesterol esterase and cholesterol oxidase onto sol-gel films for application to cholesterol biosensor. Analytical Chimica Acta , Vol.582, No.2, pp.335–343.

Song, W.; Li, D.; Li, Y. & Long, Y. (2010). Disposable biosensor based on graphene oxide conjugated with tyrosinase assembled gold nanoparticles. Biosensors and Bioelectronics, Vol.26, No. 7, pp. 3181-3186.

Song, Y.; Wang, L.; Ren, C.; Zhu, G. & Li, Z. (2006). A novel hydrogen peroxide sensor based on horseradish peroxidase immobilized in DNA films on a gold electrode. Sensors and Actuators B: Chemical, Vol.114, No.2, pp.1001-1006.

Staudt, L.M. (2001). Gene expression physiology and pathophysiology of the immune system. Trends in Immunology, Vol.22, pp.35–40.

Tan, X.; Tian, Y.; Cai, P. & Zou, X. (2005). Glucose biosensor based on glucose oxidase immobilized in sol-gel chitosan/silica hybrid composite film on Prussian blue modified glass carbon electrode. Analytical and Bioanalytical Chemistry, Vol.381, No.2, pp.500–507.

Tang, F.Q. & Jiang, L. (1998). Enhancement of Glucose Biosensor Response Ability by Addition of Hydrophobic Gold Nanoparticles. Annals of the New York Academy of Sciences, Vol.864, pp.538–543.

Tangkuaram, T.; Ponchio, C.; Kangkasomboon, T.; Katikawong, P. & Veerasai, W. (2007). Design and development of a highly stable hydrogen peroxide biosensor on screen printed carbon electrode based on horseradish peroxidase bound with gold nanoparticles in the matrix of chitosan. Biosensors and Bioelectronics, Vol.22, No.9-10, pp. 2071–2078.

Tatsuma, T. & Sato, T. (2004). Self-wiring from tyrosinase to an electrode with redox polymers. Journal of Electroanalytical Chemistry, Vol.572, No.1, pp.15–19.

Tiwari, A.; Aryal, S.; Pilla, S. & Gong, S. (2009). An amperometric urea biosensor based on covalently immobilized urease on an electrode made of hyperbranched polyester functionalized gold nanoparticles. Talanta, Vol.78, No.4-5, pp.1401-1407.

Tsai, C.Y.; Punl, C.C.; Chan, B.; Luh, T.Y.; Ko, F.H.; Chen, P.J. & Chen, P.H. (2005). Electrical detection of DNA hybridization with multilayer gold nanoparticles between nanogap electrodes. Microsystem Technologies, Vol.11, pp.1432–1858.

Tsai, Y.; Chen, S. & Lee, C. (2008). Amperometric cholesterol biosensors based on carbon nanotube-chitosan-platinum-cholesterol oxidase nanobiocomposite. Sensors and Actuators B: Chemical, Vol.135, No.1, pp.96–101.

Villalonga, R.; Cao, R. & Fragoso, A. (2007). Supramolecular Chemistry of Cyclodextrins in Enzyme Technology. Chemical Reviews, Vol.107, No.7, pp.3088–3116.

Walcarius, A. (2001). Electroanalysis with Pure, Chemically Modified and Sol-Gel-Derived Silica-Based Materials. Electroanalysis, Vol.13, No.8–9, pp.701-718.

Wang, B. & Dong, S. (2000). Sol–gel-derived amperometric biosensor for hydrogen peroxide based on methylene green incorporated in Nafion film. Talanta, Vol.51, No.3, pp.565–572.

Wang, B.; Li, B.; Deng, Q. & Dong, S. (1998). Amperometric Glucose Biosensor Based on Sol−Gel Organic−Inorganic Hybrid Material. Analytical Chemistry, Vol.70, No.15, pp. 3170–3174.

Wang, B.; Zhang, J. & Dong, S. (2000a). Silica sol-gel composite film as an encapsulation matrix for the construction of an amperometric tyrosinase-based biosensor. Biosensors and Bioelectronics, Vol.15, No.7-8, pp.397- 402.

Wang, G.; Xu, J.J.; Ye, L.H.; Zhu, J.J. & Chen, H.Y. (2002). Highly sensitive sensors based on the immobilization of tyrosinase in chitosan. Bioelectrochemistry, Vol.57, No.1, pp. 33–38.

Wanga, H.; Wanga, X.; Zhangb, X.; Qina, X.; Zhaoa, Z.; Miaoa, Z.; Huanga, N. & Chena, Q. (2009). A novel glucose biosensor based on the immobilization of glucose oxidase onto gold nanoparticles-modified Pb nanowires. Biosensors and Bioelectronics, Vol.25, No.1, pp.142–146.

Wu, B.Y.; Hou, S.H.; Yin, F.; Zhao, Z.X.;Wang, Y.Y.;Wang, X.S. & Chen, Q. (2007). Amperometric glucose biosensor based on multilayer films via layer-by-layer self-assembly of multi-wall carbon nanotubes, gold nanoparticles and glucose oxidase on the Pt electrode. Biosensors and Bioelectronics, Vol.22, No.12, pp.2854–2860.

Xiao, F.; Zhao, F.; Zhang, Y.; Guo, G. & Zeng, B. (2009). Ultrasonic Electrodeposition of Gold−Platinum Alloy Nanoparticles on Ionic Liquid−Chitosan Composite Film and Their Application in Fabricating Nonenzyme Hydrogen Peroxide Sensors. Journal of Physical Chemistry: C, Vol.113, No.3, pp.849–855.

Xiao, Y.; Ju, H. & Chen, H. (2000). Direct Electrochemistry of Horseradish Peroxidase Immobilized on a Colloid/Cysteamine-Modified Gold Electrode. Analytical Biochemistry, Vol.278, No.1, pp.22–28.

Xiao, Y.; Ju, H.X. & Chen, H.Y. (1999). Hydrogen peroxide sensor based on horseradish peroxidase-labeled Au colloids immobilized on gold electrode surface by cysteamine monolayer. Analytical Chimica Acta, Vol.391, No.1, pp.73-82.

Xiao, Y.; Patolsky, F.; Katz, E.; Hainfeld, J.F. & Willner, I. (2003). Plugging into Enzymes": Nanowiring of Redox Enzymes by a Gold Nanoparticle.Science, Vol.299, pp.1877–1881.

Xu, S. & Han, X. (2004). A novel method to construct a third-generation biosensor: self-assembling gold nanoparticles on thiol-functionalized poly(styrene-co-acrylic acid) nanospheres. Biosensors and Bioelectronics, Vol.19, No.9, pp.1117–1120.

Xue H. & Shen, Z. (2002). A highly stable biosensor for phenols prepared by immobilizing polyphenol oxidase into polyaniline–polyacrylonitrile composite matrix. Talanta, Vol.57, No.2, pp.289–295.

Yamada, M.; Tadera, T.; Kubo, K. & Nishihara, H. (2003). Electrochemical deposition ofbiferrocene derivative-attached gold nanoparticles and the morphology of theformed film. Journal of Physical Chemistry: B, Vol.107, pp.3703–3711.

Yanez-Sedeno, P. & Pingarron, J.M. (2005). Gold nanoparticle-based electrochemical biosensors. Analytical and Bioanalytical Chemistry, Vol.382, No.4, pp.884–886.

Yang, J.; Jiao, K. & Yang, T. (2007). A DNA electrochemical sensor prepared by electrodepositing zirconia on composite films of single-walled carbon nanotubes and poly(2,6- pyridinedicarboxylic acid), and its application to detection of the PAT gene fragment. Analytical & Bioanalytical Chemistry, Vol.389, pp.913–921.

Yang, M.; Yang, Y.; Liu, Y.; Shen, G. & Yu, R. (2006). Platinum nanoparticles-doped sol-gel/carbon nanotubes composite electrochemical sensors and biosensors. Biosensors and Bioelectronics, Vol.21, No. 7, pp.1125–1131.

Yang, Y.; Wang, Z.; Yang, M.; Guoa, M.; Wu, Z.; Shen, G. & Yu, R. (2006a). Inhibitive determination of mercury ion using a renewable urea biosensor based on self-assembled gold nanoparticles. Sensors and Actuators B: Chemical, Vol.114, No.1, pp.1–8.

Yin, H.; Ai, S.; Xu, J.; Shi, W. & Zhu, L. (2009). Amperometric biosensor based on immobilized acetylcholinesterase on gold nanoparticles and silk fibroin modified platinum electrode for detection of methyl paraoxon, carbofuran and phoxim. Journal of Electroanalytical Chemistry, Vol.637, pp.21-27.

Yina, H.; Aia, S; Shia, W. & Zhub, L. (2009). A novel hydrogen peroxide biosensor based on horseradish peroxidase immobilized on gold nanoparticles-silk fibroin modified glassy carbon electrode and direct electrochemistry of horseradish peroxidase. Sensors and Actuators B: Chemical, Vol.137, No.2, pp.747-753.

Yu, J.; Liu, S. & Ju, H. (2003). Mediator-free phenol sensor based on titania sol-gel encapsulation matrix for immobilization of tyrosinase by a vapor deposition method. Biosensors and Bioelectronics, Vol.19, No.5, pp.509-514.

Zhang, G.R.; Wang, X.L.; Shi, X.W. & Sun, T.L. (2000). β-Cyclodextrin-ferrocene inclusion complex modified carbon paste electrode for amperometric determination of ascorbic acid. Talanta, Vol.51, No.5, pp.1019-1025.

Zhang, T.; Tian, B.; Kong, J.; Yang, P. & Liu, B. (2003). A sensitive mediatorfree tyrosinase biosensor based on an inorganic-organic hybrid titania sol-gel matrix. Analytical Chimica Acta , Vol.489, pp.199-206.

Zhao, L.; Siu, A.C.L.; Petrus, J.A.; He, Z. & Leung, K.T. (2007). Interfacial Bonding of Gold Nanoparticles on a H-terminated Si(100) Substrate Obtained by Electro- and Electroless Deposition. Journal of the American Chemical Society, Vol.129, No.17, pp.5730-5734.

Zhaoyang, W.; Liguo, C.; Guoli, S. & Ruqin, Y. (2006). Platinum nanoparticle-modified carbon fiber ultramicroelectrodes for mediator-free biosensing. Sensors and Actuators B: Chemical, Vol.119, No.1, pp.295-301.

Zhenga, B.; Xieb, S.; Qiana, L.; Yuanc, H.; Xiaoa, D. & Choib, M. (2010). Gold nanoparticles-coated egg shell membrane with immobilized glucose oxidase for fabrication of glucose biosensor. Sensors and Actuators B: Chemical, Vol.152, No.1, pp. 49-55.

Zhu, N.N.; Chang, Z.; Heb, P.G. & Fang, Y.Z. (2005). Electrochemical DNA biosensors based on platinum nanoparticles combined carbon nanotubes. Analytical Chimica Acta, Vol.545, pp.21-26.

Zou, Y.J.; Xiang, C.L.; Sun, L.X. & Xu, F. (2008). Glucose biosensor based on electrodeposition of platinum nanoparticles onto carbon nanotubes and immobilizing enzyme with chitosan-SiO_2 sol-gel. Biosensors and Bioelectronics, Vol.23, No.7, pp.1010-1016.

Zuo, S.; Teng, Y.; Yuan, H. & Lan, M. (2008). Direct electrochemistry of glucose oxidase on screen-printed electrodes through one-step enzyme immobilization process with silica sol-gel/polyvinyl alcohol hybrid film. Sensors and Actuators B: Chemical, Vol.133, No. 2, pp.555-560.

5

Evolution Towards the Implementation of Point-Of-Care Biosensors

Veronique Vermeeren and Luc Michiels
Hasselt University
Belgium

1. Introduction

Health care, food quality control, and environmental management often rely on the detection of abnormal molecules, in the body, in food, and in the environment, respectively. More and more, these fields are moving towards point-of-care detection, since increased analysis speed, and hence, decreased cost, are becoming important determining factors for funding.

In parallel, but also to allow for this speedy and on-site analysis, the scientific world has evolved into the 'nano'-scale. This was made possible by the dawn of bio-electronics: a scientific field coupling the achievements in molecular biology with the advances in electronics. The goal of this field is to interrogate the functional activity of bioreceptor molecules, i.e. the recognition and/or metabolization of their targets, with electronics to increase the detection speed for, and sensitivity to, certain pathogens, pollutants, and genetic mutations.

To enable the electronic interrogation of these bioreceptor molecules, they need to be attached to, or embedded into, a solid support or transducer with a favourable orientation and density, ensuring the retention of their biological functionality. The resulting analytical device is called a biosensor. The transducer 'translates' the biological recognition event between the receptor molecule and its target into a readable signal.

Many biosensors have become established in the clinical and scientific world. However, still few of them have made it to point-of-care applications. The success and applicability of biosensors as point-of-care tools is based on five requirements. They need to be sensitive, specific, fast, cheap, and portable. Electronic biosensors based on (semi-)conductive transducers are hence preferred for point-of-care applications, since they are fast in signal generation and cheap to produce.

Many popular semiconductive transduction materials, such as silicon (Si) and germanium (Ge), however, are susceptible to hydrolysis, leading to a loss of bioreceptor molecules from the surface, and hence, to instability of the sensor platform. This negatively influences the sensitivity and specificity of the sensor. This explains our increased attention towards diamond, which surpasses Si and Ge on many levels. It can be made into a semiconductor, preferred for electronic applications, it is chemically and mechanically very stable, it can be functionalized with bioreceptor molecules (DNA, aptamers, antibodies, whole cells), and it is biocompatible since it is only composed of carbon (C).

For this reason, this contribution will focus on the application of diamond in the construction of different types of electronic biosensors to be used in clinical diagnostics, food industry and environmental management.

2. Biosensor types and their application areas

2.1 DNA-sensor

A DNA-sensor is constructed by immobilizing a single-stranded DNA (ssDNA) molecule with a sequence corresponding to (a part of) the gene of interest to a solid substrate. Hybridization with a perfectly complementary sequence present in the sample will lead to a specific signal.

2.1.1 Clinical diagnostics

The DNA contains the blueprint of the human body. The genes that encode our proteins make up our phenotype. However, when mutations occur in these genes, this could lead to the formation of aberrant or non-functional proteins, infringing on the normal function of the human body. Diseases, such as cancer, sickle cell anemia, Charcot Marie Tooth's disease, Duchenne's muscular dystrophy, and many more, are caused by such DNA mutations. Detection of these mutations in the DNA is therefore paramount for the correct diagnosis and therapeutic intervention.

A well-known application of a DNA-sensor principle is the microarray. In oligonucleotide microarrays, short genomic ssDNA fragments are spotted on the microarray, and all of the sequences on the array can cover an entire genome. Oligonucleotide microarrays are therefore mainly used for extensive genetic profiling and mutational analysis. The arrays are hybridized with fluorescently labeled genomic DNA and evaluated with a fluorescence microscope equipped with a CCD camera. These microarrays yield absolute values of the presence or absence of each particular gene sequence on the array and therefore, the comparison of two conditions, such as a healthy control and a cancerous patient, requires the use of two separate microarrays for the parallel genotyping or mutation analysis of multiple genes.

In cDNA microarrays, entire cDNA molecules are spotted on the microarray, and all of the sequences can cover the expressional activity of a certain cell or tissue type. cDNA microarrays are therefore mainly used for gene expression analysis. To compare two conditions, such as the gene expression level in a certain tissue of a healthy control and gene expression level in a certain tissue of a cancerous patient, mRNA is isolated from the tissue of the healthy control and from the tissue of the cancerous patient. Both mRNA sources are labeled with a different fluorescent dye, and the array is hybridized with a mixture of both mRNA sources. The fluorescence is again evaluated with a fluorescence microscope. These microarrays compare the expression level of the two conditions for each particular gene on the array. Hence, one microarray can be used for the expression analysis of two conditions.

However, the requirement of target labeling, and the associated need for very expensive complex optics for detection, make microarrays an extremely costly investment. For this reason, focus has shifted towards electronic, label-free DNA-sensors. DNA-based biosensors have been reported that exploit the intrinsic electro-activity of the bases guanine (G) and adenine (A). Probe ssDNA is attached to the electrode surface, and the G and/or A residues in the DNA participate in a redox reaction. The current that is generated during this redox reaction is detected, and it is proportional to the amount of G and/or A, being larger in double-stranded DNA (dsDNA). However, usually, direct detection of the G and/or A bases without the use of redox mediators is generally considered to be too insensitive. Cai et al. (2004) immobilized ssDNA onto Si electrodes, and demonstrated that they were able to distinguish complementary DNA from DNA containing 4-base mismatches as compared to the immobilized probe DNA (Cai et al., 2004). Gu et al. (2005) and Vermeeren et al. (2007) even succeeded in single-nucleotide polymorphism (SNP) sensitivity, the latter in real-time (Gu et al., 2005), (Vermeeren et al., 2007).

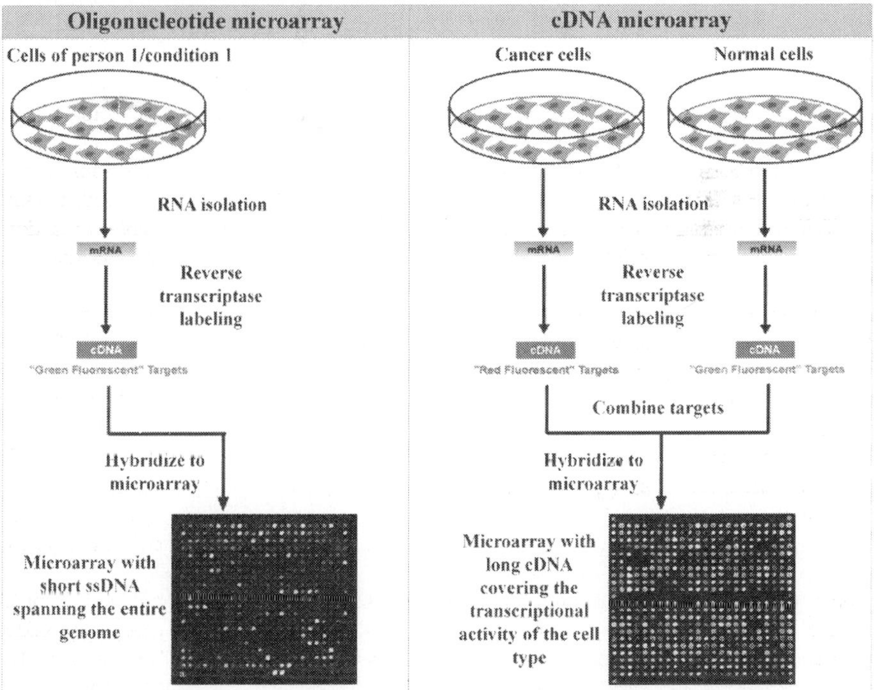

Fig. 1. Schematic diagram of an oligonucleotide microarray (left panel) and a cDNA microarray (right panel). An oligonucleotide microarray, modified with short oligonucleotide sequences covering the entire genome, gives information about the presence and absence of certain gene fragments. Each microarray is hybridized with target material of 1 condition. A cDNA microarray, modified with longer cDNA sequences covering the expressional activity of a cell type, are used for gene expression analysis. Each microarray is hybridized with target material of 2 conditions.

2.1.2 Food industry

The use of genetically modified strains of crops is becoming more and more widespread. Informing the consumers is of utmost importance. Moreover, the presence of contaminating microbial life in food and is a major health care concern. Therefore, biosensor research has focused on the detection of genetically modified organisms (GMOs) and viral and the presence of viral or bacterial DNA in food.

Tichoniuk et al. (2008) developed an electrochemical DNA-sensor that was capable of distinguishing between genetically modified and unmodified soybeans without DNA amplification. Gold (Au) electrodes were modified with ssDNA corresponding to genetically modified soybeans. Methylene blue was used as a hybridization indicator, interacting more readily with G in ssDNA than in dsDNA. Hybridization with modified soybeans was reflected by a decrease in the voltammetric peak of methylene blue, while treatment with unmodified soybeans had no effect in the peak (Tichoniuk et al., 2008). Joon-Hyung et al. (2008) constructed a label-free electrochemical DNA-sensor against Salmonella. Salmonella species are classified as bioterrorism threat agents by the Center for Disease Control and prevention (CDC). DNA from Salmonella Enterica Serovar Enteritidis was amplified by Polymerase Chain Reaction (PCR) and exposed to a nanoporous Si substrate modified with Salmonella-specific 26-mer probe ssDNA (Joon-Hyung et al., 2008).

2.1.3 Environmental management

DNA-sensors are also starting to be used to screen various environmental matrices, such as water, soil, and plant samples, for the presence of infectious agents and analytes that have binding affinities for the structure of DNA, and thus induce DNA damage.

Marrazza et al. (1999) developed two disposable electrochemical DNA-sensors, one based on DNA hybridization to detect the presence of the bacteria *Chlamydia trachomatis*, and one based on the interaction of small molecules with the DNA. For the first sensor, 21-mer ssDNA probes specific for *Chlamydia* were immobilized onto a graphite screen-printed electrode. Potentiometric Stripping Analysis (PSA) was used to detect the hybridization to complementary target DNA. The increasing oxidation peak area of daunomycin, an intercalator of dsDNA, was used as an indicator for the hybridization, and thus for the presence of *Chlamydia* in the sample. However, the sensitivity of the assay was insufficient to allow a direct detection without PCR amplification of the sample. Their second sensor was constructed by immobilizing calf thymus ssDNA onto a graphite screen-printed electrode. The decreasing oxidation peak of G was used as an indicator for the interaction between ssDNA and cisplatin and polychlorobiphenyls (PCBs). They even tested real river water samples, and succeeded in the rough categorization into toxic and non-toxic water samples. However, they were not able to distinguish between the different compounds that were present (Marrazza et al., 1999).

2.2 Immunosensor

An immunosensor is constructed by immobilizing an antibody directed against the protein target of interest to a solid support. Recognition of its target antigen will lead to a specific signal.

2.2.1 Clinical diagnostics

Since many diseases have their origin in the presence of DNA mutations in crucial genes, as explained above, these diseases are also often characterized by the presence of abnormal proteins in the body. Diagnosis is based on the detection and quantification of these proteins by using antibodies directed against the protein of interest. The state-of-the-art is the Enzyme-Linked ImmunoSorbent Assay (ELISA). There are three types of ELISA.

In a sandwich ELISA, the ELISA plate is coated with target-specific antibodies. In a next step, the sample is added, and the antigens, if present, will bind to the coated antibodies. In a third step, detection antibodies, labeled with an enzyme, will bind to a different epitope of the bound antigens. Lastly, the substrate of the enzyme label is added, which is metabolized into a colored product of which the absorption is measured. The absorption is then directly proportional to the amount of bound target.

In an indirect ELISA, the sample containing or not containing the target of interest is coated onto the ELISA plate. In the next steps, the enzymatically labeled detection antibodies and the substrate are added like in the sandwich ELISA, and the absorption is again a measure for the bound targets.

In a competitive ELISA, the enzymatically labeled detection antibodies are first pre-incubated with the target antigens. Only the detection antibodies that are still free after this pre-incubation step will be available to bind to target antigens that are coated onto the ELISA plate. Here, the absorption of the enzymatically generated product is indirectly proportional to the amount of target antigen in the sample.

Many ELISA kits exist for all sorts of applications. However, the technique requires many reaction steps, which increases the analysis time and cost. For this reason, focus has shifted towards electronic, label-free immunosensors. Fang et al. (2010) described the development of a novel immunosensor based on a sol-gel derived Barium Strontium Titanate (BST) thin film and interdigitated electrodes for the diagnosis of Dengue infection. The Dengue virus particles were immobilized onto the electrodes, to capture the Dengue antibodies present in human serum. With impedance spectroscopy and I-V measurements, it was possible to detect Dengue antibodies in human serum even after a 50 000-fold dilution. Since Dengue infection is also diagnosed using the salivary antibodies, of which the concentration is relatively close to the concentration in serum, the sensor could possibly be employed in an easy, rapid point-of-care setting (Fang et al., 2010). Pan et al. (2010) developed an amperometric immunosensor for the diagnosis of Urinary Tract Infection (UTI), using lactoferrin (LTF) as a biomarker for UTI. They immobilized biotinylated anti-LTF onto Au electrodes functionalized with self-assembled monolayers (SAMs) coupled with biotin and strepatvidin. Detection was based on a horse-radish peroxidise (HRP)-conjugated anti-LTF antibody and the HRP substrate. The current generated by the enzymatic reaction was transferred to the electrodes through the use of the redox mediator potassium ferricyanide ($K_3Fe(CN)_6$). They reached a detection limit of 145 pg/ml (Pan et al., 2010).

2.2.2 Food industry

Electrochemical immunosensors can also be applied in food analysis, for quality control. For example, Chemburu et al. (2005) developed a flow-through amperometric immunosensor to detect the presence of *E. coli*, *L. monocytogenes*, and *C. jejuni*. They immobilized antigen-specific antibodies onto carbon particles, and obtained detection limits of 50, 10, and 50 colony-forming units (CFU)/ml, respectively. They then applied this to milk and chicken extract, and observed a *L. monocytogenes* detection limit of 30 CFU/ml in chicken extract (Chemburu et al., 2005). Micheli et al. (2004) constructed an electrochemical immunosensor against domoic acid. Domoic acid is a neuroexcitatory toxin from marine diatoms, found in sea products. It is the causative agent of amnesic shellfish poisoning (ASP). Using screen-printed electrodes, the authors claim a detection limit of domoic acid of 20 μg/g in mussels, which is the maximum acceptable limit defined by the Food and Drug Administration (FDA) (Micheli et al., 2004).

2.2.3 Environmental management

Pesticides are widely used in agriculture to protect crops. However, their use has also created serious concerns regarding their effects on the environment. Hence, identification and quantification of pesticides is of utmost importance. Skládal and Kaláb (1995) developed a multichannel amperometric immunosensor for the detection of 2,4-dichlorophenoxyacetic acid (2,4-D). They used a competitive format. 2,4-D molecules conjugated with HRP competed with free 2,4-D for the anti-2,4-D antibodies immobilized onto the nitrocellulose-covered Au electrode. The substrate hydrogen peroxide (H_2O_2) and hydroquinone participated in the redox reaction catalyzed by HRP, and the generated current was detected amperometrically. They achieved a detection limit of 0.1 ng/ml in water (Skládal et al., 1995). Grennan et al. (2003) described an amperometric immunosensor for the analysis of the herbicide atrazine. The European Union Drinking Water Directive set official regulations on the maximum admissible concentration of atrazine in drinking water, namely 0.1 ng/ml. Single-chain antibodies against atrazine were immobilized in a polyaniline (PANI)/polyvinyl sulfonate (PVS) polymer layer on top of a carbon paste screen-printed electrode. Again, competition between HRP-labeled atrazine and native atrazine ensued, and the subsequent substrate reaction with H_2O_2 gave a detection limit of 0.1 ng/ml (Grennan et al., 2003).

2.3 Aptasensor

A recent new development in affinity sensing comes from aptamer molecules. Aptamers are short, synthetic ssDNA or ssRNA oligomers that obtain a specific and complex 3D structure. For this reason, they are able to bind to and recognize a certain target molecule (proteins, organic molecules, cells, …) with a high specificity. Because of their ease in selection and synthesis, and hence, their cheaper production cost, and their chemical stability in a variety of conditions, they display a great advantage compared to antibodies. For this reason, like antibodies, aptamers are becoming more and more valuable as receptor molecules in biosensors.

2.3.1 Clinical diagnostics

Yuan et al. (2010) developed a label-free electrochemical aptasensor for the detection of thrombin. Thrombin is a blood-clotting protein, and a high level of thrombin will cause thrombosis, while a low level will induce excessive bleeding. Nafion-coated Au electrodes were modified with alternating layers of the redox mediator thionine and Au nanoparticles. Thiol (SH)-modified thrombin aptamers were then immobilized onto the Au nanoparticles. The redox peak of thionine was monitored in the presence of $K_3[Fe(CN)_6]/K_4[Fe(CN)_6]$. Binding with thrombin resulted in a barrier for the electron transfer to the electrode coming from the redox reaction of thionine, leading to a decrease in current and in the thionine redox peak. When exposing the sensor to human serum samples, they obtained good recovery values with thrombin concentrations between 1 and 40 nM (Yuan et al., 2010).

2.3.2 Food industry

Bonel et al. (2010) reported an electrochemical aptasensor for the detection of ochratoxin A (OTA). OTA is one of the most important mycotoxin contaminants of food, particularly cereal grains, such as wheat and their derived products. The presence of OTA in these foods is a matter of great concern, as it is responsible for chronic diseases in humans and animals.

Biotinylated OTA aptamers were immobilized onto streptavidin-coated paramagnetic beads. Free OTA was allowed to compete with OTA-HRP conjugates for the aptamer-functionalized beads, and after the magnetic separation, the reacted beads were transferred to screen-printed carbon electrodes. H_2O_2 and hydroquinone participated in a redox reaction catalyzed by HRP, and the current was detected amperometrically. They reached a detection limit of 0.07 ng/ml, and the sensor was accurately applied to certified wheat samples (Bonel et al., 2010).

2.3.3 Environmental management

Olowu et al. (2010) developed an electrochemical aptasensor for the detection of 17β-estradiol. 17β-estradiol is an endocrine disrupting chemical (EDC), and thus interferes with the function of the endocrine system. EDCs are ubiquitous in the environment because of their widespread use in residential, industrial, and agricultural applications. Au electrodes were modified with poly(3,4-ethylenedioxythiopene) (PEDOT), onto which a layer of streptavidin was immobilized through Au nanoparticles and the linker 3,3′-dithiodipropionic acid (DPA). The biotinylated 17β-estradiol aptamers were bound to this streptavidin layer. The electrochemical signal was a decrease in current between the redox mediator $[Fe(CN)_6]^{-3/-4}$ and the PEDOT due to the interference of the bound 17β-estradiol with the electron transfer. The aptasensor was found to be sensitive at concentrations as low as 0.02 nM (Olowu et al., 2010).

2.4 Whole-cell biosensor

Whole-cell sensors provide some major advantages compared to other sensor types. Cells are able to detect effects of (complex) samples on living organisms. On the other hand, cells can also react to very low concentrations of certain molecules, making them more sensitive than other sensors using affinity molecules. The most popular format of whole-cell sensors involves the use of a reporter gene fused to a promoter that is influenced by the binding of a target analyte. Binding of the analyte to a cell receptor will set in motion a cascade of intracellular events, leading to the binding of a transcription factor to the promoter, which now controls the transcription of the reporter gene. This reporter gene usually codes for a fluorescent molecule or an enzyme generating a fluorescent molecule, which can be detected in response to the presence of the target analyte. However, some reports can be found using an electrochemical scheme.

2.4.1 Clinical diagnostics

Whole-cell sensors are not yet widespread in clinical diagnostics, although Akyilmaz et al. (2011) reported an electrochemical cell-based sensor for the detection of epinephrine. Epinephrine is one of the most important neurotransmitters in the mammalian central nervous system. It controls the nervous system in the execution of several biological reactions and chemical processes. Changes in its concentration may result in many diseases. Lyophilized White rot fungi cells in gelatine were immobilized onto a platinum (Pt) electrode through glutaraldehyde as a cross-linker. Their enzyme laccase oxidizes epinephrine to epinephrine quinine, thereby reducing its cofactor Cu^{2+} to Cu^{+}. $K_3(CN)_6$ regenerates the cofactor and it is the increase in the reduction peak of $K_3(CN)_6$ that was monitored after epinephrine exposure. The sensor showed a detection limit of 1.04 μM (Akyilmaz et al., 2011).

2.4.2 Environmental management

Whole-cell sensors are highly suitable for environmental monitoring as they can detect toxic effects of complex samples. These days, the pollution of groundwater due to rapid industrialization has prompted investigations of methods to detect water toxicity. Popovtzer et al. (2005) described the development of an electrochemical Si nano-biochip. Genetically engineered *E. coli* bacteria generated the signal. The promoter of their *lacZ* gene was deleted and replaced by the promoter of heat shock genes. In the presence of toxin, this promoter is activated and induces the production of β-galactosidase, the enzyme encoded by *lacZ*. The substrate of this enzyme, p-aminophenyl β-D-galactopyranoside (PAPG), was added and metabolized into p-aminophenol (PAP). PAP was subsequently oxidized at the Si electrode and the current was monitored. Concentrations as low as 0.5% of ethanol and 1.6 ppm of phenol could be detected within 10 minutes after exposure to the toxic chemical (Popovtzer et al., 2005).

3. Alternative transducer materials in biosensing

The advances in biosensor development ultimately depend on the perpetual search for optimal transducer materials, allowing rapid, sensitive and selective biological signal detection and translation. Most of the sensor devices described made use of screen-printed carbon paste, Au or Si as a transducer. For materials to be considered as transducers, they must possess a number of important characteristics.

First of all, they need to be able to undergo biofunctionalization. Secondly, the sensor surfaces need to yield bio-interfaces that can be manufactured with a high reproducibility. Thirdly, the biofunctionalized sensor surfaces must be stable in liquid measurement conditions. Finally, the bio-interfaces will be integrated into micro-electronics, requiring the materials to be compatible with micro-electronic processes.

Unfortunately, Au and Si are not chemically stable and the bio-interfaces degrade upon contact with aqueous electrolytes (Nebel et al., 2007), which limits their use for continuous monitoring and endows them with a disposable character, leading to environmental issues. The biggest disadvantage of carbon paste electrodes is the production reproducibility. Each carbon paste unit is an individual, and the physical, chemical and electrochemical properties may differ from one preparation to another.

Diamond has become an attractive alternative candidate for its use as a transducer material in bio-electronics. It is the only material that is compatible with processes applied in micro-electronics that does not show any degradation in electrolytes, even at fairly high potentials.

Moreover, the naturally insulating diamond can be made into a semiconductor by a process called doping. Doping involves the introduction of impurity atoms into the carbon lattice. Two types of diamond doping exist: p-type doping and n-type doping (Nebel et al., 2007). The difference between a p-type and an n-type semiconductor is graphically presented in figure 2.

Introduction of impurity atoms of group III, for instance boron (B) atoms, into diamond results in p-type doping. In the diamond lattice structure, each C atom has 4 electrons in its outer, valence shell, that are shared with 4 other C atoms. The valence band, now containing 8 electrons per C atom, is completely filled, forming a very stable crystal. B has only 3 electrons in its valence shell. When B is introduced into the lattice, an electron deficiency, or a positively charged hole, is created in the energy level directly above the valence band of diamond, called the acceptor level. This hole can be filled by the movement of an electron

from the valence shell of a neighbouring C atom into the hole of the B atom. B is thus called an acceptor atom. By filling the electron vacancy, a new hole is now created in the valence shell of the C atom that donated the electron, which itself can be filled by another neighbouring electron. The result is a movement of positively charged holes in the valence band of diamond. These holes are thus called the majority charge carriers.
Introduction of impurity atoms of group IV, such as phosphorous (P) atoms, into diamond results in n-type doping. P has 5 electrons in its valence shell. When P is incorporated into the diamond lattice, a situation is created where additional free electrons are supplied to the diamond lattice. Hence, P is called a donor atom. These electrons are very loosely bound in the diamond crystal, and occupy an energy level directly below the conduction band, termed the donor level. The result is a movement of negatively charged electrons in the conduction band of diamond. These electrons are the majority charge carriers. In 1997, Koizumi et al. (1997) were the first to succeed in producing n-type doped SCD using phosphine (Koizumi et al., 1997).

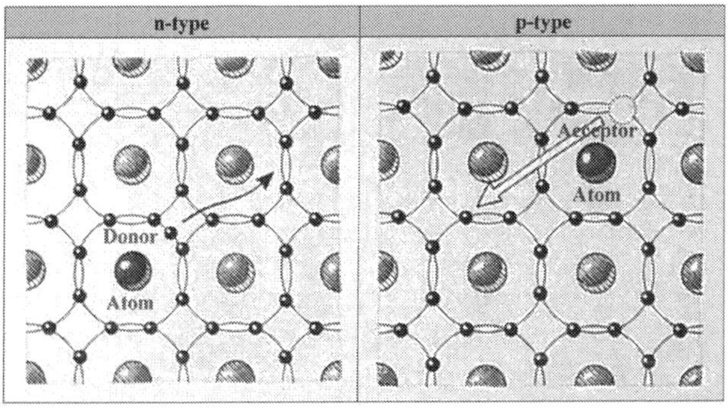

Fig. 2. Schematic diagram of an n-type and p-type semiconductor material at the atomic level.

3.1 Functionalization

3.1.1 Adsorption

Generally, physical adsorption results in significant losses of biomolecules from the surface because of the rather weak bonds involved to immobilize them. Moreover, physical adsorption leads to random orientations of the molecules, more often than not rendering the part that engages in target recognition inaccessible, thereby lowering device sensitivity. However, in some cases, adsorption is the preferred method of attachment. Some non-covalent binding approaches even yield a firmly immobilized and well-oriented biomolecule layer. Streptavidin-modified surfaces bound with biotinylated biomolecules result in the strongest non-covalent bond known. The streptavidin-biotin complexes are also extremely stable over a wide range of temperatures and pH (Gorton, 2005). On the other hand, strong hydrophobic interactions between hydrogen (H)-terminated surfaces and biomolecules are also found to be sufficient for reliable biorecognition and detection. Furthermore, when an attachment needs to be obtained between a surface and macroscopic entities, such as cells or tissues, joint forces of membrane protein interactions with each other and the surface contribute to a very stable biological meshwork.

Antibodies

Our group constructed an impedimetric immunosensor directed against C-Reactive Protein (CRP), an acute phase protein serving as a marker for cardiovascular disease, based on the physical adsorption of anti-CRP to H-terminated nanocrystalline diamond (NCD), since Silin et al. (1997) demonstrated the suitability of hydrophobic surfaces for antibody adsorption. They postulated that the protein adsorption to this type of surface was a multistep process, probably initiated by interaction of hydrophobic residues, that have temporarily become exposed at the surface of the protein, with the hydrophobic surface. This initial interaction is then followed by multipoint interactions due to various degrees of protein denaturation, making desorption from the surface extremely difficult (Silin, V et al., 1997). The experiments of our group indicated that the biological activity of the antibodies was not hampered (Bijnens et al., 2009).

Cells

Chen et al. (2009) studied the suitability of ultra-nanocrystalline diamond (UNCD) to be used as a biomaterial for the growth and differentiation of neural stem cells (NSCs). H- and oxygen (O)-terminated UNCD films were compared with for their influence on the growth, expansion and differentiation of NSCs. H-terminated UNCD films spontaneously induced cell proliferation and neuronal differentiation. O-terminated UNCD films were also shown to further improve neural differentiation, with a preference to differentiate into oligodendrocytes. Hence, controlling the surface properties of UNCD could manipulate the differentiation of NSCs for different biomedical applications (Chen et al., 2009).
Also, Smisdom et al. (2009) cultured transfected Chinese Hamster Ovary (CHO) cells on bare, H-terminated, and O-terminated NCD and microcrystalline diamond (MCD) surfaces. Optical and biochemical analyses show that compared to glass controls, growth and viability of the CHO cells were not significantly affected (Smisdom et al., 2009).

3.1.2 Covalent attachment

Covalent attachment of biomolecules to diamond is the immobilization technique of choice for biosensor fabrication. It results in a stable and long-term modification of the substrate with oriented biomolecules. The surface of the diamond can be modified to present desired functionalities. The bioreceptor molecules can subsequently be coupled to these functional groups through their own range of intrinsic or custom functionalities.

DNA and aptamers

chemical functionalization

Ushizawa et al. (2002) reported the wet-chemical modification of diamond powder (1 - 2 μm) with thymidines (T). First, the surface of the diamond powder was oxidized to its surface oxides (carboxylic acid [COOH], hydroxyl [OH], acid anhydride) by immersion into a heated mixture of sulphuric acid (H_2SO_4) and nitric acid (HNO_3). Next, the COOH-modified diamond was treated with thionyl chloride ($SOCl_2$) and T, resulting in a T-modified diamond surface. DNA molecules generated through PCR amplification could be covalently attached to the T-modified surface via a simple ligation reaction. PCR has the interesting characteristic of adding an adenine (A) base to the 3′ end of each amplified DNA molecule. These 3′A-overhangs were exploited in the ligation to the T-modified surface. Diffuse Reflectance Infrared Fourier-Transform spectroscopy (DRIFT) was used to verify the presence of DNA on the surface (Ushizawa et al., 2002). A summary of their reaction process is given in figure 3.

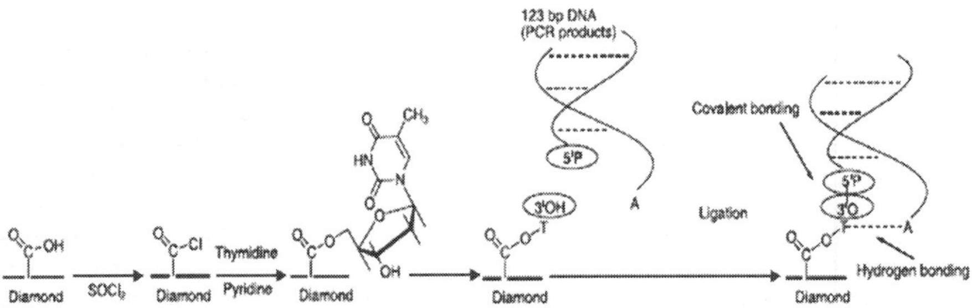

Fig. 3. Reaction process used by Ushizawa et al. (2002) for the covalent attachment of PCR-amplified dsDNA to T-modified diamond powder. Adapted from (Ushizawa et al., 2002).

electrochemical functionalization

Single-crystalline diamond (SCD) of p-type nature has been covalently modified with DNA molecules through an electrochemical procedure by Wang et al. (2004). They used a three-electrode configuration with a SCD working electrode, a Pt counter electrode and a silver/silver chloride (Ag/AgCl) reference electrode. The p-type SCD working electrode was treated with the diazonium salt 4-nitrobenzene-diazonium tetrafluoroborate. This salt was reduced in acetonitrile to nitrophenyl using Cyclic Voltammetry (CV) and attached to the SCD surface in a nitrogen gas (N_2)-purged glove-box. The nitrophenyl groups were subsequently reduced to aminophenyl groups, resulting in a NH_2-modified SCD surface. This NH_2-modified SCD could then be modified downstream with the heterobifunctional cross-linker molecule sulphosuccinimidyl-4-(N-maleimido-mehyl)cyclohexane-1-carboxylate (SSMCC). The N-hydroxy-succinimide (NHS)-ester group of SSMCC reacts with the NH_2-groups on the NCD to form amide (NH) bonds. SH-modified ssDNA could then be linked to the COOH-moiety of SSMCC at room temperature, resulting in a covalent bond (Wang et al., 2004). This procedure is outlined in figure 4.

Fig. 4. Reaction process used by Wang et al. (2004) for the covalent attachment of SH-ssDNA to aminophenyl-modified p-type SCD. Adapted from (Nebel et al., 2007).

Gu et al. (2005) functionalized p-type diamond with a PANI/polyacrylic acid (PAA) composite polymer films using CV. The p-type diamond working electrode was treated with the aniline and PAA monomeric solution, and by potential cycling the monomers were polymerized onto the electrode. In a final step, NH_2-modified ssDNA was covalently attached to the exposed COOH-groups of the PANI/PAA polymeric film by 1-ethyl-3-(3-dimethylaminopropyl)-carbodiimide (EDC) (Gu et al., 2005).

photochemical functionalization

Undoped, H-terminated NCD surfaces were covered with trifluoro-acetamide acid (TFAAD) inside a N_2-purged Teflon reaction chamber by Yang et al. (2004). This is a 10-amino-dec-1-ene molecule, protected with a trifluoro-acetic acid group at one end. The other end is terminated by a C=C double bond. The chamber was sealed with a quartz window, allowing the passage of UV-light from a low-pressure mercury lamp (0.35 $mW.cm^{-2}$ measured at the sample surface) for 12 h. This illumination process caused a covalent bond to be formed between the TFAAD and the H-terminated NCD, exposing the trifluoro-acetic acid groups at the NCD surface (Yang et al., 2002). After TFAAD attachment, the trifluoro-acetic acid groups were removed by immersion into a hydrochloric acid (HCl)/methanol solution, forming NH_2-modified NCD surfaces. These were subsequently exposed to the heterobifunctional cross-linker molecule SSMCC. SH-modified ssDNA molecules could then be linked to the SSMCC in the same way as described above. Figure 5 represents the reaction steps that were employed (Yang et al., 2004).

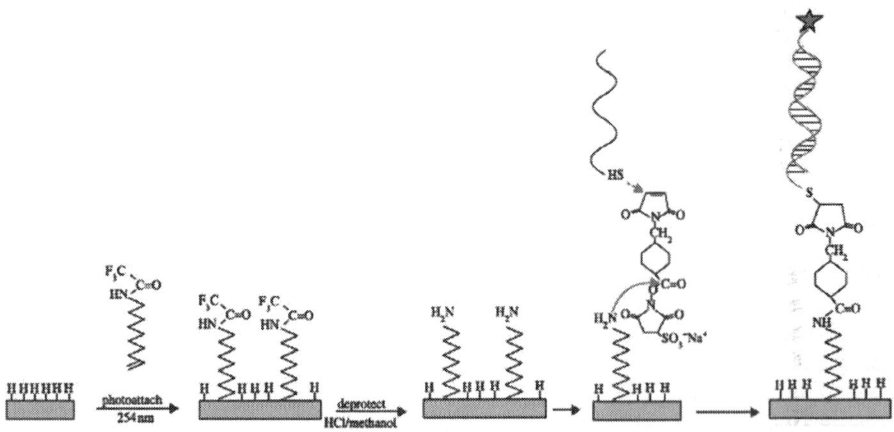

Fig. 5. Reaction process used by Yang et al. (2004) for the covalent attachment of thiolated ssDNA to photochemically activated NCD. Adapted from (Nebel et al., 2007).

Our group devized a procedure for the covalent attachment of DNA, which was a simple, two-step photochemical method using a flexible linker and a zero-length cross-linker, displayed in figure 6. Undoped, H-terminated NCD was immersed in a fatty acid molecule, 10-unedecenoic acid (10-UDA), consisting of a reactive C=C double bond on one end, and a COOH-group on the other end. A 20 h illumination with UV-light (2.5 $mW.cm^{-2}$) also caused a covalent bond to be formed between the 10-UDA and the H-terminated NCD, yielding a COOH-modified NCD surface. NH_2-modified ssDNA could then be reacted with these

COOH-groups via EDC, resulting in covalently bound ssDNA molecules to NCD through a NH bond. The presence of the 10-UDA linker molecule offers mobility to the attached DNA, increasing their availability for hybridization reactions. Moreover the EDC cross-linker did not remain present in the eventual NH bond, resulting in a smaller distance between NCD and DNA (Christiaens et al., 2006), (Vermeeren et al., 2008).

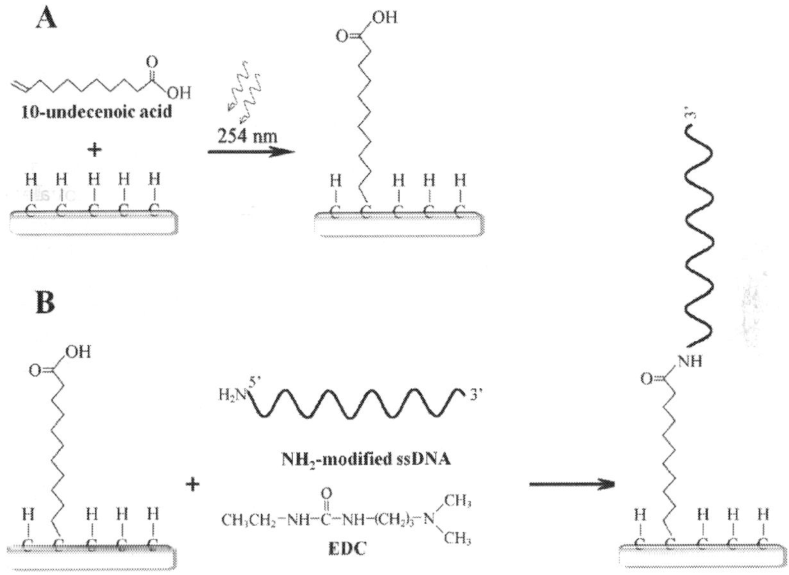

Fig. 6. Photoattachment of 10-UDA acid to the NCD surface through irradiation with 254 nm UV-light (A). Covalent attachment of NH_2-modified ssDNA to 10-UDA on an NCD suface using an EDC-mediated reaction (B).

Antibodies

Although immunosensors are often based on physical adsorption of the antibodies to the transducer, as described above, signal drift is a very common side effect associated with this manner of attachment (Carrara et al., 2008). This is the reason that a covalent attachment method is preferred in the more recent publications. Since antibodies, being proteins, possess NH_2-groups, the EDC-route described previously for the covalent attachment of NH_2-modified DNA is a very popular method. However, the procedure needs to be adjusted into a two-step process because antibodies also possess COOH-groups. The one-step procedure as described for DNA would lead to a chain formation of end-to-end attached antibodies instead of antibodies attached to the COOH-modified surface. This is the reason that, in a first step, NHS is attached to the COOH-terminated surface using EDC. In a second step, the antibodies are added, that switch places with the NHS, the latter functioning as leaving group. This way, EDC never comes into contact with the antibodies, and chain formation is avoided (Quershi et al., 2009). However, it is documented that the NH_2-terminus of antibodies are located at the antigen-binding variable regions, and not many aminoacids with NH_2-containing side groups, like lysine, are present in the constant

Fc region of the antibodies. Although a more stable molecular layer is obtained with this procedure, possibly decreasing signal drift, it is doubtful that the orientation of the attached antibodies will be optimal (Harlow et al., 1999).

For this reason, Jung et al. developed an alternative attachment procedure for antibodies. In a first step, they covalently attached a 13 aminoacid cyclic Fc binding peptide to a COOH-modified surface using the two-step EDC-NHS route. In a second step, they added the antibodies, that will be captured by their Fc regions, resolving the orientation issue (Jung et al., 2008). There is no covalent bond between the antibodies and the Fc binding proteins, but the well-organized monolayer of molecules will possibly suffice to stabilize the electronic signal.

3.2 Electrochemical characterization

Because of the increasing focus on point-of-care analyte detection, electrochemical biosensors are most popular. Considering the five requirements, electrochemical biosensors are sensitive, specific, cheap, easy to miniaturize, and can detect the analyte recognition in real-time, making them fast. Moreover, the continuous response of the electrochemical sensor allows computerized control, simplifying the electrochemical detection, and lowering the cost even more.

Electrochemical biosensors can be subdivided into amperometric, potentiometric, impedimetric, and field effect transistor (FET)-based biosensors. However, only impedimetric, and field effect transistor (FET)-based biosensors have the potential to allow for real-time and label-free target detection, which are key requirements for point-of-care application. Unfortunately, it has generally been accepted that FET-based biosensing is problematic, to say the least. The counter-ion screening effect is the main reason for this fact. Charged groups in the molecular layer on top of the electrode will be neutralized by the surrounding counter-ions that are present in the buffer solution during measurement. This will result in net uncharged molecular layers, causing the biological recognition event to go undetected with FET-based devices. Hence, only Electrochemical Impedance Spectroscopy (EIS)-based biosensing will be discussed.

3.2.1 Theory of Electrochemical Impedance Spectroscopy (EIS)

In an ideally resistive electrical circuit, the elements such as the voltage (V), current (I), and resistance (R), behave independent of the voltage frequency, and are governed by Ohm's law:

$$R = \frac{V}{I}$$

Often, however, the electrical circuit is not purely resistive, but also contains inductive (L) and capacitive (C) components. If in this case an alternating (AC) voltage is applied, I and V become out of phase, and are frequency-dependent. For this reason, the oscillating V and I will be written as complex entities, as a function of their magnitudes V_0 and I_0, respectively, the phase shift φ of I with respect to V, and the frequency ω:

$$V(t) = V_0 \exp(j\omega t)$$

$$I(t) = I_0 \exp\left[j(\omega t - \varphi)\right]$$

Consequently, the simple R is replaced by the complex impedance, Z. Being a complex entity, Z is also defined by its magnitude, Z_0, and its phase shift, φ:

$$Z = \frac{V(t)}{I(t)} = Z_0 e^{j\varphi} = Z_0(\cos\varphi + j\sin\varphi)$$

where $Z_0(\cos\varphi)$ and $Z_0(\sin\varphi)$ are the real part, $\mathrm{Re}(Z)$, and the imaginary part, $\mathrm{Im}(Z)$, of the complex impedance, Z, respectively. In other words, impedance signifies opposition to current flow in an alternating current (AC) electrical circuit.

Two popular ways exist to graphically represent the impedance data: a Bode plot and a Nyquist plot. A Bode plot depicts the magnitude of the complex impedance, Z, or the phase shift, φ, as a function of frequency, ω. Usually, a logarithmic scale is used for the magnitude and the frequency. Figure 7 shows an example of a Bode plot of the complex impedance, Z, and of the phase shift, φ, for a parallel RC circuit.

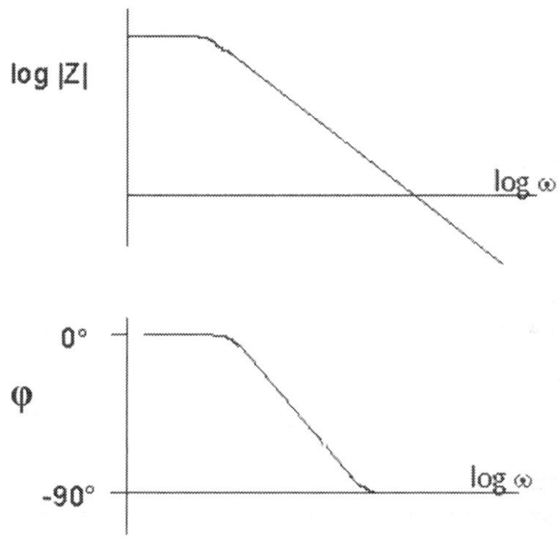

Fig. 7. Bode plot of the complex impedance, Z (upper panel), and of the phase shift, φ (lower panel), versus frequency, ω, for a parallel RC circuit. Both the X-axis and the Y-axis are represented by a logarithmic scale.

A Nyquist plot displays the imaginary part and the real part which make up the complex impedance, Z. The negative form of $\mathrm{Im}(Z)$ is plotted on the Y-axis, while $\mathrm{Re}(Z)$ is presented on the X-axis. Figure 8 shows a Nyquist plot of the same parallel RC circuit as in figure 7.

Each point in this Nyquist plot represents the complex impedance, Z, at one frequency, ω. When drawing a vector through the zero-point to this point, the magnitude, $|Z|$, and the phase shift, φ, can be deduced. The frequency, ω, decreases from right to left in the plot (Young et al., 1999).

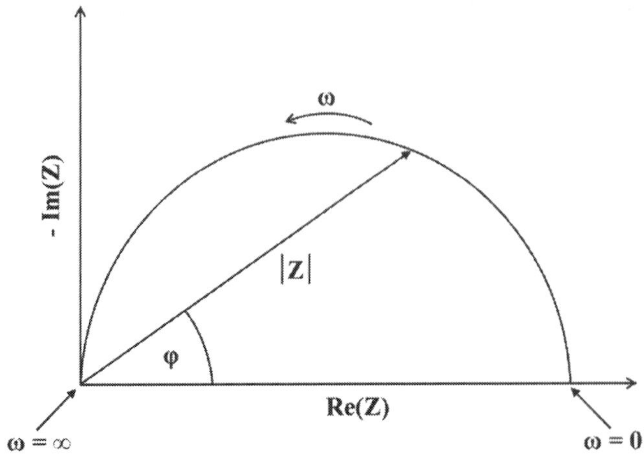

Fig. 8. Nyquist plot, displaying $-\mathrm{Im}(Z)$ versus $\mathrm{Re}(Z)$, for a parallel RC circuit.

When a semiconductor electrode is placed into contact with an electrolyte, the Fermi level, E_F, of the semiconductor and the chemical potential of the electrolyte, μ, are initially not in equilibrium. Two alternative events can occur to obtain the necessary thermodynamic equilibrium, depending on the type of semiconductor. These are shown in figure 9.

When a p-type semiconductor is placed in contact with a liquid, electrons move from the electrolyte into the semiconductor, thereby depleting the positively charged holes in the material and creating a region just below the semiconductor surface where no majority charge carriers exist. This region is called the depletion zone or the space-charge region. When no more electrons move into the semiconductor, thermodynamic equilibrium is reached between E_F and μ, resulting in a downward bending of the valence and conduction bands in the p-type semiconductor.

When an n-type semiconductor is placed in contact with a liquid, electrons move from the semiconductor into the electrolyte, also decreasing the amount of majority charge carriers in the material and creating a depletion zone or space-charge region just below the semiconductor surface. At thermodynamic equilibrium, the result is an upward band bending. These phenomena occurring in the semiconductor are called field-effects.

Any chemical modification in the electrode-electrolyte interface, for instance the binding of an antigen to an antibody-modified electrode, or the hybridization of target ssDNA to a ssDNA-modified electrode, will alter this equilibrium, and hence the degree of band bending. In other words, the depletion zone in the semiconductor can be made wider or narrower by external events. A narrowing of the depletion zone corresponds to a decrease in impedance, since the obstacle for charge carriers that want to cross this space-charge region decreases. A widening of the depletion zone corresponds to an increase in impedance, since the obstacle for charge carriers that want to cross this space-charge region increases. Since DNA is negatively charged, it will likely exert a field-effect in a semiconductor when bound to its surface. EIS is therefore often used as a mechanism to detect hybridization events.

When ssDNA is attached to the surface of a p-type semiconductor, their negative charges attract the holes in the semiconductor to the surface-DNA interface. The space-charge region becomes narrower, and the downward band bending becomes less steep. Moreover, additional negative charges brought about by hybridization will increase this effect even more. The result is a decrease in impedance.

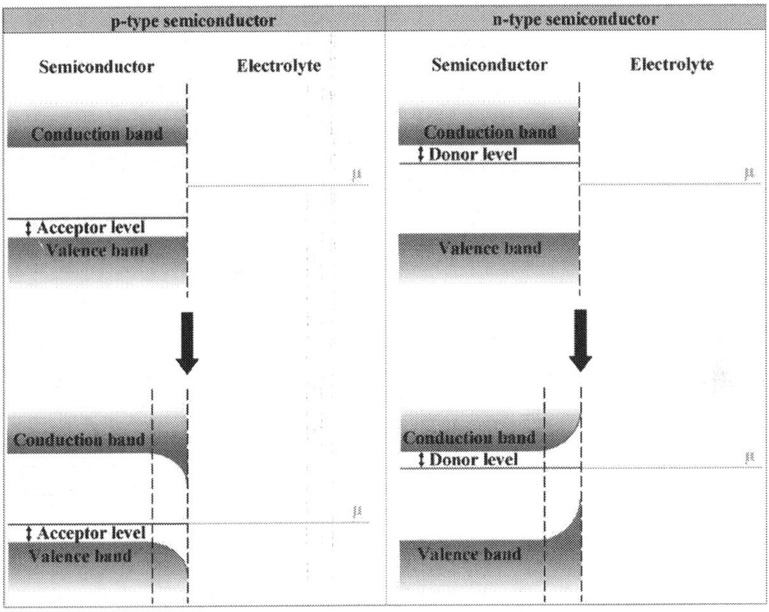

Fig. 9. Generation of thermodynamic equilibrium in p-type (left panel) and n-type (right panel) semiconductors through downward and upward band bending, respectively.

When ssDNA is attached to the surface of a n-type semiconductor, their negative charges repel the electrons in the semiconductor. The space-charge region becomes wider, and the upward band bending becomes more pronounced. This effect is again amplified by hybridization.

In EIS, an AC potential is generated over a range of frequencies between the biologically modified semiconductor working electrode and a counter electrode. The impedance is subsequently measured between these two electrodes, through the electrolyte, for each frequency in the analyzed frequency range. By modelling the observed impedance effects with an electrical circuit, one can associate certain effects with changes in electrical elements, further elucidating the events at the molecular level. It is a useful tool for label-free and real-time target detection. This decreases cost and analysis time (Nebel et al., 2006), (Young et al., 1999), (Memming, 2000), (Chakrapani et al., 2007).

3.2.2 Impedimetric DNA-sensors

Impedimetric diamond-based DNA-sensors are very popular in the literature. Yang et al. (2004) monitored selective DNA hybridization using EIS. H-terminated NCD working electrodes of p-type nature were covalently modified with SH-ssDNA molecules. A Pt foil and a Ag/AgCl wire were used as counter and reference electrode, respectively. They showed that measurements at open-circuit potential displayed a significant decrease in impedance at frequencies of >10^4 Hz, even in real-time, when the NCD electrode was exposed to complementary target ssDNA, while 4-base mismatch sequences were easily discriminated. By electrical circuit modelling, they attributed this effect to a hybridization-induced field-effect in the NCD film (Yang et al., 2004). Gu et al. (2005) covalently immobilized NH_2-modified ssDNA onto p-type diamond with a PANI/PAA composite polymer. A three-electrode system was used for EIS. The p-type diamond served as a working electrode, the counter electrode was a Pt wire and the reference electrode was Ag/AgCl. They observed an impedance decrease, this time in the lower frequency regions (10 - 100 Hz) upon complementary hybridization, and a decrease in electron-transfer resistance to the electrode. Electric circuit modelling, using the same circuit model as Yang, attributed this lower frequency region to reflect the polymer/molecular double-layer. They suggest that hybridization with complementary DNA decreases the resistance and increases the capacity of the polymer, both due to an increase in ionic density at the interface. The space-charge region of the p-type diamond electrode was reflected at frequencies of ~1000 Hz. They found that DNA hybridization also altered the electrical response of the electrode through a field-effect, resulting in a decreased impedance in this space-charge region. The linear range of target ssDNA detection was 50 to 200 nM, with a detection limit of 20 nM. They obtained SNP sensitivity (Gu et al., 2005). In our group, we investigated the possibility of SNP detection on NCD using EIS. Probe ssDNA molecules were covalently attached to COOH-modified NCD working electrodes. The frequency-dependent change in impedance was analyzed in real-time with complementary ssDNA and ssDNA containing a SNP. SNP discrimination was possible in real-time during denaturation at the highest frequency of 1 MHz within 5 minutes. This SNP sensitivity is clinically relevant since numerous genetic illnesses are caused by point mutations. It is reflected in a fast impedance decrease for the SNP-duplexes and a slower impedance decrease for the complementary duplexes. Since complementary duplexes are stable molecules, they have a rather high melting temperature, reflected in a slow impedance decrease rate. SNP-duplexes are much less stable than complementary duplexes, and hence they have a lower melting temperature. This is reflected in a faster impedance decrease rate. This exact principle of SNP differentiation based on different melting temperatures is also the basis of Denaturing Gradient Gel Electrophoresis (DGGE) used for SNP identification, but it is the first time that this is reported with an electronic technique. Like is possible with DGGE, EIS could also enable mutation identification, since different types of mutations will also yield duplexes with different melting temperatures (Vermeeren et al., 2007).

3.2.3 Impedimetric immunosensors

Impedimetric diamond-based immunosensors are also widespread, and it has been established that antigen recognition causes an increased thickness in the molecular layer, leading to a clear capacitive effect in the impedance spectrum. Yang et al. (2007) used EIS to directly detect antigen-antibody binding on diamond and Si. A Pt foil and Ag/AgCl served as a counter and a reference electrode, respectively. They covalently modified n-type and p-type Si and p-type NCD with human IgG and IgM. The Fc regions of these covalently attached IgG and IgM antibodies served as antigens for anti-human IgG and anti-human IgM. They succeeded in real-time and label-free detection of selective antigen recognition, and observed an increase in impedance at frequencies >10^4 Hz for the p-type substrates, and a decrease in impedance in the same frequency region for n-type Si. Circuit modelling showed that the frequency region sensitive for antigen recognition is dominated by the space-charge region of the electrode. When positively charged anti-IgG and anti-IgM approach a p-type surface, the holes are repelled and widen the depletion zone, increasing the impedance in the space-charge region. When positively charged anti-IgG and anti-IgM approach a n-type surface, the electrons are attracted, which narrows the depletion zone, decreasing the impedance in the space-charge region. The detection limit for real-time selective IgG detection was 42 nM in 12 minutes (Yang et al., 2007). In our group, as already mentioned, H-terminated NCD working electrodes were modified with anti-CRP by simple physical adsorption. A Au wire in contact with the reaction fluid served as a counter electrode. The selective antigen recognition was analyzed in real-time, and the detection limit was found to be 10 nM, which was in the physiologically relevant range, and could be discriminated within 10 minutes (Bijnens et al., 2009).

3.2.4 Impedimetric aptasensors

Tran et al. (2011) described an impedimetric aptasensor for the detection of human IgE. Human IgE has been demonstrated to be a mediator in allergic reactions. Allergenicity is a major health concern in both children and adults. Approximately 2% of adults and 8% of children suffer from allergenicity. Allergic reactions are caused by exposure of the skin to chemicals, or of the respiratory system to pollen or dust, and consumption of certain food products. The total IgE level in serum is therefore widely considered as a marker for atopic diseases. IgE aptamers were covalently attached to NCD electrodes, and the impedimetric response was monitored continuously during IgE incubation. They obtained a detection limit of 0.03 μg/ml in serum (Tran et al., 2011).

4. Future research

Science is focusing more and more on the development of point-of-care biosensors to diagnose diseases, assess food quality, and monitor the environment. The five requirements that need to be met are high sensitivity, high specificity, high analysis speed, low cost, and portability. Speed and low cost are obtained by analyzing in real-time and working in a label-free setting, respectively. Biosensors based on an impedimetric read-out offer the most potential to combine all of these factors.

However, an electrochemical read-out has implications on the choice of transducer material. EIS implies a semiconducting material to transducer the biological event into a readable signal, but most semiconductors are sensitive to hydrolysis when in contact with an electrolyte. This causes an unstable molecular layer, leading to signal drift. This issue becomes of less importance when a disposable, single-use application of the sensor is envisaged. However, in some circumstances, such as continuous measurements of cardiovascular markers or environmental toxins, signal stability is paramount. Semiconducting diamond could be a promising alternative, because extremely stable C-C bonds can be formed between the material and all kinds of bioreceptor molecules.

Another aspect that needs attention is the fact that no conclusion, be it in the medical, environmental, or food industry, is reached by the monitoring of one single analyte. Multiplexing is necessary to reach a reliable and well-founded diagnosis. Only few reports have mentioned the simultaneous detection of multiple markers, but rarely more than two. To extend the concept of a point-of-care sensor, that is functional under controlled conditions, into a device that is able to be used in a real application field, the transducer will need to be arrayed, and each spot will have to be read out separately, and reach the same sensitivity and specificity as the monofunctionalized version. A firm collaboration between bioelectronics and bioengineering is necessary to succeed in this task.

In order to reach higher sensitivities and lower detection limits, the use of cells as actual biosensors also merits further exploration. Because of the cell's membrane receptors, it is it's job to respond to very low concentrations of analytes. Recombinant DNA technology could allow the construction of a custom-made receptor, leading to a reporter cell with tailored specificity.

For all of the further refinements of biosensor development, it is clear that a strong interdisciplinary relationship and collaboration is necessary between bioelectronics, bioengineering, molecular biology, physics, and chemistry. Only then will we evolve towards the actual implementation of point-of-care biosensors.

5. References

Akyilmaz, E., Turemis, M., & Yasa, I. (2011). Voltammetric determination of epinephrine by White rot fungi (Phanerochaete chrysosporium ME446) cells based microbial biosensor. Biosens.Bioelectron., Vol. 26, No. 5, pp. (2590-2594)

Bijnens, N., Vermeeren, V., Daenen, M., Grieten, L., Haenen, K., Wenmackers, S., Williams, O. A., Ameloot, M., VandeVen M., Michiels, L., & Wagner, P. (2009). Synthetic diamond films as a platform material for label-free protein sensors. Phys.Stat.Sol.(a), Vol. 206, No. 3, pp. (520-526)

Bonel, L., Vidal, J. C., Duato, P., & Castillo, J. R. (2010). An electrochemical competitive biosensor for ochratoxin A based on a DNA biotinylated aptamer. Biosens.Bioelectron., in press

Cai, W., Peck, J. R., van der Weide, D. W., & Hamers, R. J. (2004). Direct electrical detection of hybridization at DNA-modified silicon surfaces. Biosens.Bioelectron., Vol. 19, No. 9, pp. (1013-1019)

Carrara, S., Bhalla, V. K., Stagni, C., Benini, L., Riccò, B., & Samorì, B. (2008). Improving probe immobilization for label-free capacitive detection of DNA hybridization on microfabricated gold electrodes. Sensors and Transducers, Vol. 88, pp. (31-39)

Chakrapani, V., Angus, J. C., Anderson, A. B., Wolter, S. D., Stoner, B. R., & Sumanasekera, G. U. (2007). Charge transfer equilibria between diamond and an aqueous oxygen electrochemical redox couple. Science, Vol. 318, No. 5855, pp. (1424-1430)

Chemburu, S., Wilkins, E., & Abdel-Hamid, I. (2005). Detection of pathogenic bacteria in food samples using highly-dispersed carbon particles. Biosens.Bioelectron., Vol. 21, No. 3, pp. (491-499)

Chen, Y. C., Lee, D. C., Hsiao, C. Y., Chung, Y. F., Chen, H. C., Thomas, J. P., Pong, W. F., Tai, N. H., Lin, I. N., & Chiu, I. M. (2009). The effect of ultra-nanocrystalline diamond films on the proliferation and differentiation of neural stem cells. Biomaterials, Vol. 30, No. 20, pp. (3428-3435)

Christiaens, P., Vermeeren, V., Wenmackers, S., Daenen, M., Haenen, K., Nesladek, M., vandeVen, M., Ameloot, M., Michiels, L., & Wagner, P. (2006). EDC-mediated DNA attachment to nanocrystalline CVD diamond films. Biosens.Bioelectron., Vol. 22, No. 2, pp. (170-177)

Fang, X., Tan, O. K., Tse, M. S., & Ooi, E. E. (2010). A label-free immunosensor for diagnosis of Dengue infection with simple electrical measurements. Biosens.Bioelectron., Vol. 25, No. 5, pp. (1137-1142)

Gorton, L. (Ed.). (2005). Comprehensive analytical chemistry: Biosensors and modern biospecific analytical techniques, Elsevier Science, 978-0444507150, Amsterdam

Grennan, K., Strachan, G., Porter, A. J., Killard, A. J., & Smyth, M. R. (2003). Atrazine analysis using an amperometric immunosensor based on single-chain antibody fragments and regeneration-free multi-calibrant measurement. Anal.Chim.Acta, Vol. 500, No. 1-2, pp. (287-298)

Gu, H., Su, X., & Loh, K. P. (2005). Electrochemical impedance sensing of DNA hybridization on conducting polymer film-modified diamond. J.Phys.Chem.B, Vol. 109, No. 28, pp. (13611-13618)

Harlow, E. & Lane, D. (1999). Using Antibodies: A Laboratory Manual. Cold Spring Harbor Laboratory Press, 978-087969544-6, Cold Spring Harbor, NY

Joon-Hyung, J., Deng, Z., Alocilja, E. C., & Grooms, D. L. (2008). Label-Free DNA Sensor on Nanoporous Silicon-Polypyrrole Chip for Monitoring Salmonella Species. Sensors Journal, IEEE, Vol. 8, No. 6, pp. (891-895)

Jung, Y., Kang, H. J., Lee, J. M., Jung, S. O., Yun, W. S., Chung, S. J., & Chung, B. H. (2008). Controlled antibody immobilization onto immunoanalytical platforms by synthetic peptide. Anal.Biochem., Vol. 374, No. 1, pp. (99-105)

Koizumi, S., Kamo, M., Sato, Y., Ozaki, H., & Inuzuka, T. (1997). Growth and characterization of phosphorous doped (111) homoepitaxial diamond thin films. Appl.Phys.Lett., Vol. 71, pp. (1065-1067)

Marrazza, G., Chianella, I., & Mascini, M. (1999). Disposable DNA electrochemical sensor for hybridization detection. Biosens.Bioelectron., Vol. 14, No. 1, pp. (43-51)

Memming, R. (2000). Semiconductor electrochemistry. (1), Wiley-VCH, 978-3527301478, Weinheim

Micheli, L., Radoi, A., Guarrina, R., Massaud, R., Bala, C., Moscone, D., & Palleschi, G. (2004). Disposable immunosensor for the determination of domoic acid in shellfish. Biosens.Bioelectron., Vol. 20, No. 2, pp. (190-196)

Nebel, C. E., Rezek, B., Shin, D., & Watanabe, H. (2006). Surface electronic properties of H-terminated diamond in contact with adsorbates and electrolytes. Phys.Stat.Sol.(a), Vol. 203, No. 13, pp. (3273-3298)

Nebel, C. E., Shin, D., Rezek, B., Tokuda, N., Uetsuka, H., & Watanabe, H. (2007). Diamond and biology. J.R.Soc.Interface, Vol. 4, No. 14, pp. (439-461)

Olowu, R. A., Arotiba, O., Mailu, S. N., Waryo, T. T., Baker, P., & Iwuoha, E. (2010). Electrochemical Aptasensor for Endocrine Disrupting 17ß-Estradiol Based on a Poly(3,4-ethylenedioxylthiopene)-Gold Nanocomposite Platform. Sensors, Vol. 10, No. 11, pp. (9872-9890)

Pan, Y., Sonn, G. A., Sin, M. L., Mach, K. E., Shih, M. C., Gau, V., Wong, P. K., & Liao, J. C. (2010). Electrochemical immunosensor detection of urinary lactoferrin in clinical samples for urinary tract infection diagnosis. Biosens.Bioelectron., Vol. 26, No. 2, pp. (649-654)

Popovtzer, R., Neufeld, T., Biran, D., Ron, E. Z., Rishpon, J., & Shacham-Diamand, Y. (2005). Novel integrated electrochemical nano-biochip for toxicity detection in water. Nano.Lett., Vol. 5, No. 6, pp. (1023-1027)

Quershi, A., Saravan, K. S., Gurbuz, Y., Howell, M., Kang, W. P., & Davidson, J. L. (2009). A new nanocrystalline diamond-based biosensor for the detection of cardiovascular risk markers, Proceedings of the Eurosensors XXIII conference, Lausanne, Switzerland, 2009

Silin, V., V, Weetall, H., & Vanderah, D. J. (1997). SPR Studies of the Nonspecific Adsorption Kinetics of Human IgG and BSA on Gold Surfaces Modified by Self-Assembled Monolayers (SAMs). J.Colloid Interface Sci., Vol. 185, No. 1, pp. (94-103)

Skládal, P. & Kaláb, T. (1995). A multichannel immunochemical sensor for determination of 2,4-dichlorophenoxyacetic acid. Anal.Chim.Acta, Vol. 316, No. 1, pp. (73-78)

Smisdom, N., Smets, I., Williams, O. A., Daenen, M., Wenmackers, S., Haenen, K., Nesládek, M., D'Haen, J., Wagner, P., Rigo, J.-M., Ameloot, M., & vandeVen, M. (2009). Chinese hamster ovary cell viability on hydrogen and oxygen terminated nano- and microcrystalline diamond surfaces. Phys.Stat.Sol.(a), Vol. 206, No. 9, pp. (2042-2047)

Tichoniuk, M., Ligaj, M., & Filipiak, M. (2008). Application of DNA Hybridization Biosensor as a Screening Method for the Detection of Genetically Modified Food Components. Sensors, Vol. 8, No. 4, pp. (2118-2135)

Tran, D. T., Vermeeren, V., Grieten, L., Wenmackers, S., Wagner, P., Pollet, J., Janssen, K. P., Michiels, L., & Lammertyn, J. (2011). Nanocrystalline diamond impedimetric aptasensor for the label-free detection of human IgE. Biosens.Bioelectron., Vol. 26, No. 6, pp. (2987-2993)

Ushizawa, K., Sato, Y., Mitsumori, T., Machinami, T., Ueda, T., & Ando, T. (2002). Covalent immobilization of DNA on diamond and its verification by diffuse reflectance infrared spectroscopy. Chem.Phys.Lett., Vol. 351, pp. (105-108)

Vermeeren, V., Bijnens, N., Wenmackers, S., Daenen, M., Haenen, K., Williams, O. A., Ameloot, M., vandeVen, M., Wagner, P., & Michiels, L. (2007). Towards a real-time, label-free, diamond-based DNA sensor. Langmuir, Vol. 23, No. 26, pp. (13193-13202)

Vermeeren, V., Wenmackers, S., Daenen, M., Haenen, K., Williams, O. A., Ameloot, M., Vande, V. M., Wagner, P., & Michiels, L. (2008). Topographical and functional characterization of the ssDNA probe layer generated through EDC-mediated covalent attachment to nanocrystalline diamond using fluorescence microscopy. Langmuir, Vol. 24, No. 16, pp. (9125-9134)

Wang, J., Firestone, M. A., Auciello, O., & Carlisle, J. A. (2004). Functionalization of ultrananocrystalline diamond films by electrochemical reduction of aryldiazonium salts. Langmuir, Vol. 20, pp. (450-456)

Yang, W., Auciello, O., Butler, J. E., Cai, W., Carlisle, J. A., Gerbi, J. E., Gruen, D. M., Knickerbocker, T., Lasseter, T. L., Russell, J. N., Jr., Smith, L. M., & Hamers, R. J. (2002). DNA-modified nanocrystalline diamond thin-films as stable, biologically active substrates. Nat.Mater., Vol. 1, No. 4, pp. (253-257)

Yang, W., Butler, J. E., Russell, J. N., Jr., & Hamers, R. J. (2004). Interfacial electrical properties of DNA-modified diamond thin films: Intrinsic response and hybridization-induced field effects. Langmuir, Vol. 20, No. 16, pp. (6778-6787)

Yang, W., Butler, J. E., Russell, J. N., Jr., & Hamers, R. J. (2007). Direct electrical detection of antigen-antibody binding on diamond and silicon substrates using electrical impedance spectroscopy. Analyst, Vol. 132, No. 4, pp. (296-306)

Young, H. D., Freedman, R. A., Sandin, T. R., & Lewis Ford, A. (1999). University Physics. (10), Addison Wesley Publishing Company, 978-0201603224, Boston

Yuan, Y., Yuan, R., Chai, Y., Zhuo, Y., Liu, Z., Mao, L., Guan, S., & Qian, X. (2010). A novel label-free electrochemical aptasensor for thrombin based on the {nano-Au/thionine}n multilayer films as redox probes. Anal.Chim.Acta, Vol. 668, No. 2, pp. (171-176)

6

GMR Biosensor for Clinical Diagnostic

Mitra Djamal[1], Ramli[2], Freddy Haryanto[1] and Khairurrijal[1]
[1]*Institut Teknologi Bandung*
[2]*Universitas Negeri Padang*
Indonesia

1. Introduction

Clinical diagnostics is a field in which new methods of laboratory analysis for faster, direct, more accurate, more selective, has a high output and less expensive than conventional methods are in high demand. Because of its small size, transduction ultrasensitive and possible integration in Microsystems lab-on-a-chip, biosensing devices are made with nano-technology is a potential candidate to meet all the requirements above.
Since last decade, many researchers have been brought their work to carry out on biomagnetism and magnetic biosensors based on molecular processes. Their works focus not only on application of magnetic nanoparticles in biomedicine (Pankhurst et al., 2009) but also on their synthesis (Roca et al., 2009), functionalization (Berry, 2009) and their detection by magnetic sensors (Megens et al., 2005). As shown in Fig.1, magnetic micro-machine has been applied in medicine. This machine is designed to move through the human body and his pathway is controlled by magnetic field.

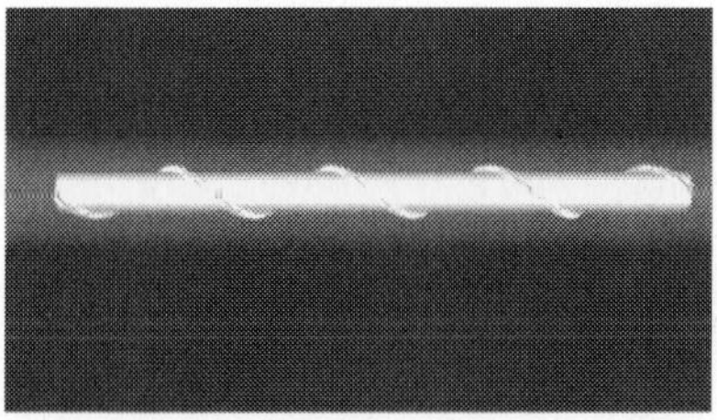

Fig. 1. Magnetic micro-machine (Adapted from Ishiyama et al., 2001)

Nowadays, accurate, rapid, cheap and selective analysis is required for clinical and industrial laboratories. Magnetoresistive biosensors seem to be among the best candidates to meet these criteria. Since the late 1990s, magnetoelectronics (Xu et al., 2008) has emerged as one of several new platform technologies for biosensor and biochip development. This technology is based on the detection of biologically functionalized micrometer or nanometer-sized magnetic labels, using high-sensitivity microfabricated magnetic-field sensors.
In recent years, giant magnetoresistance (GMR) sensors have shown a great potential as sensing elements for biomolecule detection. The resistance of a GMR sensor changes with the magnetic field applied to the sensor, so that a magnetically labeled biomolecule can induce a signal. Compared with the traditional optical detection that is widely used in

biomedicine, GMR sensors are more sensitive, portable, and give a fully electronic readout. Due to advantages of GMR materials for magnetic field measurements, such as: high sensitivity and quick response under low magnetic field, more attentions have been paid on developing GMR material for biosensors.

The chapter covers the design, fabrication and testing of both types of biosensor nanodevices. Further integration of nanosensors, microfluidics, optical and electronic functions on a single sensing circuit could lead to a complete "lab-on-chip" technological solution which could be used in medical applications. Examples of fabrication, characterization and real applications of the devices will be discussed as well as the way of their integration.

This chapter is organized as follows; an overview of the GMR sensors, a brief overview of biosensor and its potential application in clinical diagnosis, a complete description of GMR biosensors application in medical starting from a general overview and showing examples based in integrated GMR biosensor of the latest developments in this field. Finally, the future trend of this exciting GMR biosensor for medical application is discussed.

2. An overview of the GMR sensors

Magnetoresistance is defined as the change in the resistance of a material in response to an externally applied magnetic field. The first announcement of the GMR effect was reported in 1988 by Baibich (Baibich et al., 1998). They discovered that the resistance of a sandwich type multilayer with magnetizations aligned initially (in the magnetic field H = 0) antiparallel decreased more than 50% after applying an external magnetic field. Because this decrease of resistance was very large they called this effect giant magnetoresistance (GMR). Since the discovery of the giant magnetoresistance (GMR) effect in magnetic multilayer systems, sensors employing this effect have been utilized in many areas of science and technology.

The GMR material is a material that has huge magnetoresistance, good magnetic-electrical properties, so that potentially to be developed to become next generation magnetic field sensing devices like sensors. The GMR sensor has many attractive features, for example: reduction size, low-power consumption, low price as compared to other magnetic sensors and its electric and magnetic properties can be varied in very wide range.

The GMR effect is a quantum mechanical effect observed in the thin film structure consisting of ferromagnetic layers separated by nonmagnetic layers. Thin film of GMR has different structures and each structure has the effect of magnetoresistance (MR) are also different. Structure of GMR consists of a sandwich structure, the spin valve and multilayer as shown in Fig. 2.

Physics basis of the GMR effect is related to the fact that the spin of electrons has two different values (called the spin up and spin down). When these spin across the material that has been magnetized, one type of spin may be experiencing barriers (resistance) which is different than that experienced by other types of spin. This property indicates the existence of spin dependent scattering.

GMR phenomena in multilayer ferromagnetic can be explained using Mott model which was introduced as early as 1936 to explain the sudden increase in resistivity of ferromagnetic metals as they are heated above the Curie temperature (Mott, 1936). In this model: (1). electrical conductivity in metals can be described in connection with two free conduction channel in which the former relates to an electron with spin up and others associated with the electron with spin down, (2). in ferromagnetic metals the rate of scattering of spin up and spin down electrons are very different.

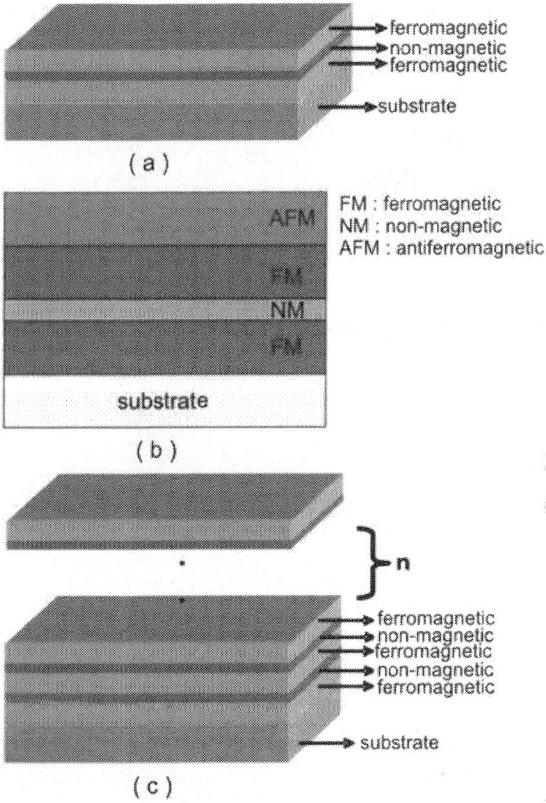

Fig. 2. Structure of GMR thin film. (a). Sandwich. (b). Spin valve. (c). Multilayer.

The GMR effect relies on the experimentally established fact that electron spin is conserved over distances of up to several tens of nanometers, which is greater than the thickness of a typical multilayer. Therefore, the electric current in the trilayer flows in two channels, one corresponding to electrons with spin projection ↑ and the other to electrons with spin projection ↓. Since the ↑ and ↓ spin channels are independent (spin is conserved) they can be regarded as two wires connected in parallel and the GMR can be explained using a simple resistor model, as shown in Fig. 3.

Consider the ferromagnetic multilayer configuration such as Fig. 3, and it is assumed that strong scattering occurs for electrons with spin antiparallel to the direction of magnetization, while the weak scattering occurs for electrons with spin parallel to the direction of magnetization. This assumption describes the asymmetry in the meetings condition at the Fermi level corresponding to Mott's second argument.

In the ferromagnetic configuration Fig. 3 (a) of the trilayer, electrons with spin ↑ are weakly scattered both in the first and second ferromagnetic layer, whereas the ↓ spin electrons are strongly scattered in both ferromagnetic layers. This is modelled by two small resistors in the spin ↑ spin channel and by two large resistors in the spin ↓ channel in the equivalent resistor network. Since the ↓ and ↑ spin channels are connected in parallel, the total resistance of the trilayer is determined by the low resistance ↑ spin channel which shorts the high-resistance ↓ spin channel. Therefore the total resistance of the trilayer in the ferromagnetic configuration is low. On the other hand, ↓ spin electrons in the antiferromagnetic configuration are strongly scattered in the first ferromagnetic layer but weakly scattered in the second ferromagnetic layer. The ↑ spin electrons are weakly scattered in the first ferromagnetic layer and strongly scattered in the second. This is modelled in Fig. 3 (b) by one large and one small resistor in each spin channel. There is no shorting and the total resistance in the antiferromagnetic configuration is much higher than in the ferromagnetic configuration.

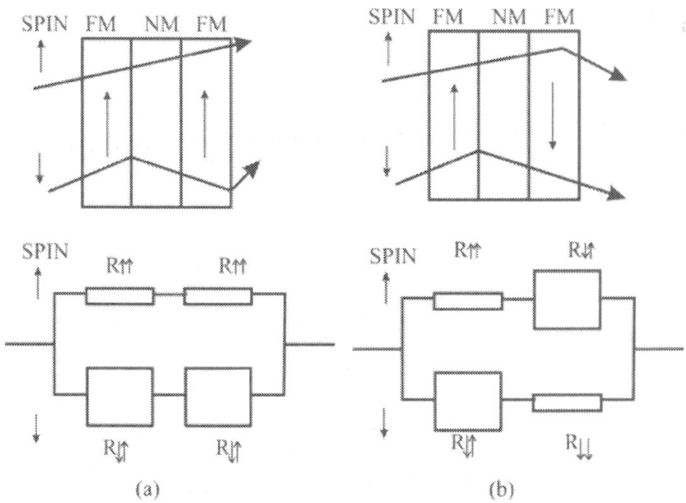

Fig. 3. Resistor model of GMR (Adapted from Mathon, 2001).

In 1988 experiments on layered thin films of ferromagnetic metal (FMs) alternated to a non-magnetic metal (NM) led to the simultaneous and independent discovery of the giant magnetoresistance (GMR) by A. Fert (Baibich et al., 1988) and P. A. Grünberg (Binasch et al., 1989). Fig. 4 shows the original results obtained by Baibich and coworkers. The (001)Fe/(001)Cr *bcc* superlattices were grown by the MBE method. The magnetoresistance was measured at 4.2 K for different thicknesses of the Cr spacer. The authors explained the GMR effect as follows. The resistivity drops when the magnetic external field overcomes the antiferromagnetic coupling and the alignment of magnetizations becomes a parallel arrangement. It was supposed that the spin-dependent scattering of the conduction electrons in the magnetic layers or at their interfaces was responsible for the GMR effect. The scattering in antiparallel alignment is much larger than in the parallel case. Complete review of the GMR can be found at (Tsymbal & Pettifor, 2001).
In this field, we also have developed GMR material with sandwich structure (Djamal et al., 2006). Recently, we have successfully developed GMR thin film with sandwich structure using dc-opposed target magnetron sputtering, and we obtained about 65 % MR value at

room temperature in NiCoFe/Cu/NiCoFe sandwich (Djamal et al., 2009a; Djamal et al., 2009b; Ramli et al., 2009; Djamal et al., 2010; Ramli et al., 2010). The GMR ratio curve for NiCoFe/Cu/NiCoFe sandwich is shown in Fig. 5, 6, 7 and 8.

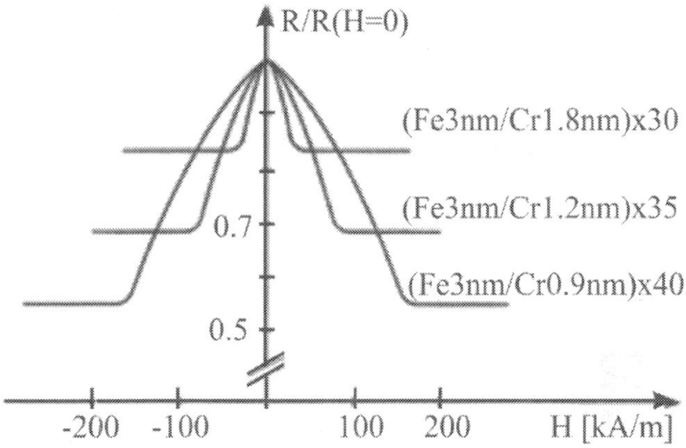

Fig. 4. The first announcement of GMR effects (Adapted from Baibich et al., 1988).

Fig. 7 shows variation of magnitude of GMR ratio versus Cu layers thickness. Their general appearance is a classical behavior of MR evolution with magnetic field that has been observed in many multilayers (Dieny et al., 1991; Tang et al., 2007; Tripathy & Adeyeye, 2007) based on ferromagnetic transition metal and a non magnetic layers. The dependence of GMR value on the non-magnetic layer thickness in magnetic multilayer and spin valves qualitatively ascribed to two factors (Parkin, 1998), ie.: (i) with increasing spacer thickness the probability of scattering increases as the conduction electrons traverse the spacer layer, which reduces the flow of electrons between the ferromagnetic layers and consequently reduces GMR; (ii) the increasing thickness of the nonmagnetic layer enhances the shunting current within the spacer, which also reduces GMR. These two contributions to GMR can be phenomenological described as the relative resistance change ΔR by the following expression:

$$\frac{\Delta R}{R} = \left(\frac{\Delta R}{R}\right)_0 \frac{exp\left(-d_{NM} / l_{NM}\right)}{\left(1 + d_{NM} / d_0\right)} \tag{1}$$

The parameter l_{NM} is related to the mean free path of the conduction electrons in the spacer layer, d_{NM} is spacer layer thickness. The parameter d_0 is an effective thickness, and $(\Delta R/R)_0$ is a normalization coefficient. The decay in GMR value with increasing Cu thickness can be described approximately:

$$\frac{\Delta R}{R} \approx \frac{1}{t_{Cu}} exp\left(-t_{Cu} / \lambda_{Cu}\right) \tag{2}$$

where t_{Cu} is the Cu thickness and λ_{Cu} describes the scattering within the Cu layer interior.

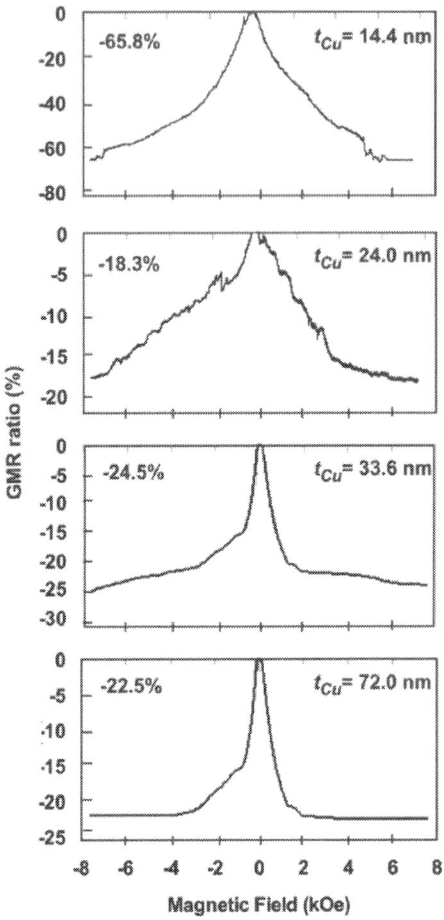

Fig. 5. The dependence of GMR ratio on the spacer layer thickness (t_{Cu}) with fixed NiCoFe layer thickness (t_{NiCoFe} = 62.5 nm).

In sandwich structure, the decrease in magnitudo of GMR ratio at low thickness of NiCoFe in Fig. 8 is due to the scattering on the outer surface like substrate or buffer layer (Dieny., 1994). This scattering significantly affects GMR, when the thickness of the ferromagnetic layer becomes smaller than the longer of the two mean-free paths associated with the spin up and spins down of electrons.

Fig. 6 shows that at the thickness of NiCoFe over 62.5 nm the magnitude GMR ratio decreases. This phenomenon could be explained by the appearance of inactive region in NiCoFe layer that shunts the current. On the other hand, the sharpness of GMR curve increases with increasing NiCoFe layer thickness, as observed in Fig. 6.

Generally, there are many sensors can be used for measuring magnetic field namely fluxgate sensor, Hall sensor, induction coil, GMR sensor, SQUID sensor and some others. Due to advantages of GMR materials for magnetic field measurements, such as: high sensitivity and quick response under low magnetic field, more attentions have been paid on developing GMR material for magnetic field sensors. Table 1 illustrates the differences between GMR and other magnetic field sensors (Han et al., 2005). Besides that, GMR material based sensors have more benefit compared to other magnetic sensors such as smaller size, lower power and lower cost (see Fig. 9).

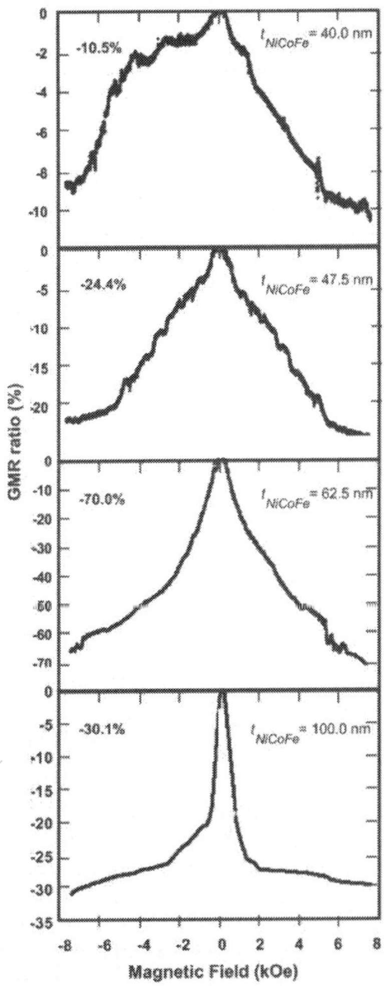

Fig. 6. The dependence of GMR ratio on the ferromagnetic layer thickness (t_{NiCoFe}) with fixed Cu layer thickness (t_{Cu} = 14.4 nm).

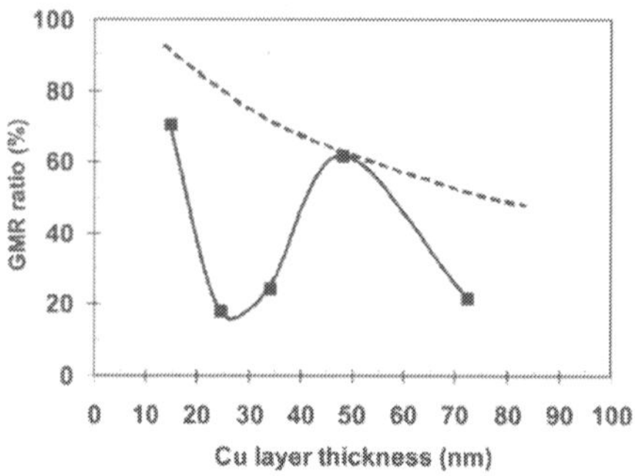

Fig. 7. Variation of magnitude of GMR ratio versus Cu layer thickness. The dotted line shows the decay of GMR ratio with increasing of Cu layer thickness as expressed in eq. (2).

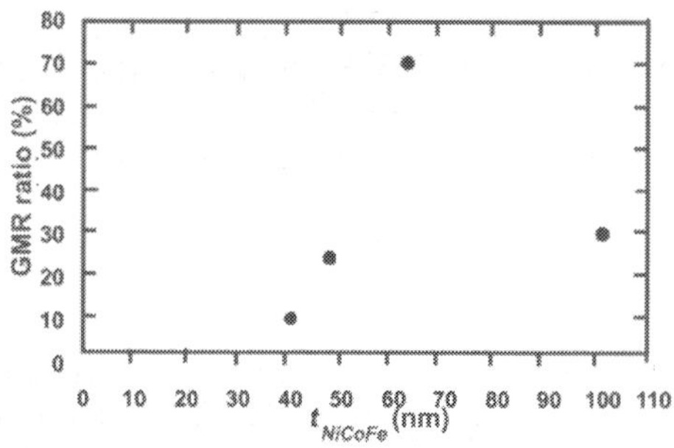

Fig. 8. Variation of magnitude of GMR ratio versus NiCoFe layer thickness.

Since the late 1990s, magnetoelectronics (Prinz, 1998) has emerged as one of several new platform technologies for biosensor and biochip development. This technology is based on the detection of biologically functionalized micrometer or nanometer-sized magnetic labels, using high-sensitivity microfabricated magnetic-field sensors. GMR biosensors seem to be among the best candidates to meet these criteria. The GMR biosensors capable of highly sensitive detection are poised to become a dominant player in the vast world of biosensors (Hall et al., 2010).

	H range (T)	Sensitivity (V/T)	Rensponse time	Power consumption	Sensor head size
GMR	10^{-12}-10^{-2}	120	1 MHz	10 mw	10-100μm
Hall	10^{-6}-10^{2}	0.65	1 MHz	10 mw	10-100μm
SQUID	10^{-14}-10^{-6}	10^{-14}	1 MHz	10 mw	10-100μm
Flux gate	10^{-12}-10^{-2}	3.2	5 kHz	1 w	10-20 mm

Table 1. Comparison of magnetic field sensors commonly used.

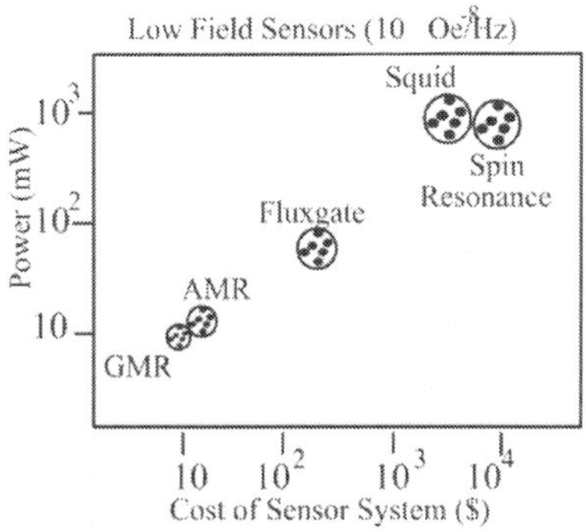

Fig. 9. Comparison of power, price and size of some magnetic sensors

3. Biosensor and its potential application in clinical diagnostic

A biosensor is generally defined as an analytical device, which makes use of a biological molecular recognition component connected to a transducer to generate a quantifiable electronic output signal, in response to a biological or chemical analyte (Li et al., 2006). Biosensors are under intense development for a wide range of applications from medical diagnostics to countering bio-terrorism.

Research in this area can be divided into three directions. The first direction focuses on the development of the synthesis of magnetic beads with desired magnetic properties that can be engaged with a high degree of specificity as microarrays. The development of high-precision on-chip electrostatic or magnetic field gradient architectures became the main mention of the second direction. This chip has capability to manipulate functionalized single magnetic beads as well as the microfluidic circuits. Fig. 10 shows one example of functionalized single magnetic beads. The third area is development of biocompatible solid-state sensors for quantitative magnetic beads. Two type of this sensor can be seen in Fig. 11.

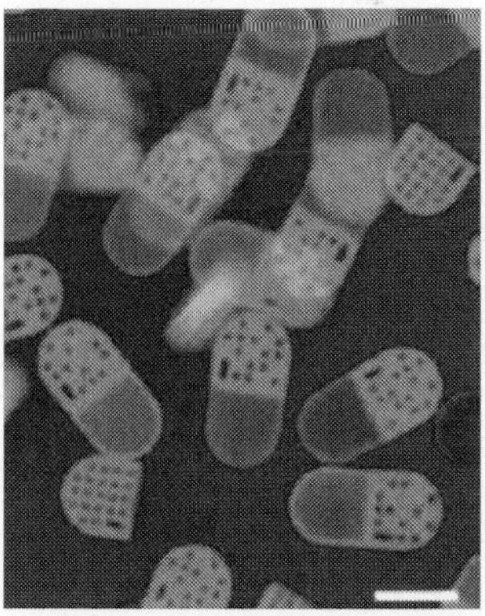

Fig. 10. Functionalized single magnetic beads fabricated by continuous-flow lithography. Scale bar represents 100 μm [Adapted from Pregibon et al, 2007].

The first sensor based on GMR effect and the other based on the Tunneling Magnetoresistance (TMR). Both of these sensors have the same structure, only the non-magnetic metal spacer in GMR sensor is replaced with a very thin insulating barrier. This insulating barrier commonly made from Al_2O_3 or MgO.

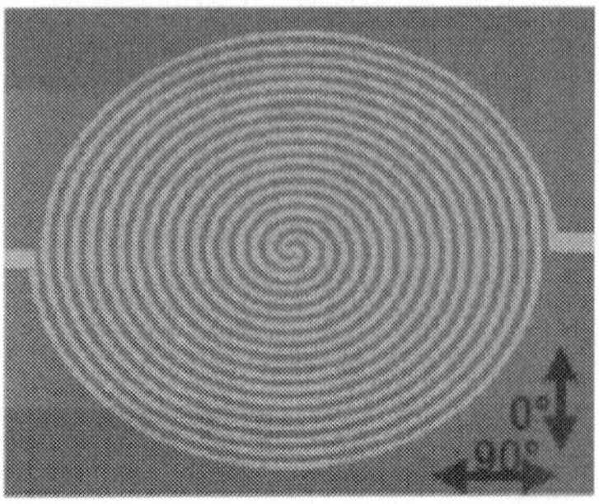

(a)

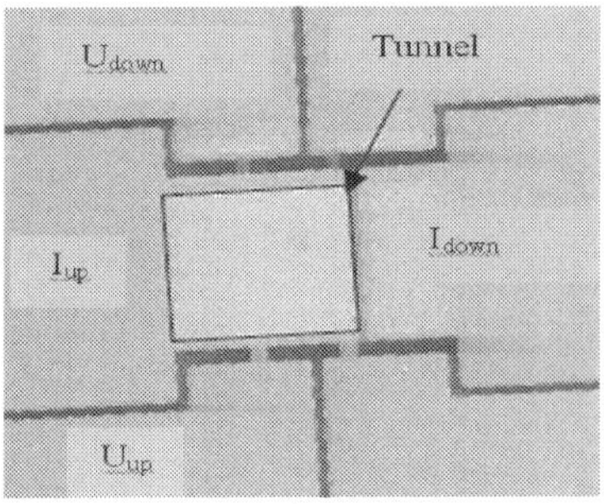

(b)

Fig. 11. (a). GMR sensor. (b). TMR (Tunnelling magnetoresistance) [Adapted from Ishiyama et al., 2001].

4. The GMR biosensor and its application in clinical diagnostic

The development of robust, versatile and high throughput biosensing platforms is expected to have far-reaching implications in medicine, point-of-care clinical diagnostics, pharmaceutical drug development, and genomic and proteomic research. Enabled by rapidly emerging nanotechnologies (nanoparticles, nanotubes, and nanowires) and microfabrication techniques (MEMS, microfluidics, and CMOS), several new sensing platforms have been proposed and tested for biomedical applications, one of them is GMR biosensors.

As we have known that the detecting elements of biosensors work in different physicochemical ways: optical, piezoelectric, electrochemical, thermometric, and magnetic. Biosensors using magnetics utilize the magnetic field created by magnetic particles that bind to target molecules in a biological assay (Fig. 12).

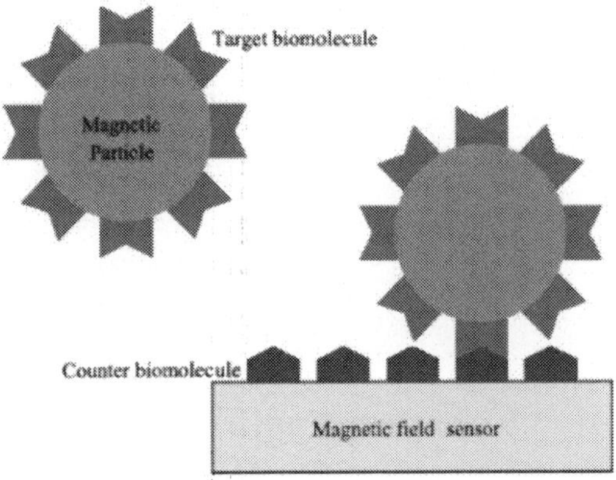

Fig. 12. Schematic of magnetically labeled biomolecule detection in a biosensor. Target biomolecules bound with a magnetic particle interact with magnetoresistive sensor-bound counter biomolecules to be detected.

A first model for the detection of magnetic markers by GMR-type magnetoresistive sensors was published by Tondra, et al., 1999 in NVE Inc. (Tondra et al., 1999). He concluded that single magnetic markers of any size can be detected as long as the sensor has about the same size as the marker and the insulating protection layer is thin enough.
Baselt et al. (1998) were the first to demonstrate using GMR sensors as biosensors and several groups have continued the research and development of magnetic biosensing technology (Ferreira et al., 2003; Rife et al., 2003; Reiss et al., 2005; Xu et al., 2008; Osterfeld et al., 2008; Koets et al., 2009; Hall et al., 2010).
The incorporation of GMR structures in bacteria sensing is illustrated in Fig. 13 by Millen, (Millen et al., 2005). Generally, the surface of the GMR sensing region is modified to allow the binding of capture antibody. When the GMR structure is exposed to a sample solution that contains target antigens, complex binding between the target antigen and antibody occurs. This is followed by the addition of antibody coated magnetic particles that subsequently labeled the target antigens and form a series of sandwich-like structures.

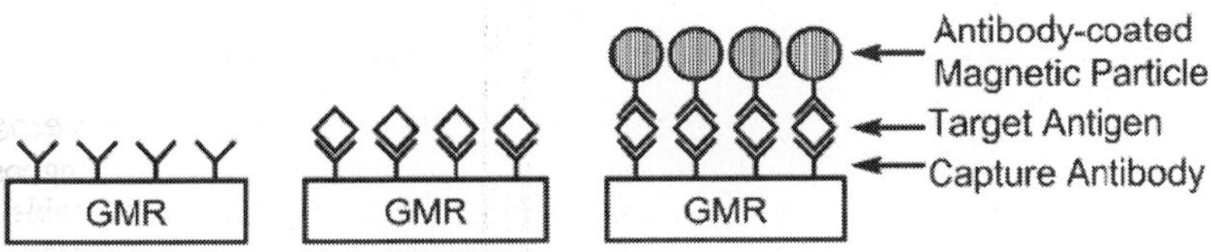

Fig. 13. Bacteria sensing using a GMR biosensor (Adapted from Millen et al., 2005).

In order to detect the magnetic particles bound on a GMR structure surface, an external magnetic field is applied in the z-direction, as illustrated in Fig. 14 (Rife et al., 2003). The GMR biosensors detect the stray field from the magnetic tag to infer the number of captured analytes. Bound magnetic particles that are exposed to a magnetic field will generate magnetic induction in the x-direction. Since the GMR structure detects only the x-component of the magnetic field, the external magnetic field in the z-direction does not have any effect on the detection.

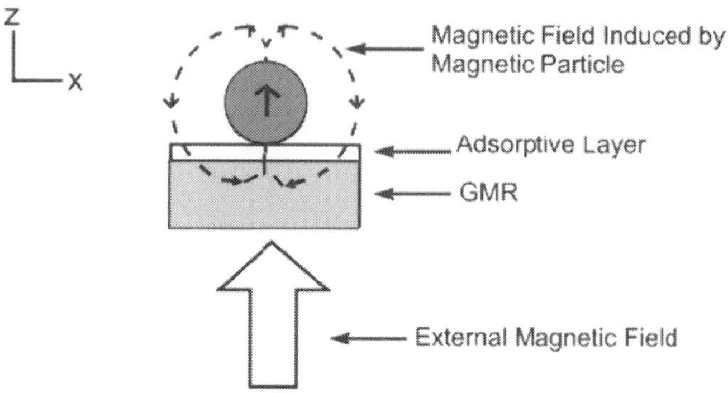

Fig. 14. Detection of magnetic particle on GMR biosensor (Adapted from Rife et al., 2003).

5. Future trend in GMR biosensor for clinical diagnostic

A number of magnetic sensors have been designed and developed as detector for magnetic markers. Although their principles have different operation, there are two kinds of type that have been developed namely mass-coverage sensors with active areas of hundred square arrays and single-bead detector. With excellent signal to noise ratio, GMR biosensor is one of mass-coverage sensors. Freitas et al. reported that they can made mass-coverage GMR sensor to detect DNA from genes associated with cystic fibrosis (Freitas et al., 2004). The other group also reported real-time measurement of the progress of binding of functionalised bead to sensor in liquid (Golub et al., 1999; Graham et al., 2003). One of mass-coverage sensors based on GMR can be seen in Fig. 15.

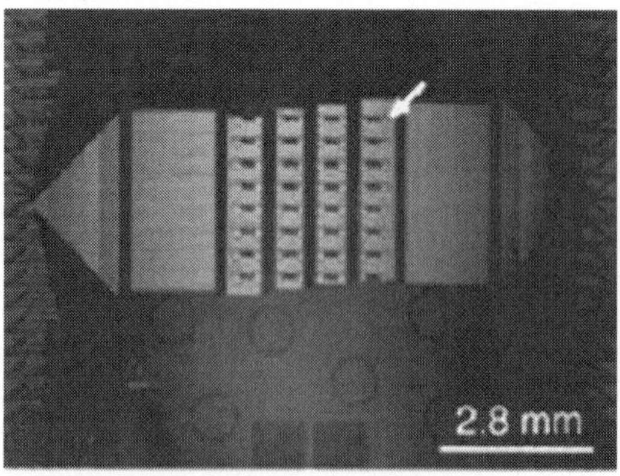

Fig. 15. Image of magnetonanosensor chip with 64 sensors in an 8 x 8 array. The arrow indicates a single chip. [Adapted from Gaster et al., 2009]

GMR biosensors rely on a magnetic tag. Biosensors utilizing magnetic tags offer several key advantages over other sensing modalities (Hall et al., 2010). First, the biological samples (blood, urine, serum, etc.) naturally lack any detectable magnetic content, providing a sensing platform with a very low background level and thus lower detection limit of analytes. Second, the sensors can be arrayed and multiplexed to perform analysis on a panel of proteins or nucleic acids in a single assay. Lastly, the sensors can be manufactured cheaply, in mass quantities, to be deployed in a one-time use disposable format. For these reasons, magnetic biosensors are an attractive and competitive alternative to optical techniques.

6. Conclusion

The GMR biosensor are best candidates for future device based on lab-on a-chip, compact and inexpensive detection units in clinical diagnostic. Compared to complex and expensive optical detection systems, the GMR biosensor measures electrical signal directly from the sensor, and makes a low-cost, highly portable device feasible. On other hand, GMR biosensors are more sensitive, portable and give a fully electronic readout.

7. Acknowledgement

This work was partially supported by Doctoral Dissertation Research Grant (Hibah Penelitian Disertasi Doktor) No: 501/SP2H/PP/ DP2M/VI/2010 and Competency Grant (Hibah Kompetensi) No: 407/SP2H/PP/DP2M/VI/2010 The Ministry of National Education Republic of Indonesia.

8. References

Baibich, M. N, Broto, J. M, Fert, A, Nguyen V. D, Petroff, F, Etienne, F, Creutz, P, Friederich, A, and Chazelas, A, (1988). Giant Magnetoresistance of (001) Fe/(001) Cr Magnetic Superlattices, *Phys. Rev. Lett.* 68 2472 - 2475.

Berry, C. C., (2009). Progress in functionalization of magnetic nanoparticles for applications in biomedicine. J Phys D 42:224,003.

Binasch, G., Grunberg, P., Saurenbach, F., Zinn, W., (1989). Enhanced magnetoresistance in layered magnetic structures with antiferromagnetic interlayer exchange, *Phys. Rev.* B 39, 4828-4830.

Dieny, B., Speriosu, V. S., Metin, S., Parkin, S. S. P., Gurney, B. A., Baumgart, P., Wilhoit, D. R., (1991). Magnetotransport properties of magnetically soft spin-valve structures. *J.Appl.Phys.* 69, 4774-4780.

Dieny, B., (1994). Giant magnetoresistance in spin-valve multilayers. *J. Magn. Magn. Mater.* 136, 335-359.

Djamal, M., Darsikin, Saragi, T., Barmawi, M., (2006). Design and development of magnetic sensors based on giant magnetoresistance (GMR) materials, *Material Science Forum*, Vol. 517, 207-211.

Djamal, M., Ramli, Yulkifli, Khairurrijal, (2009a). Effect of Cu Layer Thickness on Giant Magnetoresistance Properties of NiCoFe/Cu/NiCoFe Sandwich. Proceeding of *ICCAS-SICE* 2009 Fukuoka, Japan, August 18-21, 2009, 365-368.

Djamal, M., Ramli, Khairurrijal, (2009b). Giant Magnetoresistance Material and Its Potensial for Biosensor Applications, Proc. of ICICI-BME 2009, November 23-25, 2009, 19-24.

Djamal, M., Ramli, Yulkifli, Suprijadi, Khairurrijal, (2010). Biosensor Based on Giant Magnetoresistance Material. *International Journal of E-Health and Medical Communications*, 1(3), 1-17.

Ferreira, H. A, Graham, D. L, Freitas, P. P, Cabral, J. M. S, (2003). Biodetection using magnetically labeled biomolecules and arrays of spin valve sensors. *Journal of Applied Physics* 93, 7281–7286.

Freitas, P. P, Ferreira, H. A, Graham, D. L, Clarke, L, Amaral, M, Martins, V, Fonseca, L, and Cabral, J. S,(2004). Magnetoresistive biochips. *Europhys News* 36(6):224–226.

Gaster, R. S, Hall, D. A, Nielsen, C. H, Osterfeld, S. J, Yu, H, Mach, K. E, Wilson, R. J, Murmann, B, Liao, J. C, Gambhir, S. S, and Wang, S. X, (2009). Matrix-insensitive protein assays push the limits of biosensors in medicine. *Nat Med* 15.1327–1332.

Golub, T. R, Slonim, D. K, Tamayo, P, Huard, C, Gaasenbeek, M, Mesirov, J. P, Coller, H, Loh, M. L, Downing, J. R, Caligiuri, M. A, Bloomfield, C. D, and Lander, E. S (1999). Molecular classification of cancer: class discovery and class prediction by gene expression monitoring. Science 286:531–537.

Graham, D. L, Ferreira, H. A, Bernardo, J, Freitas, P. P, and Cabral, J. M. S, (2003). Single magnetic microsphere placement and detection on-chip using current line designs with integrated spin valve sensors: biotechnological applications. J Appl Phys 91(10): 7786–7788.

Hall, D. A, Gaster, R. S. Lin, T, Osterfeld, S. J, Han, S, Murmann, B, and Wang, S. X, (2010). GMR biosensor arrays: A system perspective. *Biosensors and Bioelectronics*. 25 (2010) 2051–2057.

Han, M., Liang, D.F., Deng, L.J., (2005). Sensors development using its unusual properties of Fe/Co-based amorphous soft magnetic wire, *Journal of Materials Science*, 40, 5573-5580.

Ishiyama. K, Sendoh, M, Yamazaki, A and Arai, K. I, (2001). Swimming micro-machine driven by magnetic torque. *Sensor and Actuator* A 91. 141-144.

Ishiyama, K., et al., (2009). Magnetic wireless actuator for medical applications., Lecutre Note of Biosensor from G.Reiss.

Koets, M., van der Wijk, T., van Eemeren, J., van Amerongen, A., Prins, M.,(2009). *Biosensors and Bioelectronics*. 24, 1893–1898.

Li, G, Sun, S, Wilson, R. J, White, R. L, Pourmand, N, and Wang, S. X, (2006). Spin valve sensors for ultrasensitive detection of superparamagnetic nanoparticles for biological applications. *Sens. Actuators* A 126, 98–106.

Mathon, J., (2001). Phenomenological Theory of Giant Magnetoresistance, In M. Ziese & M.J Thornton (Ed.), *Spin Electronics*.(pp. 71-88). Springer-Verlag, Berlin.

Megens, M, Prins, M, (2005). Magnetic biochips: a new option forsensitive diagnostics. *J Magn Magn Mater* 293:702–708.

Millen, R. L, Kawaguchi, T, Granger, M. C, and Porter, M. D, (2005). Giant Magnetoresistive Sensors and Superparamagnetic Nanoparticles: A Chip-Scale Detection Strategy for Immunosorbent Assays. *Anal. Chem.* 77, 6581–6587.

Mott. N. F, (1936). The Resistance and Thermoelectric Properties of the Transition Metals, *Proc. Royal Soc. Lond A*. 156, 368-382.

Osterfeld, S. J, Yu, H, Gaster, R. S, Caramuta, S, Xu, L, Han, S, Hall, D. A, Wilson, R, Sun, S, White, R. L, Davis, R. W, Pourmand, N, and Wang, S. X, (2008). *Proceedings of the National Academy of Sciences*. 105, 20637–20640.

Pankhurst, Q. A, Thanh, N. K. T, Jones, S. K, and Dobson, J, (2009). Progress in application of magnetic nanoparticles in biomedicine. J Phys D 42:224,001.

Parkin, S. S. P, (1998). The Magic of Magnetic Multilayers, *IBM Journal of Research and Development*; Vol.42, No.1, pp.3 -6.

Pregibon, D. C, Toner, M, and Doyle, P. S, (2007). Multifunctional encoded particles for high-throughput biomolecule analysis. *Science* 315.1393–1396.

Prinz, G. A, (1998). Device Physics-Magnetoelectronics, *Science*, 282, 1660-1663.

Ramli, Muhtadi, A. H, Sahdan, M. F, Haryanto, F, Khairurrijal and Djamal, M, (2010). Effect of Ferromagnetic Layer Thickness on the Giant Magnetoresistance Properties of NiCoFe/Cu/NiCoFe Sandwich. Proceeding *3rd Asian Physic Symposium* (APS) 2009, ISBN: 978-979-98010-5-0, Bandung, 22 - 23 July 2009. 65 - 67.

Ramli, Muhtadi, A.H., Sahdan, M.F., Haryanto, F., Khairurrijal, Djamal, M., (2010). The Preliminary Study Of Giant Magnetoresistance Sensor For Detection Of Oxygen In Human Blood. *AIP Conf. Proc.* -- December 23, 2010 -- Volume 1325. 309-312.

Reiss, G., Brueckl, H., Huetten, A., Schotter, J., Brzeska, M., Panhorst, M., Sudfeld, D., Becker, A., Kamp, P.B., Puehler, A., Wojczykowski, K., Jutzi, P., (2005). Magnetoresistive sensors and magnetic nanoparticles for biotechnology. *Journal of Materials Research*. 20, 3294–3302.

Rife, J. C, Miller, M. M, Sheehan, P. E, Tamanaha, C. R, Tondra, M, and Whitman, L. J, (2003). Design and Performance of GMR Sensors for the Detection of Magnetic Microbeads in *Biosensors Sensors and Actuators A: Physical* 107, 209–218.

Roca, A. G, Costo, R, Rebolledo, A. F, Veintemillas, V. S, Tartaj, P, Gonzalez, C. T, Morales, M. P, and Serna, C. J, (2009). Progress in the preparation of magnetic nanoparticles for applications in biomedicine. *J Phys D* 42:224,002.

Tang, X. T, Wang, G. C, and Shima, M, (2007). Layer thickness dependence of CPP giant magnetoresistance ini individual CoNi/Cu multilayer nanowires grown by electrodeposition. *Phys. Rev. B* 75 134404.

Tondra, M, Porter, M, Lipert, R. J, (1999). Model for detection of immobilized superparamagnetic nanosphere assays labels using giant magnetoresistive sensors. *J. Vac. Sci. Technol. A* 18 (4), 1125–1129.

Tripathy, D and Adeyeye, A. O, (2007). Effect of spacer layer thickness on the magnetic and magnetotransport properties of Fe_3O_4/Cu/$Ni_{80}Fe_{20}$ spin valve structures. Phys. Rev. B 75, 012403.

Tsymbal, E.Y and Pettifor, D. G, (2001). *Perspectives of Giant Magnetoresistance*, in Solid State Physics, ed. by H. Ehrenreich and F. Spaepen, Vol. 56 , Academic Press, 113-237.

Xu, L, Yu, H, Michael, S. A, Han, S. J, Osterfeld, S, White, R. L, Pourmand, N, and Wang, S. X, (2008). Giant magnetoresistive biochip for DNA detection and HPV genotyping. *Biosensors and Bioelectronics* 24, 99–103.

7

Label-free Biosensors for Health Applications

Cai Qi[1], George F. Gao[2,3] and Gang Jin[4]
[1]*Institute of Food Safety, Chinese Academy of inspection and quarantine*
[2]*Beijing Institutes of Life Science, Chinese Academy of Sciences*
[3]*CAS Key Laboratory of Pathogenic Microbiology and Immunology, Institute of Microbiology, Chinese Academy of Sciences*
[4]*Institute of Mechanics, Chinese Academy of Sciences*
China

1. Introduction

Biosensors are widely used for health applications. Indeed, the current success of biosensors is attributed to the extraordinary demands of disease diagnoses and control, as well as the ability of biosensors to offer a convenient, hygienic, rapid, and compact method for personal monitoring. Biosensors offer enormous potential for detecting a wide range of analytes in the health care and food industries and in environmental monitoring. As quoted, MicroChips president John Santini expects the technology to be used as in-the-flesh physicians within 10 years: "It's a very exciting time," he says. "Our next step is a manually, wirelessly controlled biosensor that detects and treats an acute condition, and then a biosensor that will approximate an artificial organ; it'll sense a condition and respond automatically without user intervention." In this chapter, we review applications and advances in biosensor technology, focusing on four applications in the health field: 1) investigation of the interaction of antigens with antibodies produced in healthy and diseased subjects, 2) disease markers and virus detection, 3) clinical diagnosis and control of emerging infectious diseases, and 4) market potentials. Specifically, we discuss the application of a label-free biosensor based on ellipsometry in the development of future biosensors, the current and future clinical applications of this technology, and its viability. The goal of this chapter is to provide a brief description of the role of biosensors in *in vitro* diagnostics and scientific research related to the health field. Readers interested in competing or related technologies (e.g., ellipsometry, microfluidics, and surface modification technologies) are referred to one of several excellent recent reviews (Jin et al., 2011; Qi et al., 2009a; Zhang, et al., 2005). In the following section, health applications are described using a label-free biosensor based on ellipsometry.

2. Label-free biosensor based on ellipsometry

2.1 Biomedical application history

The first publication concerning biological application of antigen and antibody is a paper by Langmuir and Schaefer dating back to 1936 (Hans, 1998, as cited in Langmuir& Schaefer, 1936). The interaction between an antigen-immobilized substrate and the corresponding antibodies was observed with an optical technique. Although this original 'immunosensor' was over 59 years old at the time, the concept of a biosensor was first brought forward in 1995 by Jin and Hans and used to study biomolecular interactions (Jin et al., 1995, 1996). A biomolecule layer composed of a common protein, such as fibrinogen, human serum albumin, or human immunoglobulin G, was spread on the surface of the sensor. The interaction between general proteins such as fibrinogen and an antibody against fibrinogen was then investigated. However, biosensor detection of clinical samples was only recently developed, such as detection of disease markers and viruses and investigation of interactions between antibodies and antigens related to clinical diagnoses (Jin et al., 2011; Qi et al., 2009a).

2.2 Technical characteristics of the biosensor based on ellipsometry

The principle of the biosensor has been discussed in several reports (Jin et al., 2011; Z.H. Wang et al., 2006). Here, we list some key technical characteristics of biosensors based on ellipsometry:

- Label-free

When the interaction between biomolecules occurs, the variation of the molecular mass surface concentration on the surface is identified by the biosensor based on ellipsometry without label (e.g., the horseradish peroxidase used in enzyme-linked immunosorbent assays).

- High-throughput

Combined with a microfluidic array reactor, which fabricates the chips, the biosensor based on ellipsometry has become an automatic and high-throughput system by adding ligand, washing, blocking, and reacting samples. Recently, an 8×6 biomolecule reactor-array was developed as a promising technique for a parallel protein assay. The 48 protein arrays in the 8×6 matrix are shown in Figure 1 (Jin, 2008). Interaction of common protein, detection of five hepatitis B virus markers in patient serum, detection of different ladder concentrations, and the detection sensitivity of CD146 (known as the melanoma cell adhesion molecule or cell surface glycoprotein MUC18) (Guezguez B, 2007) are presented on the chip.

- Rapid

Using the automatic program of the microfluidic array reactor to add ligands, washing, blocking, and reacting samples, ligands screening and detection of markers can be accomplished in 1 to 2 h.

- Low sample consumption

Consumption of ligands and samples is on the microliter level. For example, in hepatitis B virus detection, hepatitis B virus ligand consumption is 10 μl/area (The area is a small squareness area, see Figure 1.), and hepatitis B virus serum consumption is 40 μl/area (Qi, et al. 2009a). Enzyme-linked immunosorbent assays in milliliter level require a larger volume of the same concentration.

- Low damage to the biomolecules

The biosensor works via an optical, reflection-based technique that uses polarized light to determine the optical properties of a sample (Z.H. Wang, et al., 2003a). It is almost "touch-free" to read the detection result, so there is a decreased effect to bioactivity than, for instance, atomic force microscopy and surface-enhanced laser desorption/ionization.

- High sensitivity

The biosensor displays different detection sensitivity toward different samples. For example, the sensitivity of the biosensor for detecting antigen markers, such as hepatitis B virus surface antigen, reaches 1 ng/ml (Qi, et al. 2009a), while the detection sensitivity of CD146 is < 1 ng/ml (see Figure 1: F5, F6, and F7 areas).

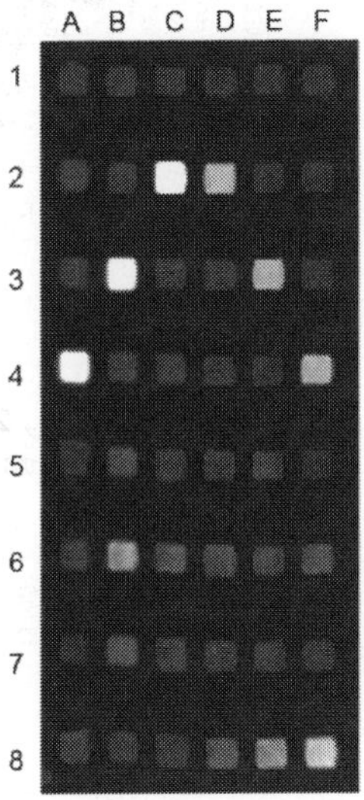

Array	Detailed reactants
C1	Ligand HBsAb
B1	HBsAg negative sample / Ligand HBsAb
A1	HBsAg standard sample (1ng/ml) / Ligand HBsAb
F1	Ligand HBsAg
E1	HBsAb negative sample / Ligand HBsAg
D1	HBsAb standard sample (1ng/ml) / Ligand HBsAg
A5, B5, C5, D5, E5	Ligand five marks of hepatitis (HBcAg,HBeAg,HBeAb,HBsAg, HBsAb)
A6, B6, C6, D6, E6	Hepatitis positive serum / Ligand five marks of hepatitis
A7, B7, C7, D7, E7	Hepatitis negative serum / Ligand five marks of hepatitis
A8, E2, F2, F3, D3, D4, E4	Ligand IgG
D2, E3, F4	Anti-IgG / Ligand IgG
B8-F8	Anti-IgG (with concentration of 1, 10, 10^3, 10^4, 10^5ng/ml) / Ligand IgG
A2, A3, B2, B4, C3, C4	Ligand FIB
C2, B3, A4	Anti-FIB / Ligand FIB
F5	Ligand CD146 (AA98)
F6,F7	CD146 positive serum (< 1ng/ml) / Ligand CD146

Fig. 1. Forty-eight protein arrays in a matrix. Left: The visual result of a protein micro-array. Right: The detailed reactants relative to the left graph (Jin, 2008).

- Automatic control

Some parameters of the microfluidic array reactor, such as the position number of the sample plate, flow velocity in the microfluidic array reactor of sample or ligand, time of immobilization or reaction, and number of cycles, can be edited in the automatic program.

- Visualization of results

Visualized gray-scale images are offered by imaging ellipsometry in several seconds, which is shown on a computer screen. The target interacting ligands on the surface can be identified by values in gray-scale with associated software.

- Quantitative detection

Combined with the calibration curve method, disease markers and viruses in samples can be detected easily and quantitatively with the label-free biosensor.

2.3 Operational process of the biosensor based on ellipsometry

The operational process of the biosensor, which includes surface modification, ligand immobilization, biomolecule interaction, and result reading, is shown in Figure 2.

Surface modification is a process by which chemical reagents for reactive groups on the silicone surface for biomolecule immobilization Surface modification has two obvious functions: one is the presentation of ligand on the biosensing surface; and the other is to prevent nonspecific binding (Jin, 2008). Presently, surface modification methods include physical adsorption, chemical covalent immobilization, and biologic modification. Physical adsorption is seldom used because the immobilized proteins suffer partial denaturation and tend to leach or wash off of the surface and compete with adsorption (Bhatia, et al., 1989).

Chemical covalent immobilization is often used to immobilize proteins due to the strong, stable linkage, and biological modification is a future direction because it provides oriented immobilization and better biological compatibility. Aldehyde modification, carboxyl modification, and biologically oriented immobilization are often used in biomedical applications (Qi, et al., 2010, 2009b; Z.H. Wang & Jin, 2004, 2003a).

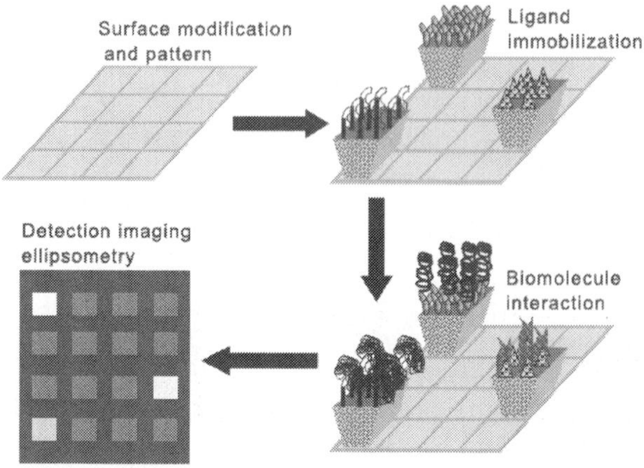

Fig. 2. Operational process of the biosensor based on ellipsometry. Antibodies (or antigens) can be immobilized as ligands to each patterned area as a bio-probe on the modified surface of a silicon substrate. Each bio-probe can capture its corresponding antigens (or antibodies) in a test sample pumped by microfluidic reactor. When the corresponding antigens (or antibodies) in the solution interact with the bio-probes, forming a complex, the surface concentration becomes higher than the initial bio-probe layer. The distribution of the lateral protein layer pattern is simultaneously detected by imaging ellipsometry, which may further point to the existence of antigens (or antibodies) in the tested solution (Jin, 2008).

3. Applications in the health field

In the field of human health, there is an increasing demand for inexpensive and reliable sensors to quickly detect and analyze various and rapidly changing disease markers. For example, patients frequently display rapid variations in biochemical levels of disease markers such as C-reactive protein that require instant assays to detect. Indeed, early detection and diagnosis can be used to greatly reduce the cost of patient care associated with the advanced stages of many diseases. More than a hundred types of proteins recognized as diseases markers can be detected by traditional analytical techniques such as enzyme-linked immunosorbent assays. However, based on the above features of the ellipsometry-based biosensor, it has also been widely used to detect and monitor biomolecule interactions, especially for biomedical applications. A sample focusing on tumor marker detection is shown in Figure 3.

The ability to detect pathogenic and physiologically relevant biomolecules in the body with high sensitivity and specificity offers the opportunity for early diagnosis and treatment of diseases.

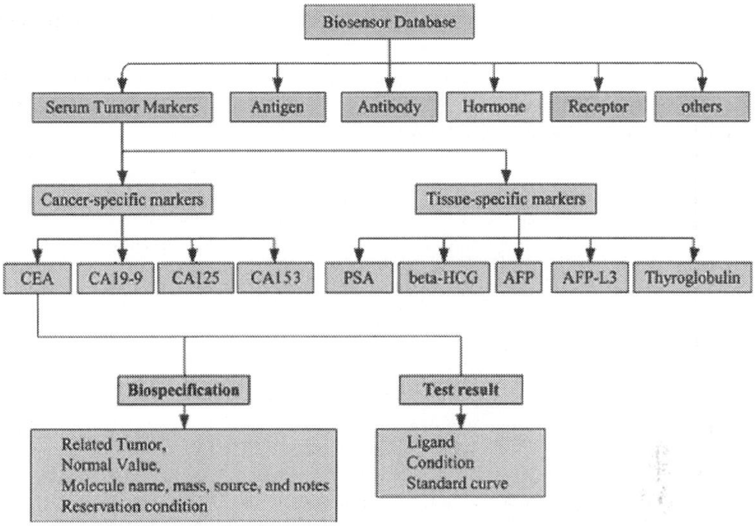

Fig. 3. Application of the biosensor. The use of biosensors to detect tumor markers in serum has spread widely (Jin, 2011).

3.1 The interaction of antigens with antibodies in healthy and diseased subjects

The initial impetus for advancing biosensors based on ellipsometry came from detection of the interaction of general antibodies and antigens, and some basic methods have been established, such as the ligand immobilization, high specificity probe screening, protein delivery, biomolecule affinity presentation on a chip, specific interactions, the influence of nonspecific binding, detection sensitivity, sample consumption, and calibration curves for quantitative detection.

3.1.1 Detection of antigen-antibody interactions

In biomedicine, human fibrinogen, hepatitis B surface antigen, human immuoglobulin G, and human serum albumin are often used as mode proteins. Using the aforementioned proteins as models with the biosensor, the feasibility is shown in Figure 4. Significant increases of gray-scale value appear in the square areas exposed to the corresponding target (Jin, et al., 2003). These results demonstrate that target samples can be identified by the ellipsometry-based biosensor.

3.1.2 Real-time detection of the antibody-antigen interaction

The biosensor based on ellipsometry can monitor protein interactions in situ and in real time to provide protein interaction kinetics information, such as association rate, dissociation rate, and affinity constants. Some special operation details of real-time detection are shown.

- Model proteins were prepared and immobilized on the substrate;
- The chip was inserted into the reaction cell;
- A mixture of antiserum containing corresponding antibody was poured into the reaction cell;

- A series of images (in gray-scale) of several binding processes between antibodies in solution and antigens were recorded by the biosensor; and
- The surface concentrations of analytes in the analytical areas of each image were measured and plotted versus time to determine the real-time binding curves.

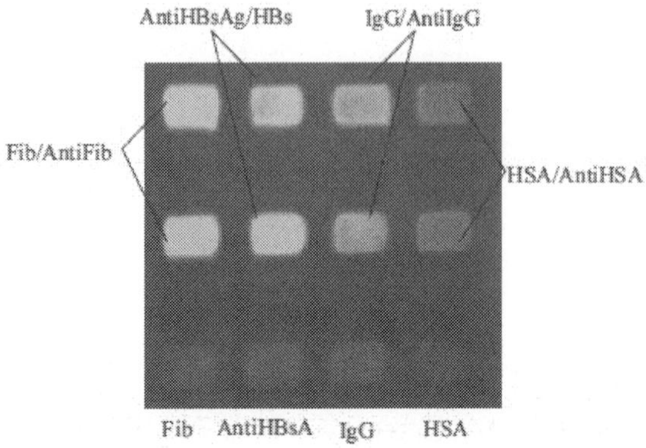

Fig. 4. Detection of several model proteins using the biosensor based on ellipsometry. Model proteins Fib, AntiHBsA, IgG and HSA were immobilized in four different columns, respectively. Phosphate-buffered saline was added to one area as a reference control. Corresponding target was then added to the other two areas in the column. (Z.H. Wang & Jin, 2003b)

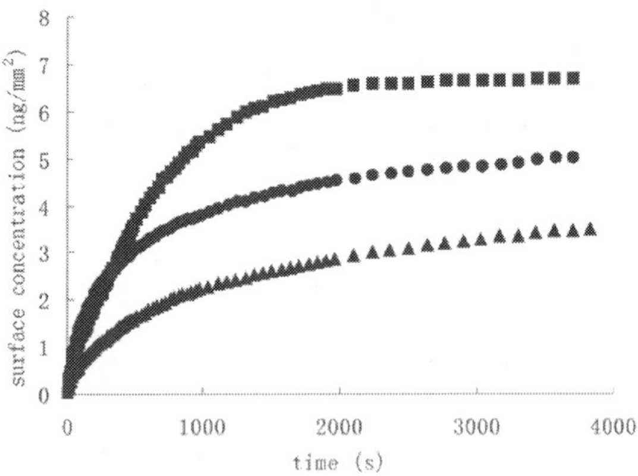

Fig. 5. Binding curves of anti-fibrinogen/fibrinogen (■), anti-human immunoglobulin/human immunoglobulin (●), and anti-human serum albumin/human serum albumin (▲) obtained by the biosensor (Z.H. Wang & Jin, 2003b).

The real-time binding curves are shown in Figure 5. Detailed data processing and kinetics analysis was performed according to the method described in the literature (Malmborg, et al., 1992). In a clinical setting, a patient's serum is a mixture similar to that used to generate

Figure 5, containing antibodies against fibrinogen, human serum albumin, and human immunoglobulin. A chip contains many immobilized ligands that bind to the same marker in serum but with different binding affinities. The biosensor offers a convenient way to compare these ligands' binding affinities under the same conditions, and ligands with high affinity can be screened. The convenient way comparing these ligands' binding affinities might compare the effectiveness of drug and screen drug, so the ability to sense multiple interactions in real-time makes the biosensor particularly well suited for monitoring disease progress, screening for highly effective drugs, and understanding disease mechanisms.

The interaction of antigens and antibodies produced in healthy and diseased subjects (e.g., hepatitis B markers antibodies and antigens (Qi, et al., 2009a), severe acute respiratory syndrome virus particles and antibodies (Qi, et al., 2006a), ricin antibody screening (ricin found in castor beans is one of the most potent plant toxins) (Niu, et al., 2010), and others) has been studied by the biosensor based on ellipsometry. These studies demonstrate the biosensor's use for health applications.

3.2 Disease markers and virus detection

Protein markers should be specific and sensitive and have prognostic value. Efforts to discover disease markers have focused on elucidating serum molecules that have diagnostic and prognostic value (Schena, 2005). High-throughput biosensors, including the biosensor based on ellipsometry, may shorten the time required to find disease markers. In this respect, biosensors are the best choice among the current techniques.

3.2.1 Qualitative detection of five hepatitis B virus markers

Hepatitis B virus is a human hepadnavirus that causes acute and chronic hepatitis and hepatocellular carcinoma (Bai, et al., 2003). The detection of hepatitis B virus markers is clinically important for the diagnosis of infection with this virus (Chen, et al., 2006). Five markers of hepatitis B virus (including hepatitis B surface antigen, the hepatitis B surface antibody, hepatitis B e antigen, hepatitis B e antibody, and hepatitis B core antibody) are a group of general markers used in the monitoring of hepatitis B virus infection. Following key steps of detection markers were operated for clinical application:

- Screening for highly effective probes;
- Detection sensitivity; and
- Optimization of detection conditions.

Presently, several probes can be simultaneously compared by the biosensor on one chip, which is shown in Figure 6. For the same target, different probes present different values in the grayscale, which indicates that the various probes have different bioactivities. Thus, highly effective probes were found for sensitive clinical diagnosis.

Sensitivity is important for hepatitis B marker detection. Hepatitis B surface antibody and hepatitis B surface antigen national positive reference samples (from the National Institute for the Control of Pharmaceutical and Biological Products (China)) were detected by the biosensor in 2009. The detection sensitivity of hepatitis B surface antigen is 1 ng/ml, and the detection sensitivity of hepatitis B surface antibody is > 1 IU/ml. Thus, the sensitivity has already reached clinical standards.

The biosensor based on ellipsometry permits multiplexed analysis. It can detect the five Hepatitis B markers of several patients simultaneously in about 1 h, proving its feasibility in clinical diagnosis. High affective probes increase sensitivity and resolving power. Other biosensor advantages, such as higher sensitivity, a simplified process, and short test time, are also significant for rapid diagnosis.

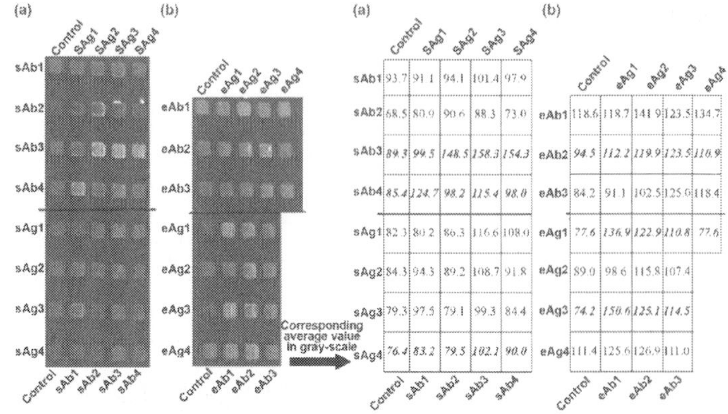

Fig. 6. Screening of hepatitis B ligands. (a) Screening of hepatitis B surface antibody and hepatitis B surface antigen. Different lots of hepatitis B surface antibody (sAb) and antigen (sAg) ligands were first immobilized in different rows. After blocking with BSA, the first row was used as a control. Different lots of hepatitis B surface antigen and hepatitis B surface antibody markers were detected in different rows. (b) Screening for hepatitis B e antibody and hepatitis B e antigen. The *italics* indicate results with the largest variation in gray-scale values, which in turn indicate that the ligands had higher bioactivity (Qi, et al., 2009a).

3.2.2 Quantitative detection of breast cancer marker: Carbohydrate antigen 15-3

In 2008, an estimated 636,000 cases of breast cancer were diagnosed in high resource countries, while an additional 514,000 cases were diagnosed in low and middle resource countries, where it has now become the most common female cancer (El Saghir, et al., 2011). Carbohydrate antigen 15-3 is frequently measured as a breast cancer marker test using the biosensor based on ellipsometry (Zhang, et al., 2005). According to Figure 2, quantitative analysis of carbohydrate antigen 15-3 was performed using the calibration curve method:

- A serum sample with a known concentration of carbohydrate antigen 15-3 was serially diluted;
- These various concentrations were detected;
- A calibration curve was drawn using the 15-3 concentration as the abscissa and the gray-scale value as the vertical axis;
- An unknown sample was analyzed; and
- The concentration of 15-3 in the unknown sample was determined with the calibration curve.

The concentration of carbohydrate antigen 15-3 in a serum sample had been determined by an electrochemiluminescence immunoassay. The serum sample with known concentration is used as standard sample to make a calibration curve of the biosensor. The calibration curve of carbohydrate antigen 15-3 detection is shown in Figure 7. The index period of the curve is 0~20 kIU/L, corresponding to gray-scale values of 58~99. If the concentration exceed the detection scope (0~20 kIU/L), the unknown test samples must be diluted; the lower limit of detection is 1 kIU/L. The realization of quantitative label-free detection of a cancer marker may aid in earlier diagnosis, monitoring the course of the disease, even exploring the mechanism of cancer.

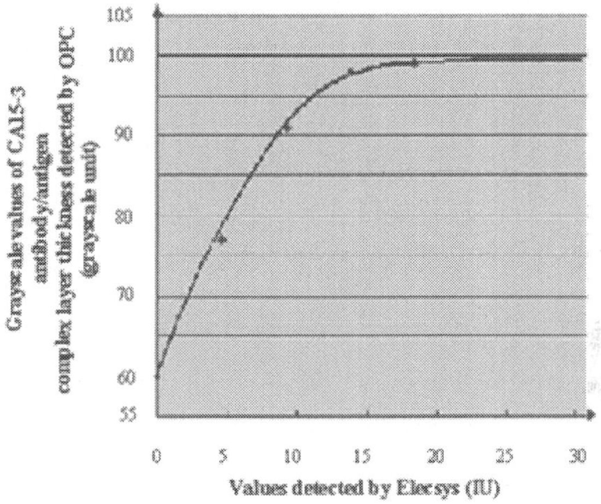

Fig. 7. Calibration curve for carbohydrate antigen 15-3 concentration detection (Zhang, et al., 2005).

3.2.3 Detection of tumor markers

Analyzing only one tumor marker is insufficient to diagnose cancer in 2010, a review exhibited a novel co-detection of three common tumor markers: alpha-fetoprotein, alpha-L-fucosidase, and ferritin (Jin, 2011). Thus, quantitative analysis was performed by the biosensor with the following calibration curve method:

- A chip was designed to simultaneously detect three markers in a sample;
- A calibration curve for the biosensor was plotted;
- A cut off value was determined by the receiver operating characteristic; and
- The three markers in a clinical serum sample were examined on a chip.

Detection results of several patients' markers were compared and analyzed. Sensitivity reached the ng/ml or U/L level. Thirty-two normal sera and 24 liver cancer patient sera were quantitatively analyzed. The realization of simultaneous detection of several markers by the biosensor may increase diagnostic specificity in a clinical setting.

3.2.4 Detection of phage M13KO7 for building virus a detection model

Phages are estimated to be the most widely distributed and diverse entities in all reservoirs populated by bacterial hosts. In 2009, Phage M13KO7 was detected by the biosensor based on ellipsometry as a model for virus detection. A highly versatile and powerful virus detection platform has been established (Qi, et al., 2009b). Based on common antibody/antigen or disease marker detection, three key steps (e.g., ligand immobilization, sensitivity detection, and microscopic confirmation) were optimized.

The avidin/biotin method (Fig. 8) was chosen to immobilize the antibody bio-GP3 against phage M13KO7. The avidin/biotin immobilization method is often used in other immunoassays (Vijayendran & Leckband, 2001). It has several advantages: 1) ligands are strongly immobilized because biotin and avidin can specifically interact with stronger affinity (~$10^{15}M^{-1}$) than the antibody-antigen interaction (~10^{5}-$10^{12}M^{-1}$) (Friguet, et al., 1985; Malmborg, et al., 1992); 2) immobilization is oriented, which helps antibody display its Fab domain for improved sensitivity; and 3) it may offer a more physiological environment.

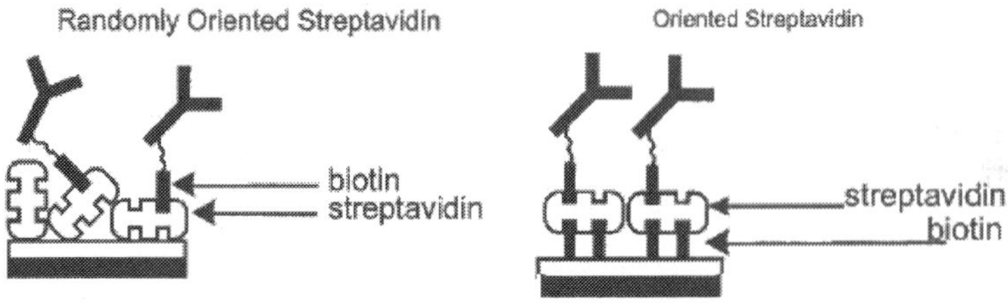

Fig. 8. Avidin/biotin immobilization method (Vijayendran & Leckband, 2001).

The sensitivity of phage M13KO7 detection can reach 10^9 plaque forming units/ml. Phage detection results by the biosensor have been confirmed with atomic force microscope. Imaging indicates that the biosensor can capture whole viruses, not just fragments. Thus, the virus detection biosensor platform has potential applications for human health.

3.2.5 Detection of avian influenza virus

According to World Health Organization statistics, the number of cases of avian influenza virus H5N1 directly crossing barriers and infecting humans was 534, causing 316 deaths by March 2011 (World Health Organization, 2011). Avian influenza virus subtype H5 can be detected with the biosensor based on ellipsometry using the above virus detection platform.
The oriented immobilization of probe was realized using protein A and antibody for avian influenza virus detection. Figure 9 (A) shows the probe immobilization method. This is a kind of biological immobilization, which also offers a more physiologically relevant environment to maintain the bioactivity of the probe (Qi, et al., 2010). The results show that 4A4 antibody can react specifically with avian influenza virus subtype H5N1, while CAM4 can interact with both H5N1 and H9N2.
The sensitivity of H5N1 detection is 2.56×10^{-3} tissue culture infectious dose/ml, which is more sensitive than a lateral-flow immunoassay (Remel Inc.). The corresponding areas were scanned with near-field optical microscopy. The microscopic evidence is presented in Figure 10, showing that intact avian influenza virus particles were bound. Direct virus detection may help with earlier diagnosis than disease marker detection.

3.2.6 Detection of other disease markers and viruses

C-reactive protein (Zhu, et al., 2007), soluble angiopoietin receptor Tie-2 (C.L. Wang, et al., 2009), thymidine phosphorylase (Li, et al., 2004), Alzheimer's disease tau protein (Qi, et al., 2006b), and others had also been detected using the biosensor. These diseases markers are closely related to human health. Thus, qualitative or quantitative detection with the biosensor can aid in earlier disease diagnosis and improve health.

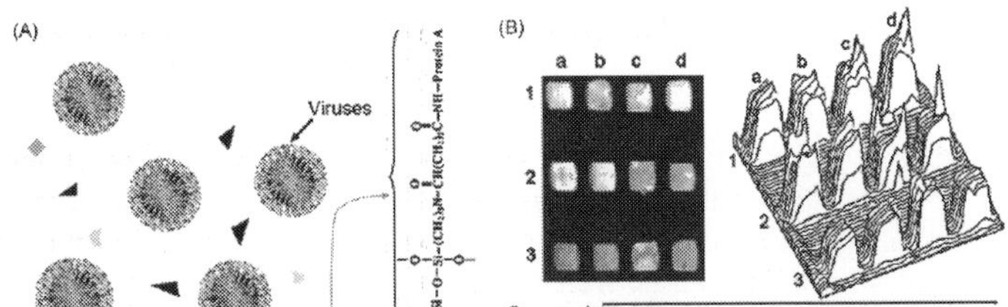

Gray-scale value	a	b	c	d
1	169.5±6.9	154.6±6.9	191.3±26.9	193.4±8.0
2	156.7±10.6	170.0±8.0	137.9±2.0	137.8±1.6
3	130.1±5.3	130.2±5.8	129.3±3.2	135.0±2.4

Fig. 9. Detection of avian influenza virus samples using the biosensor based on ellipsometry. (A) Schematic illustration. Avian influenza virus antibody is immobilized on the substrate. (B) Experimental image in gray-scale and a 3-D gray-scale distribution map. Antibody CAM4 was immobilized in columns 'a' and 'b'; 4A4 in columns 'c' and 'd'; H5N1, H9N2 and the control are shown in rows '1', '2', and '3', respectively (Qi, et al., 2010).

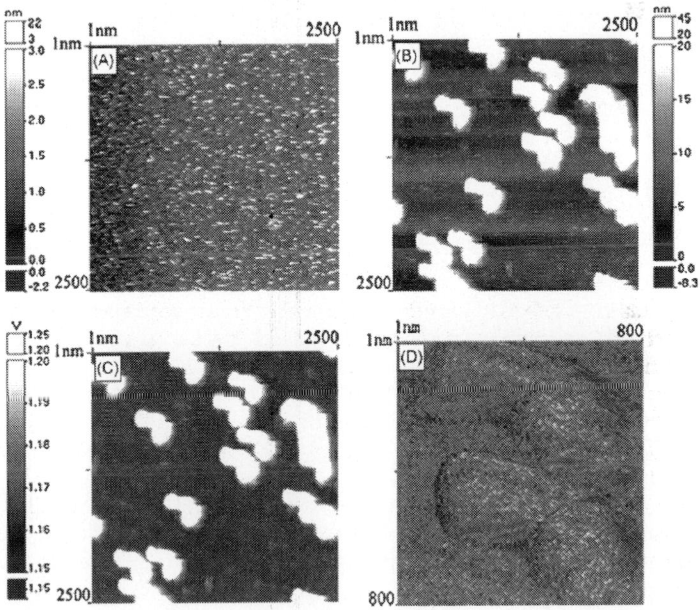

Fig. 10. Near-field optical microscopy images of H5N1. (A) and (B) Shear force mode images for H9N2 and H5N1, respectively. (C) Reflection mode image of H5N1. (D) 3-D reflection mode image of H5N1 (Qi, et al., 2010).

3.3 Clinical diagnosis and control of emerging infectious diseases

The ability of the biosensor based on ellipsometry to detect antibodies or antigens, disease markers, and viruses from patient samples with high sensitivity and specificity offers a powerful opportunity in early diagnosis and treatment of diseases. Related clinical applications have begun.

3.3.1 Clinical diagnosis of hepatitis B patients' sera

Hepatitis B virus infection is the most common cause of chronic liver diseases; an estimated 350 million people are chronically infected with hepatitis B virus worldwide (Sun, et al., 2002). Further, hepatitis B virus infection plays an important role in the development of hepatocellular carcinoma (De Mitri, et al., 2010). A rapid, simple, and direct method is urgently needed for clinical hepatitis B diagnosis. In section 3.2.1, the screening probe, standard national reference sample detection, and highly sensitive hepatitis B detection results demonstrated that the biosensor based on ellipsometry is feasible for clinical diagnosis of the disease (Z.H. Wang, et al., 2006; Jin, et al., 2004). Thus, the application of the biosensor based on ellipsometry could greatly enhance hepatitis B detection speed.

Cut-off values are important for clinical diagnosis of hepatitis B and it detection by the biosensor based on ellipsometry. The cut-off value can help us to distinguish between strong positive, near cut-off, and negative samples. Other diagnosis techniques, such as enzyme-linked immunosorbent assays, have cut-off value instructions included in the assay kits (Qi, et al., 2009a). The cut-off value of the biosensor was determined with a receiver operating characteristic curve. With the cut-off value, the detection of five hepatitis B virus markers by the biosensor was consistent with enzyme-linked immunosorbent assays.

Sera from 169 patients were analyzed with the biosensor for the purpose of clinical diagnosis. Samples from 60 patients included clinical information of hepatitis B from Shandong Provincial Hospital from qualitative enzyme-linked immunosorbent assay detection results (the assay kit was produced by Shanghai Rongsheng Biotech Co. Ltd). The remaining samples were from patients from the Tientsin Blood Disease Hospital and also included clinical information of hepatitis B (the assay kit was produced by Beijing Wantai Co Ltd.) Figure 11 shows the detection results of 109 hepatitis B patients' sera samples from

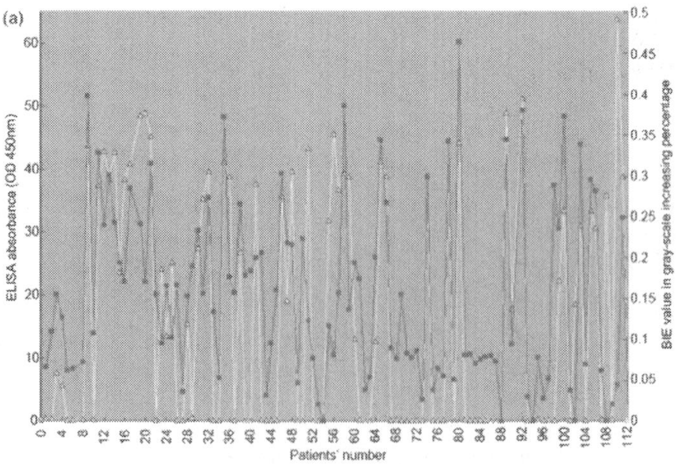

Fig. 11. Comparison of hepatitis B surface antigen detection by the biosensor based on ellipsometry (■) and by enzyme-linked immunosorbent assays (Δ) (Qi, et al., 2009a).

the Tientsin Blood Disease Hospital. The hepatitis B surface antigen detection results using the biosensor are compared with those of enzyme-linked immunosorbent assays. Regression analysis revealed that the results are in good agreement between the two methods ($r=0.67>r_{0.01}=0.247$).

The biosensor based on ellipsometry allows the multiplexed analysis and detection of five hepatitis B virus markers in clinical samples. The biosensor has a simplified process and short test time, which can detect the five markers from several patients simultaneously in about 1 h. The higher throughput of the biosensor may enable improved setup for detection sensitivity, time, and accuracy in the future.

3.3.2 Quantitative detection of clinical sera from breast cancer patients

Breast cancer incidence rates vary widely across the world, from 19.3 per 100,000 women per year in Eastern Africa to 89.9 per 100,000 women per year in Western Europe (Ferlay, et al., 2010). Carbohydrate antigen 15-3 is particularly valuable for treatment monitoring in patients that have breast cancer that cannot be evaluated using existing radiological procedures. Carbohydrate antigen 15-3 is also used during the postoperative surveillance of asymptomatic women who have undergone surgery for invasive breast cancer.

Using the quantitative calibration curve in section 3.2.2, 60 clinical patients' serum samples were quantitatively analyzed with the biosensor, including 24 women with intraductal carcinoma, 15 with mucinous carcinoma, 5 with in situ lobular carcinoma, 2 with medullary carcinoma, and 14 with breast diseases but no evidence of cancer (Zhang, et al., 2005). Thirty healthy sera were also collected. The median patient age was 48.5 years. These clinical sera samples were examined with both the biosensor based on ellipsometry and electrochemiluminescence immunoassays (Elecsys 2010 system, Roche Diagnostics) via the double-blinded method. The electrochemiluminescence immunoassay is the gold standard of breast cancer marker carbohydrate antigen 15-3 detection. A receiver operating characteristic plot curve (Handley, et al., 1982) was used to determine the result of the biosensor based on ellipsometry, which is shown in Figure 12.

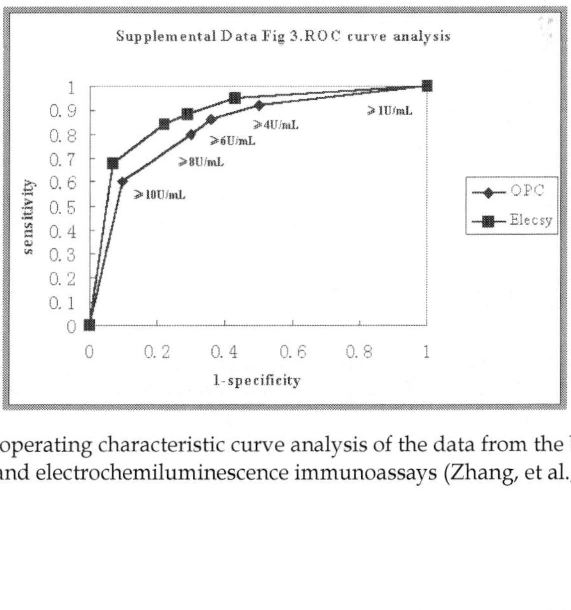

Fig. 12. Receiver operating characteristic curve analysis of the data from the biosensor based on ellipsometry and electrochemiluminescence immunoassays (Zhang, et al., 2005).

The result of this analysis proved that the biosensor results are consistent with those of the electrochemiluminescence immunoassay, reaching the clinical diagnosis standard level.

3.3.3 Clinical detection of sera from severe acute respiratory syndrome coronavirus (SARS-CoV)-infected patients

The outbreak of SARS in late 2002 in southeast China spread rapidly to over 30 countries and resulted in more than 800 deaths (Poutanen, et al., 2003; Feng & Gao, 2007). In 2003, the biosensor based on ellipsometry was used to detect the infectious pathogens.

Before analyzing clinical SARS patients' sera, some antibodies from a phage-display library were identified by the biosensor. SARS-CoV virions were used as a probe by the biosensor to assess the efficiency of the antibodies b1 and h12. The identification of new and effective antibodies is significant for more accurate diagnosis of the illness and the development of a vaccine.

Ten SARS patients and 12 healthy volunteers (controls) were tested with the biosensor. SARS-CoV virions were immobilized on the surface as the probe to detect antibodies in the patients' sera (Figure 13). From the analysis of the results, different patients had different antibody contents, which might help doctors estimate disease progress. The entire detection process only requires approximately 40 min.

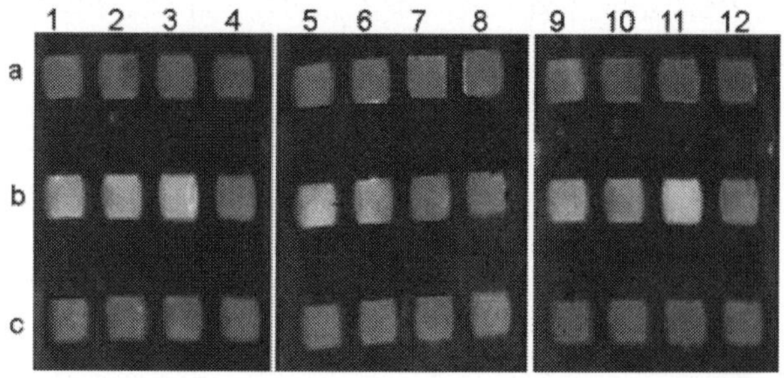

Fig. 13. Analysis of SARS patients' serum samples using the biosensor based on imaging ellipsometry. a1~12 are negative samples; b1~12 are SARS patients; and c1~12 are blank controls (Qi, et al., 2005).

The real-time function of the biosensor was mentioned above in section 3.1.2. The kinetic process of interaction between the antibodies and SARS virus was analyzed with the biosensor. The affinity of antibodies b1 and h12 for SARS virus are 9.5×10^6 M^{-1} and 1.36×10^7 M^{-1}, respectively. Real-time detection revealed that antibody h12 has a higher affinity for the virus than antibody b1.

As a label free method, the biosensor based on ellipsometry is a competent mechanism for analyzing clinical serum samples from SARS patients and the affinity between these antibodies and the SARS coronavirus. Compared with surface plasmon resonance (SPR), a fairly widely applied optical detection method for real-time detect interaction of biomolecules (Hall, et al., 2010), the biosensor also allows label-free samples and crude samples to be used directly without previous purification. The biosensor based on ellipsometry has advantages such as: 1) lower cost (e.g., a piece of the biosensor based on ellipsometry silicon wafer is about $1, while a piece of surface plasmon resonance glass slide costs about $70-80); 2) the biosensor can provide 24 real-time curves simultaneously, allowing high-throughput detection; and 3) multiplex microarray was imaged and offered an image.

3.4 Market potential for scientific research related to the health field

The continual development of the biosensor based on ellipsometry shows both market potential for scientific research related to the health field and an increasing number of applications for basic biology research. The following are two applications of the biosensor on vesicular membrane proteins, demonstrating its value to general biology.

3.4.1 Detection of interaction among vesicular membrane fusion proteins

Membrane-associated proteins provide the minimal fusion machinery necessary for cellular vesicles to fuse to target organelle membranes in eukaryotic cells (Jahn & Scheller, 2006). The qualitative and quantitative identification of membrane-associated proteins interactions is the key to understanding the mechanisms of membrane fusion, which is vital for cell division, cellular structure organization, and biological information processing (Zhang, et al., 2009). To investigate the characteristics of these newly discovered membrane-associated protein pairs such as: Sec22, Ykt6, Sso2 and Sso1, the biosensor based on ellipsometry was used to detect the interactions among soluble N-ethylmaleimide-sensitive factor attachment protein receptors (SNAREs, a kind of protein that assembles into coiled-coil tetramers to promote membrane fusion). The interactions among several SNAREs (i.e., Sec22, Ykt6, Sso1, and Sso2) were analyzed by the biosensor based on ellipsometry. The in vitro detection results from the biosensor are consistent with the results of yeast two-hybrid assays at the domain level in vivo (Zhang, et al., 2009; Jin et al., 2011). Further, the kinetic binding process of two SNAREs (Ykt6 and Sso2) was measured using the real-time function of the biosensor. The rapid detection and identification of vesicular protein–protein interactions is essential for understanding vesicle trafficking and for understanding the system-level organization of cellular structure, biological information processing, and molecular mechanisms.

3.4.2 Vesicle adsorption visualization

Recently, a type of total internal reflection imaging ellipsometry was developed for real-time detection of biomolecular interactions (Jin, et al., 2011). This method was used to visualization the of vesicles adsorption process. Non-specific adsorption and desorption on a poly-L-lysine-modified gold surface was analyzed with real-time curves by the biosensor. The biosensor results were consistent with a phase contrast microscopy (NIKON, TI-U, Japan) results. The vesicle adsorption and desorption processes visualized by the biosensor are significant to the study of cell membrane properties. Micron target detection is the future aim of the biosensor based on total internal reflection imaging ellipsometry. Therefore, we expect that the biosensor based on ellipsometry has a yet-unexploited huge market potential for application in biological basic research related to the health field.

4. Summary

In the human health field, the biosensor based on ellipsometry is widely used to monitor or detect biological molecules for applications ranging from common infectious diseases to cancers. Some adaptations of this system for biomedical and clinical applications (e.g., disease marker detection, virus detection, and real-time monitoring) have been developed.

With recent progress on vesicular membrane proteins, the biosensor based on ellipsometry technology also shows significant promise in basic biological research. Furthermore, through miniaturization, it is possible to fabricate the biosensors that are portable, low-cost, high-throughput, and highly sensitive for diseases such as HIV/AIDS. As the biosensor based on ellipsometry becomes simpler and more widely available, we expect to see a proliferation of uses in conjunction with telecommunications equipment. Wide application of the biosensor based on ellipsometry will be explored in monitoring personal health, the food we consume, and our environment in the future.

5. Acknowledgements

Work in GFG's laboratory is supported by China Ministry of Science and Technology (MOST Project 973, Grant No. 2011CB504703). GFG is a leading principal investigator of Innovative Research Group of National Natural Science Foundation of China (NSFC, Grant No. 81021003). JG and QC acknowledges financial support from the National Basic Research Program of China 2009CB320300, the National Basic Research Program (Project 973) of China (2007CB310505) Chinese Academy of Sciences (KJCX2-YW-Mo3 and -M04), Nature Science Foundation of Shandong Province (Q2007C07), the Basic Scientific Research Special Foundation of Chinese Academy of Inspection and Quarantine (2010JK002).

6. References

Bai, Y.J.; Zhao, J.R.; Lv, G.T.; Zhang, W.H.; Wang, Y. & Yan, X.J. (2003). Rapid and high throughput detection of HBV YMDD mutants with fluorescence polarization. *World J Gastroenterol* 9(10): 2344-2347.

Bhatia, S.K.; Shriver-Lake, L.C.; Prior, K.J.; Georger, J.H.; Calvert, J.M.; Bredehorst, R. & Ligler, F.S. (1989). Use of thiol-terminal silanes and heterobifunctional crosslinkers for immobilization of antibodies on silica surfaces. *Anal Biochem* 178(2): 408-413.

Chen, Y.; Wu, W.; Li, L.J.; Lou, B.; Zhang, J. & Fan, J. (2006). Comparison of the results for three automated immunoassay systems in determining serum HBV markers. *Clin Chim Acta* 372(1–2): 129–133.

De Mitri, M.S.; Cassini, R, & Bernardi, M. (2010). Hepatitis B virus-related hepatocarcinogenesis: molecular oncogenic potential of clear or occult infections. *Eur J Cancer* 46(12): 2178-2186.

El Saghir, N.S.; Adebamowo, C.A.; Anderson, B.O.; Carlson, R.W.; Bird, P.A.; Corbex, M.; Badwe, R.A.; Bushnaq, M.A.; Eniu, A.; Gralow, J.R.; Harness, J.K.; Masetti, R.; Perry, F.; Samiei, M.; Thomas, D.B.; Wiafe-Addai, B.& Cazap, E.(2011). Breast cancer management in low resource countries (LRCs): Consensus statement from the Breast Health Global Initiative. *Breast.* Pressing

Feng, Y. & Gao, G.F. (2007). Towards our understanding of SARS-CoV, an emerging and devastating but quickly conquered virus. *Comp Immunol Microbiol Infect Dis* 30(5-6): 309-327.

Ferlay, J.; Shin, H.R.; Bray, F.; Forman, D.; Mathers, C. & Parkin, D.M. (2010). Estimates of worldwide burden of cancer in 2008: GLOBOCAN 2008. *Int J Cancer* 127(12): 2893-2917

Friguet, B.; Chaffotte, A.F.; Djavadi-Ohaniance, L. & Goldberg, M.E. (1985). Measurements of the true affinity constant in solution of antigen-antibody complexes by enzyme-linked immunosorbent assay. *J Immunol Methods* 77(2): 305-19.

Guezguez, B.; Vigneron, P.; Lamerant, N.; Kieda, C.; Jaffredo, T. & Dunon, D. (2007). Dual role of melanoma cell adhesion molecule (MCAM)/CD146 in lymphocyte endothelium interaction: MCAM/CD146 promotes rolling via microvilli induction in lymphocyte and is an endothelial adhesion receptor. *J Immunol* 179(10):6673-6685.

Hall, K. & Aguilar, M.I. (2010). Surface plasmon resonance spectroscopy for studying the membrane binding of antimicrobial peptides. *Methods Mol Biol* 627(2): 13-23.

Handley, J.A. & McNeil, B.J. (1982). The meaning and use of the area under a receiver operating characteristic (ROC) curve. *Radiology* 143(1): 29–36.

Jahn, R.& Scheller, RH. (2006). SNAREs--engines for membrane fusion. *Nat Rev Mol Cell Biol* 7(9):631-43.

Jin, G.; Tengvall, P.; Lundstrom, I. & Arwin, H. (1995). Abiosensor concept based on imaging ellipsometry for visualization of biomolecular interactions. *Anal Biochem* **232**(1):69–72.

Jin, G.; Jansson, R. & Arwin, H. (1996). Imaging ellipsometry revisited: developments for visualization of thin transparent layers on silicon substrates. *Rev Sci Instrum* 67(8): 2930-2936.

Jin,G.; Wang,Z.H.; Qi,C.; Zhao,Z.Y.; Chen,S.; Meng,Y.H.; Ying,P.Q.; Xia, L.H.& Wan,L.J. (2003). Immune-microassay with optical proteinchip for protein detection. *Proceedings of the 25th annual international conference of the IEEE EMBS,* Cancun Mexico, 3575-3577. Sep 17-21, 2003.

Jin, G.; Zhao, Z.Y.; Wang, Z.H.; Meng, Y.H.; Ying, P.Q.; Chen, S.; Chen, Y.Y.; Qi, C.& Xia, L.H. (2004). The development of biosensor with imaging ellipsometry. *Proceedings of 26th Annual International Conference of the IEEE Engineering in Medicine and Biology Society*, ISSN: 05891019. San Francisco, CA, United states. September 1-5, 2004.

Jin, G. (2008). Development of biosensor based on imaging ellipsometry. *Phys Stat Sol* 205(4): 810–816.

Jin, G.; Meng, Y.H.; Liu, L.; Niu, Y.; Chen, S.; Cai, Q.& Jiang, T.J. (2011). Development of biosensor based on imaging ellipsometry and biomedical applications. *Thin Solid Films* 519(9): 2750-2757.

Langmuir, I & Schaefer, VJ. (1936). Optical measurements of the thickness of a film adsorbed from a solution. *J Am Chem Soc* 59: 1406

Li, A.L.; Li, H.W.; Zhang, J. & Xiu, R.J. (2004). Initial Study on Thymidine Phosphorylase in Breast Cancer Tissue by Optical Protein Chip. *J of Chinese Microcirculation* 8(4): 257-260.

Malmborg, A.C.; Michaëlsson, A.; Ohlin, M.; Jansson, B. & Borrebaeck, C.A. (1992). Real time analysis of antibody-antigen reaction kinetics. *Scand J Immunol* 35(6): 643-650.

Niu, Y.; Zhuang, J.; Liu, L.; Yan, X.Y. & Jin, G. (2011). Two kinds of anti-ricin antibody and ricin interaction evaluated by biosensor based on imaging ellipsometry. *Thin Solid Films* 519(9): 2768-2771.

Poutanen, S.M.; Low, D.E.; Henry, B.; Finkelstein, S.; Rose, D.; Green, K.; Tellier, R.; Draker, R.; Adachi, D.; Ayers, M.; Chan, A.K.; Skowronski, D.M.; Salit, I.; Simor, A.E.; Slutsky, A.S.; Doyle, P.W.; Krajden, M.; Petric, M.; Brunham, R.C.; McGeer, A.J.; National Microbiology Laboratory, Canada.& Canadian Severe Acute Respiratory

Syndrome Study Team.(2003).Identification of severe acute respiratory syndrome in Canada. *N Engl J Med* 348(20):1995-2005.

Qi, C. Duan, JZ. Wang, Z.H., & et al. (2006a). Investigation of interaction between two neutralizing monoclonal antibodies and SARS virus using biosensor based on imaging ellipsometry. Biomed Microdevices 8(3): 247–253.

Qi, C.; Hao, R.Q. & Jin, G. (2006b) Detection Alzheimer's disease (AD) tau protein using protein chip biosensor. *Acta Biophysica Sinica* 22: 17

Qi, C.; Zhu, W.; Niu, Y.; Zhang, H.G.; Zhu, G.Y.; Meng, Y.H.; Chen, S.& Jin, G. (2009a). Clinical HBV markers detection with biosensor based on imaging ellipsometry. *J Viral Hepat* 16(11):822-832.

Qi, C.; Lin, Y.; Feng, J.; Wang,Z.H.; Zhu, C.F.; Meng, Y.H.; Yan, X.Y.; Wan, L.J.& Jin, G. (2009b). Phage M13KO7 detection with biosensor based on imaging ellipsometry and AFM microscopic confirmation. *Virus Res* 140(1-2): 79-86.

Qi, C.; Tian, X.S.; Chen, S.; Yan, J.H.; Cao, Z.; Tian, K.G.; Gao, G.F.& Jin, G. (2010) . Detection of avian influenza virus subtype H5 using a biosensor based on imaging ellipsometry. *Biosens Bioelectron* 25(6): 1530-1534.

Schena, M. (2005). *Protein microarrays*. Jones and Bartlett Publishers,Inc. ISBN 0-7637-3127-7. Canada.

Sun, Z.; Ming, L.; Zhu, X. & Lu, J. (2002). Prevention and control of hepatitis B in China. *J Med Virol* 67(3): 447-450.

Vijayendran, R.A. & Leckband, D.E. (2001). A quantitative assessment of heterogeneity for surface- immobilized proteins. *Anal Chem* 73(3): 471-480.

Wang, C.L.; Li, J.Q.; Li, H.W.; Jin, G; Wang, Z.H.; Meng, Y.H. & Xiu, R.J. (2009). Soluble angiopoietin receptor Tie-2 in patients with acute myocardial infarction and its detection by optical protein-chip. *Artif Cells Blood Substit Immobil Biotechnol* 37(4): 183-186.

Wang, Z.H. & Jin, G. (2003b). A label-free multisensing immunosensor based on imaging ellipsometry. *Anal chem* 75(22):6119-6123.

Wang, Z.H. & Jin, G. (2003a). Feasibility of protein A for the oriented immobilization of immunoglobulin on silicon surface for a biosensor with imaging ellipsometry. *J Biochem Biophys Methods* 57(3): 203-211.

Wang, Z.H. & Jin, G. (2004). Covalent immobilization of proteins for the biosensor based on imaging ellipsometry. *J Immunol Meth* 285(2): 237-243.

Wang, Z.H.; Meng, Y.H.; Ying, P.; Qi, C. & Jin, G. (2006). A label-free protein microfluidic array for parallel immunoassays. *Electrophoresis* 27(20):4078–4085.

World Health Organization [WHO]. (2011). Available from: March 2011. http://www.who.int/csr/disease/avian_influenza/country/cases_table_2011_03_16/en/index.html

Yan X, Lin Y, Yang D, & et al. (2003). A novel anti-CD146 monoclonal antibody, AA98, inhibits angiogenesis and tumor growth. Blood 102(1):184-191.

Zhang, H.; Chen, J.; Wang, Y.; Peng, L.; Dong, X.; Lu, Y.; Keating, A.E. & Jiang, T. (2009). A computationally guided protein-interaction screen uncovers coiled-coil interactions involved in vesicular trafficking. *J Mol Biol* 392(1): 228-241.

Zhang, H.G.; Qi, Cai.; Wang, Z.H.; Jin, G.& Xiu, R.J. (2005). Evaluation of a New CA15-3 Protein Assay Method: Optical Protein-Chip System for Clinical Application. *Clinical Chemistry* 51(6): 1038-1040.

Zhu, W.; Sun, H.L.; Jin, G.; Qi, C. & Zhao, Z.Y. (2007). Study on ellipsometry-imaging protein-chip for CRP quantitative detection. *Int J Lab Med* 28(7): 577-582.

8

Preparation and Characterization of Immunosensors for Disease Diagnosis

Antonio Aparecido Pupim Ferreira, Cecílio Sadao Fugivara, Hideko Yamanaka and Assis Vicente Benedetti
Instituto de Química, UNESP - Univ Estadual Paulista
Brazil

1. Introduction

The antigens are viruses, bacteria or part of, toxin or any molecules (organic or inorganic) that is antigenic (may induce an immunological response and can be recognized by antibody). The antibody is a glycoprotein which is produced in response of antigenic attack. Reaction between antigen and antibody by structural complementation is the base of immunoassay. If the immunological receptor is immobilized on a transducer for detecting a target analyte the device is called immunosensor. Either antibody or antigen could be immobilized on the transducer which converts the biological signal into electrical signal. The immunosensor is classified as optical, mass-sensitive or electrochemical according to the technique. The electrochemical immunosensor, according to the transducer, is classified as amperometric, potenciometric, impedimetric, condutometric.
The cells or organs release trace levels of specific glicoprotein, enzymes and hormones into health patients' serum but the concentrations increase when they are injured. It means that the methodology for clinical diagnosis must be sensitive and with high reproducibility and repeatability. The interaction between antibody and antigen is usually selective presenting high affinity constant (around 10^{15}). Therefore immunosensors are being applied for diagnosis of various diseases states and also to improve effective drug administration.
Studies on immunosensors like potenciometric (Tang et al., 2005), condutometric (Lu et al., 2009), piezeletric (Ren et al., 2008, Sener et al., 2010, Pohanka et al., 2007), fiber optic (Kwon et al., 2002), scanning tunnelling microscopy (Lee et al., 2009) have been published for disease diagnosis. State of immunoassay technologies for tumor diagnosis (Wu et al., 2007) and environmental analysis have been reviewed recently (Farre´ et al., 2009).
The results obtained by immunosensor must have reproducibility and repeatability in order to diagnose the disease or to monitor the disease treatment. Such properties are reached when the system is well optimized and characterized. On this chapter the amperometric and impedimetric devices will be focused on the preparation and characterization of the immunosensor in order to improve its performance.
Usually the complex formed by the affinity reaction between the antigen-antibody is not electrochemically active. It is possible to monitor the reaction by amperometric technique by using an enzyme as tracer like classical ELISA (enzyme-linked immunesorbed assay); in this case instead of absorbance the current intensity is measured. The immunosensor where the affinity reaction is monitored by tracer is indirect and the format could be classified as

sandwich, competitive or indirect (Tijssen, 1985). On the other hand, the impedimetric immunosensor is based on impedance measurement of the electrical equivalent circuit of the oscillator. Consequently no label is necessary to monitor the affinity reaction.

The kind of electrochemical transducer and technique of receptor immobilization play an important role on the selectivity of the immunosensor. For instance, gold screen printed electrode was used for *Trypanosoma cruzi* (*T. cruzi*) protein immobilization through self assembled monolayer (SAM) in order to diagnose Chagas disease (Ferreira et al., 2005). Anti-human cardiac myoglobin antibody immobilized on carbon screen printed electrode by passive adsorption (O'Regan, et. al, 2002) was applied as biochemical marker for acute myocardial infarction (myoglobin) detection; carbon screen printed electrode modified by multiwall carbon nanotubes (MWCNT) and gold nanoparticles was the platform to immobilize the antibody *P. falciparum* for malaria diagnose (Sharma et al., 2008). Glassy carbon electrode (GCE) was modified by Nafion® for competitive detection of anti-schistosoma japonicum antibody (Zhou et al., 2003); modified with multiwall carbon nanotubes integrated with microfluidic systems for quantification of prostate specific antigen in human serum samples (Panini et al., 2008); Fe_3O_4 magnetic nanoparticles/chitosan composite film modified GCE for ferritin determination (Wang & Tan, 2007); GCE functionalized Au nanoparticles for cancer cells detection (Wang & Tan, 2007); bi-layer nano-Au and nickel hexacyanoferrates nanoparticles modified GCE for determination of carcinoembryonic antigen (Yuan et al., 2009). Phenylboronic acid conjugated thiol-mixed monolayer on gold wire (Wang et al., 2008) was proposed for alfa fetoprotein (AFP) detection; such antigen was also detected by microfluidic cell (Maeng et al., 2008); gold nanowire to differentiate between lung and colon cancer (Patil et al., 2008). Graphite-epoxy composite (GEC) electrodes as a platform to immobilize tissue transglutaminase were employed for the autoimmune disorder celiac disease (Pividori et al., 2009), silver epoxy-graphite composite for cardiac troponins detection (Silva et al., 2010).

Cellular products over-expressed by malignant cells have been used as tumor markers but one marker could not be specific to a particular tumor. In this case an array of immunosensor could be the solution (Wu et al., 2007).

Electrochemical impedance spectroscopy (EIS) has been used as a technique for characterization of electrode surface modification but the analysis of interfacial property changes is useful also to monitor the biorecognition events involving antibody-antigen interaction for disease diagnosis. Silver electrodes for interleukin-12 correlated to the diagnosis of multiple sclerosis (La Belle et al., 2007); electropolymerized nanocomposite film containing polypyrrole, polypyrrolepropylic acid and Au nanoparticles was developed for Interleukin 5 which is associated with several allergic diseases (Chen et al., 2008). Gold and platinum electrodes were investigated to diagonose Chagas disease (Diniz et al., 2003) as well as gold screen printed electrodes (Ferreira et al., 2010). The transglutaminase was immobilized on gold screen printed electrode through polyelectrolyte to diagnose celiac disease (Balkenhohl &Lisdat 2007); the impedance signal after the interaction between the Ag and Ab was amplified by using secondary HRP-labelled antibody; the main advantage of impedimetric methodologies (direct immunosensor) was not applied.

Most of amperometric and impedimetric immunosensors published on the literature have no detailed electrode surface characterization which is important for the reproducibility and stability of the device.

2. Preparation and handling of electrodes

Conventional gold and graphite electrodes, screen-printed electrodes (SPE), electrodes prepared from CD-Rs (CDtrodes), gold and magnetic nanoparticles, carbon-on-metal, carbon nanotubes, carbon paste and others substrates have been used as support matrices (transducers) to immobilize biological compounds. The manner of preparation and handling of electrodes are very important for the stability and packing of self-assembled monolayers (SAM) or films and subsequent modifications steps of the analytical methodology.

On cleaning screen-printed electrodes for sensors some recommendations, before the first modification step, were previously described in the literature: washing the SPE gold-based electrode with ethanol or acetone (Ferreira et al., 2010; Navrátilová & Skaládal, 2004; Kaláb & Skládal, 1995), or surface pretreatments for the immunosensors development (Escamilla-Gomez et al., 2009). Carpini et al. gave the following information about pretreatment of SPE gold-based electrodes: "*Although mechanical or electrochemical cleaning of the gold surface is usually recommended, both thiol-tethered DNA probe immobilization and naphthol electrochemistry are not significantly affected by surface pretreatments. Thus, screen-printed gold electrodes were used as produced*" (Carpini et al., 2004); Xu et al. also used as received SPE gold-based electrode for HRP immobilization (Xu et al., 2003).

Recently, García-González et al. characterized different SPE-gold electrodes used for sensors preparation and the electrodes were used without pretreatment (García-González et al., 2008). Escamilla-Gomez et al. used gold screen-printed electrodes (AuSPEs) pretreated with acid solution (H_2SO_4) for impedimetric immunobiosensors. AuSPES were obtained from different manufacturers, then various cyclic voltammograms were recorded and the electrodes washed with deionized water (Escamilla-Gomez et al., 2009). The SPE gold-based electrode, depending on the manufacturing, is not exactly a gold electrode, so the acid treatment used for cleaning their surfaces cannot be applied. Sometimes modifications may occur mainly on the surface of the reference electrode and for this reason aggressive medium cannot be used for cleaning this type of SPE electrodes (Ferreira et al., 2010).

It is important to know that the SPE used in the immunosensors construction must be in an aluminum sealed package in which each electrode is individually isolated from the atmosphere, or in special boxes also protected from the atmosphere. In the case of the locked package of one electrode, it should only be opened just before use and the surface must be protected against any contamination. Obviously, if this care is not taken in consideration the SPE electrodes are improper to use for sensors preparation and even for electrochemical studies. SPE electrodes stored in aluminum sealed package or in other way can sometimes undergo oxidation and then they must be rejected. Another important factor to be considered on the SPE use for one specific study is the utilization of electrodes which belong to the same manufacturing batches. Differences between batches are linear. It means that different batches result in different output signal by scale not by shape. If the response is calibrated by internal standard, such calibration will be valid for all batches (production in series). Using different batches absolute reproducibility of the immunosensors cannot be ensured.

When conventional gold surface is used, the pretreatment procedures can be mechanical, chemical and electrochemical (Campuzano et al., 2002, 2006; Hoogvliet et al., 2000). The influence of the different surface pretreatments on the immunosensor response of a polycrystalline gold electrode should be studied (Carvalhal et al., 2005). Gold transducers

are very often used because of the facility to obtain a stable assembled layer. Thiol and disulphide groups quickly adsorb on gold surfaces, and over longer periods covalent bonds are formed (Godínez, 1999). Cysteamine ($HS-CH_2-CH_2-NH_2$), for example, a thiol with a short chain length, has two functional groups that can be used as a bridge between the electrode and other kinds of layers. The stability and organization of monolayer depend on the length of the chains between the terminal and free groups and also on the lateral interactions between chains. Short chains can lead to the formation of a less stable and more disorganized layer (Mendes et al., 2008). SBZA (4-(methylmercapto)-benzaldehyde) can also be used to produce self-assembled monolayers to prepare gold surfaces for further modification and presents the advantage that it substitutes, for instance, cysteamine and glutaraldehyde since both S-H and CHO groups are present in this molecule. However, special care is needed with its incubation due to its high solubility in ethanol, and also the monolayer must be formed under refrigeration and humid atmosphere (Conoci et al., 2002).
Many other kinds of molecules may form self-assembled monolayers to immobilize biological molecules or materials in order to develop immunosensors: fullerene-C_{60}, ferrocene, ionic liquid (1-siobutyl-3-methylimidazolium bis(trifluoromethylsulfonyl)amine) (Xiulan et al., 2011), electropolymerized thionine (Tang et al., 2008), lysine (Wang et al., 2010), hydroquinone (Xuan et al., 2003), aminosilane (Parker et al., 2009).
Biological molecules or materials can be immobilized on the SAMs or modified SAMs or, in some cases directly on the electrode surface. In the latest case, special attention should be given to the loss of activity due to some steric impediment involving electroactive sites.
The influences of the immobilization processes on the immunossensor performance were evaluated with different transducers, antigens and antibodies. Considering the various steps involved in the immunosensor construction, very important details must be considered in the analytical procedure of antigen incubation. The results obtained for shorter antigen incubation times may be a consequence of some partial leaching of antigen due to an unstable self-assembled monolayer formation, while those for longer incubation times may indicate a possible degradation of the modified electrode surface, with loss of layer integrity. Therefore, a detailed study to optimize the incubation time of antigen in the development of biosensors is strongly recommended (Ferreira et al., 2010).
The immobilization of antibodies on solid-phase materials has been used for the development of the immunosensor and different procedures were described in the literature. Problems associated with biological activity of the antibodies on immobilization have been observed in many cases (Lu et al., 1996). The interactions antigen-antibody are complexes by nature and the reproducible response characteristic of immunosensors requires that the affinity reaction is minimally disturbed by the fabrication procedure. The random orientation of the asymmetric macromolecules on transducers is one of the main reasons for such loss. Protein A, produced by *Staphylococcus aureus,* is a highly stable receptor capable of binding to the Fc fragment of immunoglobulins and the Fab binding sites of IgG antibody are thus oriented for immuassays reactions (Sjoquist et al., 1972; Lee et al., 2004). Therefore, these binding characteristics of the protein A can be used as an affinity surface in immunosensors construction (Campanella et al., 1999).
Magnetic nanoparticles as substrate for biomolecules immobilization are a special alternative used in recent years for the construction of immunosensors (Wang & Tan, 2007; Tang et al., 2008). Due to their attractive properties, magnetic nanoparticles have been used in immunology (Ao et al., 2006), cell separation processes or purging processes (Bittencourt

et al., 2006; Sonti & Bose, 1995). Several applications of magnetic nanoparticles in the immobilization of immunoglobulines have also been reported (Pham & Sim, 2010; Smith et al., 2006).

Other conditions affecting the immunosensor response characteristics must be critically examined: they include the purity of the reagents, incubation temperature in different steps of immunoassay, ionic strength and solution composition, working pH range, condition of the electrode surface and the oxygen content of the solution.

3. Techniques for surface control and immunosensor characterization

The preparation and control of the substrate surface and its modification constitute critical steps of the immunosensor development since they must permit the immobilization of biological molecule or material on the electrode surface and the interaction between the modified surface and the sample. The optimization of the incubation time is very critical on the different steps of the immunosensor development.

A detailed characterization of the various steps involved in the immunosensor development can be useful for understanding the contribution of each step on the behavior of the global system, and for further improvement of the analytical process. So, it is strongly recommended that each step of the immunosensor construction be carefully evaluated using different electrochemical and non-electrochemical techniques.

The interpretation of the results obtained by applying, in an adequate manner, appropriate experimental techniques can provide information on the distribution of structural defects, redox properties and the kinetics and mechanism of the monolayer formation or other modifications introduced on the surface, such as ions incorporation, water uptake and so on. The different electrochemical techniques can help understanding the electron transfer and mass transfer processes after each different step of immunosensor building. The non-electrochemical ones may inform on the morphology and topography of the bare and modified surface, on the interaction between the modifier and the surface, on the chemical nature of the bonds and molecules attached on the surface and on the interaction of energy (special by light) with the different entities constituting the system which is being studied, allowing their identification and the knowledge and applications of their properties.

3.1 Electrochemical techniques

Electrochemical techniques are largely used by researchers of different scientific fields due to the fact that the equipment used is of low cost, simple, and easy to utilize and have the advantage of being *in situ* techniques, which allows monitoring the studied system in real time. Many different electrochemical techniques have been used to monitor the response of different surfaces such as gold, graphite, carbon nanotubes, gold nanowires, gold nanoparticles, metallic oxide nanoparticles, spin-on glass surfaces, carbon paste, which can be modified with different modifiers to form SAMs and composites to incorporate active materials and built the desired immunosensor. Each step of this process may be carefully characterized using cyclic voltammetry (CV), electrochemical impedance spectroscopy (EIS), quartz crystal microbalance, chronoamperometry and amperometry, square wave voltammetry (SWV), differential pulse voltammetry (DPV), ellipsometry, and measurements of electrical resistances.

3.1.1 Cyclic voltammetry

For a better understanding of cyclic voltammetry and its general applications the readers can refer to some text books (Noel & Vasu, 1990; Gasser Jr., 1993; Compton & Banks, 2009). As indicated above, cyclic voltammetry (CV) is the electrochemical technique most frequently used to get the first information on the nature of the electrode surface, such as its purity (Angerstein-Kozlowska et al., 1973), stability (Cabot et al., 1991; Benedetti et al., 1991), reproducibility and repeatability (Horta et al., 2009). Sometimes CV is used for cleaning the electrode surface (Calvo et al., 2004); for activating (Tang et al., 2006); and for reconstructing the electrode surface, or to determine the electrode active surface area for small molecules (hydrogen, methanol, CO, ethanol, etc.), which adsorb on the electrode surface (Biegler et al., 1971; Godoi et al., 2009). Cyclic voltammograms obtained for large molecules can be used to determine the real surface area of an electrode, resulting in an area similar to the geometric one (Noel & Vasu, 1990). Such large molecules can be coordination and other inorganic compounds (ferro/ferricyanide, ferrocene/ferrocinium, etc.) and highly solvated ions which may stay in solution without adsorbing on the electrode surface. CV is very often to help establish the global mechanism of an electrochemical process occurring in solution (Naal et al., 1994) or occurring at a surface as nucleation (Noel & Vasu, 1990).
This technique may also indicate some contamination of the electrolyte used as in the case of a phosphate buffer solution, pH 7.4, containing the redox pair $Fe(CN)_6^{-3}/Fe(CN)_6^{-4}$ which was used to characterize the gold electrodes prepared from CDs (CDtrodes). This was observed in our laboratory. Fig. 1 shows the cyclic voltammograms of this system obtained using the same experimental conditions except that the phosphate buffer solution for recording the cyclic voltammogram of Fig. 1b was changed. It is clearly seen that the cyclic voltammogram in Fig. 1a was distorted probably by some impurity that came from the solution that adsorbed on the electrode surface and partially blocked it. This conclusion was drawn after testing all the other possibilities, such as checking cables and all electrical connections, cleaning the electrochemical cell and its components, recording CVs in other equipment, trying several CDtrodes and changing both ferro/ferricyanide salts. The conclusion was that phosphate salts of the buffer solution had been contaminated.
However, it is possible that the main reasons for the large use of cyclic voltammetry is the simplicity of equipment, facilities to scan a large energy range and also a large potential scan rate (from microvolt to hundreds of megavolts per second) which can be coupled with changes in the temperature of the electrochemical cell to study the kinetic of chemical coupled reactions, and mainly its didactical presentation. But sometimes the results of CV are misinterpreted causing some confusing regarding the irreversibility generated by fast chemical coupled reaction or by slow charge transfer reaction. This confusion can be normally distinguished experimentally by changing the scan rate (v) and / or the temperature of the system. Another common misinterpretation is related to the effect of ohmic drop on the anodic and cathodic peak potentials separation since the ohmic drop presents similar effect as a quasi-reversible process (Taconni et al., 1973). In this case it is important, after checking the position of the electrodes in the cell and the Luggin capillary position respect to the surface of the working electrode, to increase the solution conductivity in order to diminish the uncompensated solution resistance.
A simple example of uncompensated resistance effect (ohmic drop effect) can be observed in Fig. 2 for 4×10^{-3} mol L^{-1} $Fe(CN)_6^{4-}$ ion in KCl aqueous solution where the concentration of the supporting electrolyte was 0.5 or 0.05 mol L^{-1} at different scan rates. Typical E/I profile

can be seen for the redox couple studied with anodic (E_{ap}) and cathodic (E_{cp}) current peaks well-defined. Also, no current peaks appear in the absence of potassium ferrocyanide. The experimental conditions were the same except for the supporting electrolyte concentration, which varied.

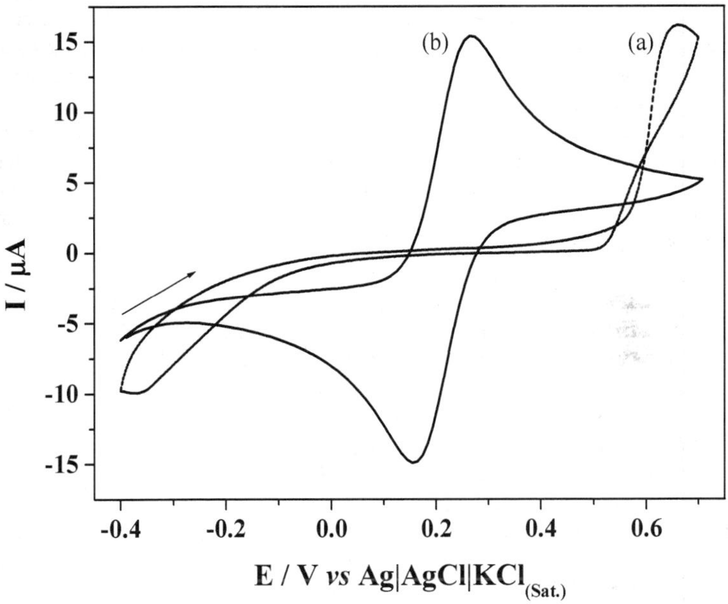

Fig. 1. Cyclic voltamograms of gold CDtrode in 1.0×10^{-3} mol L^{-1} $Fe(CN)_6^{3-/4-}$ phosphate buffer solution 0.1 mol L^{-1}, pH 7.4, at 50 mV s^{-1}. The CDtrode was cycled in 2.0 mol L^{-1} H_2SO_4 solution at 50 mV s^{-1}: (a) contaminated phosphate buffer solution; (b) cleaned phosphate buffer solution (Reproduced by permission of M.V. Foguel).

The main differences between these cyclic voltammograms were the separations between the anodic and cathodic peaks (ΔE_p) and the difference between the anodic or cathodic current peaks. For 0.5 mol L^{-1} KCl the values of ΔE_p were around 60 mV in 0.5 mol L^{-1} KCl (Fig. 2a) for all scan rates measured, while in 0.05 mol L^{-1} KCl, ΔE_p varied from 80 to 120 mV for $5 \geq v/\text{mV s}^{-1} \geq 100$ (Fig. 2b). CVs recorded in 0.05 mol L^{-1} KCl aqueous solution present all the characteristics of an increase in the uncompensated solution resistance as v increases: augment in the peak potential separation, decrease in current peaks and rounding of the peaks. The effect of current migration is very low for 0.05 mol L^{-1} KCl and completely negligible for 0.5 mol L^{-1} KCl in aqueous solution (Bard & Faulkner, 1980). In a parallel experiment, CVs were recorded for a solution containing 2.0×10^{-2} mol L^{-1} $Fe(CN)_6^{3-}$ + 2.0×10^{-2} mol L^{-1} $Fe(CN)_6^{4-}$ in the absence of KCl salt. The peak potentials were separated by more than 150 mV at 50 mV s^{-1} and the peak current was lower than the current measured when KCl was present. It means that the sum of migration and diffusion currents was unable to overcome the influence of the ohmic drop, leading to a lower instead of a higher total current. The decrease in the peak current was caused by the solution resistance.

Feldberg (Feldberg, 2008) simulated the effect of uncompensated resistance on the cyclic voltammetric response of an electrochemically reversible surface-attached redox couple assuming an uniform current and potential distribution across the electrode surface. The similarity of the effect of voltammetric responses for a slow electrochemical reaction and the uncompensated resistance is evident, which may cause misinterpretation of the mechanism of the electrode process. It is also common to attribute the linear current peak, I_p - $v^{1/2}$ relationship to diffusion, but sometimes nucleation or other processes can follow the same relationship (Noel & Vasu, 1990).

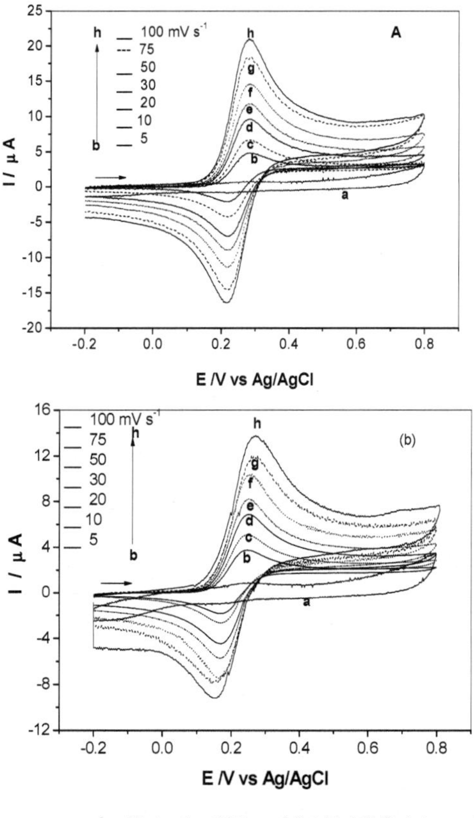

Fig. 2. Cyclic voltammograms for Pt in 4 x 10^{-3} mol L^{-1} $Fe(CN)_6^{4-}$ ion + KCl aqueous solution (**a**) 0.5 and (**b**) 0.05 mol L^{-1}, at 25 °C, geometric area of the working electrode of 0.027 cm^2 and at different scan rates.

As seen above, the CV has been often used to characterize immunosensors and many times a phosphate-based buffer solution is used, which may present effect of uncompensated resistance due to its low conductivity, resulting in cyclic voltammograms for $Fe(CN)_6^{3-}$ /$Fe(CN)_6^{4-}$ redox couple away from that expected for a one-electron reversible process under diffusion control. For this reason, phosphate buffer saline solution shows cyclic voltammograms with a better definition since it shows lower effect of uncompensated solution resistance maintaining all other parameters and conditions constant. For instance, Figure 3 shows two cyclic voltammograms for screen printed electrode and gold electrode in 1.0×10^{-2} mol L^{-1} $Fe(CN)_6^{4-}$, 0.1 mol L^{-1} phosphate buffer solution, pH 6.9, at 50 mV s^{-1} and 25 °C. The anodic and cathodic peak potential separation (ΔE_p) values are higher than 59.15 mV/n and therefore the electrode process cannot be described as one-electron charge transfer under diffusion control. It is well known that phosphate buffer solutions pH near 7 and salts concentrations around 0.1 mol L^{-1} present no classical response expected for a completely reversible process. The main reasons for that are the deviation of a reversible process, which leads to a response of a quasi-reversible system, and the influence of ohmic drop. Both of them increase the (ΔE_p) values. It is probable that both effects are present in the CVs of Fig. 3.

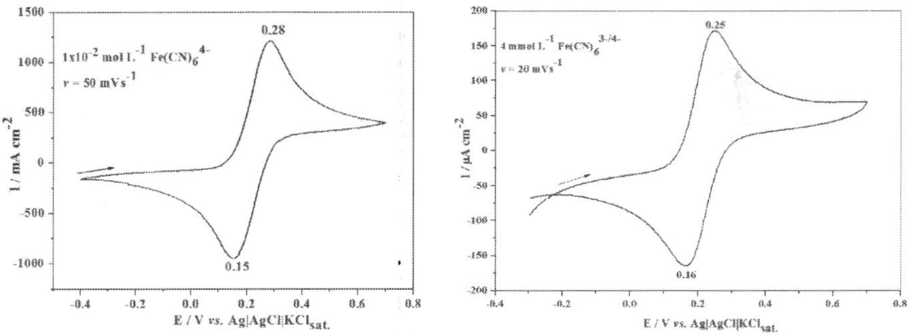

Fig. 3. Cyclic voltammograms for bare (a) gold-CDtrode ($A_{geom.}$ =0.071 cm^2) and (b) gold electrode ($A_{geom.}$ =0.0227 cm^2) in 0.1 mol L^{-1} phosphate buffer solution, pH 6.9, containing potassium forrocynide, at 25°C.

Cyclic voltammograms for a bare gold electrode recorded in 2.0×10^{-3} mol L^{-1} $Fe(CN)_6^{3-/4-}$, 0.1 mol L^{-1} phosphate buffer solutions, pH ≃ 7, at 25 mV s^{-1} resulted in ΔE_p = 90 mV (Campuzano et al., 2006), while in 2.5×10^{-3} mol L^{-1} $Fe(CN)_6^{3-/4-}$, 0.01 mol L^{-1} phosphate buffer, 0.1 mol L^{-1} KCl, pH 7.0, at 50 mVs^{-1}, a ΔE_p = 65 mV was measured (Pei et al., 2001). It is evident that the phosphate buffer saline (PBS) solution presents higher conductivity and is recommended whenever possible.

When 0.5 mol L^{-1} $NaClO_4$ plus 1×10^{-3} mol L^{-1} $Fe(CN)_6^{4-}$ was used, at 100 mV s^{-1} a ΔE_p = 70 mV was measured (Janeck et al., 1998). The idea that ohmic drop effect is present at lower concentrations of supporting electrolyte can be also inferred from the following results: 0.1 mol L^{-1} $NaClO_4$ and 0.1 mol L^{-1} KCl with 2×10^{-3} mol L^{-1} $Fe(CN)_6^{3-/4-}$, pH 7.0, at 25 mV s^{-1}: ΔE_p = 140 mV and 150 mV, respectively (Campuzano et al. 2006). However, recently Cho et al. (Cho et al., 2008) measured a ΔE_p = 100 mV for 2.5×10^{-3} mol L^{-1} $Fe(CN)_6^{3-/4-}$, 0.5 mol L^{-1} KCl at 50 mV s^{-1}. When CVs were recorded for different screen printed gold electrodes (SPE) in 1×10^{-3} mol L^{-1} $Fe(CN)_6^{3-}$ ion + 0.1 mol L^{-1} H_2SO_4 aqueous solution at 100 mV/ s ΔE_p = 62 to 76 mV and at 2000 mV s^{-1} ΔE_p = 78 to 231 mV were obtained, suggesting some influence of SPEs, mainly at higher potential scan rates (García-González et al., 2008). It is important to note that the conductivity of the sulfuric acid solution is higher than phosphate buffer and 0.1 mol L^{-1} KCl or $NaClO_4$ resulting in a lower ΔE_p value.

When an electrode is modified with self-assembled monolayer, or other modifiers, a barrier may be formed on the electrode surface, which in some extension hinders the charge transfer reaction. So, this effect can be studied by analyzing the changes in the electrochemical response of a reversible or quasi-reversible redox reaction of some electroactive species present in solution. Cyclic voltammetry of electroactive species such as $Fe(NC)_6^{3-/4-}$, ferrocinium/ferrocene, and others which can be used as markers, is a valuable and convenient tool for monitoring the barrier effect of the modified electrode, since the electron transfer between the electrode and species in solution must occur by tunneling either through the barrier or through the defects in the barrier. The tunneling electron transfer is expected to occur when the surface is completely covered by the modifier and an electron transfer via pinholes when it occurs at the defects of the modifier layer, situation where the microelectrode approach could be used. Having in mind a barrier effect, the surface coverage can be estimated from CVs resulting in a semi-quantitative analysis of this effect. So, in general, slight distortions on CVs compared to the bare electrode are expected when the modifiers produce a low surface coverage, which means that the access to the electroactive species from the solution to the electrode occurs without significant impediment. A great distortion on CVs suggests a strong barrier effect, limiting the access of the electrode surface by the markers present in the solution. Based on these ideas the surface coverage could be estimated from cyclic voltammograms assuming linear diffusion to bare areas by the equation (Janeck et al., 1998):

$$\theta_{CV} = 1 - (I_{p,mod}/I_{p,bare}) \tag{1}$$

where $I_{p,mod}$ and $I_{p,bare}$ represent the peak currents for the marker on the modified and bare electrodes, respectively. Different factors influence the cyclic voltammetric response: surface roughness, dominance of radial diffusion near each defect site (Janeck et al., 1998), the presence of positive or negative charge on the modifier can electrostatically interact with the marker increasing or decreasing the interaction strength, i.e., facilitating or making the charge transfer more difficult, or influence the lateral interaction by repulsion between the modifiers species (Calvo et al., 2004; Doblhofer et al., 1992; Ferreira et al., 2009). On a surface coverage, $\theta \leq 0.98$ at intermediates scan rates can give peak current intensity almost the same as the one obtained for a bare electrode, and a $\theta = 0.9945$ may show only 30% of decreasing in the peak current (Sabatani & Rubinstein, 1987).

Attention must be paid in using equation (1) to estimate the surface coverage, and generally, its values are lower than those obtained by other techniques including electrochemical impedance spectroscopy. Amatore et al. (Amatore et al., 1983) demonstrated that equation (1) is inappropriate for describing the fractional coverage of electrode surface due to the dominance of radial diffusion near each pinhole or defect site, and also the charge transfer reaction occurs without significant impediment. For instance, when cysteamine (CYS) and CYS and glutaraldehyde (GA) are used to form SAMs on gold-based electrodes, the surface coverage is low, around 0.10 for CYS-SPE and 0.35 for GA-CYS-SPE, and the charge transfer reaction involving the marker occurs similarly as in the bare electrode, with very low impediment (Ferreira et al., 2009). In this case tunneling of electron through the film can be ruled out (Porter et al., 1987) and probably the electroactive species reached the electrode through the large SAM free space of the electrode surface.

However, in the immunosensor characterization, CV was used to choose the better working potential for amperometric analysis (Stefan & Aboul-Enein, 2002; Zhou et al., 2003) and also to detect the presence of SAM and other modifiers on the electrode surface. CV was also used to evaluate if the SAM of hydroquinone on the gold electrode acted as a mediator of the redox reaction with pyruvate in phosphate buffer saline (PBS) solution, pH 7.4. Anodic and cathodic peak currents depending on the pyruvate solution concentration were observed after 5 min of dropping pyruvate solution on the pyruvate oxidase-adsorbed nylon membrane placed on the top of a gold electrode. The result allowed to conclude that SAM of hydroquinone acted as a good electron mediator for charge transport between pyruvate oxidase-adsorbed nylon membrane and the gold electrode (Xuan et al., 2003). It is easy to denote the presence of the SAM, for instance, on gold electrode since it can be oxidized to form gold oxides which are reduced to metallic gold again. A fresh gold electrode was evaluated before and after thiol deposition by means of a triangular potential scanning (Tlili et al., 2004) and it was observed that the oxidation reaction was reduced and no cathodic current peak was observed after the SAM formation of thiol. The stability of o-quinone produced on glassy carbon electrode modified with single-walled carbon nanotubes was confirmed by CV (Panini et al., 2008). Calvo et al. (Calvo et al., 2004) synthesized the redox polymer $Os(byp)_2ClPyCH_2NH$ poly(allylamine) (PAH-Os) and deposited on the thiolated (SAM of sodium 3-mercapto-1-propanesulfonate) gold electrode forming a bilayer, which was modified with antibiotin IgG and a supramolecular structure was constructed layer-by-layer. This structure responded catalytically to the presence of hydrogen peroxide when HRP is attached to PAH-Os/IgG multilayer. The cyclic voltammetry was used to confirm the presence of osmium in the PAH-Os/IgG multilayer self-assembled structure on gold and evaluate the electrode process involving the redox Os(III)/Os(II) pair in the presence and absence of hydrogen.

Cyclic voltammetry can also be used to increase the performance of the electrode surface, as in the case of highly oriented antibody on gold nanoparticle surface, which has its activity strongly influenced by the surface properties of the transducer (Lu et al., 1995). In this case, the existence of multiple states of adsorbed proteins involving multipoint hydrophobic, electrostatic, and hydrogen bond was assumed for the different surfaces and protein interactions caused by the unfolding of adsorbed proteins. It means that the surface can be treated in such way in order to change its activity. The influence of a chemical/electrochemical treatment of nanoparticles of gold/thionine-modified carbon paste interface can also be verified using repetitive cyclic voltammetry, which allows observing the evolution of the electrode surfaces along the potential excursion. Repetitive cyclic voltammograms of gold-thionine-carbon paste electrode in acetic/acetate buffer solution, pH 7.0 behaved in a completely different way when recorded before and after electrode treatment with 10%HNO_3 + 2.5%$K_2Cr_2O_7$ for 90 s and applying +1.5 V/SCE. The oxidation and reduction peaks decrease or disappear as the number of cycles increases for the electrode without treatment probably due to the removal of the hydrophilic gold nanoparticles and thionine molecules from the electrode. The authors also reported that the solution gradually passed from transparent to opaque. On the contrary, for the treated electrode the cyclic voltammograms improved with the number of cycles, probably because of the thionine molecules could be firmly attached to carbon surface via -Co-NH- structure. It is also possible that some electropolymerization occurs, constructing a third-generation network which could give higher stability to the thionine. The treatment also modified the carbon particles which underwent oxidation to form -COOH groups which can react with -NH_2 of thionine to form new -CO-NH- groups. Gold nanoparticles synthesized on multiwall carbon nanotube screen printed electrodes were also evaluated using cyclic voltammetry before and after modifications having $Fe(CN)_6^{3-/4-}$ as redox probe (Sharma et al., 2008). The MWCNTs were treated with acid solution to produce COOH-MWCNT/SPE and these MWCNTs were mixed in a Nafion® solution. The influence Nafion® concentrations deposited on bare SPE was studied in the presence of the redox probe. The greatest anodic peak current was obtained with 0.1 % Nafion® solution, which was chosen for further experiments. Higher concentrations, mainly 1% of Nafion®, blocked the electrode surface. A series of unmodified and modified SPE with gold nanoparticles (Nano-Au/SPE), MWCNTs (MWCNT/SPE), or gold nanoparticles plus MWCNTs (Nano-Au/MWCNTs/SPE) were studied in 1×10^{-3} mol L^{-1} $Fe(CN)_6^{3-/4-}$, 0.1 mol L^{-1} KCl at 50 mV s^{-1}. All modified electrodes showed a peak current higher than the bare one, which was attributed to the increase of the effective electrode surface area. This result is interesting because the active area increased, but in general, the modification of the electrode leads to a decrease in the anodic or cathodic peak current of the redox probe, except when some catalytic or immunosensor reaction occurs.

Gold nanoparticles and agar-agar solution deposited on graphite SPE generates Nano-gold/SPE and they can be evaluated by cyclic voltammetry performed in a thionine solution as redox probe (Zhao et al., 2007). For instance, in acetate buffer solution the CV behavior of thionine showed that the pair of current peaks decreased and shifted in a negative direction as the pH increased from 4 to 7, indicating that H^+ favored the redox reaction of thionine. To demonstrate the stability of the SPE nine parallel tests were done at pH 5.5 and the anodic potential for thionine was 0.796 ± 0.042 V/Ag|AgCl|KCl (KCl concentration not mentioned), and the peak current was 0.276 ± 0.003 μA, showing good reproducibility. The enzymatic catalysis, which indicates that the system works, was clearly demonstrated when H_2O_2 was added to the thionine solution since the cathodic peak greatly increased and the anodic one disappeared. However, the cathodic current greatly diminished when the immunoreaction (*Vibrio parahaemolyticus*, VP + anti-VP → immunocomplex) was permitted to occur. A similar study was also developed with immunologically-sensitive elements for prostate-specific antigen (PSA) detection using a self-assembled phenylboronic acid monolayer on gold (Liu et al., 2008), and CV together with photometry was applied to detect the formation of imunocomplexes of HRP-conjugated anti-PSA and its antigen.

An interesting application of cyclic voltammetry to characterize immunosensors was recently reported (Parker et al., 2009) for aflotoxin M1 detection using an array of 35 microsquares gold electrodes with 20 μm × 20 μm dimensions and edge-to-edge spacing of 200 μm, which avoids overlapping diffusion layers between neighboring microelectrodes in the array. The marker was 1.0×10^{-3} mol L^{-1} ferrocene monocarboxylic acid in 0.01 mol L^{-1} PBS solution at 5 mV s^{-1}, and a sigmoid response characteristic of steady-state CVs as expected for microelectrodes with a sufficient separation between two adjacent electrodes was obtained. The microelectrode interspacing was made of silicon nitride modified with aminosilane and cross-linked with 1,4-phenylene diisothiocyanate to give a larger modified area and to reduce the effect of surface modification on the electrode surface (microelectrodes). It leads to a signal less attenuated by the immobilized reagents. Afterwards, DNA was incubated and it was thought that only the surface covered with silicon nitride modified by aminosilane and 1,4phenylene diisothiocyanate had been modified with DNA. However, when microsquare platinum electrodes were used the current diminished in comparison to the bare electrode, suggesting that some silane attached to platinum surface allowing DNA interaction; this reduced the active area for $Fe(CN)_6^{3-/4-}$ reaction. When microsquares of gold were used the current was the same for both bare and DNA-modified electrodes, suggesting that the modification procedure has not significantly covered the gold surface. Certain shielding of $Fe(CN)_6^{3-/4-}$ reaction can be due to the physical coverage of the electrode by DNA and electrostatic repulsion between the negatively charged redox couple ions and the DNA phosphate backbone.

Lately, many other studies were developed using gold nanoparticles attached on a modified glassy carbon electrode, which is normally treated by applying a potential perturbation to produce hydroxyl groups on the surface, and cyclic voltammetry was used to characterize the changes caused by the different surface treatment and modification steps up to the construction of the immunosensor (Yuan et al., 2009; Lai et al., 2009).

In these cases as in many others, in general, cyclic voltammetry was used to identify the presence of modifiers on the surface by analyzing the response of a redox couple on the distortions of the CVs such as separation of peak potentials and blocking of the current. Rarely, cyclic voltammetry was used to estimate the surface coverage, θ, values in immunosensors characterization, which were also compared with those estimated from EIS studies (Ferreira et al., 2009). From CV studies, the values of θ for CYS-SPE, GA-CYS-SPE, Tc85 protein-GA-CYS-SPE were 0.10, 0.35 and 0.84, respectively, while from EIS they were 0.32, 0.34 and 0.99, respectively.

3.1.2 Electrochemical impedance spectroscopy

Electrochemical impedance spectroscopy is a very useful technique to study almost all phenomena occurring at an interface since it can explore a large frequency range covering a vast interval of time constant values. It allows to separate different processes such as capacitive, charge transfer, mass transfer, adsorption/desorption, and so on. For this reason, EIS is a powerful tool for investigating the mechanisms of electrochemical reactions, measuring transport properties of materials, measuring dielectric properties of materials, exploring properties of porous electrodes, investigating passive surfaces, investigating modified electrodes and, more recently, it has often been used to monitor the properties of SAMs, mainly in the presence of a redox couple in the electrolyte solution. It is important to note that the studies in the absence of a redox couple in the working solution are also of great significance to understand the stability, the electrical and physicochemical properties of the modified surface, but are rarely performed in the immunosensors field. The possibilities of using EIS are shown in Fig. 4.

Even considering that EIS is a powerful tool for studying many phenomena, as in the case of other electrochemical techniques, it does not allow the identification of chemical species. For this reason, many non-electrochemical techniques must be used to understand the global process operating on the interface which is being studied.

Where does the power of the EIS technique come from? It is a linear technique and as consequence the results are directly interpreted based on the Linear Systems Theory; if an infinite frequency range is explored, the impedance or admittance contains all of the information that can be obtained from the system by linear electrical perturbation/response techniques; the experimental efficiency is extraordinarily high, it means that a high quantity of information is transferred to the observer compared to the quantity produced by the experiment; the validity of the data is readily determined using integral transform techniques that are independent of the physical processes involved. So, what is the main

problem of using impedance? In general, the major problem resides in the models and mathematics involved in the data interpretation (MacDonald, 2006).
To review the fundamentals and to get more details and applications of impedance electrochemical spectroscopy some text books are recommended (Orazem & Tribollet, 2008; Macdonald, 1987; Gabrielli, 1980).

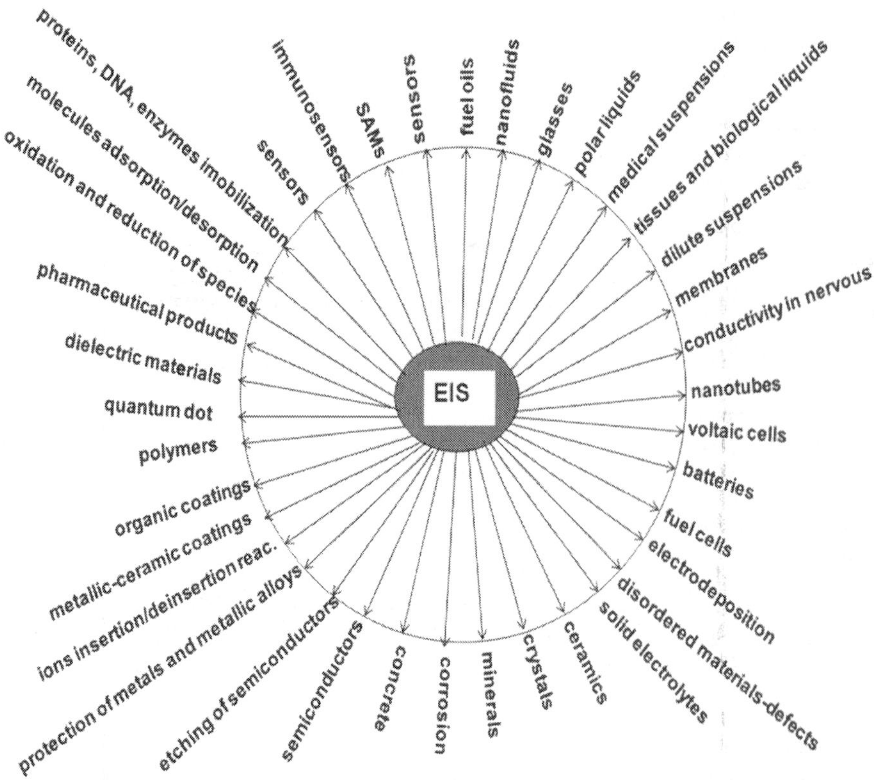

Fig. 4. Some systems that can be studied using EIS.

A great advantage of using EIS is that due to the small amplitude of the sine wave (current or potential) applied to perturb the system respect to its equilibrium or steady state, a sinusoidal perturbation of certain frequency results in a sinusoidal response with the same frequency, although the amplitudes of the entry and exit signals may be different and may present a phase shift. If the perturbation is appropriate the response can be analyzed using the theory of electrical circuits, which can be represented by a proper arrangement of resistors, capacitors and inductors, assuming a linear system. These equivalent electrical circuits (EEC) are models developed to explain the electrochemical impedance data and they must obey at least two conditions (Bonora et al., 1996): all elements of the EEC must have a clear physical meaning and associated to a property of the system which should be able to

produce that electrical response; the EEC must be as simple as possible and generate impedance spectra which are different from the experimental one only by a small defined quantity. The error must be low, not periodical or regular as a function of the frequency.
However, one needs to know that the electrochemical systems are not linear systems, and their response can only approximate of a linear system if, for instance, an enough small perturbation in relation to the equilibrium or steady state is applied to the system. On the other hand, a very small perturbation produces, generally, only a very small response signal, which can be affected by the noise, with a low signal-to-noise ratio. Thus, some requirements must be followed or observed to have a trustful impedance experiment such as linearity, stability and causality (Orazem & Tribollet, 2008, Gabrielli, 1980). It is possible that more than one EEC fits well to the experimental data and the choice by one of them must be based on the knowledge of the physical and physical-chemical phenomena occurring at the interface and on experiments under other conditions.
The obedience to the linearity principle depends on the amplitude of the sine wave, which is governed by the compromise between the desire to minimize the nonlinear response by using small amplitude, and to minimize noise by using a large amplitude perturbation. Therefore, choose the appropriate amplitude value of the sine wave perturbation is always very important to guarantee the best response of the system at each frequency applied and that the system is still exhibiting a linear behavior, which must be experimentally demonstrated. Note that all equipment gave the amplitude of the potential sine wave as rms (root mean square) that is defined as: amplitude $_{rms}$ (mV) = amplitude (mV) × $(\sqrt{2})^{-1}$. To evaluate if the system is or not in a linear regime one can record several impedance diagrams applying different amplitudes keeping all other parameters constant. Afterwards the modulus of impedance (|Z|) values are obtained from the impedance diagrams at certain frequencies (choose one or more frequency values but it is very important to examine the low frequency region since this region is more susceptible to a non-linearly response). The |Z|/|Z| ratio values measured at certain frequency (denominator obtained at 5 mV (rms)) are plotted against the amplitude (rms). Fig. 5 shows the |Z|/|Z| ratio values *vs.* amplitude plot for a carbon paste electrode in 0.1 mol L^{-1} phosphate buffer saline (PBS) solution pH 7.4 containing 1 × 10^{-3} mol L^{-1} $Fe(CN)_6^{3-/4-}$ ions. This figure clearly indicates that the system responds non-linearly for amplitude (rms) higher than 10 mV at the frequency of 50 mHz.
The stability means that the system should be stable at least during the time course of the experiment. It should be important at the end of an EIS experiment reproduces it beginning the impedance recording from the low to the high frequency, just the opposite that the experiment is normally performed. The causality is another important aspect in electrochemical impedance measurement: it means that no variation in the system can be observed before applying the perturbation. Also, the measured impedance must be finite.
If one compares a simulating with an experimental data set the interpretation of experimental results are rarely simple and further attention is needed. The difficulty may arise from the formation of adsorbed intermediates, which can lead to an adsorption pseudo-capacitance, two separately or partially overlapped semicircles can be shown meaning that the reaction can be more complex than the model; surface heterogeneities are equal to different charge transfer resistances, and also capacitances in a smaller extension; a range of time constants near each other can be a result of differences in the charge transfer kinetic from site to site, producing overlapping of time constants; and surface roughness. All these factors led to a depression of the semicircle causing its center to be below the real impedance axis (Gileadi, 1993; Jorcin et al., 2006) and then a constant phase

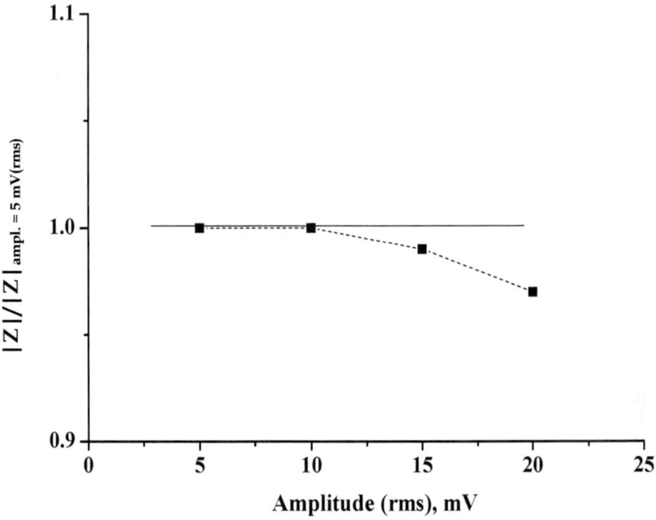

Fig. 5. Modulus of impedance (|Z|) vs. amplitude (rms) for a carbon paste electrode in 0.1 mol L^{-1} phosphate buffer solution pH 7.4 containing 1 × 10^{-3} mol L^{-1} $Fe(CN)_6^{3-/4-}$ ions at 25°C and 50 mHz.

element (CPE) substitutes a capacitor in EECs (Barsoukov & Macdonald, 2005). For the case that a CPE is parallel with a charge transfer resistance (R_{CT}) to form a "classical" semicircle, the following equation allows to calculate the capacitance value (Hsu & Mansfeld, 2001):

$$C=CPE(\omega_{max})^{n-1}=Y_o(\omega_{max})^{n-1} \quad (2)$$

In this equation Y_o is the canstant phase element parameter, ω_{max} represents the frequency at which the imaginary component reaches a maximum value and n is the exponent. Figure 6 shows the simulation of an EEC with a CPE parallel with a charge transfer resistance with different values of n. The results demonstrated that the depression of the semicircle increases as the n values increase.

Other complications come from the experiment such as non-uniform current distribution caused by the geometry of the cell as a whole or by an excessive approximation of the Luggin capillary of the reference to the working electrode in an effort to minimize the ohmic drop; solution creeping in the crevice formed between the working electrode and its non-conducting holder; changes occurring on the surface during measurement, for instance, corrosion of the working electrode (Gileadi, 1993). It is very important to note that the equations for EIS are based on the assumption that the surface is invariant during the frequency sweeping. It is worse if one scans up to very low frequencies.

All researchers using electrochemical techniques and mainly EIS must be careful and adopt very simple but very important cautions: use shielded cables and cables as short as possible; put the measuring system (electrochemical cell and equipment) in a Faraday cage; connect the electrical systems to a stabilized voltage; use no-break and excellent ground with wires separated from the electricity cables; do not connect to the stabilized electricity line equipment which can cause noise; avoid working near equipment with significant magnetic field; avoid using a plug located near distribution electricity lines; check switch on and off and other electric switches, electric contacts of electronic plates, cables and alligators clips (sometimes nickel or silver deposition or even metallic welding is recommended); be attentive with other sources of noise like electronic ballast for fluorescent lamp, radio waves, etc.; choose appropriate noise filters; test the potentiostat/galvanostat with a dummy cell (this test does not work for open circuit measurements because of filters only work when the equipment is on, meaning that some potential or current is applied, not at open circuit potential); check if the Luggin capillary is not blocked and so on.

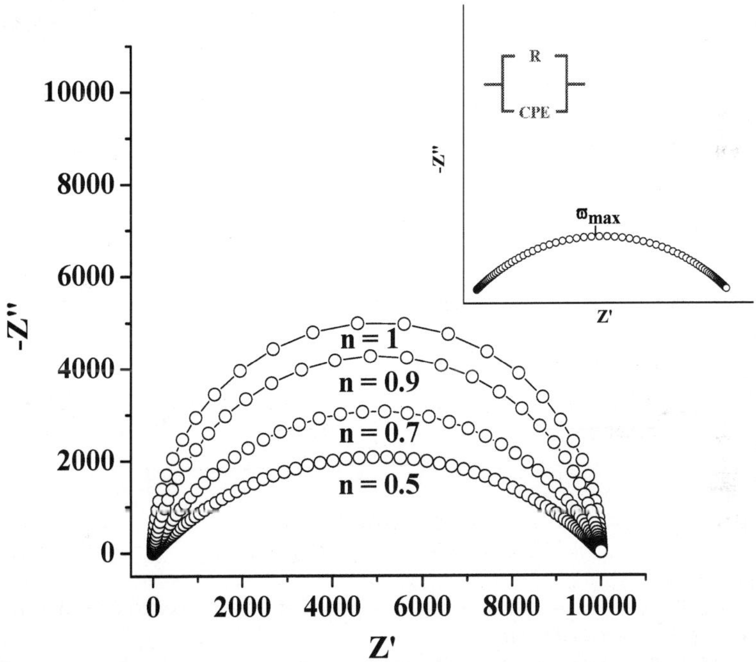

Fig. 6. Simulating impedance diagrams for the ECC showed in the figure for R_{CT} = 10.000 Ω, CPE = 1 × 10^{-5} μF cm^{-2} s^{n-1} and different n values.

An important aspect to be considered in impedance measurement is the working/counter electrodes areas ratio. Considering that both working and auxiliary electrodes are connected in series the capacitance measured of the cell corresponds to the sum of the inverse of both capacitances (C) (Orazem & Tribollet, 2008). The impedance of the cell is given by $Z_{cell} = Z_{WE} + Z_{CE}$ where Z_{WE} is the impedance of the working electrode and Z_{CE} is the counter electrode one. As both electrodes are good electrical conductors the real part of impedance is negligible and the imaginary part is $1/j\omega C$ where ω is the frequency and j is equal $\sqrt{-1}$.

However, if the area of the counter electrode is 20 times (or more) greater than the working electrode its capacitance is much higher than the capacitance of the working electrode. Therefore, the term $1/j\omega C_{CE}$ is much lower, and the capacitance of the electrochemical cell can be considered as that of the working electrode. Also, the impedance measured is normally not influenced by the one of the reference electrode due to the following facts: a) in terms of resistance or impedance the contribution of the reference is negligible since the entering impedance of the potentiostat is generally equal or greater than 10^{12} Ω, which is much higher than the impedance of the reference; b) in terms of capacitance the contribution of the reference can also be neglected considering the very low current passes through the reference and a Pt wire connected to the reference via a 0.1 μF non electrolytic capacitor can also be used.

These very simple recommendations which seem naïve are mainly for people who are being introduced in electrochemical techniques especially in electrochemical impedance spectroscopy as it is very sensitive to the experimental arrangement.

For each frequency applied only one impedance value is given in the impedance diagram for the system and it is recommended to read 10 to 12 points/decade which should be obtained for a less stable system using a low integration time and for more stable systems a higher integration time. The experimental points of a impedance diagram cannot be connected each other. The integration time means the necessary time to read each point of the impedance diagram with the precision chosen. This time is inserted in EIS acquisition software in different ways depending on the instrument. Therefore, each point in the impedance diagram represents a mean value of a certain numbers of reading and when the instrument cannot read an impedance value at the applied frequency with the precision established by the operator a dispersed point is obtained or the time required is too long to get a point in the impedance diagram. At low frequencies it is more common observe dispersed points due to the long time of measuring.

The impedance measurement represents the response of all components of the system: instrument of measuring, electrochemical cell and connection cables. In this case the limits of the instrument mainly at extreme frequencies or impedance must be considered. The response of an ideal electrochemical cell consisting of resistors and capacitors can be evaluated in an Accuracy Contour plot (Gamry Instruments, 2006) where the following parameters are established: the maximum measurable impedance, the lowest measurable capacitance, the maximum measurable frequency, the low impedance at high frequencies and the lowest measurable impedance. The impedance of an electrochemical cell can also be measured with some accuracy using this type of plot if the data are collected following the EIS theory: linear stationary system without current fluctuation and using an appropriate electrochemical cell.

The maximum impedance that the equipment can measure with accuracy at low frequencies is limited by the current fluctuation in the cell, fluctuation in the current measuring by the instrument and internal resistance. Under this condition the current values measured are very low, for instance, for an impedance of 10^{12} and 10 mV_{rms} the current will be 10^{-14} A, and the noise can significantly influence the measuring, making it important to use of a Faraday cage. This inconvenience can partially be removed by increasing the perturbation amplitude which is limited by the linearity of the system.

The capacitance of the instrument is important for systems like semiconductors, dielectrics and organic coatings (paintings) deposited on metallic substrates. For coatings the capacitance decreases as its thickness increases, situation in which the capacitance of the instrument can be important.

In general the maximum frequency is limited by the slow response of the components of the potentiostat, its instability, and the slow response of the reference electrode, which can be solved coupling a platinum wire (fast response) to the reference by a non-electrolytic capacitor. The capacitance of this capacitor must be chosen according to the system which is being studied. Systems with low impedance values (batteries and fuel cells) are normally studied at high frequencies where an inductive signal can be obtained. This inductive signal may originate from a physical chemistry process or can be an artifact caused by the inductance of the cell cables.

In the case of low frequencies and low impedances the measurement can be limited by the ability of the potentiostat in allowing the passage of high currents (an amplitude of 10 mV_{rms} with an impedance of 0.01 Ω generates a current of 1 A).

Experimental and simulated data are frequently represented in different formats such as complex plane (Nyquist) plot (Z″ *vs.* Z′ where Z″ is the imaginary and Z′ the real impedance), complex plane admittance plot (-Y″ *vs.* Y′ where Y″ represents the imaginary part of admittance and Y′ the real part), complex plane capacitance plot (C″ *vs.* C′ where C″ represents the imaginary part of capacitance and C′ the real part), Bode impedance modulus *vs.* frequency (log |Z| *vs.* log (f /Hz)) and Bode phase angle *vs.* frequency (-θ or -ϕ *vs.* log (f /Hz)). All complex plane plots must be isometrically represented. Sometimes it is convenient to subtract from the real part of impedance data the solution resistance before plotting the complex plane plots or normalize all complex plane plots to the same values of solution resistance. If the complex plane plots at high frequency show very different values a correction of the Bode phase plot is also recommended. This correction must result in the same values for both real and imaginary values at high frequency (choose a frequency in a stable region).

Regarding immunosensors, the study of the electrochemical impedance response of each step of the electrode modifications, which can be related to the nature of the different surfaces generated, may inform about the charge transport through the layers, surface coverage, and on the influence of antigen or antibody incubation time on the layer stability, mainly distinguishing physical and chemical interactions. EIS can also be used to develop impedimetric sensors.

For the major part of the studies in which the EIS technique was used to characterize each step of an electrode modification $Fe(CN)_6^{3-/4-}$ redox couple was employed as a marker and the data were qualitatively analyzed (Xiulan et al. 2011; Wang & Tan, 2007; Yuan et al., 2009; Wang et al., 2008; Liang et al., 2008). In the Nyquist plot a semicircle at high or middle frequencies followed by a straight line at lower frequencies were frequently observed. The semicircle was attributed to the redox process involving the oxidation and reduction of the marker and the straight line was related to the diffusion-limited process of the species in solution. The amplitude of the semicircle corresponds to the charge transfer resistance (R_{CT}) of the marker oxidation and reduction, the real impedance at highest frequency corresponds to the solution resistance, and the capacitance of the electrical double layer can be obtained from the frequency value at the maximum of the semicircle or from the value of the CPE. The values of the elements of the ECC are obtained by fitting the experimental data with an appropriate EEC which generally corresponds to the Randles circuit where a CPE substitutes the ideal element. The values of R_{CT} generally increased with the modification steps since the access of marker species to the electrode surface became more difficult and the semicircle overlapped the straight line which may disappear depending on how the electrode surface has been blocked. The values of EEC elements obtained in the simulation must be compared with those previously reported for the same or similar systems (Ferreira et al., 2009).

In some cases the stepwise process of the immunosensor construction was studied by EIS (Yuan et al., 2009)] and the real impedance measured in $Fe(CN)_6^{3-/4-}$ redox couple PBS solution (pH 7.0) was higher for the bare glassy carbon electrode than for the electrode modified with gold nanoparticles due to the increase in the active area of the electrode. In the next step the electrode was modified with nickel hexacianoferrate the charge transfer resistance increased due to the partial blocking of the electrode surface. However, the R_{CT} value decreased again when gold nanoparticles were incorporated to this modified electrode. The decrease of R_{CT} can be related to the increase of the conductivity of the system. When more modifications with organic molecules were performed the R_{CT} increased as expected.

Recently, more detailed studies on the surface modification using EIS with (Ferreira et al., 2009) and without (Ferreira et al., 2010) a redox marker $(Fe(CN)_6^{3-/4-}$ in the solution were performed. In the first study diffusion coefficients of the marker, R_{CT} and C_{dl} values were obtained and compared with data of literature for the bare gold-based SPE. The values of apparent R_{CT} and surface coverage of SPE with CYS, CYS-GA and CYS-GA-Tc85 protein were determined based on a treatment of impedance previously developed for θ values lower (Gueshi et al., 1978; Matsuda et al., 1979) and higher (Finklea et al., 1993) than 0.9. The modified electrode was interpreted as a perforated layer with the transfer reaction occurring at the uncovered regions of the electrode surface which represent defects on the SAM. The changes observed in the cyclic voltammograms and complex plane plots were analyzed considering that the defects are disc-like shapes uniformly distributed over the surface. Therefore the modified electrodes could behave as microarray electrodes with the redox species diffusing to the bottom of the pinholes to undergo charge transfer reaction. For $\theta >$ 0.9 the equations for the impedance were derived for microarray electrodes based on the nonlinear diffusion (Amatore et al., 1983) and from the real faradaic impedance, Z'_f *vs.* $\omega^{-1/2}$ and the appropriate equations R_{CT} and σ (Warburg coefficient) can be obtained when $\omega \to 0$. The faradaic impedance can be obtained by subtracting the solution resistance from the real part of impedance values (Janeck et al., 1998). The σ value is used to obtain the diffusion coefficient value using equation (3):

$$\sigma = \sqrt{2}\, RT/(n^2F^2CA\sqrt{D}) \quad (3)$$

where R, T and F have their usual meaning, C is the concentration of redox species, A is the geometric area of the electrode, n the number of electrons transferred per molecule or ion, D the diffusion coefficient. From the intersection of the lines at high and low frequency domains the nearest spacing between pinholes can be estimated, and then the values of r_a (mean radii of active area, i.e. pinholes) and r_b (mean radii of inactive area, space between neighbor pinholes). From impedance data the surface coverage were estimated to be around 0.32 for CYS-SPE, 0.34 for GACYS-SPE, and 0.99 for Tc85 protein-GA-CYS-SPE. For $\theta = 0.32$, the radii of individual active regions, and of surrounding inactive regions, were estimated to be 17 and 22 μm, respectively, for both CYS-SPE and GA-CYS-SPE. For the Tc85 protein-GA-CYS-SPE system ($\theta = 0.99$) the estimated radii of pinholes (r_a) and inactive areas (r_b) were 10

and 98 μm, respectively, and the distance between two adjacent pinholes, $2r_b$, was 196 μm. These distances are important to allow and facilitate immunoreactions to occur, and can also be regulated by producing SAMs with molecules of different chain length.
In the second study, electrochemical impedance spectroscopy was used to investigate each step of the procedure employed to modify a screen-printed electrode in pH 6.9 phosphate buffer in the absence of a marker in the solution (Ferreira et al., 2010). The SPE was modified with self-assembled monolayers of CYS followed by GA. Afterwards, the *T. cruzi* antigenic protein Tc85 was immobilized for 2 to 18 hours and bovine serum albumin, BSA, was used to avoid non-specific reactions. The complex plane plots were much more complicated to analyze when compared to the electrodes subjected to the same modification having a redox marker in the working solution. Different EECs have been used to fit the complex plane plots depending on the step of modification. It was demonstrated that phosphate ions adsorb on the electrode surface and the presence of oxygen altered the response of the bare one when compared to the one obtained in its absence. The real impedance values for each step of modification were much higher than those obtained in the presence of the redox marker and increased after each step of surface modification. The modulus of impedance obtained at 10 mHz from the log $|Z|$ vs. log f (not shown) increased in the following order: bare SPE (32 kΩ cm^2) < SPE-CYS (48 kΩ cm^2) < SPE-CYS–GA (53 kΩ cm^2) << SPE-CYS–GA-Tc85 protein (105 kΩ cm^2) << SPE-CYS-GA-Tc85 protein blocked with BSA (575 kΩ cm^2). A very significant result that originated from this investigation using EIS was the influence of the incubation time on the stability of the GA-CYS-SPE incubated with Tc85 protein. The impedance response was extremely dependent of the incubation time. The best incubation time of the Tc85 protein was 6-8 hours.
The total real impedance was very low (around 2 kΩ cm^2) for 2 and 4 h of incubation. A small capacitive semi-circle, followed by an incomplete capacitive arc was observed for 2 h, while an inductive loop was observed for 4 h at low frequencies. The real impedance increased considerably (from around 2 kΩ cm^2 to more than 120 kΩ cm^2) for 6 and 8 h of incubation and for 15 and 18 h incubation the real impedance decreased drastically. For 18 h of incubation an inductive loop was clearly observed, followed by a capacitive arc at lower frequencies. Bode phase plots showed three time constants for curves obtained for 2, 4 and 18 hours of protein incubation while two time constants for curves were recorded after 6, 8 and 15 hours. The interpretation of impedance data was based on physical and chemical adsorption, degradation of the layer at high and middle frequencies and charge transfer reaction involving mainly the reduction of oxygen at low frequencies. In the absence of a redox maker in an aerated phosphate buffer solution, these time constants were interpreted based on physical and chemical adsorption and degradation of the layer at high and middle frequencies, and charge transfer reaction involving mainly the reduction of oxygen at low frequencies (Ferreira et al., 2010). In conclusion, it was demonstrated that the electrochemical impedance spectroscopy is a powerful tool to evaluate the different stages and the integrity of the surface modifications and to optimize the incubation time of protein in the development of immunosensors.
By plotting the differences in R_{CT} values of a redox probe for a modified electrode before and after the assay procedure as a function of the antigen or antibody concentration an impedimetric immunosensor can be developed (Balkenhohl, T. & Lisdat, 2007; Barton et al., 2008; Vig, et al., 2009; Xiulan, et al., 2011). Navrátilová and Skládal (Navrátilová & Skládal, 2004) demonstrated the possibility of monitoring the immunoreaction of

dichlorophenoxyacetic acid herbicide (acid 2,4-D) on SPEs modified with SAMs at a fixed frequency. EIS were also used to study the regeneration of the immunosensor (Liu et al., 2008;Xiulan et al., 2011) by comparing the impedance diagrams and parameters obtained for immnusensors and after removing the antigen or antibody from the surface and following the next steps of immunosensor construction and analysis using the same protocol as before. In general, the first regeneration causes insignificant changes in the immunosensor response, but second and further regenerations diminished the immunosensor efficiency.

3.1.3 Other electrochemical techniques

Quartz crystal microbalance (QCM), ellipsometry, chronoamperometry, amperometry, square wave voltammetry (SWV), diferential pulse voltametry (DPV) and measurements of electrical resistance or conductance have also been used to study the characterization and the assay immunosensors.

The QMC technique has received special attention in the latest years and is based on the application of an antibody coating or an enzyme on a quartz crystal resonator with a cleaning gold surface which will capture a specific pathogen. The capture of the target pathogen increases the mass or viscosity of the environment of the gold surface changing the frequency resonance of the crystal. The impedance of the oscillating quartz crystal exposed to different concentrations of *Salmonella* was measured (Kim et al., 2003). An antibody-coated paramagnetic microspheres captured the *Salmonella* cells and the complex was magnetically moved to the sensing crystal and then captured by immobilized antibodies. The magnetic force was useful to enhance the response of the sensor. Many other studies were developed using the QMC technique to confirm the deposition of biological molecules on self-assembled superstructures and immunosensor assay (Shen et al., 2001; Calvo et al., 2004; Tlili et al., 2004; Mutlu et al., 2008; Boujday et al., 2009). A deep discussion on the use of QMC technique on the step-by-step immunosensor characterization and on immunosensor assay can be found in another specific chapter in this book.

In the immunosensors field the ellipsometry technique is generally used to characterize and understand antibody Langmuir-Blodgett films immobilized on immunoassay surfaces and determine the mean thickness of the films (Tengvall et al., 1998; Preininger et al., 2000; Nagare & Mukherji, 2009).

Chronoamperometry and amperometry techniques were largely used to measure the current and catalytic current generated by applying certain potentials and time during the immunosensors construction and immnunosensors assay (Martins et al., 2003; Ferreira et al., 2005; Zacco et al., 2006; Panini et al., 2008; Pividori et al., 2009).

Square wave voltammetry (SWV) and differential pulse voltammetry (DPV) as analysis techniques are much more sensitive than cyclic voltammetry and amperometry mainly due to the elimination of the background current during the experiment course and for this reason they are frequently used in immunosesors assay (Arias et al., 1996; Wang & Tan, 2007; Tang & Xia, 2008; Yang et al., 2009).

The measurements of electrical resistances or conductance (Tang & Xia, 2008; Maeng et al., 2008) have also been used to characterize immunosensors and in immunosensors assay. In the first case less labor and expensive and shorter time consuming immunosensor than conventional one was developed and in the second case a biosensor system that can be used for simultaneous screening of multiple pathogens in a sample was fabricated and characterized.

3.2 Non-electrochemical techniques

Surfaces modified with SAMs and by the different steps of immunosensors construction have also been characterized using infrared-based techniques including diffuse-reflectance infrared Fourier transform spectroscopy (DRIFTS), Fourier transform infrared spectroscopy (FTIR) and Fourier transform infrared attenuated total reflectance spectroscopy (FTIR-ATR). Infrared-based techniques have successfully been used in many surfaces characterization as adjunct to more well-known spectroscopic methods and are often useful where traditional techniques fail. Transducers modified with SAMs and biological molecules exhibit the conditions required for analysis, otherwise the molecules are diluted with non-absorbing powder such as KBr (Tengvall et al, 1998; Pradier et al., 2002).

Others techniques have been used as X-ray photoelectron spectroscopy (XPS) (Yam et al., 2001), Auger electron spectroscopy (AES) (Yang et al., 2009; Huang & Lee, 2008), contact angle measurements (Martins et al, 2003), surface plasmon resonance (Sigal et al., 1998; Silin et al., 1997), radiolabelling (Tidwell et al., 1997) for immunosensors characterization.

Atomic force microscopy (AFM) has been utilized to analyze the presence of the biological layer on the transducer and to obtain information on the surface morphology of the biological element of the sensor (topography images) or to immobilize the antigen or antibody-coated cantilever as immunosensor transducer, (Takahara et al., 2002; Ferreira et al., 2006; Grogan et al., 2002; Ferreira & Yamanaka, 2006).

The scanning electron microscopy (SEM) and transmission electron microscopy (TEM) were also used (Gan et al., 2010; Lu et al., 2010) since they can inform about the morphology of the unmodified and modified surfaces and on the nature of the nanoparticles used to construct the first step of an immunosensor or added after the end of some specific step to enhance the immunosensor response.

Enzyme-linked immunosorbent assay (ELISA) is a classical method employed in the optimization of the methodology to determine the presence of an immobilized active antibody or antigen and to monitor the lifetime and stability of the immobilized biological molecule and is also used to characterize the steps of immunosensors construction. The spectrophotometric method is used to detect the products of a reaction involving antigen and antibody with enzyme-linked and is essentially important to consider the principle of ELISA methodology on the surface transducer (Grogan et al., 2002; Ferreira et al., 2005)

4. Concluding remarks

The immobilization of antibodies on solid-phase materials has been used for the development of the immunosensor and different procedures were described in the literature. The potentiality of the methodology for disease diagnosis could be transformed into tools for clinical laboratories if the device would be repetitive, reproducible and sensible enough to distinguish the health from the sick person. The stable immobilization of biological compound on the transducer surface and then the surface characterization through electrochemical and non-electrochemical techniques will improve the real application of such devices.

Several electrochemical techniques such as potentiometry, amperometry, differential pulse voltammetry, square wave voltammetry, quartz crystal microbalance and electrochemical impedance have been used to determine the performance of the immunosensors and for analytical applications. However, it was also demonstrated in this chapter that some of these techniques such as cyclic votammetry and mainly electrochemical impedance based on the microelectrodes theory can be used to have a better idea about the surface coverage and also to estimate the size of pinholes and the mean distance between two adjacent pinholes. This distance is important to allow and facilitate the immunoreactions, and can also be regulate by producing SAMs with molecules of different chain length. It was also suggested that electrochemical impedance can satisfactorily be used to choose the best incubation time of each step of immunosensor construction. EIS may also help to a better understand the changes in the electrochemical response of each step of the immunosensor construction in the absence and presence of a marker since it is a high sensitivity technique and allows separating the contribution of the solution resistance from the other processes occurring at the electrode and solution interface.

The tendency in the immunosensor development seems indicate studies involving microfluidics, immunoarrays, transducers modified with nanoparticles, nanotubes and nanocones to produce devices with high sensitivity and able to be used for simultaneous screening of multiple pathogens.

The challenge is to develop immunosensor with a good performance to allow the point-of-care testing (POCT) it means a clinical results conveniently and immediately to the physician.

5. Acknowledgment

The authors wish to thank FAPESP and CNPq (Proc. 300728/2007-7 and 313307/2009-1).

6. References

Amatore, C.; Saveant, J.M. & Tessler, D.J. (1983). Charge transfer at partially blocked surface. A model for the case of microscopic active and inactive sites. *J. Electroanl. Chem.*, 147, 39-51.

Angerstein-Kozlowska, H; Conway, B.E. & Sharp, W.B.A. (1973). The real condition of electrochemically oxidized platinum surfaces. Part I. Resolution of component processes. *J. Electroanal. Chem.*, 43, 9-36.

Ao, L.; Gao, F.; Pan, B.; He, R & Cui, D. (2006). Fluoroimmunoassay for antigen based on fluorescence quenching signal of gold nanoparticles. *Anal. Chem.*, 78, 1104-1106.

Arias, F.; Godínez, L.A.; Wilson, S.R.; Kaifer, A.E. & Echegoyen, L. (1996). Interfacial hydrogen bonding. Self-assembly of a monolayer of a fullerene-crown ether derivative on gold surfaces derivatized with an ammonium-terminated alkanethiolate. *J. Am. Chem. Soc.*, 118, 6086–6087.

Balkenhohl, T. & Lisdat, F. (2007). Screen-printed electrodes as impedimetric immunosensors for the detection of anti-transglutaminase antibodies in human sera. *Anal. Chim. Acta*, 597, 50–57.

Bard, A.J. & Faulkner, L.R. (1980). Electrochemical methods, John Wiley & Sons, N.Y.

Barsoukov, E. & Macdonald, J. R. (2005). Impedance spectroscopy theory, experiment, and applications, John Wiley & Sons, USA.

Barton, A.C.; Davis, F. & Higson, S. P. J. (2008). Labeless immunosensor assay for the stroke marker protein neuron specific enolase based upon an alternating current impedance protocol. *Anal. Chem., 80,* 9411-9416.

Benedetti, A.V.; Nakazato, R.Z.; Sumodjo, P.T.A.; Cabor, P.L.; Centellas, F.A. & Garrido, J.A. (1991). Potentiodynamic behaviour of Cu-Al-Ag alloys in NaOH: A comparative study related to the pure metals electrochemistry. *Electrochim. Acta*, 36, 1409-1421.

Biegler, T.; Rand, D.A.J. & Woods, R. (1971). Limiting oxygen coverage on platinized platinum; relevance to determination of real platinum area by hydrogen adsorption. *J. Electroanal. Chem.*. 29, 269-277.

Bittencourt, R.A.C.; Pereira, H.R.; Felisbino, S.L.; Murador, P.; Oliveira, A.P.E & Deffune, E. (2006). Isolation of bone marrow mesenchymal stem cells. *Acta Ortop. Bras.*, 14, 22-24.

Bonora, P.L.; Defrorian, F. & Fedrizzi, L. (1996). Electrochemical impedance spectroscopy as a tool for investigating underpaint corrosion. *Electrochim. Acta*, 41, 1073-1082.

Boujday, S.; Méthivier, C.; Beccard, B. &Pradier, C.-M. (2009). Innovative surface characterization techniques applied to immunosensor elaboration and test: Comparing the efficiency of Fourier transform–surface plasmon resonance, quartz crystal microbalance with dissipation measurements, and polarization modulation–reflection absorption infrared spectroscopy. *Anal. Biochem.*, 387, 194–201.

Cabot, P.L.; Centellas, F.A.; Garrido, J.A.; Sumodjo, P.T.A.; Benedetti, A.V. & Nakazato, R.Z. (1991). The influence of the electrochemical treatment on copper-aluminum-silver alloys in deaerated 0.5M sodium hydroxide. *J. Appl. Electrochem.*, 21, 446-451.

Calvo, E.J.; Danilowicz, C.; Lagier, C.M.; Manrique, J. & Otero, M. (2004). Characterization of self-assembled redox polymer and antibodies molecules on thiolated gold electrodes. *Biosens. Bioelectron.*, 19, 1219-1228.

Campanella, L.; Attioli, R.; Colapicchioni, C. & Tomassetti, M. (1999). New amperometric and potentiometric immunosensors for anti-human immunoglobulin G determinations. *Sensors Actuators B*, 55, 23-32.

Campuzano, S.; Gálvez, R.; Pedrero, M.; Villena, F.J.M. & Pingarrón, J.M. (2002). Preparation, characterization and application of alkanethiol self-assembled monolayers modified with tetrathiafulvalene and glucose oxidase at a gold disk electrode. *J. Electroanal. Chem.*, 526, 92-100.

Campuzano, S.; Pedrero, M.; Montemayor, C.; Fatás, E. & Pingarrón, J.M. (2006). Characterization of alkanethiol-self-assembled monolayers-modified gold electrodes by electrochemical impedance spectroscopy. *J. Electroanal. Chem.*, 586, 112-121.

Carpini, G.; Lucarelli, F.; Marrazza, G. & Mascini, M. (2004). Oligonucleotide-modified screen-printed gold electrodes for enzyme-amplified sensing of nucleic acids. *Biosens. Bioelectron.*, 20, 167-175.

Carvalhal, R.F.; Freire R.S. & Kubota, L.T. (2005). Polycrystalline gold electrodes: a comparative study of pretreatment procedures used for cleaning and thiol self-assembly monolayer formation. *Electroanalysis*, 17, 1251-1259.

Chen, W.; Lu, Z. & Li, C. M. (2008). Sensitive human interleukin 5 impedimetric sensor based on polypyrrole-pyrrolepropylic acid-gold nanocomposite. *Anal. Chem., 80,* 8485–8492.

Cho, S.H.; Kim, D. & Park, S.-M. (2008). Electrochemistry of conductive polymers 41. Effects of self-assembled monolayers of aminothiophenols on polyaniline films. *Electrochim. Acta*, 53, 3820-3827.

Choa, H.; Parameswaran, M. &Yu, H-Z. (2007). Fabrication of microsensors using unmodified office inkjet printers. *Sensors Actuators B*, 123, 749-756.

Compton, R.G. & Banks, C.E. (2009). Understanding voltammetry, World Scientific. London.

Conoci, S.; Valli, L.; Rella, R.; Compagnini, G. & Cataliotti, R.S. (2002). A SERS study of self-assembled (4-methylmercapto)benzaldehyde thin films. *Mater. Sci. Eng. C*, 22, 183-186.

Diniz, F.B.; Ueta, R.R.; Pedrosa, A.M.C.; Areias, M.C.; Pereira, V.R.A.,; Silva, E.D.; Silva Jr.; J.G., Ferreira A.G.P. & Gomes, Y.M. (2003). Impedimetric evaluation for diagnosis of Chagas' disease: antigen-antibody interactions on metallic eletrodes. *Biosens. Bioelectron.*, 19, 79-84.

Doblhofer, K.; Figura, J. & Fuhrhop, J.-H. (1992). Stability and electrochemical behavior of "self-assembled" adsorbates with terminal ionic groups. *Langmuir*, 8, 1811–1816.

Escamilla-Gomez, V.; Campuzano, S.; Pedrero, M. & Pingarron, J.M. (2009). Gold screen-printed-based impedimetric immunobiosensors for direct and sensitive *Escherichia coli* quantization. *Biosens. Bioelectron.*, 24, 3365-3371.

Farre´, M.; Kantiani, L.; Pérez, S. & Barcelo, D. (2009). Sensors and biosensors in support of EU Directives. *Trends in Anal. Chem.*, 28, 170-185.

Feldberg, S.W. (2008). Effect of uncompensated resistance on the cyclic voltammetric response of an electrochemically reversible surface-attached redox couple: Uniform current and potential across the electrode surface, *J. Electroanal. Chem.*, 624, 45-51.

Ferreira, A.A.P. & Yamanaka, H. (2006). Microscopia de força atômica aplicada em imunoensaios, *Quim. Nova*, 29, 137-142.

Ferreira, A.A.P.; Alves, M.J.M.; Barrozo, S.; Yamanaka, H. & Benedetti, A.V. (2010). Optimization of incubation time of protein Tc85 in the construction of biosensor: Is the EIS a good tool? *J. Electroanal. Chem.*, 643, 1-8.

Ferreira, A.A.P.; Colli, W.; Costa, P.I. & Yamanaka, H. (2005). Immunosensor for the diagnosis of Chagas' disease. *Biosens. Bioelectron.*, 21, 175–181.

Ferreira, A.A.P.; Fugivara, C.S.; Barrozo, S.; Suegama, P.H.; Yamanaka, H. & Benedetti, A.V. (2009). Electrochemical and spectroscopic characterization of screen-printed gold-based electrodes modified with self-assembled monolayers and Tc85 protein. *J. Electroanal. Chem.*, 634, 111–122.

Ferreira, A.A.P.; Colli, W.; Alves, M.J.M.; Oliveira, D.R.; Costa, P.I.; Güell, A.G.; Sanz, F.; Benedetti, A.V. & Yamanaka, H. (2006). Investigation of the interaction between Tc85-11 protein and antibody anti-*T. cruzi* by AFM and amperometric measurements. *Electrochim. Acta*, 51, 5046-5052.

Finklea, H.O.; Snider, D.A.; Fedyk, J.; Sabatani, E.; Gafni, Y. & Rubinstein, I. (1993). Characterization of octadecanethiol-coated gold electrodes as microarray electrodes by cyclic voltammetry and ac impedance spectroscopy. *Langmuir*, 9, 3660–3667.

Gabrielli, C. (1980). Identification of electrochemical processes by frequency response analysis, Solartron instrumentation group monograph, The Solartron Electronic group Ltd., Farnborough, England.

Gamry Instruments (2006). Accuracy contour plots - Technical Note, PA, USA.

Gan, N.; Hou, J.; Hu, F.; Zheng, L.; Ni, M. & Cao, Y. (2010). An amperometric immunosensor based on a polyelectrolyte/gold magnetic nanoparticle supramolecular assembly—modified electrode for the determination of HIV p24 in serum. *Molecules*, 15, 5053-5065.

García-González; R., Fernández-Abedul, M.T.; Pernía, A. & Costa-García, A. (2008). Electrochemical characterization of different screen-printed gold electrodes. *Electrochim. Acta*, 53, 3242-3249.

Gasser Jr., D.K. (1993). Cyclic voltammetry - Simulation and analysis of reaction mechanisms, VCH Publishers. Germany.

Gileadi, E. (1993). Electrode kinetics for chemists, chemical engineers, and materials scientists. VCH Publishers, Inc., N.Y.

Godínez, L.A. (1999). Substratos modificados con monocapas autoensambladas: dispositivos para fabricar sensores y estudiar procesos químicos y fisicoquímicos interfaciales. *J. Mexican Chem. Soc.*, 43, 219-229.

Godoi, D. R. M.; Perez, J. & Mercedes Villullas, H. (2009). effects of alloyed and oxide phases on methanol oxidation of Pt-Ru/C nanocatalysts of the same particle size. *J. Phys. Chem.*, C 113, 8518–8525.

Grogan, C.; Raiteri, R.; O'Connor, T.G.M.; Glynn, J.; Cunningham, V.; Kane, M.; Charlton, M. & Leech, D. (2002). Characterisation of an antibody coated microcantilever as a potential immuno-based biosensor. Biosens. Bioelectron., 17, 201-207.

Gueshi, T.; Tokuda, K. & Matsuda, H. (1978). Voltammetry at partially covered electrodes. Part I. Chronopotentiometry and chronoamperometry at model electrodes. *J. Electroanal. Chem.*, 89, 247–260.

He, F.; Shen, Q.; Jiang, H.; Zhou, J.; Cheng, J.; Guo, D.; Li, Q.; Wang, X.; Fu, D. & Chen, B. (2009).Rapid identification and high sensitive detection of cancer cells on the gold nanoparticle interface by combined contact angle and electrochemical measurements. Talanta, 77, 1009–1014.

Hoogvliet, J.C.; Dijksma, M.; Kamp, B. & van Bennekom, W.P. (2000). Electrochemical pretreatment of polycrystalline gold electrodes to produce a reproducible surface roughness for self-assembly: a study in phosphate buffer pH 7.4. *Anal. Chem.*, 72, 2016-2021.

Horta, D.G.; Bevilaqua, D.; Acciari, H.A.; Garcia Jr., O. & Benedetti, A.V. (2009). Optimization of the use of carbon paste electrodes (CPE) for electrochemcial studies of chalcopyrite. *Quím. Nova*, 32, 1734-1738.

Hsu, C.H. & Mansfeld, F. (2001). Technical note. Concerning the conversion of constant phase element Y_0 into capacitance. *Corrosion*, 57, 747-748.

Huang, I.Y. & Lee, M.C. (2008). Development of a FPW allergy biosensor for human IgE detection by MEMS and cystamine-based SAM technologies. *Sensors Actuator* B, 132, 340-348.

Janeck, R.P.; Fawcett, W.R. & Ulman, A. (1998). Impedance spectroscopy on self-assembled monolayers on Au(111): sodium ferrocyanide charge transfer at modified electrodes. *Langmuir*, 14, 3011-3018.

Jorcin, J.-B;Orazem, M.E.; Pébère, N. & Tribollet, B. (2006). CPE analysis by local electrochemical impedance spectroscopy. *Electrochim. Acta*, 51: 1473-1479.

Kaláb T. & Skládal, P. (1995). A disposable amperometric immunosensor for 2,4-dichlorophenoxyacetic acid. *Anal Chim Acta*, 304, 361-368.

Kim, G.-O.; Garth, A. & Letcher, S.V. (2003). Impedance characterization of a piezoelectric immunosensor part II: Salmonella typhimurium detection using magnetic enhancement. *Biosens. Bioelectron.*, 18, 91-99.

Kwon, H.J.; Balcer, H.I. & Kang, K.A. (2002). Sensing performance of protein C immuno-biosensor for biological samples and sensor minimization. *Comparative Biochemistry and Physiology Part A*, 132, 231–238.

La Belle, J.T.; Bhavsar, K.; Fairchild, A.; Das, A.; Sweeney, J.; Alford T.L.; Wang, J.; Bhavanandan V.P. & Joshi, L. (2007).A cytokine immunosensor for multiple sclerosis detection based upon label-free electrochemical impedance spectroscopy. *Biosens. Bioelectron.*, 23, 428–431.

Lee, J.; Kang, D.; Kim, S.; Yea, C.; Oh, B. & Choi, J. (2009). Electrical detection of b-amyloid(1-40)using scanning tunnelling microscopy. *Ultramicroscopy*, 109, 923–928.

Lee, W.; Lee, D.-B.; Oh, B.-K; Lee, W.H. & Choi, J.-W. (2004). Nanoscale fabrication of protein A on self-assembled monolayer and its application to surface plasmon resonance immunosensor. *Enzyme Microb. Tech.*, 35, 678-682.

Liang, R.; Peng, H. & Qiu, J. (2008). Fabrication, characterization, and application of potentiometric immunosensor based on biocompatible and controllable three-dimensional porous chitosan membranes. *J. Coll. Interf. Sci.*, 320, 125-131.

Liu, S.; Zhang X.; Wu, Y.; Tu, Y. & He, L. (2008). Prostate-specific antigen detection by using a reusable amperometric immunosensor based on reversible binding and leasing of HRP-anti-PSA from phenylboronic acid modified electrode *Clin. Chim. Acta*, 395, 51–56.

Liu, Y.; Gore, A.; Chakrabartty, S. & Alocilja E.C. (2008). Characterization of sub-systems of a molecular biowire-based biosensor device. *Microchim. Acta*, 163, 49-56.

Lu, B.; Smyth, M.R. & O´Kennedy, R. (1996). Oriented immobilization of antibodies and its applications in immunoassays and immunosensors. *Analyst*, 121, 29R-32R.

Lu, B.; Xie, J.M.; Lu, C.L.; Wu, C. & Wei, Y. (1995). Luminescence quenching behavior of an oxygen sensor based on a Ru(II) Complex dissolved in polystyrene. *Anal. Chem.*, 67, 83-87.

Lu, M.; Lee, D.; Xue W. & Cui, T. (2009). Flexible and disposable immunosensors based on layer-by-layer self-assembled carbon nanotubes and biomolecules. *Sensors and Actuators A*, 150, 280–285.

Macdonald J.R. Editor (1987). Impedance spectroscopy: emphasizing solid materials and systems. John Wiley & Sons, N. Y.

MacDonald, D.D. (2006). Reflections on the history of electrochemical impedance spectroscopy. *Electrochim. Acta*, 51, 1376-1388.

Maeng, J.-H.; Lee, B.-C.; Ko, Y.-J.; Cho, W.; Ahn, Y.; Cho, N.-G.; Lee, S.-H. & Hwang, S. Y. (2008). A novel microfluidic biosensor based on an electrical detection system for alpha-fetoprotein. *Biosens. Bioelectron.*, 23, 1319–1325.

Martins, M.C.L.; Fonseca, C.; Barbosa, M.A. & Ratner, B.D. (2003). Albumin adsorption on alkanethiols self-assembled monolayers on gold electrodes studied by chronopotentiometry. *Biomaterials*, 24, 3697–3706.

Mendes, R.K.; Carvalhal, R.F. & Kubota, L.T. (2008). Effects of different self-assembled monolayers on enzyme immobilization procedures in peroxidase-based biosensor development. *J. Electroanal. Chem.*, 612, 164-172.

Mutlu, S.; Çökeliler, D.; Shard, A.; Goktas, H.; Ozansoy, B. & Mutlu, M. (2008). Preparation and characterization of ethylenediamine and cysteamine plasma polymerized films on piezoelectric quartz crystal surfaces for a biosensor. *Thin Solid Films*, 516, 1249–1255.

Naal, Z.; Tfouni, E. & Benedetti, A.V. (1994). Electrochemical behaviour of (N-R-4-Cyanopyridinium)-pentaamminruthenium(II) derivatives in acidic medium. Hydrolysis of coordinated nitriles. *Polyhedron*, 13, 133-142.

Nagare, G.D. & Mukherji, S. (2009). Characterization of silanization and antibody immobilization on spin-on glass (SOG) surface. *Appl. Surf. Sci.*, 255, 3696–3700.

Navrátilová, I. & Skládal, P. (2004). The immunosensors for measurement of 2,4-dichlorophenoxyacetic acid based on electrochemical impedance spectroscopy. *Bioelectrochem.*, 62, 11–18.

Noel, M. & Vasu K.I. (1990). Cyclic voltammetry and the frontiers of electrochemistry, Cambridge University Press. England.

O'Regan, T.M.; O'Riordan, L.J.; Pravda, M.; O'Sullivan, C.K. & Guilbault, G.G. (2002). Direct detection of myoglobin in whole blood using a disposable amperometric immunosensor. *Anal. Chim. Acta*, 460, 141–150.

Orazem, M.E. & Tribollet, B. (2008). Electrochemical impedance spectroscopy.John Wiley & Sons, Inc., Hoboken, N. J.

Panini, N.V.; Messina, G.A.; Salinas, E.; Fernández, H. & Raba, J. (2008). Integrated microfluidic systems with an immunosensor modified with carbon nanotubes for detection of prostate specific antigen (PSA) in human serum samples. *Biosens. Bioelectron.*, 23, 1145–1151.

Parker, C.O.; Lanyon, Y.H.; Manning, M.; Arrigan, D.W.M. & Tothill, I.E. (2009). Electrochemical immunochip sensor for aflatoxin M1 detection. *Anal. Chem.*, 81, 5291-5298.

Patil, S.J.; Zajac, A.; Zhukov, T. & Bhansali, S. (2008). Ultrasensitive electrochemical detection of cytokeratin-7, using Au nanowires based biosensor. *Sensors and Actuators B*, 129, 859–865.

Pei, R.; Cheng, Z.; Wang, E. & Yang, X. (2001). Amplification of antigen–antibody interactions based on biotin labeled protein–streptavidin network complex using impedance spectroscopy. *Biosens. Bioelectron.*, 16, 355-361.

Pham, T.T-H. & Sim, S. J. (2010). Electrochemical analysis of gold-coated magnetic nanoparticles for detecting immunological interaction. *J. Nanopart. Res.*, 12, 227-235.

Pividori, M.I.; Lermo, A.; Bonanni, A., Alegret, S. & del Valle, M. (2009).Electrochemical immunosensor for the diagnosis of celiac disease. *Anal. Biochem.* 388, 229–234.

Pohanka M.; Pavlis, O. & Skládal, P. (2007). Diagnosis of tularemia using piezoelectric biosensor technology. *Talanta* 71, 981–985.

Porter, M.D.; Bright, T.B.; Allara, D.L. & Chidsey, C.E.D. (1987). Spontaneously organized molecular assemblies. 4. Structural characterization of n-alkyl thiol monolayers on gold by optical ellipsometry, infrared spectroscopy, and electrochemistry. *J. Am. Chem. Soc.*, 109, 3559-3568.

Pradier, C.-M.; Salmain, M.; Zheng, L. & Jaouen, G. (2002). Specific binding of avidin to biotin immobilized on modified gold surfaces Fourier transform infrared reflection absorption spectroscopy analysis. *Surf. Sci.*, 502–503, 193–202.

Preininger, C.; Clausen-Schaumann, H.; Ahluwalia, A. & Rossi, D. (2000). Characterization of IgG Langmuir–Blodgett films immobilized on functionalized polymers. *Talanta*, 52, 921–930.

Ren, J.; He, F.; Yi, S. & Cui, X. (2008). A new MSPQC for rapid growth and detection of *Mycobacterium tuberculosis*. *Biosens. Bioelectron.*, 24, 403–409.

Sabatani, E. & Rubinstein, I. (1987). Organized self-assembling monolayers on electrodes. 2. Monolayer-based ultramicroelectrodes for the study of very rapid electrode kinetics. *J. Phys. Chem.*, 91, 6663–6669.

Sener, G.; Ozgur, E.; Yılmaz, E.; Uzun, L.; Say, R. & Denizli, A. (2010).Quartz crystal microbalance based nanosensor for lysozyme detection with lysozyme imprinted nanoparticles. *Biosens. Bioelectron.*, 26, 815–821.

Sharma, M.K.; Rao, V.K.; Agarwal, G.S.; Rai, G.P.; Gopalan, N.; Prakash, S.; Sharma, S.K. & Vijayaraghavan, R. (2008). Highly sensitive amperometric immunosensor for detection of *Plasmodium falciparum* histidine-rich protein 2 in serum of humans with malaria: comparison with a commercial kit. *J. Clin. Microbiol.*, 46, 3759–3765.

Shen, D.; Huang, M.; Chow, L. & Yang, M. (2001). Kinetic profile of the adsorption and conformational change of lysozime on self-assembled monolayers as revealed by quartz crystal resonator. *Sensor Actuators* B, 77, 664–670.

Sigal, G.B.; Mrksich, M. & Whitesides, G.M. (1998). Effect of surface wettability on the adsorption of proteins and detergents. *J. Am. Chem. Soc.*, 120, 3464–3473.

Silin, V.; Weetall, H. & Vanderah, D. (1997). SPR studies of the nonspecific adsorption kinetics of human IgG and BSA on gold surfaces modified by self-assembled monolayers (SAMs). *J. Colloid Interface Sci.*, 185, 94–103.

Silva, B.V.M.; Cavalcanti, I. T.; Mattos, A. B.; Moura, P.; Sotomayor, M.T. & Dutra, R. F. (2010). Disposable immunosensor for human cardiac troponin T based on streptavidin-microsphere modified screen-printed electrode. *Biosens. Bioelectron.*, 26, 1062–1067.

Sjoquist, J.; Meloun, B. & Hjelm, H. (1972). Protein A isolated from Staphylococcus aureus after digestion with lysostaphin. *Eur. J. Biochem.*, 29, 572-578.

Smith, J.E.; Wang, L. & Tan, W. (2006). Bioconjugated silica-coated nanoparticles for bioseparation and bioanalysis. *Trends Anal. Chem.*, 25, 848-855.

Sonti, S.V. & Bose, A. (1995). Cell separation using protein-A-coated magnetic nanoclusters. *J. Colloid Interface Sci.*, 170, 575-585.

Stefan, R.-I. & Aboul-Enein, H.Y. (2002). The construction and characterization of an amperometric immunosensor for the thyroid hormone (+)-3,3′,5,5′-tetraiodo-L-thyronine (L-T4). *J. Immunoassay & Immunochem.*, 23, 429–437.

Taconni, N.R.; Calandra, A.J. & Arvía, A.J. (1973). A contribution to the theory of the potential sweep method: charge transfer reactions with uncompensated cell resistnace. *Electrochim. Acta*, 18, 571-577.

Takahara, A.; Hara, Y.; Kojio, K. & Kajiyama, T. (2002). Plasma protein adsorption behavior onto the surface of phase-separated organosilane monolayers on the basis of scanning force microscopy. *Colloid Surf. B: Biointerfaces*, 23, 141–152.

Tang, D. & Xia, B. (2008). Electrochemical immunosensor and biochemical analysis for carcinoembryonic antigen in clinical diagnosis. *Microchim. Acta*, 163, 41-48.

Tang, D.; Yuan, R. & Chai, Y. (2006). Electrochemical immuno-bioanalysis for carcinoma antigen 125 based on thionine and gold nanoparticles-modified carbon paste interface. *Anal. Chim. Acta*, 564, 158-165.

Tang, D.; Yuan, R. & Chai, Y. (2008). Magneto-controlled bioelectronics for the antigen-antibody interaction based on magnetic-core/gold-shell nanoparticles functionalized biomimetic interface. *Bioprocess Biosyst Eng.*, 31, 55-61.

Tang, D.; Yuan, R.; Chai,Y. & Fu, Y. (2005). Study on electrochemical behavior of a diphtheria immunosensor based on silica/silver/gold nanoparticles and polyvinyl butyral as matrices. *Electrochem. Comm.*, 7, 177–182.

Tengvall, P.; Lundstrom, I. & Liedberg, B. (1998). Protein adsorption studies on model organic surfaces: an ellipsometric and infrared spectroscopic approach. *Biomaterials*, 19, 407–422.

Tidwell, C.D.; Ertel, S.I. & Ratner, B.D. (1997). Endothelial cell growth and protein adsorption on terminally functionalized, self-assembled monolayers of alkanethiolates on gold. *Langmuir*, 13, 3404–3413.

Tijssen, P. (1985). Practice and theory of enzyme immunoassays, Laboratory techniques in biochem. and molecular biology v.15, R.H.Burdon, P.H.van Knippenberg (ed.), Elsevier Science Publishers.

Tlili, A.; Abdelghani, A.; Hleli, S. & Maaref, M.A. (2004). Electrical characterization of a thiol SAM on gold as a first step for the fabrication of immunosensors based on a quartz crystal microbalance. *Sensors*, 4, 105-114.

Tokuda, K.; Gueshi, T. & Matsuda, H. (1979). Voltammetry at partially covered electrodes. Part III.Faradaic impedance measurements at model electrodes. *J. Electroanal. Chem.*, 102, 41–48.

Vig, A.; Muñoz-Berbel, X.; Radoi, A.; Cortina-Puig, M. & Marty, J.-L. (2009). Characterization of the gold-catalyzed deposition of silver on graphite screen-printed electrodes and their application to the development of impedimetric immunosensors. *Talanta*, 80, 942–946.

Wang, J.; Zhang, S. & Zhang, Y. (2010). Fabrication of chronocoulometric DNA sensor based on gold nanoparticles/poly(L-lysine) modified glassy carbon electrode. *Anal. Biochem.*, 396, 304-309.

Wang, S.-F. & Tan, Y.-M. (2007). A novel amperometric immunosensor based on Fe_3O_4 magnetic nanoparticles/chitosan composite film for determination of ferritin. *Anal. Bioanal. Chem.*, 387, 703-708.

Wang, Z.; Tu, Y. & Liu, S. (2008). Electrochemical immunoassay for α-fetoprotein through a phenylboronic acid monolayer on gold. *Talanta*, 77, 815–821.

Wu, J.; Fu, Z.; Yan, F. & Ju, H. (2007).Biomedical and clinical applications of immunoassays and immunosensors for tumor markers. Trends in Anal. Chem., 26, 679-688.

Xiulan, S.; Zaijun, L.; Yan, C.; Zhilei, W.; Yinjun, F.; Guoxiao, R. & Yaru, H. (2011). Electrochemical impedance spectroscopy for analytical determination of paraquat in meconium samples using an immunosensor modified with fullerene, ferrocene and ionic liquid. *Electrochim. Acta*, 56, 1117-1122.

Xu, X.; Liu, S. & Ju, H. (2003). A novel hydrogen peroxide sensor via the direct electrochemistry of horseradish peroxidase immobilized on colloidal gold modified screen-printed electrode. *Sensors*, 3, 350-360.

Xuan, G.S.; Oh, S.W. & Choi, E.Y. (2003). Development of an electrochemical immunosensor for alanine aminotransferase. *Biosens. Bioelectron.*, 19, 365-371.

Yam, C.-M.; Pradier, C.-M.; Salmain, M.; Marcus, P. & Jaouen, G. (2001). Binding of biotin to gold surfaces functionalized by self-assembled monolayers of cystamine and cysteamine: Combined FT-IRRAS and XPS characterization. *J. Coll. Interface Sci.*, 235, 183–189.

Yang, X.; Yuan, R.; Chai, Y.; Zhuo, Y.; Hong, C.; Liu, Z. & Su, H. (2009). Porous redox-active Cu_2O–SiO_2 nanostructured film: Preparation, characterization and application for a label-free amperometric ferritin immunosensor. *Talanta*, 78, 596-601.

Yuan, Y.-R.; Yuan, R.; Chai, Y.-Q.; Zhuo, Y. & Miao, X.-M. (2009). Electrochemical amperometric immunoassay for carcinoembryonic antigen based on bi-layer nano-Au and nickel hexacyanoferrates nanoparticles modified glassy carbon electrode. *J. Electroanal. Chem.*, 626, 6–13.

Zacco, E.; Pividori, M.I. & Alegret, S. (2006). Electrochemical biosensing based on universal affinity biocomposite platforms. *Biosens. Bioelectron.*, 21, 1291–1301.

Zhao, G.; Xing, F. & Deng, S. (2007). A disposable amperometric enzyme immunosensor for rapid detection of Vibrio parahaemolyticus in food based on agarose/nano-Au membrane and screen-printed electrode. *Electrochem. Comm.*, 9, 1263-1268.

Zhou, Y.-M.; Wu, Z.-Y.; Shen, Z.-L & Yu, R.-Q. (2003). An amperometric immunosensor based on Nafion-modified electrode for the determination of *Schistosoma japonicum* antibody. *Sensors & Actuators* B, 89, 292-298.

Biosensors for Detection of Low-Density Lipoprotein and its Modified Forms

Cesar A.S. Andrade[1], Maria D.L. Oliveira[2], Tanize E.S. Faulin[3], Vitor R. Hering[4] and Dulcineia S.P. Abdalla[3]
[1]*Centro Acadêmico de Vitória, Universidade Federal de Pernambuco Vitória de Santo Antão*
[2]*Departamento de Bioquímica, Universidade Federal de Pernambuco Recife*
[3]*Departamento de Análises Clínicas e Toxicológicas, Faculdade de Ciências Farmacêuticas, Universidade de São Paulo*
[4]*Departamento de Bioquímica, Instituto de Química, Universidade de São Paulo Brazil*

1. Introduction

Low-Density Lipoprotein (LDL) is the major carrier of cholesterol in the blood and plays important physiological roles in cellular function and regulation of metabolic pathways. Nevertheless, there are unquestionable evidences that increased plasma levels of LDL, especially their modified particles, are associated with atherosclerosis (Miller et al., 2010; Levitan et al., 2010). Atherosclerosis is a chronic disease that develops progressively through the continuous evolution of arterial wall lesions centered on the accumulation of cholesterol-rich lipids, several types of cells and an accompanying immune-inflammatory response (Libby et al., 2009). This disease begins in childhood, progresses relatively silently during adolescence and early adulthood but becomes clinically evident in the middle age or later leading to events such as myocardial infarction and stroke (McGill et al., 2000). The atherosclerotic cardiovascular disease is a major health problem worldwide and the most common cause of death in westernized countries, leading to a substantial economic burden. Whereas the levels of LDL and modified LDL circulating forms in the plasma are important predictive markers to gauge risk of cardiovascular events, there is need to develop reliable rapid assays for quantifying LDL and its modified forms, such as, the biosensors.

In general, biosensor is a measuring system that is composed by two major parts: a recognition part and a transducer part. The recognition part involves biological sensing elements or receptor molecules that lend the sensor specific to a target analyte (Chunta et al., 2009; Cooper & Cass, 2004; Fowler et al., 2008). A variety of biological substances can be used including antibodies, affinity ligands, isolated receptors, enzymes, organelles, microorganisms, cells, tissues, oligonucleotides, and lipoproteins. When biological substances interact with the target analytes, there is a change in one or more physicochemical parameters such as generation of ions, gases, electrons, second messenger formation, increase or decrease in enzyme activity, heat or mass. The transducer can be used to convert these properties into electrical signal.

There are three main types of transducers applied to LDL detection: piezoelectric (mass sensitive), optical and electrochemical. Among all types of transducers, the piezoelectric device has been used like LDL sensor. Piezoelectric device, often named quartz crystal microbalance (QCM), shows a very high sensitivity for detecting the target analyte that is placed on the surface of the device and generates the resonant frequency change. A piezoelectric biosensor device has important attractive properties such as small size, rapidity with high throughput, high sensitivity, and specificity. Lipoprotein immunosensors based on piezoelectric technology have been applied to capture and detect ligands on lipoprotein particles (Snellings et al., 2003). At the same time to explore monoclonal LDL antibodies (MAbs) in the interaction with the main protein constituent of human low density lipoprotein (apoB-100) a surface plasmon resonance (SPR)-based biosensor has been employed. Using this technique it is possible to measure the multimolecular complex between MAbs and epitopes of the apoB-100 in real time (Matharu et al., 2009a). The SPR detects and measures changes in refractive index due to the binding and dissociation of interacting molecules at or in proximity to the gold surface. This change of the refractive index is proportional to the concentration of the interacting molecule and causes a shift in the angle of incidence at which the SPR phenomenon occurs.

Electrochemical methods associated with nanomaterials have been employed to develop electrochemical biosensors for the detection of LDL. Cyclic voltammetry (CV) can be used to monitor the biomolecular interaction and explore association between antibody and LDL based on the modification at anodic and cathodic peaks (Stura et al., 2007). CV is an analytical technique to study the electro-activity of compounds, to characterize the redox properties and to provide information about the kinetics of electron transfer reaction of any coupled chemical reaction. Therefore, the advantage of electrochemical impedance spectroscopy (EIS) over other electrochemical techniques is that only small-amplitude perturbations from steady state are needed, and information concerning the interface can be provided (Bockris et al., 2000; Bard & Faulkner, 2001; Macdonald, 1987). In general, this system has been utilized to fabricate label-free high-sensitivity immunosensors with highly sensitive response to LDL (Yan et al., 2008). Hence, further studies based on LDL biosensors have been directed to diminish the detection time and develop new ways of detecting LDL and modified LDL.

2. LDL and its modified forms

The major lipids present in the blood plasma are cholesterol, fatty acids, triglycerides and phospholipids. Cholesterol is present in dietary fat, and can be synthesized in the liver by a mechanism that is under close metabolic regulation. Cholesterol, like all lipids, is not water soluble and thus, it is transported in the plasma in association with proteins (apolipoproteins), forming complexes known as lipoproteins. Lipoproteins are classified on the basis of their densities, which increases from chylomicrons through lipoproteins of very low density (VLDL), intermediate density (IDL) and low density (LDL) to high density lipoproteins (HDL) (Marshall & Bangert, 2008). The physiological function of LDL particles is to provide cells with the cholesterol they need mainly for steroid hormone synthesis and membrane formation. LDL particles assume a globular shape with an average diameter of about 22 nm and they are organized into two major compartments. An apolar core comprised primarily of cholesteryl esters, minor amounts of triglycerides and some free unesterified cholesterol surrounded by an amphipathic shell. This outer shell is composed of a phospholipid monolayer containing most of the free unesterified cholesterol and one single molecule of apolipoprotein B-100 (apoB-100) (Prassl & Laggner, 2009). However, LDL particles can undergo *in vivo* modification by oxidation, glycation, nitration and carbamylation, among other reactions. The extent of LDL modification can range from minimal modification, resulting minimally modified particles, such as the electronegative LDL subfraction (Damasceno et al., 2006), to extensive oxidation. Oxidized LDL is a generic term that describes a variety of modifications of both the lipid and protein components of LDL. Transition metal ions, lipoxygenases, myeloperoxidase, peroxynitrite and other reactive nitrogen and oxygen species derived from this enzyme, among others, have been suggested to be responsible for *in vivo* oxidative modification of LDL in humans (Stocker & Keaney, 2004; Malle, et al., 2006). Reactive oxygen species induce fragmentation of apoB-100. The polyunsaturated fatty acids in cholesteryl esters, phospholipids and triglycerides are also subjected to free radical-initiated oxidation to yield a broad array of smaller fragments (Matsuura et al., 2008). This results in a variety of reactive aldehyde products, including (E)-4-hydroxynon-2-enal (HNE) and malondialdehyde (MDA), which form covalent adducts with amino acid residues of LDL, generating HNE-LDL and MDA-LDL, respectively (Annangudi et al., 2008; Viigimaa et al., 2010). Glycated LDL is formed by the nonenzymatic covalent binding of reactive aldehydes (from glucose or related species) to a reactive amine (e.g., lysine and arginine side chains) on apoB-100 (Brown et al., 2007). The initial Schiff base undergoes subsequent rearrangement into Amadori products. The Amadori sugar–amino acid adducts can undergo progressive nonenzymatic reactions, leading to the formation of advanced glycation end (AGE) products, resulting in AGE-LDL (Basta et al., 2004; Hodgkinson et al., 2008). LDL can even be modified by urea-derived cyanate. Patients with kidney disease have elevated plasmatic levels of urea. Urea undergoes a spontaneous nonenzymatic transformation to cyanate in aqueous solutions and cyanate can react irreversibly with N-terminal groups of amino acids from LDL by a process known as carbamylation, forming carbamylated LDL (Asci et al., 2008).

The modified LDL forms, independent of the type of modification, triggers various biological responses, including pro-inflammatory reactions potentially involved in atherogenesis, promoting endothelial cell injury, expression of adhesion molecules on endothelium and vascular smooth muscle cell proliferation. Moreover, the modified LDL is uptaken by macrophages via scavenger receptors resulting in the accumulation of cholesterol within the macrophages and the formation of foam cells in the arterial intima. This continuous process lead to advanced lesions in arteries with a core of lipids and necrotic tissue covered by a fibrous cap. Disruption of the cap can lead to thrombosis and many of the adverse clinical outcomes associated with atherosclerosis (Hansson & Libby, 2006). As the LDL modified forms are proinflammatory and proatherogenic, studies have been done to develop a method to quantify the modified LDL subfraction as a blood biomarker to diagnose cardiovascular diseases and perhaps predict clinical outcomes. Plasma biomarkers have the advantage of being non-invasive and, if abnormal, allow opportunities of early stage intervention.

3. Methods for measurement of LDL and modified LDL

A classic method for measurement of LDL is the beta-quantification, which involves ultracentrifugation and a chemical precipitation step (Bachorik, 1997). Because beta-quantification is cumbersome and requires sophisticated equipment, in most clinical laboratories LDL is usually estimated by Friedewald equation (Friedewald et al., 1972), an indirect method, which estimates the LDL from measurements of total cholesterol (TC), triglycerides (TG), and HDL (Eq. 1).

$$LDL(mg / dL) = TC - HDL - TG / 5 \tag{1}$$

Despite the simplicity and lack of cost, the error of determining LDL through that estimation comprises the addition of the analytical errors of the three parameters used in the calculus. In addition, the use of that formula has severe limitations and cannot be applied to samples containing TG levels > 400 mg/dL or in samples with chylomicrons, as occurs in non-fasting samples. Because of the limitations of the Friedewald calculation, some clinical laboratories use enzymatic colorimetric methods for quantification of LDL, which are direct, relatively simple, can be used in automated systems (Cordova et al., 2004; Esteban-Salan et al., 2008) and LDL values are not affected by the presence of increased levels of triglycerides (Rifai et al., 1998). The aforementioned methods quantify the total LDL (modified and unmodified fractions). In the last two decades, aiming to determine the modified LDL subfraction in the blood circulation, ELISAs (Enzyme-Linked Immunosorbent Assay) using monoclonal antibodies were developed. There are ELISAs used in research to measure oxidized LDL (Itabe & Ueda, 2007) and electronegative LDL (Faulin et al., 2008). ELISA is a method that has high sensitivity and specificity, low cost, technical simplicity, versatility and ability to adapt to different degrees of automation, however, it is a time-consuming test consisting of several steps.

4. Biosensors

A biosensor is a physicochemical analytical device for the detection of an interaction of the analyte that combines with a biological component, which recognizes a chemical or physical change, with a detector component that produces a measurable signal in response to the environmental change (Chunta et al., 2009; Cooper & Cass, 2004; Fowler et al., 2008). The characteristic trait of a biosensor is the direct spatial contact between the biological recognition element (or bioreceptor) and the transducing element (Thevenot et al., 1999). Therefore, biosensor is a measurement device or system that is composed of two major parts: a recognition part and a transducer part (Fig. 1).

A biosensor is an integrated receptor-transducer device, which is capable of providing selective quantitative or semi-quantitative analytical information (Jambunathan & Hillier, 2003). The biosensor consists, on the one hand, of a biological recognition element, which acts upon a biochemical mechanism, and of a transducer relying on electrochemical, mass, optical or thermal principles.

Typical bioreceptors in biosensors are enzymes, antibodies, lectins, microorganisms and nucleic acids. In addition, the use of biosensors offer several benefits over conventional diagnostic tools as simplicity, specificity, speed, low-cost, portable instrumentation and capability for continuous monitoring in real-time (Freire et al., 2002; Malhotra et al., 2006; Zhao & Ju, 2006). LDL sensors (lipoprotein sensors) are a new promising group or bioreceptors, because of their outstanding selectivity and stability in responses that provides an evaluation about biomedical diagnosis in plasma LDL levels (Matharu et al., 2009a, 2009b, 2010). New methods for diagnosis of LDL employing biosensors are the current demand to evaluate the risk factors for atherosclerosis. Thus, the basic principles of the quartz crystal microbalance (QCM), surface plasmon resonance (SPR), cyclic voltammetry (CV) and electrochemical impedance spectroscopy (EIS) are discussed with the purpose of showing their importance in quantitative or qualitative LDL analysis.

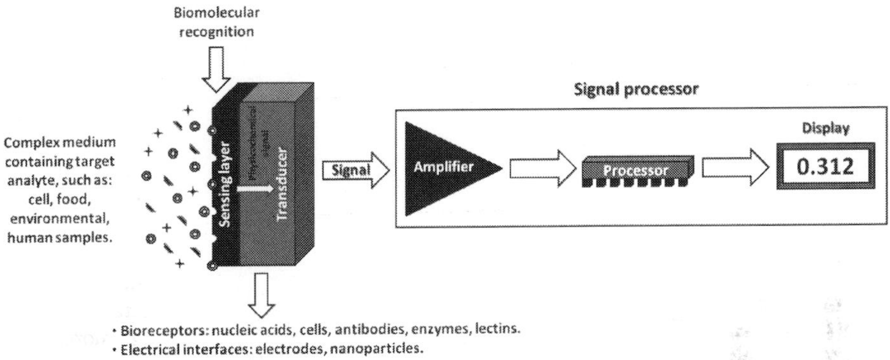

Fig. 1. Schematic diagram of a biosensor. A biosensor consists of a bioreceptor for the specific detection of the respective analyte in spatial contact to a transducer for converting the signal into an electrically manageable format and a signal processing unit.

5. Quartz crystal microbalance

Among biosensor devices, piezoelectric has been highly recognized due to their small size, low cost, use of a small volume of sample, high sensitivity, high specificity, rapid response, reproducibility and ease of portable multiple specific sensor array fabrication (Chunta et al., 2009). The QCM is an ultra-sensitive weighing device (to measure or detect a small mass change) that utilizes the mechanical resonance of piezoelectric single-crystalline quartz (Höök & Rudh, 2005). The piezoelectricity was discovered by Jacques and Pierre Curie in 1880 (Curie J. & Curie P., 1880a,b) as a potential difference generated across two surfaces of a crystal (including quartz, Rochelle salt and tourmaline) under strain, whose magnitude of electrical potential was proportional to the applied stress (Chunta et al., 2009; Höök & Rudh, 2005; Smith, 2008). Therefore, piezoelectricity is defined as electric polarization produced by mechanical strain in certain crystals, the polarization being proportional to the strain (Smith, 2008).

Quartz crystals (Fig. 2a) are generally used as weighing devices. Quartz crystal can be cut in different angles which gives different quartz crystal types with specific properties. Typically for piezoelectric analytical work, quartz crystals are cut in the AT form, at a +35°15′ angle from the Z-axis (Bunde et al., 1998). This geometry has a zero temperature coefficient which provides a stable oscillation with almost no temperature fluctuation in frequency in wide temperature range (Höök & Rudh, 2005). In addition, quartz is the most commonly crystal used, due to its strong piezoelectric response, abundance, processability, and anisotropy.

QCM is an important technique that has unique advantages for addressing the problems and issues involved in developing these new measurement methodologies (Marx, 2003). The use of the crystal resonator has been extended to numerous applications in different fields like electrochemistry and biology (Arnau, 2008). According to Smith (2008) the resonance frequency depends upon the angles with respect to the optical axis at which the wafer was cut from a single crystal and inversely on the crystal thickness.

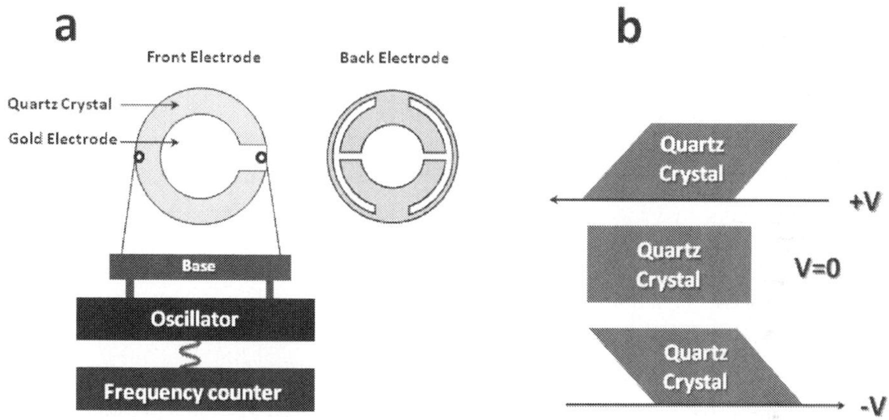

Fig. 2. Experimental apparatus for a piezoelectric system (a) and piezoelectric effect for shear motion (b).

5.1 Principles of mass measurement

When an alternating-current (AC) voltage is applied across of AT-cut quartz crystal (Fig. 2b), through opposing electrodes deposited on its surfaces, the resonance is excited if the frequency of the applied voltage corresponds to the resonance frequency (f_0) of the crystal (Arnau, 2008; Chunta et al., 2009; Höök & Rudh, 2005; Smith, 2008). It generates a transversal acoustic wave propagating through the quartz to the contacting media and this condition occurs when the thickness of the disc is an odd integer number of half-wavelengths of the standing wave induced between the electrodes, causing the mechanical oscillation to have its anti-nodes at each electrode interface (Höök & Rudh, 2005). The resonance frequency of the crystal is thus directly proportional to the total mass of the crystal. The frequency range for the fundamental mode of quartz is between 5 and 20 MHz (Marx, 2003). Although, most applications have used QCM devices operating in the 5-10 MHz range.

A method for correlating changes in the oscillation frequency of a piezoelectric crystal with the mass deposited on it was developed by Günter Sauerbrey (Sauerbrey, 1959). Sauerbrey developed a method for measuring the frequency and its changes by using the crystal as the frequency determining component of an oscillator circuit. The Sauerbrey equation is defined as:

$$\Delta f = \frac{-2\Delta m f_0^2}{A\sqrt{\rho_q \mu_q}} = -C\Delta m \tag{2}$$

where Δf is the change in the fundamental frequency (Hz), Δm is mass change (g), f_0 is the resonant frequency of crystal (Hz), A is piezoelectrically active crystal area (area between

electrodes in cm^2), ρ_q is density of quartz crystal (ρ_q = 2.648 g/cm^3), μ_q is shear modulus of quartz for AT-cut crystal (μ_q = 2.947x10^{11} g/cm.s^2), and C is the mass sensitivity constant (based on type of crystal used) (s.g^{-1}).
According to Bunde and collaborators (1998), Sauerbrey's equation is based on the deposition of rigid layers that are infinitesimally thin and, thus, dampen the propagation of the bulk shear wave in a fashion identical to quartz itself. Since the film is treated as an extension of thickness, this approach only applies to systems in which the some conditions are present, as follow: deposited mass must be rigid, uniformly distributed and frequency change $\Delta f/f < 0.02$ (Srivastava & Sakthivel, 2001).
This approach was developed for oscillation in air and only applies to rigid masses attached to the crystal. In the beginning of 80's, scientists have been shown that quartz crystal microbalance measurements can be performed in Newtonian liquid. Kanazawa and collaborators (1985) showed that the change in the resonant frequency of quartz crystal that contacted with the liquid is expressed by:

$$\Delta f = -f_0^{3/2}\left(\frac{\rho_L \eta_L}{\pi \rho_q \mu_q}\right)^{1/2} \quad (3)$$

where ρ_L is the density of liquid in contact with the crystal and η_L is the viscosity of liquid in contact with the crystal (Kanazawa & Gordon II, 1985).

5.2 Piezoelectric LDL biosensors

Lipoprotein biosensors based on piezoelectric technology have been employed to capture and detect ligands on lipoprotein particles. The critical step in LDL detection is the selective separation of LDL from the other lipoprotein fractions (Snellings et al., 2003). A specific ligand for the LDL receptor is apoB-100 (Schumaker et al., 1994), a major apolipoprotein of LDL and a very large glycoprotein consisting of a single polypeptide chain of 4536 amino acid residues with a molar mass of 514 kDa (Yang et al., 1986). The entrapment of LDL in the arterial intima is mainly due to the specific interaction between the lysine-rich sites on apoB-100 and the extracellular matrix (ECM) components such as collagen, proteoglycans (PGs), and glycosaminoglycans (GAGs) (D'Ulivo et al., 2010). Valuable techniques already exist for studies on apoB-100 and ECM interactions (D'Ulivo et al., 2009, 2010). In addition, other techniques as affinity chromatography and capillary electrochromatography are available for apoB-ECM interaction studies (D'Ulivo et al., 2009), but new microsystems and miniaturized instrumental tools are desirable to provide complementary information. D'Ulivo and collaborators (2010) explored the applicability of the QCM for interaction studies between apoB-100 peptide fragments and various components of the ECM. They selected three peptide residues from the apoB-100 sequence that are responsible for the binding of LDL with PGs (Skålén et al., 2002). One of these is a water-soluble peptide residue with 19 amino acids, positively charged (net charge of +6) that interacts selectively with the LDL receptor (Camejo et al., 1998). The second positive peptide, consisting of 42 amino acids, has a net charge of +3. This peptide is fairly hydrophobic and soluble only in pure dimethyl sulfoxide and in lipids. Neutral peptide fragment with 11 amino acids was selected as control fragment, since it should not interact with the ECM components (D'Ulivo et al., 2009). Functionalized carboxyl and polystyrene sensor chips were used in this study to evaluate the interactions between apoB-100 peptide fragments and components of the ECM. D'Ulivo and collaborators (2010) showed that apoB-100 peptides interact with ECM components via electrostatic interactions, most likely involving their positive residues, lysine and arginine, and that the binding is selective for GAGs.

Others reports describe the use of QCM for on-line monitoring of the adsorption of LDL onto cholesterol-modified dextran (CMD) (Liu et al., 2007). Because LDL particles are the main carries of cholesterol transfer and metabolism, accumulation of LDL is regarded as the first stage of atherosclerotic lesions. These researchers have been engaged in evaluatin the hydrophobic adsorbent, CMD, to investigate the kinetic adsorption curves. Experimental results showed that this system was capable to predict the adsorption capacities and concentrations at ng/µl. Many researchers have been involved in development of different kinds of adsorbents including non-specific, selective adsorbents and immuno-adsorbent according to the molecular structure of LDL (Behm et al., 1989; Bosch et al., 1997).

Piezoelectric technique can be associated to SPR technique to obtain new immunosensor devices. Immunosensors are affinity ligand-based biosensing devices that involve the coupling of immunochemical reactions to appropriate transducers. In recent decades, immunosensors have received rapid development and wide applications with various detection formats (Luppa et al., 2001; Stefan et al., 2000). The general working principle of the immunosensors is based on the fact that the specific immunochemical recognition of antibodies (antigens) immobilized on a transducer to antigens (antibodies) in the sample media can produce analytical signals dynamically varying with the concentrations of analytes of interest. Matharu et al. (2009a) obtained an accurate and specific human plasma LDL immunosensor based on SPR and QCM by immobilizing anti-apolipoprotein B (AapoB) onto self-assembled monolayer of 4-aminothiophenol (AT). The AapoB/AT/Au immunosensor detected LDL up to 0.252 µM (84 mg/dl) and 0.360 µM (120 mg/dl) with sensitivity of 475.39 Hz/µM and 977.96 m°/µM by QCM and SPR techniques, respectively. The analysis of the values of association constants at different temperatures and the enthalpy of adsorption (ΔH_{ads}) indicated the AapoB-LDL interaction to be endothermic in nature. The positive value of entropy ($T\Delta S_{ads}$) was found to be greater than ΔH_{ads} indicating the adsorption process to be entropy driven. Kinetic, thermodynamic, and sticking probability studies revealed that desorption of water from LDL and AapoB surfaces play the most important role in the binding of LDL to AapoB which enhances with increase in the temperature. In addition, a label-free and reusable AapoB/AT/Au immunosensor was fabricated for estimation of LDL.

6. Surface plasmon resonance

Due to the introduction of sensitive bench top instruments and the expansion in the range of strategies for studying biological or biochemical systems (Green et al., 2000; Oliveira et al., 2011) in more recent times, SPR based techniques have found expanded use and recently they have been introduced in clinical studies (Matharu et al., 2009a, 2009b). The competitive advantages of such techniques include the fact that SPR can be applied to a wide range of biomedically relevant interfaces and allows both real-time qualitative and quantitative assessments of the prevailing biomolecular interactions while eliminating the need of labeling reagents and without any complex sample preparation. The use of SPR technique to probe ligand-ligate surface interactions is advantageous, since it is able to rapidly monitor dynamic process, such as adsorption or degradation. SPR provides further information on the rate and extent of adsorption, enabling the determination of dielectric properties, association/dissociation kinetics and affinity constants of specific ligand-ligate interactions (Green et al., 2000). In addition, the SPR signal is highly sensitive to even small changes in the refractive index at the interface with a thin noble metal film (Helali et al., 2008). The phenomenon of anomalous diffraction on diffraction gratings due to the excitation of surface plasma waves was first described by Wood (1902). Otto (1968) and Kretschmann & Raether (1968) demonstrated the method of attenuated total reflection (ATR) for optical excitation of surface plasmons (SP). In the Otto setup, the light is shone on the wall of a prism and totally reflected. In this system a thin metal layer is positioned close enough, that the evanescent waves can interact with the plasma waves on the surface and excite the plasmons. In the case of Kretschmann configuration - widely used within the designs of most SPR instruments - relies on the phenomenon of ATR (Fig. 3). This phenomenon occurs when light travelling through an optically dense medium (e.g. glass) reaches an interface between this medium and a medium of a lower optical density (e.g. air), and is reflected back into the dense medium, and an evanescent wave penetrates through the noble metal layer (Green et al., 2000). The plasmons are excited at the outer side of the film.

6.1 Theoretical background

SPR is a quantum electromagnetic phenomenon arising from the interaction of light with free electrons at metal-dielectric interface, i.e., a charge-density oscillation propagating wave along the interface of two media with dielectric constants of opposite signs (Abdulhalim et al., 2008; Green et al., 2000; Homola et al., 1999; Lundstrom, 1994). A gold film in contact with a water interface is the most common system used in SPR experiments, since gold has a negative dielectric function (ε) in the infrared and visible regions of the electromagnetic spectrum, whereas water has a positive dielectric function (Johnson & Christy, 1972). The energy carried by photons of light is transferred to collective excitations of free electrons, called SP, at that interface and this transfer of energy occurs only at a specific resonance wavelength of light when the momentums of the photon and the plasmon are matched (Abdulhalim et al., 2008). This condition is only satisfied at distinct angles of incidence, appearing as a drop in the reflectivity of incident light (Daghestani & Day, 2010; Novotny & Hecht, 2006). The field vectors of electromagnetic wave reach a maximum at the interface and decay evanescently with distance normal into a metal (typically gold or silver) and dielectric media. The SP propagates as an electromagnetic surface wave, which is a transverse magnetic-polarized wave (TM-PW). TM-PW can be defined as a magnetic vector perpendicular to the direction of propagation of the ESW and parallel to the plane of interface. Correlating the relationship between the wave vector along the interface and the angular frequency ω, the surface plasmons can have a range of energies that depends on the complex dielectric function of the metal (ε_m) and the dielectric function of the adjacent medium (ε_d), as shown by the following equation:

$$k_{sp} = \frac{\omega}{c}\sqrt{\frac{\varepsilon_m \varepsilon_d}{\varepsilon_m + \varepsilon_d}} \tag{4}$$

where k_{sp} is the wave vector of the SP, ω is the angular frequency, c is the speed of light in a vacuum, and ε_m and ε_d are the permittivity of a metal and a dielectric material, respectively (Raether, 1988). In the Eq. 4, the real part determines the SP wavelength and the imaginary part determines the propagation length of the SP along the interface, which is responsible for the evanescent field (Daghestani & Day, 2010).

According to Smith & Corn (2003) SP can be directly excited by electrons; however, they cannot be excited directly by light because they have a longer wave vector than light waves of the same energy ($k_{light} = \omega/c$). The wave vector of a photon must be increased to convert the photon into SP. A monochromatic p-polarized light source is used in SPR measurements and the interface between the two optically dense media is coated with a thin metal film (Fig. 3). The Eq. 4 under conditions of ATR (Kretschmann configuration) becomes,

$$k_{ATR} = \frac{\omega}{c}\sin\theta\sqrt{\varepsilon_p} \tag{5}$$

where ε_p is the dielectric constant of the prism, and θ is the angle of incidence of the light on the metal film (Raether, 1988).

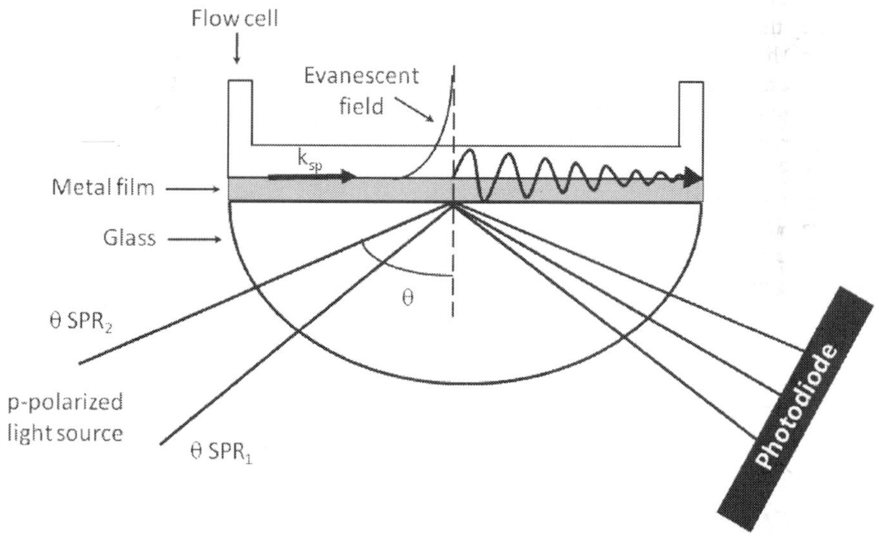

Fig. 3. Schematic diagram of SPR Kretschmann configuration. θSPR_1 and θSPR_2 represents the relation of SPR angle in the absence and presence of species on the metallic surface, respectively.

When the parallel component of the incident light is equivalent to the SP propagation constant, i.e., $k_{SP} = k_{ATR}$ (Eq. 4 and 5) a drop in reflectance will be found, due to the formation of an evanescent wave, that propagates through the metallic surface and interacts with the external medium (Damos et al., 2004), as follow:

$$\frac{\omega}{c}\sqrt{\frac{\varepsilon_m\varepsilon_d}{\varepsilon_m+\varepsilon_d}} = \frac{\omega}{c}\sin\theta\sqrt{\varepsilon_p} \tag{6}$$

which can be rewritten as

$$\theta = \arcsin\left(\sqrt{\left(\frac{\varepsilon_m \varepsilon_d}{\varepsilon_m + \varepsilon_d} x \frac{1}{\varepsilon_p}\right)}\right) \quad (7)$$

In this last expression it can be seen that the system optical properties, like the metal, prism and matrix dielectric constants, induce changes in the resonance angle, making it possible to apply the SPR phenomenon to monitor changes in the sensor surface (Damos et al., 2004). SPR technique relies on the principle that any changes on the dielectric sensing surface will cause a shift in the angle of reflectivity, followed by a detector, in order to satisfy the resonance condition (Daghestani & Day, 2010).

6.2 SPR measurement

In a simple SPR measurement, a target component or analyte is captured by the capturing element or so-called ligand and this ligand is permanently immobilized on the sensor surface previous to the measurement. The direct detection is the event of capturing the analyte by the ligand gives rise to a measurable signal. For each measurement, the surface is primed with a suitable buffer solution to create a baseline on the SPR curve (Green et al., 2000). It is of vital relevance to have a reliable baseline before the capturing event starts (Tudos & Schasfoort, 2008). Once the biomolecule comes into contact with the surface, rapid adsorption occurs resulting in an increase in the SPR angle and is followed by a plateau in the adsorption profile due to saturation of the surface (Fig. 3a). Finally, the biomolecule solution is replaced with a buffer to remove loosely bound material. The difference between the θSPR_1 to θSPR_2 gives an indication on the extent of adsorption (Fig. 3b), and the positive gradient of the SPR adsorption curve determines the rate of adsorption (Damos et al., 2004; Green et al., 2000; Tudos & Schasfoort, 2008).

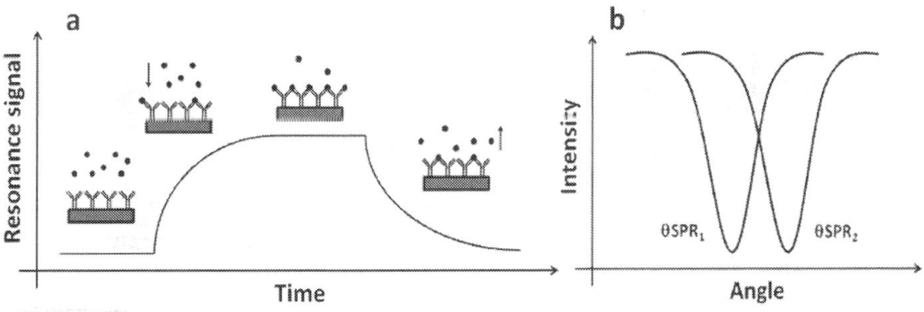

Fig. 3. Sensorgram showing the steps of an analysis cycle of association and dissociation steps (a). A change in refractive index at the surface of the metal film will cause an angle shift from θSPR_1 to θSPR_2 (b).

Often SPR measurements are carried out to determine the kinetics of a binding process. For realistic results it is vital to prevent immobilization from changing the ligand in a way that would influence its strength or affinity towards the target component (Tudos & Schasfoort, 2008).

6.3 Optical LDL biosensor

The SPR detects and measures changes in refractive index due to the binding and dissociation of interacting molecules at or in proximity to the gold surface. This change of the refractive index is proportional to the concentration of the interacting molecule and causes a shift in the angle of incidence at which the SPR phenomenon occurs. In addition, to explore monoclonal LDL antibodies in the interaction with the main protein constituent of human LDL (apoB-100) is possible to use a SPR-based biosensor to measure the multimolecular complex between MAbs and epitopes of the apoB-100 in real time.

Robbio and collaborators (2001) using a SPR-based biosensor, studied the interaction of ten different murine MAbs (all IgG_1), raised against apoB-100. These MAbs identify distinct domains on apoB-100, relevant to LDL-receptor interaction: epitopes in the amino-terminal region and in the middle region of native apoB-100. A multisite binding analysis was performed to further characterize the epitopes recognized by all these MAbs. The capacity of each MAb to interact with the entrapped apoB-100 in a multimolecular complex was monitored in real time by SPR. The results achieved were comparable to those obtained by western immunoblotting using the same reagents. However, SPR ensures a more detailed epitope identification, demonstrating that SPR technology can be successfully used for mapping distinct epitopes on apoB-100 protein in solution dispensing with labels and secondary tracers.

In another study, some authors (Gaus & Hall, 2003) have been investigating the use of peptides for the development of new LDL biosensor. Gaus & Hall (2003) selected short peptides sequences that showed binding selectivity towards native and oxidized LDL. Peptides were investigated for application in atherosclerosis risk monitoring using SPR technique. The peptides were immobilized on a gold SPR surface and LDL binding detected as a shift in the resonance. 3.7×10^7 ($\pm 5.6 \times 10^6$) LDL/mm^2/μg/ml solution LDL were bound on GlySerAspGlu-OH and 6.8×10^7 ($\pm 9.2 \times 10^6$) LDL/mm^2/μg/ml on GlyCystineSerAspGlu, compared with $\sim 10^8$ LDL/mm^2/μg/ml on LDL receptor ligand repeat peptide. They found a good correlation between LDL binding on these ligands and residual amino groups on the apoprotein of the LDL, which is an indicator of oxidation level. A very small sample (20 μl) could be taken for analysis and diluted 1:20 with physiological buffer prior to assay (giving total volume 0.4 ml). In addition to the obvious advantage in the required sample size, this has the effect of diluting potential plasma protein interference to levels where they no longer gave a significant background SPR response.

According to Laffont et al. (2002) glycation is responsible for disruption of lipoprotein functions leading to the development of atherosclerosis in diabetes. Glycation is the result of the irreversible attachment of sugar moieties to NH_2-protein groups, and is believed to play an important role in cardiovascular disease development among diabetic population through an impairment of lipoprotein functions. Glycation of lipoproteins as VLDL and HDL also affects their functional activities. Glycated VLDL display a higher residence time in plasma, are poorer substrates for lipoprotein lipase than non-glycated VLDL (Mamo et al., 1990), and glycation impairs paraoxonase activity in HDL (Hedrick et al., 2000). Laffont et al. (2002) also studied the effect of the early-glycation of apoE2, apoE3 and apoE4 on their binding to receptors. Glycated apoE binding to heparin and heparan sulfates (HS) was assessed by SPR technology (Laffont et al., 2002). Site-directed mutagenesis was then performed on Lys-75, the major glycation site of the protein. The prepared mutant protein proved to be useful as a tool to study the role of Lys-75 in apoE glycation. The results showed that, although glycation has no effect on apoE binding either to the LDL receptor

(LDL-R) or to scavenger receptor A (SR-A), it impairs its binding to immobilized heparin and HS. The glycation of Lys-75 was found to proceed rapidly and contributed significantly to total protein glycation. Laffont et al. (2002) showed that the glycation of Lys-75, a major glycation site in apoE, is a rapid process which contributes significantly to total apoE glycation. Although the glycation of apoE has no effect on its binding either to LDL-R or to SR-A, it impairs all three common apoE isoforms that bind to HS.

Some authors (Kudo et al., 2001) have previously shown that Asp-hemolysin binds to oxidized LDL (OxLDL) in a concentration-dependent manner. They investigated the relationship between the oxidation extent of LDL and its binding activity to Asp-hemolysin, to assess the binding specificity of Asp-hemolysin for OxLDL with several scavenger receptor ligands and to attempt the real-time kinetic measurement of the Asp-hemolysin-OxLDL interactions and calculations of the kinetic constants from SPR results. They showed that Asp-hemolysin has high affinity binding protein for OxLDL, and its binding specificity is distinct from any receptor for OxLDL. SPR studies revealed that OxLDL binds with high affinity (K_D = 0.63 μg/ml) to Asp-hemolysin. These studies suggest that Asp-hemolysin may bind to OxLDL using a mechanism different from the scavenger receptors.

The self-assembly of molecular building blocks into ordered nanostructures is not only a key to various biological phenomena, but also an attractive route for fabricating novel biosystems. Choi et al. (2004) developed an antibody-based immunoassay system to detect LDL. The self-assembled monolayer of 11-mercaptoundecanoic acid (11-(MUA)) and hexanethiol mixture was fabricated to form the stable protein G layer. 3-[(cholamidopropyl)dimethyl-ammonio]-1-propane sulfonate (CHAPS) was used for the regulation of protein G aggregate immobilized on the 11-(MUA) surface. The generic property of CHAPS made it possible to regulate the amount of protein immobilized on the surface. The anti-LDL layer on self-assembled protein G using CHAPS was applied to SPR immunosensor for detection of LDL and its detection limit was 100 pM. The relation with the change of SPR minimum angle and surface structure of fabricated layers with respect to the introduction of CHAPS implicate the importance of molecular control for the enhancement of immunosensor performance.

Although, some authors (Snellings et al., 2003) have fabricated an acoustic wave biosensor for detection of lipoprotein fractions using dextran sulfate (DS) modified self-assembled monolayer of 11-mercapto-1-undecanol on gold (Au) surface, it has been found that DS coating is more selective to LDL fraction as compared to other lipoprotein fractions. However, the authors could not achieve reproducibility for coating DS onto a similar surface and the sensor lacked specificity.

Lectin-like OxLDL receptor 1 (LOX-1) is the major OxLDL receptor of vascular endothelial cells and is involved in an early step of atherogenesis (Sawamura et al., 1997). LOX-1 is a membrane protein with a type II orientation consisting of four domains and the extracellular part of LOX-1 comprises an 82-residue stalk region (NECK) and a C-type lectin-like ligand-binding domain (CTLD). The CTLD is connected to the NECK domain that has a coiled-coil sequence, which promotes LOX-1 homodimerization (Ishigaki et al., 2007). Ohki and collaborators (2010) revealed the functional significance of the clustered organization of the ligand-binding domain of LOX-1 with SPR. They have been used biotinylated CTLD immobilized on a streptavidin sensor chip to make CTLD clusters on the surface. Their results showed that a single homodimeric LOX-1 extracellular domain had lower affinity for OxLDL in the supramicromolar range of dissociation constant (K_D). Single LOX-1 receptor per se does not exert the full binding ability to OxLDL. Monomeric CTLD has shown rather marginal binding to OxLDL. A multivalent interaction between the clustered LOX-1 and OxLDL should be essential to gain biologically significant binding activity. The experiment with the W150A (W150 residue locates at the dimer interface) mutant suggested that each LOX-1 in the cluster must retain the proper CTLD dimer; otherwise, LOX-1 loses the binding activity to OxLDL. Regarding the reduced activity of W150A, Ohki et al. (2010) cannot rule out the possible contribution of the "hydrophobic tunnel" that runs through the dimer interface of the CTLD. This tunnel is proposed to be engaged in OxLDL recognition. Ohki et al. (2010), in combination with the analyses on the loss-of-binding mutant W150A, concluded that the clustered organization of the properly formed homodimeric CTLD is essential for the strong binding of LOX-1 to OxLDL. It was important to evaluate and understand the mode of LOX-1 binding to OxLDL to explain the initial step of atherogenesis.

7. Electrochemical techniques

An important point to electrochemical sensor design lies in the molecular understanding of the relationship between surface structure and reactivity. The fabrication of sensor materials with unique response characteristics has created a pressing need to understand their chemical and physical properties. Understanding the fundamental process that govern sensor response in most cases leads to the development of electroanalytical devices with superior selectivity, excellent chemical stability, higher sensitivity, and lower detection limits. In order to meet these needs, it has been necessary to study various electrical processes that occur at the surface of the sensor or inside the sensor matrix itself. Electrochemical biosensors constitute a rapidly growing area of interest to biotechnologists. These devices combine the analytical power of electrochemistry with the specificity of biological molecules for particular substrates.

7.1 Cyclic voltammetry

Voltammetry belongs to a category of electro-analytical methods, through the information about an analyte that is obtained by varying a potential and then measuring the resulting current (Brett & Brett, 1993). It is, therefore, an amperometric technique. Since there are many ways to vary a potential, there are also any forms of voltammetry, such as: polarography, linear sweep, differential staircase, normal pulse, reverse pulse and more (Brett & Brett, 1993; Bard & Faulkner, 2001).

Cyclic voltammetry (CV) measurements are the current signals based on the electrochemical species consumed and/or generated during a biological and chemical interaction process of a biologically active substance and substrate (Oliveira et al., 2009; Oliveira et al., 2011). CV is one of the most widely used forms and it is useful to obtain information about the redox potential and electrochemical reaction (e.g. the chemical rate constant) of analyte solutions (Brett & Brett, 1993). In this case, this voltage is swept between two values at a fixed rate, however, when the voltage reaches V_2 the scan is reversed and the voltage is swept back to V_1, as is illustrated in Fig. 4a. The scan rate, $(V_2-V_1)/(T_2-T_1)$, is a critical factor, since the duration of a scan must provide sufficient time to allow for a meaningful chemical reaction to occur. Varying the scan rate, therefore, yields correspondingly varied results (Bard & Faulkner, 2001).

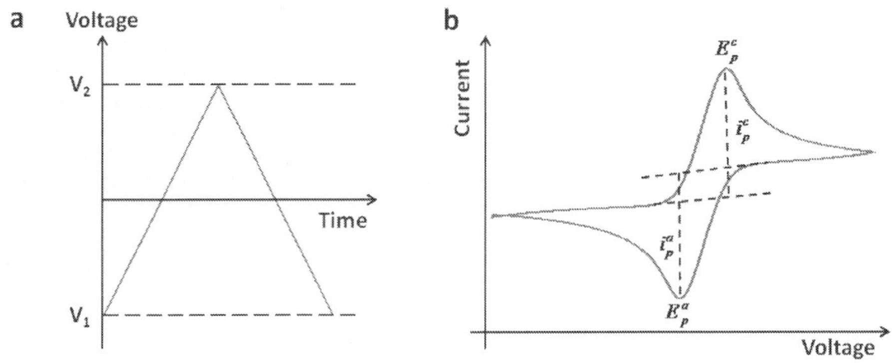

Fig. 4. Cyclic voltammetry waveform (a) and typical cyclic voltammogram (b). E_p^c (E_p^a) and i_p^c (i_p^a) are the potential and current at cathodic (anodic) peak, respectively.

The voltage is measured between the reference electrode and the working electrode, while the current is measured between working electrode and the counter electrode. The obtained measurements are plotted as current vs. voltage, also known as a voltammogram. As the voltage is increased toward the electrochemical reduction potential, the current will also increase. With increasing voltage toward V_2 past this reduction potential, the current decreases, having formed a peak as the analyte concentration near the electrode surface diminishes, since the oxidation potential have been exceeded (Brett & Brett, 1993). As the voltage is reversed to complete the scan toward V_1, the reaction will begin to reoxidize the product from the initial reaction. This produces an increase in current of opposite polarity as compared to forward scan, but again decreases, having formed a second peak as the voltage scan also provides information about the reversibility of a reaction at a given scan rate (Bard & Faulkner, 2001). There are two components to the current: (a) a capacitive component resulting from re-distribution of charged and polar species at the electrode surface (non-Faradaic process) and (b) a component resulting from exchange of electrons between the electrode and redox species immobilized at the electrode surface, or free in solution (Faradaic process) (Bard & Faulkner, 2001). At sufficiently oxidizing or reducing potentials, where the ratio of electron transfer between the electrode and the redox species in solution is sufficiently fast, the Faradaic current is controlled by the rate of diffusion to the electrode. Hence, for the reversible reduction of redox species O:

$$O + ne \leftrightarrow R \tag{8}$$

With a redox potential E^0, the Faradaic current, i_f, will depend on the concentration gradient of O at the electrode surface:

$$i_f = nFAD_0\left(\frac{d[O]}{dx}\right)x = 0 \tag{9}$$

where, A is the area of the electrode, D_0 is the diffusion coefficient of O, n is the number of electrons transferred and F is Faraday's constant. By holding the working electrode at a positive potential and then sweeping towards and beyond E^0, the surface concentration of O will change in accordance with the Nernst equation:

$$\frac{[O]}{[R]} = \exp[\frac{nF}{RT}(E - E^0)] \tag{10}$$

where, E is the electrode potential, R is the gas constant and T is the temperature in Kelvins. The shape of the voltammogram for a given compound depends not only on the scan rate and the electrode surface, which is different after each adsorption step, but also depends on the catalyst concentration. For example, increasing the concentration of reaction specific enzymes at a given scan rate will result in a higher current compared to the non-catalyzed reaction (Tan et al., 2005).

The waveform of the voltage applied to a working electrode in CV is triangular shaped (i.e., the forward and reverse scan). Since, this voltage varies linearly with the time the scan rate is the slope (V/s). An example, of a CV for the reduction of ferricyanide to ferrocyanide ($K_4[Fe(CN)_6]^{4-}/K_3[Fe(CN)_6]^{3-}$) is shown in Fig. 4b. The peak shape of the reductive and reverse oxidative current vs. electrode potential curve (i-E) in Fig. 4b is typical of an electrode reaction in which the rate is governed by diffusion of the electroactive species to a planar electrode surface. That is the rate of the electron transfer step is fast compared to the rate at which ferricyanide is transported (diffuses) from the bulk solution to the electrode surface due to a concentration gradient, as ferricyanide is reduced to ferrocyanide. In such a case peak current, i_p, is governed by the Randle-Sevcik relationship:

$$i_p = Kn^{3/2}AD^{1/2}c^b v^{1/2} \tag{11}$$

where the constant $K = 2.72 \times 10^5$, n is the number of moles of electrons transferred per mole of electroactive species (e.g., ferricyanide), A is the area of the electrode in cm^2, D is the diffusion coefficient in cm^2/s, c^b is the solution concentration in mole/l, and v is the scan rate of the potential in V/s.

The i_p is linearly proportional to the bulk concentration, c^b, of the electroactive species, and the square root of the scan rate, $v^{1/2}$. Thus, an important diagnostic is a plot of the i_p vs. $v^{1/2}$. If the plot is linear, it is reasonably safe to say that the electrode reaction is controlled by diffusion, which is the mass transport rate of the electroactive species to the surface of the electrode across a concentration gradient. The thickness (δ) of the diffusion layer can be approximated by $\delta \sim [Dt]^{1/2}$, where D is the diffusion coefficient and t is time in seconds. A quiet (i.e., unstirred solutions) is required. The presence of supporting electrolyte, such as KNO_3 in this example, is required to prevent charged electroactive species from migrating in the electric field gradient (Bard & Faulkner, 2001).

7.2 Electrochemical impedance spectroscopy

Electrochemical impedance spectroscopy (EIS) has long been established as a sensitive technique to monitor the electrical response of a solid/liquid system subjected to the application of a periodic small amplitude AC signal. Analysis of the system response provides information concerning the solid/liquid interface and on the eventual occurrence of reactions at this local region (MacDonald, 1987). EIS is a non-destructive steady-state technique that is capable of probing the relaxation phenomena over a range of frequencies (Bockris et al., 2000; Bard & Faulkner, 2001; Macdonald, 1987).

The power of EIS lies in its ability to provide in situ information on relaxation times over the frequency range 10^6 to 10^{-4} Hz. It is a tool that has been used to identify and separate different contributions to the electric and dielectric responses of the biosystems.

Impedance spectroscopy is a powerful method of analysing the complex electrical resistance of a system and is sensitive to surface phenomena and changes of bulk properties. The impedance Z of a system is generally determined by applying a voltage perturbation with small amplitude and detecting the current response. From this definition, the impedance Z is the quotient of the voltage-time function V(t) and the resulting current-time function I(t):

$$Z = \frac{V(t)}{I(t)} = \frac{V_0 \sin(2\pi ft)}{I_0 \sin(2\pi ft + \phi)} = \frac{1}{Y} \tag{12}$$

where V_0 and I_0 are the maximum voltage and current signals, f is the frequency, t the time, ϕ the phase shift between the voltage-time and current-time function, and Y is the complex conductance or admittance. The impedance is a complex value, since the current can differ not only in terms of the amplitude but it can also show a phase shift ϕ compared to the voltage-time function. Thus, the value can be described either by the modulus $|Z|$ and the phase shift ϕ or alternatively by the real part Zr and the imaginary part Zi of the impedance. This is illustrated in Fig 5.

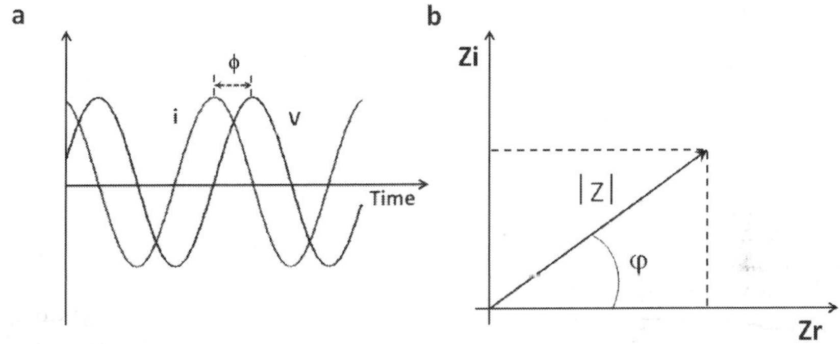

Fig. 5. Impedance is a complex value that is defined as the quotient of the voltage (time) and current (time) functions. It can be expressed as the modulus $|Z|$ and the phase angle ϕ, or it can be specified by the real (Zr) and the imaginary (Zi) parts of the impedance.

Therefore, the results of an impedance measurement can be illustrated in two different ways: using a Bode plot which plots log $|Z|$ and ϕ as a function of log f, or a Nyquist plot which plots Zr and Zi. On the Nyquist plot the impedance (Fig. 6a) can be represented as a vector (arrow) of length $|Z|$. The angle between this vector and x-axis, commonly called the phase angle, is ϕ (=argZ).

Nyquist plots have one mayor shortcoming. When you look any data point on the plot, you cannot tell what frequency was used to record that point. This plot results from electrical circuit of Fig. 6b. Another popular representation method is the Bode plot. The impedance is plotted with log frequency on the x-axis and both the absolute values of the impedance ($|Z| = Z_0$) and the phase-shift on the x-axis.

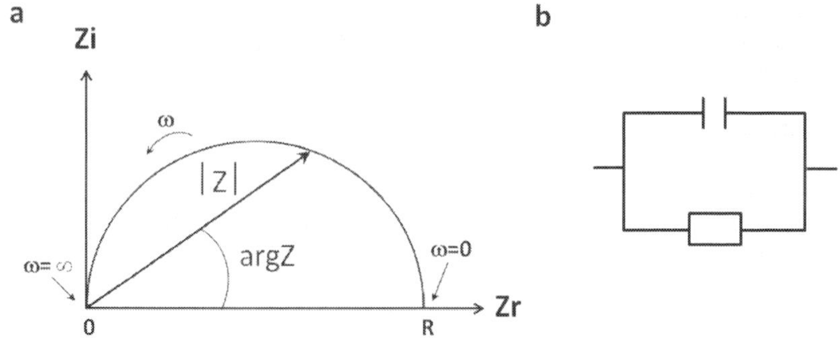

Fig. 6. Nyquist plot with impedance vector (a) and simple equivalent circuit with one time constant (b).

In the typical biosensor application of EIS, the biological component is immobilized on the working electrode and the interaction with an analyte molecule is detected. The impedance of the sensing electrode (the working electrode modified with the biological component) controls the overall impedance. Like all electrochemical biosensors, impedimetric sensors are bioelectronic devices that make use of the interactions of biomolecules with a conductive (or semiconducting) transducer surface. The detection process involves the formation of the recognition complex between the sensing biomolecule and the analyte at the interface electronic transducer, which directly or indirectly alters the electrical properties of the recognition surface.

7.3 Electrochemical LDL biosensors

Cyclic voltammetry can be used to monitor the molecular interaction and explore association between biomolecules and LDL based on the modification at anodic and cathodic peaks. Nicolini's group (Stura et al., 2007) improve the mechanical stability of electrodes based on P450scc for LDL-cholesterol detection and measure, using anodic porous alumina (APA). They have been shown, by means of CV measurements, that the sensitivity of the APA+P450scc system was slightly reduced with respect to the pure P450scc system, the readout was stable for a much longer period of time, and the measures remained reproducible inside a proper confidentiality band. To optimize the adhesion of P450scc to APA, a layer of poly-l-lysine, a poly-cation, was successfully implemented as intermediate organic structure. They obtained an optimization of the electron transfer's stability leading to the optimal detection of cholesterol in the clinical range concentration for longer times of use.

In another work, Nicolini's group (Antonini et al., 2004) employed Cytochrome P450sccK201E, mutated form of cytochrome P450scc native recombinant (P450sccNR), to study the enzyme–substrate interaction. The biochemical analysis was realized to observe the electrochemical responses of the engineerized enzyme to three different forms of cholesterol: free, LDL and high-density lipoproteins (HDL). The detection of the cholesterol was performed by electrochemical method using CV and chronoamperometry measurements. Compared to cytochrome P450sccNR, the cytochrome P450sccK201E displays a different behavior in the interaction with the substrate detection. The experimental data have shown that the mutation has improved the affinity between the cytochrome P450 and the substrates; in particular, the best responses were found in the detection of cholesterol in HDL. CV and chronoamperometry results showed that electrochemical response of the mutant P450sccK201E and P450sccNR can be utilized for the cholesterol detection.

Electrochemical methods associated with nanomaterials have been employed to develop electrochemical biosensor for the detection of LDL. More recently, a novel, sensitive, label-free, LDL electrochemical biosensor was fabricated by adsorption of antibody to apoB-100. Yan et al. (2008) developed silver chloride/polyaniline (PANI) core-shell nanocomposites (AgCl/PANI) combined with gold nanoparticles (AuNPs) to prepare the AuNPs-AgCl/PANI hybrid material. Yan et al. (2008) have been used a highly specific antibody, anti-apoB, that acts as a LDL receptor and fabricated an electrochemical biosensor by adsorption of anti-apoB on AuNPs-AgCl-polyaniline-modified glassy carbon electrode. The hybrid material could provide surface for high antibody loading due to its large surface-to-volume ratio. Since each LDL has an apoB-100 on its phospholipids coat, they could be bonded to the electrode surface through the specific antibody-antigen reaction. EIS was used to characterize the recognition of LDL. The negative charges carried by LDL phospholipids coat would block the electron transfer of the $K_4[Fe(CN)_6]^{4-}/K_3[Fe(CN)_6]^{3-}$ redox couple severely. In addition, the conductivity of LDL is very poor, so small amounts of LDL on the electrode could result in great change in the electron-transfer resistance. The biosensor exhibited a highly sensitive response to LDL with a detection limit of 0.34 pg/ml.

In others studies, Langmuir-Blodgett (LB) films of polyaniline (PANI) were utilized for the fabrication of impedimetric immunosensor for detection of human plasma LDL by immobilizing anti-apoB via EDC-NHS coupling. Anti-apoB/PANI-stearic acid LB films immunoelectrodes studied by EIS spectroscopy revealed detection of LDL in the wide range of 0.018 μM (6 mg/dl) to 0.39 μM (130 mg/dl), covering the physiological range in blood, with a sensitivity of 11.25 kΩ μM^{-1} (Matharu et al., 2010). Therefore, from the different types of biosensors discussed above we showed that the possibility to detect LDL and modified LDL by piezoelectric, optical or electrical techniques such as QCM, SPR, VC and EIS are strategic in clinical diagnostics.

8. Conclusion and future trend

Studies based on LDL biosensors have been directed to decrease the detection time and develop new ways of detecting LDL and modified LDL. The techniques discussed here can provide information on the steady state or dynamics of real time events. Therefore, the combined application of QCM, SPR, VC and EIS is a powerful tool to the development of new biosensors for LDL and modified LDL. The trend in the clinical laboratory is the development of biosensors for multiplex detection targets. A biosensor that simultaneously measures multiple analytes (e.g., HDL, LDL, VLDL, modified LDL, total cholesterol, triglycerides, C-reactive protein and others) in a single assay and gives information about the cardiovascular risk profile in few minutes is a great challenge and warrants more studies in this field.

9. Acknowledgment

The authors acknowledge the financial support of Fundação de Amparo à Ciência e Tecnologia do Estado de Pernambuco (FACEPE, grant to M.D.L.O.); Fundação de Amparo à

Pesquisa do Estado de São Paulo (FAPESP, grant to D.S.P.A. and scholarship to V.R.H.); Conselho Nacional de Pesquisa e Desenvolvimento Científico (CNPq, grant to D.S.P.A.), Rede ELINOR de Nanobiotecnologia/CAPES (grant to M.D.L.O. and C.A.S.A.) and INCT-if/CNPq (grant to D.S.P.A.).

10. References

Abdulhalim, I., Zourob, M. & Lakhtakia, A. (2008). Surface Plasmon Resonance for Biosensing: A Mini-Review. *Electromagnetics*, Vol.28, Issue3, (April 2008) p.p. 214–242, ISSN 0272-6343.

Annangudi, S.P., Deng, Y., Gu, X., Zhang, W., Crabb, J.W. & Salomon, R.G. (2008). Low-density lipoprotein has an enormous capacity to bind (E)-4-hydroxynon-2-enal (HNE): detection and characterization of lysyl and histidyl adducts containing multiple molecules of HNE. *Chemical Research in Toxicology*, Vol.21, No.7, (June 2008), p.p. 1384–1395, ISSN: 0893-228X.

Antonini, M., Ghisellini, P., Paternolli, C. & Nicolini, C. (2004). Electrochemical study of the interaction between cytochrome P450sccK201E and cholesterol. *Talanta*, Vol.62, Issue5, (April 2004), p.p. 945–950, ISSN 0039-9140.

Arnau, A. (2008). A Review of Interface Electronic Systems for AT-cut Quartz Crystal Microbalance Applications in Liquids. *Sensors*, Vol.8, (March 2008), p.p. 370-411, ISSN 1424-8220.

Asci, G., Basci, A., Shah, S.V., Basnakian, A., Toz, H., Ozkahya, M., Duman, S. & Ok, E. (2008). Carbamylated low-density lipoprotein induces proliferation and increases adhesion molecule expression of human coronary artery smooth muscle cells. *Nephrology*, Vol.13, No.6, (June 2008), p.p. 480–486, ISSN: 0931-041X.

Bachorik, P.S. (1997). Measurement of low density lipoprotein cholesterol, In: *Handbook of Lipoprotein Testing*, Rifai, N., Warnick, G.R. & Dominiczak, M.H. (Eds.), 145-160, AACC Press, ISBN 978-189-0883-35-5,Washington.

Bard, J. & Faulkner, L.R. (2001). *Electrochemical Methods: Fundamentals and Applications*, 2nd edition, John Wiley and Sons, Inc., ISBN 978-047-1043-72-0, New York, United States of America.

Basta, G., Schmidt, A.M. & De Caterina, R. (2004). Advanced glycation end products and vascular inflammation: implications for accelerated atherosclerosis in diabetes. *Cardiovascular Research*, Vol.63, No.4, p.p. 582–592, ISSN: 1755-3245.

Behm, E., Ivanovich, P. & Klinkmann, H. (1989). Selective and Specific Adsorbents for Medical Therapy. *The International Journal of Artificial Organs*, 12, Issue1, (January 1989), p.p. 1-10, ISSN 0391-3988.

Bockris, J.O.M., Reddy, A.K.N. & Gamboa-Aldeco, M. (2000). *Modern Electrochemistry 2A: Fundamentals of Electrodics*, 2nd edition, Vol.2, Klumer Academic/Plenum Publishers, ISBN 978-030-6461-67-5, New York, United States of America.

Bosch, T., Schmidt, B., Kleophas, W., Gillen, C., Otto, V., Passlick-Deetjen, J. & Gurland, H.J. (1997). LDL Hemoperfusion-A New Procedure for LDL Apheresis: First Clinical Application of an LDL Adsorber Compatible with Human Whole Blood. *Artificial Organs*, Vol.21, Issue9 (June 1997), 977-982, ISSN 1525-1594.

Brett, C.M.A. & Brett, A.M.O. (1993). *Electrochemistry: Principles, Methods, and Applications*, Oxford University Press, ISBN 978-019-8553-88-5, New York, United States of America.

Brown, B.E., Rashid, I., Van Reyk, D.M. & Davies, M.J. (2007). Glycation of low-density lipoprotein results in the time-dependent accumulation of cholesteryl esters and apolipoprotein B-100 protein in primary human monocyte-derived macrophages. *FEBS Journal*, Vol.274, No.6, (March 2007), p.p. 1530–1541, ISSN: 1742-464X.

Bunde, R.L., Jarvi, E.J. & Rosentreter, J.J. (1998). Piezoelectric Quartz Crystal Biosensor. *Talanta*, vol.46, (August 1998), pp.1223-1236, ISSN 0039-9140.

Camejo, G., Hurt-Camejo, E., Wiklund, O. & Bondjers, G. (1998). Association of apo B Lipoproteins with Arterial Proteoglycans: Pathological Significance and Molecular Basis. *Atherosclerosis*, Vol.139, (August 1998), p.p. 205–222, ISSN 0021-9150.

Choi, J.-W., Park, K.-S., Lee, W., Oh, B.-K., Chun, B.-S. & Paek, S.-H. (2004). Regulation of anti-LDL Immobilization on Self-Assembled Protein G Layer using CHAPS and its Application to Immunosensor. *Materials Science and Engineering C*, Vol.24, Issues1-2, (October 2003), p.p. 241–245, ISSN 0928-4931.

Chunta, S., Promptmas, C. & Cherdchu, C. (2009). Lipoprotein Sensor: A Piezoelectric Quartz Crystal Device. *International Journal of Applied Biomedical Engineering*, Vol.2, No.1, (July 2009), p.p. 24-32, ISSN 0973-4562.

Cooper, J.M. & Cass, A.E.G. (2004). *Biosensors - Pratical Approach*, Oxford University Press, ISBN 978-019-9638-46-8, Oxford, Great Britain.

Cordova, C.M., Schneider, C.R., Juttel, I.D. & Cordova, M.M. (2004). Comparison of LDL-cholesterol direct measurement with the estimate using the Friedewald formula in a sample of 10,664 patients. *Arquivos Brasileiros de Cardiologia*, Vol.83, No.6, Issue482-7, (January 2004), p.p. 476-81, ISSN: 0066-782X.

Curie J. & Curie P. (1880a). Développement, par Pression, de L'électricité Polaire dans les Cristaux Hémièdres à Faces Inclines. *Comptes Rendus de l'Académie des sciences*, Vol.91, p.p. 294-295, ISSN 0764-4469.

Curie J. & Curie P. (1880b). Sur L'électricité Polaire dans les Cristaux Hémièdres à Faces Inclinées. *Comptes rendus de l'Academie des Sciences*, Vol.91, p.p. 383–386, ISSN 0764-4469.

D'Ulivo, L., Saint-Guirons, J., Ingemarsson, B. & Riekkola, M.-L. (2010). Quartz Crystal Microbalance, a Valuable Tool for Elucidation of Interactions between apoB-100 Peptides and Extracellular Matrix Components. *Analytical and Bioanalytical Chemistry*, Vol.396, (December 2009), p.p. 1373–1380, ISSN 1618-2642.

D'Ulivo, L., Witos, J., Öörni, K., Kovanen, P.T. & Riekkola, M.-L. (2009). Capillary Electrochromatography: a Tool for Mimicking Collagen Surface Interactions with Apolipoprotein B-100 Peptides. *Electrophoresis*, Vol.30, (October 2009), p.p. 3838–3845, ISSN 0173-0835.

Daghestani, H.N. & Day, B.W. (2010). Theory and Applications of Surface Plasmon Resonance, Resonant Mirror, Resonant Waveguide Grating, and Dual Polarization Interferometry Biosensors. *Sensors*, Vol.10, Issue10, (November 2010) p.p. 9630-9646, ISSN 1424-8220.

Damasceno, N.R., Sevanian, A., Apolinario, E., Oliveira, J.M., Fernandes, I., & Abdalla, D.S.P. (2006). Detection of electronegative low density lipoprotein (LDL^-) in plasma and atherosclerotic lesions by monoclonal antibody-based immunoassays. *Clinical Biochemistry*, Vol.39, No.1, (November 2005), p.p. 28-38, ISSN: 0009-9120.

Damos, F.S., Mendes, R.K. & Kubota, L.T. (2004). Applications of QCM, EIS and SPR in the Investigation of Surfaces and Interfaces for the Development of (Bio)Sensors, *Química Nova,* Vol.27, No.6, (December 2004) p.p. 970-979, ISSN 1678-7064.

Esteban-Salan, M., Aguilar-Doreste, J.A., Arranz-Pena, M.L., Juve-Cuxart, S., Gich-Salarich, I., Zapico-Muniz, E. & Ordonez-Llanos, J. (2008). Multicentric evaluation of the homogeneous LDL-cholesterol Plus assay: comparison with beta-quantification and Friedewald formula. *Clinical Biochemistry,* Vol.41, No.16-17, (August 2008), p.p. 1402-1409, ISSN: 0009-9120.

Faulin, T.E.S., Sena, K.C.M., Telles, A.E.R., Grosso, D.M., Faulin, E.J.B. & Abdalla, D.S.P. (2008). Validation of a novel ELISA for measurement of Electronegative LDL. *Clinical Chemistry and Laboratory Medicine,* Vol.46, No.12, (August 2008), p.p. 1769-1775, ISSN: 1434-6621.

Fowler, J.M., Wong, D.K.Y., Halssal, H.B. & Heineman, W.R. (2008). Recent Developments in Electrochemical Immunoassays and Immunosensors, In: *Electrochemical Sensors, Biosensors and their Biomedical Applications,* Zhang, X., Ju, H. & Wang, J. (Eds.), 115-140, Academic Press Elsevier Inc., ISBN 978-012-3737-38-0, United States of America.

Freire, R.S., Thongngamdee, S., Duran, N., Wang, J. & Kubota, L.T. (2002). Mixed Enzyme (Laccase/Tyrosinase)-based Remote Electrochemical Biosensor for Monitoring Phenolic Compounds. *Analyst,* Vol.127, Issue2, p.p. 258–261, ISSN 0003-2654.

Friedewald, W.T., Levy, R.I. & Fredrickson, D.S. (1972). Estimation of the Concentration of Low-Density Lipoprotein Cholesterol in Plasma, without use of the Preparative Ultracentrifuge. *Clinical Chemistry,* Vol.18, (March 1972), p.p. 499–502, ISSN 1530-8561.

Gaus, K. & Hall, E.A.H. (2003). Short Peptide Receptor Mimics for Atherosclerosis Risk Assessment of LDL. *Biosensors and Bioelectronics,* Vol.18, (March 2003), p.p. 151-164, ISSN 0956-5663.

Green, R.J., Frazier, R.A., Shakesheff, K.M., Davies, M.C., Roberts, C.J. & Tendler, S.J.B. (2000). Surface Plasmon Resonance Analysis of Dynamic Biological Interactions with Biomaterials. *Biomaterials,* Vol.21, Issue18, (September 2000) p.p. 1823-1835, ISSN 0142-9612.

Hansson, G.K., & Libby, P. (2006). The immune response in atherosclerosis: a double-edged sword. Nature Reviews Immunology, Vol.6, No.7, (July 2006), p.p. 508-519, ISSN: 1474-1733.

Miller, Y.I., Choi, S.H., Fang, L. & Tsimikas, S. (2010). Lipoprotein modification and macrophage uptake: role of pathologic cholesterol transport in atherogenesis, In: *Cholesterol binding and cholesterol transport proteins. Structure and function in health and disease,* Harris, J.R., pp. 229-251, Springer, ISBN 978-90-481-8621-1, Dordrecht, Heidelberg, London and New York.

Hedrick, C.C., Thorpe, S.R., Fu, M.-X., Harper, C.M., Yoo, J., Kim, S.-M., Wong, H. & Peters, A.L. (2000). Glycation Impairs High-Density Lipoprotein Function. *Diabetologia,* Vol.43, (March 2000), p.p. 312–320, ISSN 0012-186X.

Helali, S., Ben Fredj, H., Cherif, K., Abdelghani, A., Martelet, C. & Jaffrezic-Renault, N. (2008). Surface Plasmon Resonance and Impedance Spectroscopy on Gold Electrode for Biosensor Application. *Materials Science and Engineering: C,* Vol.28, Issue5-6, (July 2008) p.p. 588-593, ISSN 0928-4931.

Hodgkinson, C.P., Laxton, R.C., Patel, K. & Ye, S. (2008). Advanced glycation end-product of low density lipoprotein activates the Toll-like 4 receptor pathway implications for diabetic atherosclerosis. *Arteriosclerosis, Thrombosis, and Vascular Biology,* Vol.28, No.12, (September 2008), p.p.2275–2281, ISSN: 1079-5642.

Homola, J., Yee, S.S. & Gauglitz, G. (1999). Surface Plasmon Resonance Sensors: Review. *Sensors and Actuators B,* Vol.54, Issues1-2, (January 1999) p.p. 3–15, ISSN 0925-4005.

Höök, F. & Rudh, M. (2005). Quartz Crystal Microbalances (QCM) in Biomacromolecular Recognition. *Biotech International,* Vol.2, (March 2005), p.p. 1-5, ISSN 2032-2887.

Ishigaki, T., Ohki, I., Utsunomiya-Tate, N. & Tate, S.-I. (2007). Chimeric Structural Stabilities in the Coiled-Coil Structure of the NECK Domain in Human Lectin-Like Oxidized Low-Density Lipoprotein Receptor 1 (LOX-1). *The Journal of Biochemistry,* Vol.141, Issue6, (March 2007), p.p. 855-866, ISSN 0021-924X.

Itabe, H. & Ueda, M. (2007). Measurement of plasma oxidized low-density lipoprotein and its clinical implications. *Journal of atherosclerosis and thrombosis,* Vol.14, No.1, (February 2007), p.p. 1-11, ISSN: 1340-3478.

Jambunathan, K. & Hillier, A.C. (2003). Measuring Electrocatalytic Activity on a Local Scale with Scanning Differential Electrochemical Mass Spectrometry. *Journal of the Electrochemical Society,* Vol.150, No.6, (June 2003), E312-E320, ISSN 0013-4651.

Johnson, P.B. & Christy, R.W. (1972). Optical Constants of the Noble Metals, *Physical Review B,* Vol.6, Issue12, (December 1972) p.p. 4370-4379, ISSN 1098-0121.

Kanazawa, K.K. & Gordon II, J.G. (1985). Frequency of a Quartz Microbalance in Contact with Liquid. *Analytical Chemistry,* Vol.57, Issue8, (July 1985), p.p. 1770-1771, ISSN 1177-3901.

Kretschmann, E. & Raether, H. (1968). Radiative Decay of Non-Radiative Surface Plasmons Excited by Light. *Zeitschrift für Naturforschung B,* Vol.23A, p.p. 2135–2136, ISSN 0932-0776.

Kudo, Y., Fukuchi, Y., Kumagai, T., Ebina, K. & Yokota, K. (2001). Oxidized Low-Density Lipoprotein-Binding Specificity of Asp-hemolysin from Aspergillus fumigates. *Biochimica et Biophysica Acta,* Vol.1568, (December 2001), p.p. 183-188, ISSN 0304-4165.

Laffont, I., Shuvaev, V.V., Briand, O., Lestavel, S., Barbier, A., Taniguchi, N., Fruchart, J.-C., Clavey, V. & Siest, G. (2002). Early-Glycation of Apolipoprotein E: Effect on its Binding to LDL Receptor, Scavenger Receptor A and Heparan Sulfates. *Biochimica et Biophysica Acta,* Vol.1583, (June 2002) p.p. 99– 107, ISSN 0304-4165.

Levitan, I., Volkov, S. & Subbaiah, P.V. (2010). Oxidized LDL: Diversity, Patterns of Recognition, and Pathophysiology. *Antioxidants & Redox Signaling,* Vol.13, No.1, (July 2010), p.p. 39-75, ISSN: 1523-0864.

Libby, P., Ridker, P.M., & Hansson, G.K. (2009). Leducq Transatlantic Network on Atherothrombosis. Inflammation in atherosclerosis: from pathophysiology to practice. *Journal of the American College of Cardiology,* Vol.54, No.23, (December 2009), p.p. 2129-2138, ISSN: 0735-1097.

Liu, D., He, B., Han, S., Wang, S., Liu, Q., Jun-ichic, A., Osa, T. & Chen, Q. (2007). An Adsorption Behavior of low-Density Lipoprotein onto Cholesterol-Modified Dextran Studied by a Quartz Crystal Microbalance. *Materials Science and Engineering: C,* Vol.27, Issue4, (May 2007), p.p. 665-669, ISSN 0928-4931.

Lundstrom I. (1994). Real-Time Biospecific Interaction Analysis. *Biosensors and Bioelectronics*, Vol.9, Issues9-10, (January 2002), pp. 725-736, ISSN 0956-5663.

Luppa, P.B., Sokoll, L.J. & Chan, D.W. (2001). Immunosensor principles and applications to clinical chemistry. *Clinica Chimica Acta*, Vol.314, Issue1-2, (December 2001), p.p. 1-26.

Macdonald, J.R. (1987). *Impedance spectroscopy: emphasizing solid materials and systems*, John Wiley and Sons, Inc., ISBN 978-047-1831-22-8, New York, United States of America.

Malhotra, B.D., Chaubey, A. & Singh, S.P. (2006). Prospects of Conducting Polymers in Biosensors. *Analytica Chimica Acta*, 2006, Vol.578, Issue1, (September 2006), p.p. 59–74, ISSN 0003-2670.

Malle, E., Marsche, G., Arnhold, J. & Davies, M.J. (2006). Modification of low-density lipoprotein by myeloperoxidase-derived oxidants and reagent hypochlorous acid. *Biochimica et Biophysica Acta*, Vol.1761, No.4, (April 2006), p.p. 392–415, ISSN: 0304-4165.

Mamo, J.C.L., Szeto, L. & Steiner, G. (1990). Glycation of Very Low Density Lipoprotein from Rat Plasma Impairs its Catabolism. *Diabetologia*, Vol.33, No.6, (June 1990), p.p. 339–345, ISSN 0012-186X.

Marshall, W.J. & Bangert, S.K. (2008). *Clinical chemistry*, Mosby Elsevier, ISBN 9780723434559, Philadelphia.

Marx, K.A. (2003). Quartz Crystal Microbalance: A Useful Tool for Studying Thin Polymer Films and Complex Biomolecular Systems at the Solution-Surface Interface. *Biomacromolecules*, Vol.4, No.5, (October 2002), p.p. 1099-1120, ISSN 1525-7797.

Matharu, Z., Bandodkar, A.J., Sumana, G., Solanki, P.R., Ekanayake, E.M., Kaneto, K., Gupta, V. & Malhotra, B.D. (2009a) Low Density Lipoprotein Detection Based on Antibody Immobilized Self-Assembled Monolayer: Investigations of Kinetic and Thermodynamic Properties. *The Journal of Physical Chemistry B*, Vol.29, No.118, Issue43, (October 2009), p.p. 14405-14412, ISSN 1089-5647.

Matharu, Z., Sumana, G., Gupta, V. & Malhotra, B.D. (2010). Langmuir–Blodgett films of polyaniline for low density lipoprotein detection. *Thin Solid Films*, Vol.519 (August 2010) p.p. 1110–1114, ISSN 040-6090.

Matharu, Z., Sumana, G., Pandey, M.K., Gupta, V. & Malhotra, B.D. (2009b) Low Density Lipoprotein Sensor Based on Surface Plasmon Resonance. *Thin Solid Films*, Vol.518, Issue2, (November 2009) p.p. 719-723, ISSN 0040-6090.

Matsuura, E., Hughes, G.R. & Khamashta, M.A. (2008). Oxidation of LDL and its clinical implication. *Autoimmunity* Reviews, Vol.7, No.7, (July 2008), p.p. 558–566, ISSN: 1568-9972.

McGill, H.C. Jr, McMahan, C.A., Herderick, E.E., Malcom, G.T., Tracy, R.E. & Strong, J.P. (2000). Origin of atherosclerosis in childhood and adolescence. *The American Journal of Clinical Nutrition*, Vol.72, No.5, (November 2000), p.p. 1307S-1315S, ISSN: 0002-9165.

Novotny, L. & Hecht, B. (2006). *Principles of Nano-Optics*, Cambridge University Press, ISBN 978-052-1832-24-3, Cambridge, UK.

Ohki, I., Amida, H., Yamada, R., Sugihara, M., Ishigaki, T. & Tate, S.-I. (2011). Surface Plasmon Resonance Study on Functional Significance of Clustered Organization of Lectin-like Oxidized LDL Receptor (LOX-1). *Biochimica et Biophysica Acta*, in press, ISSN 1570-9639.

Oliveira, M.D.L., Correia, M.T.S. & Diniz, F.B. (2009). Concanavalin A and Polyvinyl Butyral use as a Potential Dengue Electrochemical Biosensor. *Biosensors and Bioelectronics*, Vol.25, Issue4, (December 2009), pp. 728-732, ISSN 0956-5663.

Oliveira, M.D.L., de Melo, C.P., Glaucius, O. & Andrade, C.A.S. (2011). Development of Impedimetric and Optical Calcium Biosensor by Using Modified Gold Electrode with Porcine S100A12 protein. *Colloids and Surfaces B - Biointerfaces*, Vol.82, Issue2, (February 2011), p.p. 365-370, ISSN 0927-7765.

Otto, A. (1968). Excitation of Surface Plasma Waves in Silver by the Method of Frustrated Total Reflection. *Zeitschrift für Physik*, Vol.216, p.p. 398–410, ISSN 0340-2347.

Prassl, R. & Laggner, P. (2009). Molecular structure of low density lipoprotein: current status and future challenges. *European Biophysical Journal*, Vol.38, No.2, (September 2008), p.p. 145-158, ISSN: 0175-7571.

Raether, H. (1988). *Surface Plasmons on Smooth and Rough Surfaces and on Gratings*, Springer-Verlag, ISBN 978-038-7173-63-4, Berlin.

Rifai, N., Iannotti, E., DeAngelis, K. & Law, T. (1998). Analytical and clinical performance of a homogeneous enzymatic LDL-cholesterol assay compared with the ultracentrifugation-dextran sulfate-Mg2+ method. *Clinical Chemistry*, Jun;Vol.44, No.6, p.p. 1242-1250, ISSN: 1530-8561.

Robbio, L.L., Uboldi, P., Marcovina, S., Revoltella, R.P. & Catapano, A.L. (2001). Epitope Mapping Analysis of Apolipoprotein B-100 using a Surface Plasmon Resonance-Based Biosensor. *Biosensors and Bioelectronics*, Vol.16 (February 2001), p.p. 963–969, ISSN 0956-5663.

Sauerbrey, G. (1959). Verwendung von Schwingquarzen zur Wägung dünner Schichten und zur Mikrowägung. *Zeitschrift für Physik*, Vol.155, Issue2, (April 1959), p.p. 206–222, ISSN 0340-2347.

Sawamura, T., Kume, N., Aoyama, T., Moriwaki, H., Hoshikawa, H., Aiba, Y., Tanaka, T., Miwa, S., Katsura, Y., Kita, T. & Masaki, T. (1997). An Endothelial Receptor for Oxidized Low-Density Lipoprotein. *Nature*, Vol.386, (March 1997), p.p. 73–77, ISSN 0028-0836.

Schumaker, V.N., Phillips, M.L. & Chatterton, J.E. (1994). Apolipoprotein B and Low-Density Lipoprotein Structure: Implications for Biosynthesis of Triglyceride-Rich Lipoproteins, In: *Advances in Protein Chemistry*, Anfinsen, C.B., Edsall, J.T., Richards, F.M. & Eisenberg, D.S. (Eds.), 205-248, Calif. Academic Press, ISBN 978-012-0342-47-1, San Diego.

Skålén, K., Gustafsson, M., Rydberg, E.K., Hultén, L.M., Wiklund, O., Innerarity, T.L. & Borén, J. (2002). Subendothelial Retention of Atherogenic Lipoproteins in Early Atherosclerosis. *Nature*, Vol.417, (June 2002), p.p. 750–754, ISSN 0028-0836.

Smith, A. (2008). The Quartz Crystal Microbalance, In: *Handbook of Thermal Analysis and Calorimetry*, Brown, M. & Gallagher, P. (Eds.), 133-169, Vol.5, Elsevier B.V., ISBN 978-044-4531-23-0, Amsterdam.

Smith, E.A. & Corn, R.M. (2003). Surface Plasmon Resonance Imaging as a Tool to Monitor Biomolecular Interactions in an Array Based Format, *Applied Spectroscopy*, Vol.57, No.11, (November 2003), p.p. 320A-332A, ISSN 0003-7028.

Snellings, S., Fuller, J., Pitner, M. & David, P.W. (2003). An Acoustic Wave Biosensor for Human Low-Density Lipoprotein Particles: Construction of Selective Coatings.

Biosensors and Bioelectronics, Vol.19, Issue4, (December 2003), p.p. 353-363, ISSN 0956-5663.

Srivastava, A.K. & Sakthivel, P. (2001). Quartz-Crystal Microbalance Study for Characterizing Atomic Oxygen in Plasma Ash Tools. *Journal of Vacuum Science & Technology A*, Vol.19, Issue1, (January 2001), p.p. 97-100 ISSN 1520-8567.

Stefan, R.I., van Staden, J.F. & Aboul-Enein, H.Y. (2000). Immunosensor in clinical analysis. *Fresenius Journal of Analytical Chemistry*, 366 (December 1999) p.p. 659-668, ISSN 0937-0633.

Stocker, R. & Keaney, J.R. (2004). Role of oxidative modifications in atherosclerosis. *Physiological Reviews*, Vol.84, No.4, (October 2004), p.p. 1381–1478, ISSN: 0031-9333.

Stura, E., Bruzzese, D., Valerio, F., Grasso, F., Perlo, P. & Nicolini, C. (2007). Anodic Porous Alumina as Mechanical Stability Enhancer for LDL-Cholesterol Sensitive Electrodes. *Biosensors and Bioelectronics*, Vol.23, (July 2007), p.p. 655–660, ISSN 0956-5663.

Tan, X., Li, M., Cai, P., Luo, L. & Zou, X. (2005). An Amperometric Cholesterol Biosensor Based on Multivalent Carbon Nanotubes and Organically Modified Sol-Gel/Chitosan Hybrid Composite Film. *Analytical Biochemistry*, Vol.337, Issue1, (February 2005), p.p. 111-120, ISSN 1096-0309.

Thevenot, D.R., Toth, K., Durst, R.A. & Wilson, G.S. (1999). Electrochemical Biosensors: Recommended Definitions and Classification. *Pure and Applied Chemistry*, Vol.71, No.12, (January 2001), p.p. 2333-2348, ISSN 1365-3075.

Tudos, A.J. & Schasfoort, R.B.M. (2008). Introduction to Surface Plasmon Resonance, In: *Handbook of Surface Plasmon Resonance*, Tudos, A.J. & Schasfoort, R.B.M. (Eds.), 1-14, RSC Publishing, ISBN 978-085-4042-67-8, Cambridge UK.

Viigimaa, M., Abina, J., Zemtsovskaya, G., Tikhaze A, Konovalova, G., Kumskova, E. & Lankin, V. (2010). Malondialdehyde-modified low density lipoproteins as biomarker for atherosclerosis. *Blood Pressure*, Vol.19, No.3, (June 2010), p.p. 164–168, ISSN: 0803-7051.

Wood, R.W. (1902). On a Remarkable Case of Uneven Distribution of Light in a Diffraction Grating Spectrum. *Proceedings of the Physical Society of London*, Vol.18, No.1, p.p. 269-275, ISSN 0370-1328.

Yan, W., Chen, X., Li, X., Feng, X. & Zhu, J.-J. (2008). Fabrication of a Label-Free Electrochemical Immunosensor of Low-Density Lipoprotein. *The Journal of Physical Chemistry B*, Vol.112, No.4, (January 2008), p.p. 1275–1281, ISSN 1089-5647.

Yang, C.Y., Chen, S.H., Gianturco, S.H., Bradley, W.A., Sparrow, J.T., Tanimura, M., Li, W.H., Sparrow, D.A., DeLoof, H., Rosseneu, M., Lee, F.S., Gu, Z.W., Gotto, A.M.Jr. & Chan, L. (1986). Sequence, Structure, Receptor-Binding Domains and Internal Repeats of Human Apolipoprotein B-100. *Nature*, Vol.323, (October 1986), p.p. 738-742, ISSN 0028-0836.

Zhao, H. & Ju, H. (2006). Multilayer Membranes for Glucose Biosensing via Layer-by-Layer Assembly of Multiwall Carbon Nanotubes and Glucose Oxidase. *Analytical Biochemistry*, Vol.350, Issue1, (March 2006), p.p. 138–144, ISSN 1096-0309.

10

Multiplexing Capabilities of Biosensors for Clinical Diagnostics

Johnson K-K Ng and Samuel S Chong
National University of Singapore
Singapore

1. Introduction

The detection of biomolecules, be it proteins or nucleic acids such as DNA or RNA, is a critical process in biomedical research and clinical diagnostics. With the former, it helps us to unravel the complexity of our human body, and provides important information down at the cellular and sub-cellular level that allows us to better understand what our bodies are comprised off, how they function, how they respond to disease and aging, or why they fail to respond. This information, when applied to clinical diagnostics, help better manage our health and enhance the quality of life.

To generate any meaningful or conclusive information for clinical diagnostics, it is often needed to detect several targets simultaneously. Therefore technologies for performing biomolecular detection must be able to interrogate several targets at one time i.e. perform multiplexing. These targets can be proteins or nucleic acid targets from different cellular species, such as for infectious disease diagnosis, or from the same species i.e. along the same genome, such as single-nucleotide polymorphisms (SNPs) genotyping for pharmacogenomics. It can also be for identifying aberrant biomolecules from normal ones, such as mutation detection in cancer diagnostics and prognostics. Therefore having a platform capable of performing multiplexed biological detection is an indispensable tool for accurate clinical diagnostics.

Through advancement in molecular biology as well as in areas such as microelectronics, microfabrication, material science, and optics, there have been a proliferation of miniaturized platforms, or biosensors, for performing biological analysis based on a variety of multiplexing technologies. These ranged from those capable of detecting a few targets to those capable of interrogating hundreds or even thousands of targets. Here we attempt to provide a concise overview of such technologies, as well as provide some insight into a simple technology that we developed in-house. Due to the enormous amount of progress in this area, this is by no means a comprehensive overview.

2. Review of current technologies

2.1 Solution-based

One of the most widely used technologies for multiplexed detection involves performing the detection within a single homogeneous solution. The best example of this is the multiplexed polymerase chain reaction (PCR). PCR, which is one of the most common techniques used in molecular biology, involves using a pair of primers to amplify a certain fragment of a target DNA or RNA manifold, until there is sufficient amount for detection or further downstream analysis. In multiplex PCR, several pairs of primers are used to simultaneously amplify different fragments. It is relatively easy to perform multiplexing in PCR, because the primers can first be designed to amplify fragments of different sizes, and these fragments can then be detected based on their size differences, either using gel electrophoresis or high-resolution melting on real-time PCR systems. Alternatively, the different fragments can also be targeted by different probes conjugated to fluorescent dyes of a specific color. Upon hybridizing to the targets, the probes emit an optical signal corresponding to their dye, which is detected in a real-time PCR system.

Multiplex PCR is one of the most common techniques used in clinical diagnostics because the technology has matured significantly since its invention almost three decades ago. This is also rather easy to implement on biosensors, as the process can be carried out in microchambers (Merritt , 2010), or coupled to a capillary electrophoretic module (Thaitrong, 2009). The ability to perform multiplexed detection in PCR results from (a) the unique feature in PCR that allows primers to be designed to amplify fragments of different sizes, (b) the ability of the gel electrophoresis or real-time PCR system to differentiate the fragments by size as a result of their difference in electrophoretic mobility or melting temperature, and (3) the ability to differentiate the probes through color-emitting dyes. Probes used in multiplex PCR are conjugated with fluorescent dyes that emit different wavelengths of light, allowing them to be differentially detected. As a result, there is always a need for powerful optical detection, being capable of exciting and detecting one or multiple wavelengths of light. Due to limitations in the number of different wavelengths of light that can be excited and detected, the number of different multiplexed targets that can be detected in a single reaction is generally not high. One way to overcome this limitation is to combine multiplex PCR with other technologies, such as microarrays.

2.2 2-D microarray

The development of microarrays is driven by the demand for high throughput multiplexed analysis, such as the mapping of the human genome. This platform enables hundreds of thousands of proteins or DNA probes to be precisely immobilized onto designated locations within a microscopic area of a silicon or glass substrate (Ramsay, 1998; Schena *et al*, 1995), with the different probes identified through their unique locations. The proteins or oligonuleotides can be immobilized onto the surface using a high precision robotic arrayer or synthesized *in-situ* using light-directed chemistry. With such high density chips, it becomes possible to perform massively parallel interrogation of a large number of targets, making microarrays a platform of choice for applications such as gene expression analysis (Rahmatpanah, 2009), SNP genotyping (Wang *et al*, 1998; Lindroos *et al*, 2001) and transciptome analysis (Li *et al*, 2006).

Since the inception of the microarrays about two decades ago, there has been a host of companies offering the technology commercially. United States-based Affymetrix is one of the first companies to offer commercial oligonucleotide microarrays, with its GeneChip one of the most widely-used microarrays in a variety of applications, such as in prediction of tumour relapse in hepatocecullar carcinoma patients (Roessler, 2010). Other companies include Agilent, which uses inkjet printing for oligo synthesis on its 2D microarrays (Fig. 1), Applied Microarrays and Roche NimbleGen. CombiMatrix's CMOS arrays have addressable electrodes that have been developed for both DNA detection and immunoassays (Gunn, 2010; Cooper, 2010). With the advent of microfabrication technology and with increased competition, the prices of these microarrays have come down significantly over the years, making the technology more accessible to the research and clinical diagnostics community.

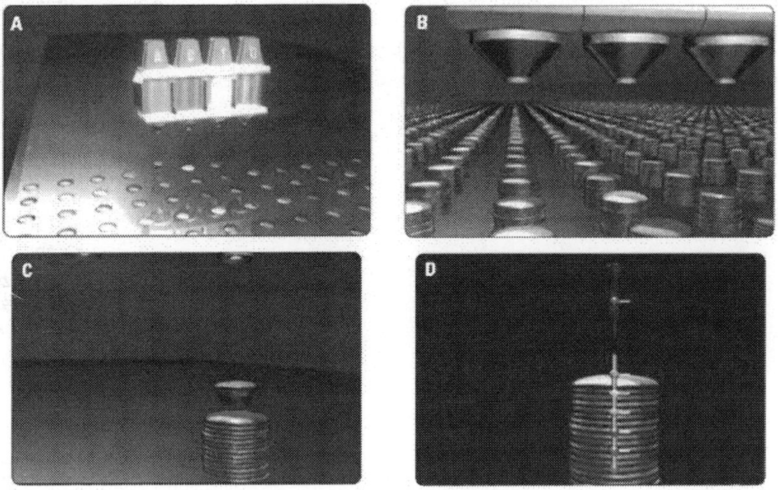

Fig. 1. Agilent's inkjet printing technology for oligonucleotide synthesis on 2D microarrrays A: the first layer of nucleotides is deposited on the activated microarray surface. B: growth of the oligos is shown after multiple layers of nucleotides have been precisely printed. C: close-up of one oligo as a new base is being added to the chain, which is shown in figure D. (Courtesy of Agilent Technologies. All rights reserved).

2.3 3-D microarray

Despite its high-throughput potential, the 2-D microarray format is restricted by the diffusion-limited kinetics, and electrostatic repulsion between the solution-phase targets and the densely localized solid-phase probes. Furthermore, the amount of probes that can be immobilized on the planar substrate, and hence the sensitivity and signal-to-noise ratio (SNR), is also somewhat limited. The introduction of 3-D microarrays go some way toward overcoming these limitations. These 3-D microarrays comprised of additional microstructures that are fabricated onto planar substrates to provide a high surface-density platform that increases the immobilization capacity of capture probes, enhances target accessibility and reduces background noise interference in DNA microarrays, leading to improved signal-to-noise ratios, sensitivity and specificity.

An example of an early 3-D microarray is the gel-based chip (Kolchinsky & Mirzabekov, 2002). The use of an array of nanoliter-sized polyacrylamide gel pads on a glass slide provides distinct 3D microenvironments for the immobilization of oligonucleotides. Compared to planar glass substrates, the gel-based format can be applied with a higher probe concentration of up to 100 fold, thereby increasing the SNR. The near solution-phase interaction between targets and probes within individual gel pads can also potentially alleviate the problems associated with diffusion-limited kinetics. These gel-based microarrays have been successfully demonstrated for the detection of SNPs associated with β-thalassemia mutations (Drobyshev *et al*, 1997), and for the identification of polymorphisms in the human mu-opioid receptor gene (LaForge *et al*, 2000).

Other 3-D structures fabricated onto planar surfaces include conical dendrons as well as micropillars (Hong *et al*, 2005). By fabricating conical dendrons, nano-controlled spacings can be created to provide enough room for the target strand to access each probe, thereby creating a reaction format resembling that in a solution (Fig. 2). As a result, the hybridization time can be reduced to significantly to allow effective discrimination of single-nucleotide mismatches (Hong *et al*, 2005).

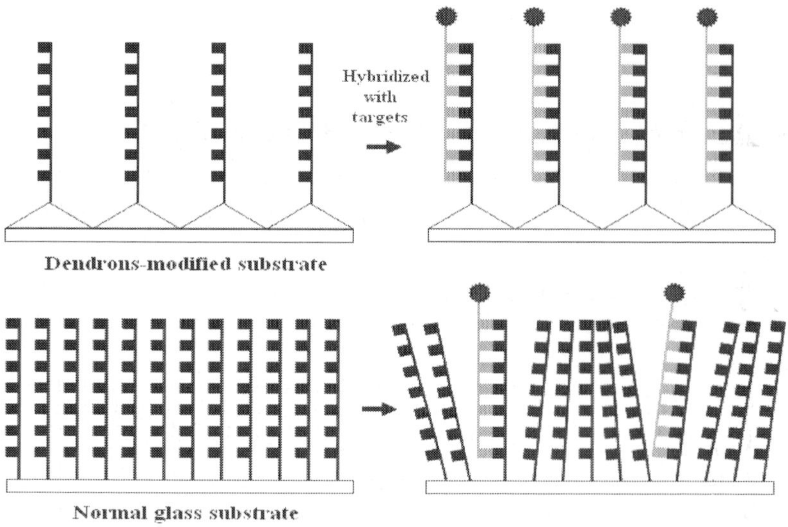

Fig. 2. Schematic diagram showing improved DNA hybridization onto a dendron-modified substrate as compared to that of a normal substrate.

Ramanamurthy *et* al (2008) reported the fabrication of ordered, high-aspect ratio nanopillar arrays on the surface of silicon-based chips to enhance signal intensity in DNA microarrays (Fig. 3). These 150-nm diameter nanopillars were found to enhance the hybridization signals by up to 7 times as compared to flat silicon dioxide substrates. In addition, hybridization of synthetic targets to capture probes that contained a single-base variation showed that the perfect matched duplex signals on dual-substrate nanopillars can be up to 23 times higher than the mismatched duplex signals. The Z-Slides microarray from United States-based company Life Bioscience comprises micropillars and nanowells to enhance spot morphology and eliminate cross-talk between probe sites. By detecting only the pillar surfaces which are several hundred microns from the base, background noise is removed from the microarray scan.

A 3-D microarray which is markedly different from the above-mentioned approaches involves immobilizing oligonucleotide probes onto a single thread instead of a planar substrate (Stimpson *et al*, 2004). The thread is subsequently wound around a core to form a compact, high-density SNP detection platform. Hybridization can be carried out by immersing the thread-and-core structure into a target solution, and completed within approximately 30 min. This platform has been demonstrated for the analysis of SNPs in CYP2C19, an important cytochrome P450 gene (Tojo *et al*, 2005).

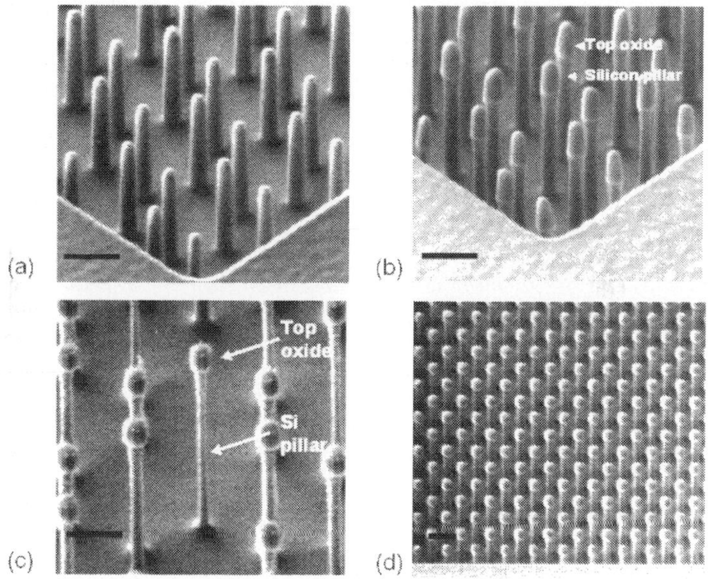

Fig. 3. SEM images of the nanopillars fabricated on silicon-based biosensors. (a) Single-substrate nanopillars consisting SiO_2. (b) Dual-substrate nanopillars consisting SiO_2 layer atop the Si pillar. (c) Very high-aspect ratio dual-substrate nanopillars. (d) Dense array of ordered dual-substrate nanopillars. Scale bars are all 500 nm.

2.4 Bead microarray

One of the best examples of 3-D microarrays, and perhaps also one of the most successful commercially available platforms, is the bead microarray. Unlike 2-D microarrays, the high surface-to-volume ratio of beads allows a larger amount of probes to be immobilized to improve the detection signals and signal-to-noise ratios. The small size of beads can further reduce the reaction volume, and the use of microfluidics in bead arrays can shorten the hybridization time to < 10 min, a 50 to 70-fold reduction as compared to conventional microarrays (Ali *et al*, 2003). Unlike 2-D or the 3-D microarrays discussed, probes are usually conjugated onto the beads prior to them being immobilized onto the microarrays. The major challenge, therefore, in developing bead arrays is to identify the identities or their corresponding immobilized probes of those randomly assembled beads in multiplexed analyses.

The most common strategy is to encode beads with colorimetric signatures using semiconductor nanocrystals, visible dyes or fluorophores, and subsequently decode them

through visual or fluorescence detection (Mulvaney *et al*, 2004). Color-encoded beads are produced by embedding them with semiconductor nanocrystals, visible dyes, or fluorophores and subsequently decoded through visual or fluorescence detection. For example, Li *et al* (2001) mixed blue, green and orange fluorophores to yield 39 different codes for encoding 3.2 μm-diameter polystyrene beads assembled onto a wafer. Alternatively, two fluorophores can be mixed in different proportions to yield 100 distinguishable bead types that are subsequently decoded using two laser beams, as in the Luminex xMAP technology (Dunbar, 2006) (Fig. 4). The emission characteristics of organic fluorescent dyes are affected by changes in temperature, which may result in some bias when used in temperature-dependent studies (Liu *et al*, 2005). The fluorescent dyes also suffer from photobleaching and this can significantly affect the discriminability between color codes, particularly if they are distinguished by the difference in their intensities.
Quantum dots, which are photostable, have size-tunable emission wavelengths, and can be excited by a single wavelength to emit different colors at one time, are widely used to distinguish beads. Han *et al.* (2001) incorporated quantum dots at different intensities and colors to yield spectrally distinguishable polymeric beads of up to 10 distinct types (Fig. 4). Using 5-6 colors, each at 6 intensity levels, it is possible to achieve up to 40 000 codes using this approach, although this has yet to be demonstrated. These techniques for color encoding beads are straightforward in that the color-emitting agents are directly impregnated into the beads. However, this also means that the encoder signals cannot be removed, resulting in possible interference between the encoder and reporter signals. To avoid this, the number of reporter dyes available for use would inadvertently be reduced. Also, encoding the beads into unique color codes is challenging as the color-emitting agents must be mixed in precise proportions. The difficulty in distinguishing a large number of color codes further means that only up to 100 color codes have been demonstrated so far, limiting them to low or medium throughout applications (Xu *et al*, 2003; Li *et al*, 2004).

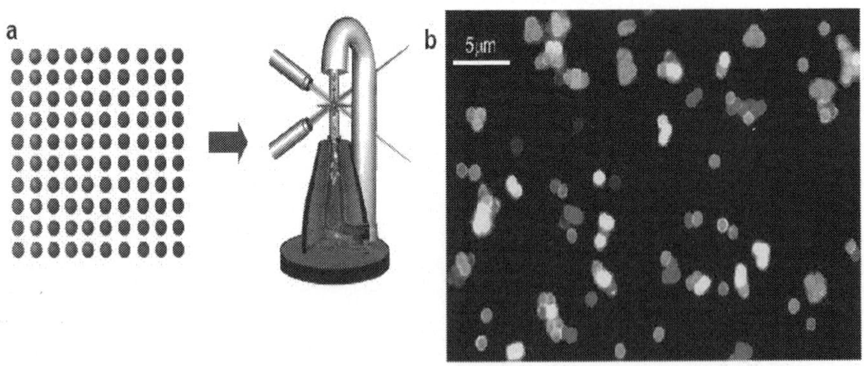

Fig. 4. (a) A set of 100 distinguishable bead types can be created by mixing precise proportions of two fluorescent dyes, and subsequently detected using a flow cytometer with two laser beams. (Courtesy of Luminex Corporation. All rights reserved). (b) Quantum dot nanocrystals of 10 different emission colors incorporated into the beads to create spectrally distinguishable types. (Adapted by permission from Macmillan Publishers Ltd: Nature Biotechnology, copyright 2001).

Beads within an array can also be individually addressed using barcodes. A graphical barcode can also be written inside fluorescently dyed beads through a technique termed "spatial selective photobleaching of the fluorescence" (Braeckmans, 2001). Using a specially adapted laser scanning confocal microscope, any sort of pattern can be photobleached at any depth inside the fluorescently dyed bead. This technique was used to photobleach a barcode of different band widths onto 45 µm-diameter fluorescent beads. The advantages of this technique are that only a single fluorescent dye is needed in the encoding scheme, and the number of codes achievable is virtually unlimited. However, there is still the problem of interference between the encoder and reporter fluorescence signals, while the effects of photobleaching during the decoding stage might alter or degrade the barcode.

A widely used bead microarray platform for biological detection and clinical diagnostics is the commercial BeadArray from Illumina, a market leader in high-throughput bead microarrays. It assembles 3-micron silica beads onto a fiber optic of planar silica slides, for a range of DNA and RNA analyses. There is also the Veracode technology, which uses digital holographic barcode to identify the beads (Lin *et al*, 2009) (Fig. 5). When excited by a laser, each microbead, which has a pillar-like rather than spherical shape, emits an image resembling a barcode. Using this method, it becomes possible to have virtually unlimited number of different bead types. The platform can be applied to both protein-based or DNA-based assays.

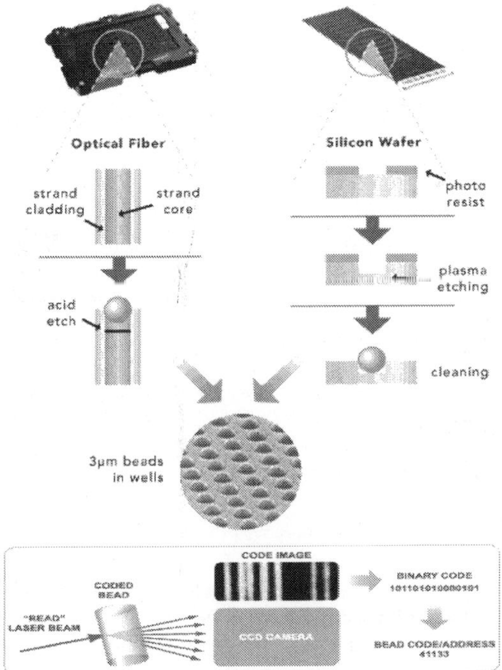

Fig. 5. Illumina's BeadArray (top panel) and Veracode technology (bottom panel). (Courtesy of Illumina. All rights reserved)

3. A simple spatially addressable bead-based biosensor

We describe here some of our own work in developing a biosensor that allow different bead types to be incorporated and addressed with minimal efforts for encoding and decoding, simplifying the development and usage of such devices (Ng *et* al, 2010). To achieve that, different bead types are incorporated and identified based on their spatial addresses (akin to microarrays) without the need for color-coding (Fig. 6). Beads of a certain type are spotted onto a polymeric micro-matrix (or gel pad) fabricated on the surface of the biosensor. The natural immobilization of the beads by the gel pad allows each bead to be anchored within the gel pad on a unique location, acquiring spatial addresses that can be easily recorded via an acquired image. Beads of a second type spotted over the same gel pad take up spatial addresses distinct from those of the first bead type, allowing the two bead types to be easily distinguished. This is repeated for immobilizing and distinguishing further bead types on the gel pad, obviating the need for prior encoding and tedious decoding of beads. The throughput can be increased by further spotting many different bead types onto the hundreds of gel pads on each biosensor. We demonstrate the use of this bead-based biosensor for detection of six common South-east Asian beta-globin gene mutations within 30 min, demonstrating its potential as a simple tool for rapid beta-thalassemia carrier screening.

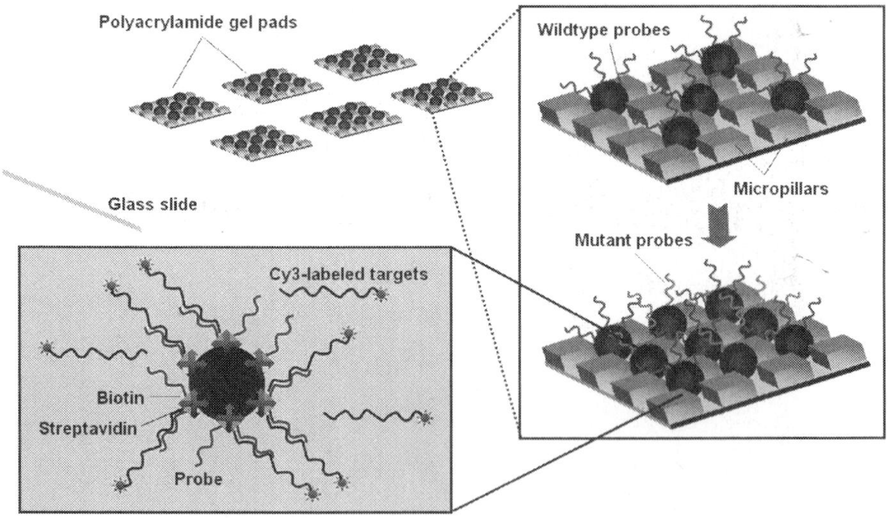

Fig. 6. Schematic representation of the spatially addressable bead-based biosensor (Adapted from Ng et al, 2010, copyright Elsevier Inc).

3.1 Biosensor fabrication

The biosensor consisted an array of 19 x 24 polyacrylamide gel pads fabricated on a glass slide (Corning, Corning, NY) pre-treated with Bind Silane (GE Healthcare, Piscataway, NJ).

The gel pads had horizontal and vertical pitch of 300 µm, and each gel pad further comprised a 10 x 10 array of micropillars (10x10x10 µm) with horizontal and vertical pitch of 10 µm (Fig. 7). A photopolymerization process described previously was used to create the array of gel pads (Proudnikov et al., 1998), after which the glass slide was treated in 0.1M $NaBH_4$ for 30 min to reduce gel pads auto-fluorescence.

The Biochip Arrayer (PerkinElmer, Boston, MA) was used to spot beads onto singular gel pads on the device. Each gel pad was spotted with about 5 nL of a particular bead solution (~ 9000 beads/µL), and then left to dry at room temperature for 2-3 min to allow beads immobilization to the gel. Beads can also be spotted manually using a pipette, although this required a larger amount of bead solution (0.25 µL) per spot and the beads usually covered 2-4 gel pads simultaneously. Positions of each spotted bead type were then recorded via autofluorescence images for determining their spatial addresses. This was repeated until all bead types for detecting a particular target were immobilized on the same gel pad. The device can then be capped with a microfluidic module for sample flow-through, or the buffer can also be applied over the spotted beads without the module. The polydimethylsiloxane (PDMS) module was fabricated using common soft lithographic techniques (Duffy et al., 1998).

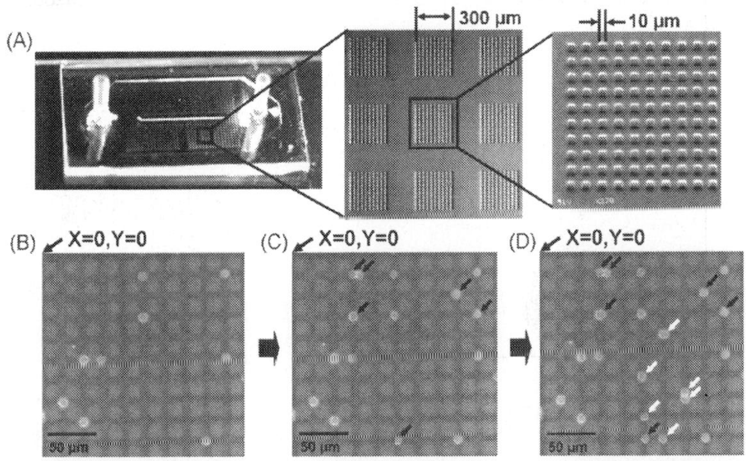

Spatial addresses

	X	Y
Bead 1-1	127	29
Bead 1-2	230	26
Bead 1-3	128	79
Bead 1-4	53	131
Bead 1-5	76	131
Bead 1-6	231	128
Bead 1-7	26	183
Bead 1-8	53	207
Bead 1-9	207	230

Spatial addresses

	X	Y
Bead 2-1	74	26
Bead 2-2	82	26
Bead 2-3	202	49
Bead 2-4	74	76
Bead 2-5	228	72
Bead 2-6	131	229

Spatial addresses

	X	Y
Bead 3-1	155	100
Bead 3-2	127	150
Bead 3-3	181	170
Bead 3-4	181	179
Bead 3-5	130	199
Bead 3-6	154	226

Fig. 7. The bead-based biosensor. (A) The device comprised an array of polyacrylamide gel pads on a glass slide. Each gel pad further comprised an array of micropillars. (B) Image after spotting the first bead type onto the gel pad. The spatial address for each bead is recorded in terms of their x, y coordinates. (C) Image after spotting a second bead type (black arrows) and finally (D) a third bead type (white arrows). (Adapted from Ng et al, 2008, copyright Elsevier Inc).

3.2 Oligonucleotide probes and targets

The six common South-east Asian beta-globin gene mutations selected for this study were -28 A→G, -29 A→G, IVSI5 G→C, IVSI1 G→T, Cd26 GAG→AAG, and IVSII654 C→T. For each mutation, allele-specific probes were designed to hybridize with perfect complementary to either the wildtype or mutant variant (Table 1). A biotin moiety was added to the 5′ end of each probe, and conjugation of probes to 9.95 μm streptavidin-modified polystyrene beads was carried out according to previously described protocol (Ng *et al.*, 2008).

PCR was carried out to amplify two fragments of the beta-globin gene, with the first fragment (319 bp) encompassing the Exon 1 which incudes all the targeted mutations other than IVSII654 C→T, which was contained in the second fragment (128 bp). Primer sequences were: Frag1-F: 5′-Cy3-ACggCTgTCATCACTTAgAC-3′ (Genbank HUMHBB sequence 62010-62029); Frag1-R: 5′-CCCAgTTTCTATTggTCTCC-3′ (HUMHBB sequence 62328-62309); Frag2-F: 5′- Cy3-TgTATCATgCCTCTTTgCACC-3′ (HUMHBB sequence 63227-63247); and Frag2-R: 5′-CAATATgAAACCTCTTACATCAg-3′ (HUMHBB: 63354-63332).

Genomic DNA (100 ng) was amplified in a total volume of 50 μL containing 0.5 μM each of the two sets of primers, 200 μM of each deoxynucleotide triphosphate, and 1 U of HotStarTaq DNA polymerase in 1× supplied PCR buffer (Qiagen). Amplification was carried out in an iCycler thermal cycler (BioRad) with an initial denaturation at 95 °C for 15 min, followed by 35 cycles at 98 °C for 30 s, 55 °C for 30 s, and 72 °C for 30 s, and a final extension at 72 °C for 5 min. Products were then re-amplified with only the forward primers to generate ssDNA for allele-specific hybridization.

Probe name	Mutation targeted	Sequence (5′-3′)
-28,-29_WT	-28/-29 WT	CCTgACTTTTATgCCCAg
-28_MT	-28 MT	CCTgACTTCTATgCCCAg
-29_MT	-29 MT	CCTgACTTTCATgCCCAg
IVSI5,1_WT	IVSI5/1 WT	CTTgATACCAACCTgCCC
IVSI5_MT	IVSI5 MT	CTTgATAgCAACCTgCCC
IVSI5_WT	IVSI1 MT	CTTgATACCAAACTgCCC
Cd26_WT	Cd26 WT	gggCCTCACCACCAAC
Cd26_MT	Cd26 MT	gggCCTTACCACCAAC
IVSII654_WT	IVSII654 WT	TTgCTATTgCCTTAACCC
IVSII654_MT	IVSII654 MT	TTgCTATTACCTTAACCC

WT: wild-type, MT: mutant

Table 1. Probe sequences for targeting each of the beta-globin gene mutations selected for this study. (Adapted from Ng et al, 2010, copyright Elsevier Inc).

3.3 Hybridization and signal detection

Re-amplified PCR products were purified using the Microcon YM-30 filter device (Millipore) before being diluted to a 10 μL hybridization solution containing 500 mM NaCl and 30% formamide. Hybidization was carried out by pipetting the solution over the spotted beads. After 30 min incubation, the device was rinsed briefly with a solution containing only 500 mM NaCl and 30% formamide, and signal capture was carried out by fluorescence imaging. The imaging system comprised an epifluorescence microscope (BX51, Olympus), 100 W mercury lamp and fluorescence filter set 41007 (Chroma Technology). MetaMorph 5.0 (Molecular Devices) was used to control acquisition of 12-bit monochrome bead images at 2 s exposure from a SPOT-RT Slider cooled-CCD camera (Diagnostic Instruments), and bead signals were quantitated using the modified version of a software developed in-house previously (Ng and Liu, 2005).

3.4 Results and discussion

To demonstrate detection of the six beta-globin gene mutations, six human samples heterozygous for -28 A→G, -29 A→G, IVSI5 G→C, IVSI1 G→T, Cd26 GAG→AAG, and IVSII654 C→T, and one homozygous for IVSII654 C→T were analyzed using the bead-based biosensor. All samples were genotyped previously by direct sequencing or multiplexed minisequencing (Wang et al., 2003). Wildtype and mutant probes targeting each mutation were conjugated to distinct bead sets, spotted onto a particular gel pad on the device, and distinguished based on their spatial addresses (Fig. 8A). Probes were designed with the targeted mutation as near as possible to its centre region, in order to increase the discrimination between matched and mismatched duplexes. Due to the proximity between the -28 and -29 mutations, as well as between the IVSI1 and IVSI5 mutations, each pair of mutations must be detected simultaneously on a single gel pad by four sets of probes to cover all possible genotypes. However, due to the lack of samples compound heterozygous for -28/-29 and IVSI1/IVSI5, only three sets of probes were required in this study for each pair of mutations.

Fig. 8B shows the signal intensity from the wildtype and mutant probes used to target each mutation. All seven different samples were correctly genotyped using the device. For heterozygous mutations, signal intensities from the wildtype probes did not differ significantly from that of the mutant probes, attaining student t-test p-values > 0.05 for all except IVSII654 which had a slightly lower p-value of about 0.01. In the absence of a mutation, the wildtype probe intensities were significantly higher than that of the mutant probes, with p-values far lower than 0.001. For the homozygous IVSII654 mutation, the mutant probe intensity was significantly higher than the wildtype probe, attaining a p-value < 0.0001. This similarity or significant difference between wildtype and mutant probe intensities allowed correct identification of the heterozygous mutant and homozygous wildtype (or mutant) samples respectively.

The spatially addressable bead-based biosensor offers an alternative tool for simple yet efficient and rapid detection of beta-thalassemia mutations. The device is comprised simply of a glass slide fabricated with a thin polyacrylamide matrix on its surface using a photopolymerization process that is faster (~ 45 min) and far less complicated than conventional photolithographic techniques for making silicon chips. The main advantage of the device is its ability to distinguish different bead types without the need for prior time-consuming and laborious techniques such as color-encoding (Braeckmans et al., 2002). This is due to the natural immobilization of the beads to the polyacrylamide gel pads, thus allowing the beads to acquire unique spatial addresses. Detection is achieved by applying the solution of PCR-amplified targets over the region of the spotted beads for passive hybridization to occur, which obviates the need for microfluidic mixing and thus microchannels. This further simplifies the fabrication process, lowers the cost of the device,

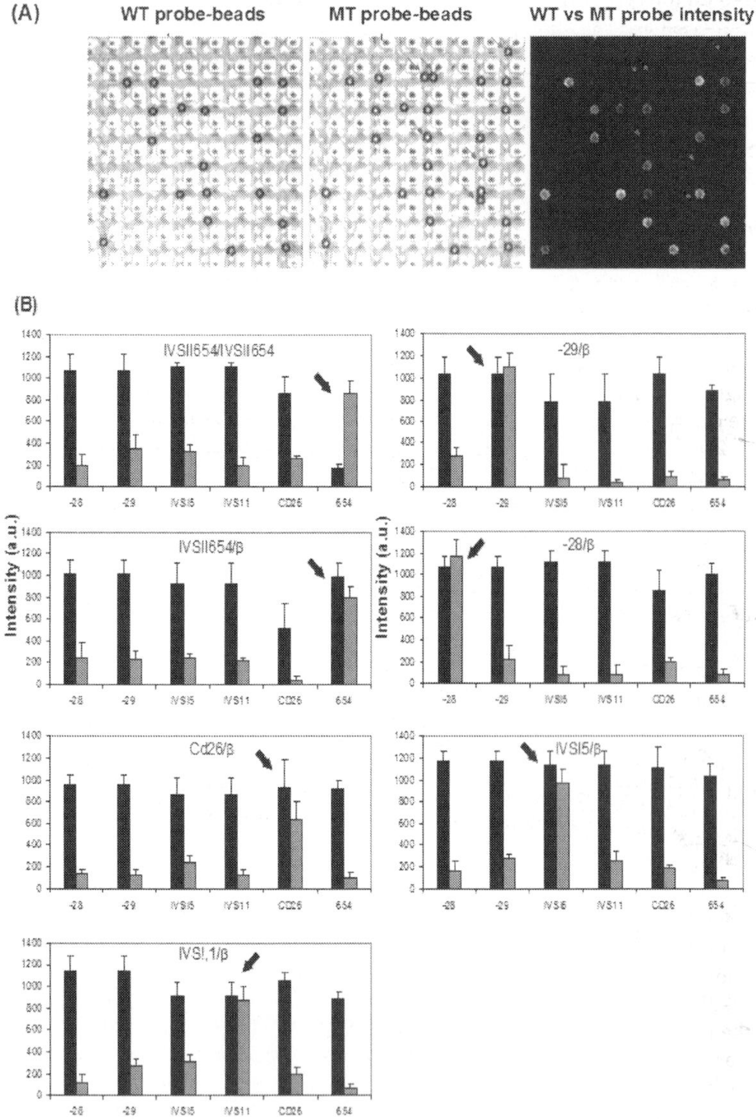

Fig. 8. Allele-specific hybridization on the device. (A) Typical example of the beads spotted onto a gel pad. Probe-beads targeting Cd26 wildtype variant were spotted onto a gel pad, followed by those targeting the mutant variant (red arrows). Difference in probe intensities showed sample to be of homozygous Cd26 normal genotype. (B) Signal intensity from the wide-type (■) and mutant (■) probe-bead targeting each of the six mutations selected for this study. (Adapted from Ng et al, 2010, copyright Elsevier Inc).

and reduces the sample volume required (< 10 μL). Despite the lack of microfluidic mixing, detection is achieved in 30 min, although this might possibly be even faster, given that we have achieved hybridization on this device within 10 min, albeit with synthetic targets (Ng et al., 2008).

4. Conclusion

The advent of biosensors has allowed biomedical research and clinical diagnostics to leverage upon the advantages of miniaturization, such as reduced sample volumes, faster reaction times, and the possibility of multiplexed detection. The last point is of particular importance, since the simultaneous detection of multiple targets at once has resulted in significant time savings, particularly for applications requiring high-throughput. Often, multiple targets must be detected in order to draw any meaningful conclusion in clinical diagnosis. So much progress has been made in this field such that it is now possible to utilize high throughput platforms such as microarrays to interrogate thousands of targets at once. The crucial role played by these technologies, such as multiplex PCR and the various forms of 2D, 3D and bead-based microarrays, in the past decades is indisputable, and will continue to be so. However several challenges exist.

First, it is important to reduce the cost of some of these technologies so as to make it more affordable, particularly for clinical diagnostics. For example, systems for real-time PCR can be quite costly, due in part to the high precision optical detection modules found within. With advances in optics, both light sources (e.g. LEDS) and detectors (e.g. digital cameras) are getting more affordable, which would help to bring down the costs of such systems. Also, part of the costs are attributable to the licensing issues. Manufacturers of real-time PCR systems and reagents have to pay a license fee including royalties to the original patent owners. With time, some of the patent protections will expire soon, so prices should also come down, as in the case of the patent expiry of the Taq polymerase in 2006. The manufacturing costs for microarrays and its bead-based counterpart are also high. Hopefully with advances in manufacturing technologies, the cost can eventually be reduced.

Second, it is important for these technologies to be of sufficient sensitivity and specificity in order to meet the standards required in clinical diagnostics. Real-time PCR has no problems with that, since it is not uncommon for it to achieve a sensitivity and specificity close to 100%. 2-D microarrays, on the other hand, might face more of a challenge. The diffusion-limited kinetics, steric hindrances and high noise contributed by the planar surface might somewhat affect sensitivity and specificity. It is important to ascertain that the microarrays can reproducibly meet the required levels of sensitivity and specificity before its application to clinical diagnostics.

Third, the reaction times for some applications can still be rather high, particularly for the microarrays. It is desirable to reduce these times further since clinical diagnostics often require a fast turn around time to minimize patient anxiety and to aid decision making in disease management.

Finally, with the advent of modern technologies, some of the multiplexing technologies discussed here might find themselves being slowly displaced. Sequencing is a method used to decipher the order of bases along a DNA. Traditionally slow, it is now possible to perform massively parallel sequencing on high-throughput platforms to speed up its rate. Known as next generation sequencing, thousands of sequences can now be generated at once, using commercial sequencers from companies such as Illumina (Solexa), Roche (454) and Applied Biosystems. Some of these platforms, like the SOLiD system from Applied Biosystems, can generate up to 60 gigabases of DNA sequence per run. With these advances in next generation sequencing comes the race for rapid and low cost full genome sequencing. The Archon X Prize for Genomics was established in October 2006 to award US$10 million to "the first Team that can build a device and use it to sequence 100 human genomes within 10 days or less, with an accuracy of no more than one error in every 100,000 bases sequenced, with sequences accurately covering at least 98% of the genome, and at a recurring cost of no more than $10,000 per genome". As of January 2011, the prize is yet unclaimed. However, the possibility of being able to sequence an entire human genome accurately, cheaply and rapidly in future might supplant some of today's multiplexing technologies like the DNA microarray.

In summary, multiplexing capabilities in biosensors have come a long way and will continue to advance rapidly in the next decade, with a large number of companies pouring in large sums of monies into research and development. The ideal platform will be one offering high-throughput, rapid and low cost diagnostics. Whether that can be realised in the near future remains to be seen.

5. References

Ramsay, G. (1998). DNA chips: State-of-the art. *Nat Biotech* 16, 40.

Ali, M.F., Kirby, R., Goodey, A.P., Rodriguez, M.D., Ellington, A.D., Neikirk, D.P. & McDevitt, J.T. (2003). DNA hybridization and discrimination of single-nucleotide mismatches using chip-based microbead arrays. *Anal Chem* 75, 4732-4739.

Braeckmans, K. (2001). A new generation of encoded microcarriers. *Drug Discovery Technology 12-17 Aug, Boston*

Chen, J., Iannone, M.A., Li, M.-S., Taylor, J.D., Rivers, P., Nelsen, A.J., Slentz-Kesler, K.A., Roses, A. & Weiner, M.P. (2000). A Microsphere-Based Assay for Multiplexed Single Nucleotide Polymorphism Analysis Using Single Base Chain Extension. *Genome Res.* 10, 549-557.

Cooper, J., Yazvenko, N., Peyvan, K., Maurer, K., Taitt, C.R., Lyon, W. & Danley, D.L. (2010). Targeted deposition of antibodies on a multiplex CMOS microarray and optimization of a sensitive immunoassay using electrochemical detection. *PLoS One.* 19, e9781.

Daelemans C, Ritchie ME, Smits G, Abu-Amero S, Sudbery IM, Forrest MS, Campino S, Clark TG, Stanier P, Kwiatkowski D, Deloukas P, Dermitzakis ET, Tavaré S, Moore GE, Dunham I. (2010). High-throughput analysis of candidate imprinted genes and allele-specific gene expression in the human term placenta. *BMC Genet.* 19, 25

Drobyshev, A., Mologina, N., Shik, V., Pobedimskaya, D., Yershov, G. & Mirzabekov, A. (1997). Sequence analysis by hybridization with oligonucleotide microchip: identification of beta-thalassemia mutations. *Gene* 188, 45-52.

Duffy, D.C., McDonald, J.C., Schueller, O.J.A. & Whitesides, G.M. (1998). Rapid Prototyping of Microfluidic Systems in Poly(dimethylsiloxane). *Anal. Chem.* 70, 4974-4984.

Dunbar, S.A. (2006). Applications of Luminex(R) xMAP(TM) technology for rapid, high-throughput multiplexed nucleic acid detection. *Clinica Chimica Acta* 363, 71.

Gunn, S., Yeh, I.T., Lytvak, I., Tirtorahardjo, B., Dzidic, N., Zadeh, S., Kim, J., McCaskill, C., Lim, L., Gorre, M., Mohammed, M. (2010). Clinical array-based karyotyping of breast cancer with equivocal HER2 status resolves gene copy number and reveals chromosome 17 complexity. *BMC Cancer.* 28, 396

Han, M., Gao, X., Su, J.Z. & Nie, S. (2001). Quantum-dot-tagged microbeads for multiplexed optical coding of biomolecules. *Nat Biotechnol* 19, 631-635.

Hong, B.J., Oh, S.J., Youn, T.O., Kwon, S.H. & Park, J.W. (2005). Nanoscale-controlled spacing provides DNA microarrays with the SNP discrimination efficiency in solution phase. *Langmuir* 21, 4257-4261.

Hong, B.J., Sunkara, V. & Park, J.W. (2005). DNA microarrays on nanoscale-controlled surface. *Nucl. Acids Res.* 33, e106.

Iannone, M.A., Taylor, J.D., Chen, J., Li, M.S., Rivers, P., Slentz-Kesler, K.A. & Weiner, M.P. (2000). Multiplexed single nucleotide polymorphism genotyping by oligonucleotide ligation and flow cytometry. *Cytometry* 39, 131-140 .

Kolchinsky, A. & Mirzabekov, A. (2002). Analysis of SNPs and other genomic variations using gel-based chips. *Hum Mutat* 19, 343-360 .

LaForge, K.S., Shick, V., Spangler, R., Proudnikov, D., Yuferov, V., Lysov, Y., Mirzabekov, A. & Kreek, M.J. (2000). Detection of single nucleotide polymorphisms of the human mu opioid receptor gene by hybridization or single nucleotide extension on custom oligonucleotide gelpad microchips: potential in studies of addiction. *Am J Med Genet* 96, 604-615.

Li, A.X., Seul, M., Cicciarelli, J., Yang, J.C. & Iwaki, Y. (2004). Multiplexed analysis of polymorphisms in the HLA gene complex using bead array chips. *Tissue Antigens* 63, 518-528.

Li, Y., Elashoff D., Oh, M., Sinha, U., St John, M.A., Zhou, X., Abemayor, E., & Wong, D.T. (2006). Serum circulating human mRNA profiling and its utility for oral cancer detection. *J Clin Oncol.* 24, 1754.

Lin, C.H., Yeakley, J.M., McDaniel, T.K. & Shen, R. (2009). Medium- to high-throughput SNP genotyping using VeraCode microbeads. *Methods Mol Biol.* 496, 129-42

Lindroos, K., Liljedahl, U., Raitio, M. & Syvanen, A.C. Minisequencing on oligonucleotide microarrays: comparison of immobilisation chemistries. *Nucleic Acids Res* 29, E69-69 (2001).

Liu, W.-T., Wu, J.-H., Li, E.S.-Y. & Selamat, E.S. (2005). Emission Characteristics of Fluorescent Labels with Respect to Temperature Changes and Subsequent Effects on DNA Microchip Studies. *Appl. Environ. Microbiol.* 71, 6453-6457.

Merritt, A.J., Keehner, T., O'Reilly, L.C., McInnes, R.L. & Inglis, T.J. (2010). Multiplex amplified nominal tandem-repeat analysis (MANTRA), a rapid method for genotyping Mycobacterium tuberculosis by use of multiplex PCR and a microfluidic laboratory chip. *J Clin Microbiol.* 48, 3758-61

Mulvaney, S.P., Mattoussi, H.M. & Whitman, L.J. (2004). Incorporating fluorescent dyes and quantum dots into magnetic microbeads for immunoassays. *Biotechniques* 36, 602-606, 608-609.

Ng, J.K. & Liu, W.T. (2005). LabArray: real-time imaging and analytical tool for microarrays . *Bioinformatics.* 21, 689-690.

Ng, J.K., Selamat, E.S. & Liu, W.T. (2008). A Spatially Addressable Bead-based Biosensor for Simple and Rapid DNA Detection. *Biosens Bioelectron.* 23, 803-810.

Ng, J.K., Wang, W., Liu, W.T., & Chong, S.S. (2010). Spatially addressable bead-based biosensor for rapid detection of beta-thalassemia mutations. *Anal Chim Acta.* 658: 193-196.

Proudnikov, D., Timofeev, E. & Mirzabekov, A., (1998). Immobilization of DNA in polyacrylamide gel for the manufacture of DNA and DNA-oligonucleotide microchips. *Anal Biochem*. 259, 34-41.

Rahmatpanah, F.B., Carstens, S., Hooshmand, S.I., *et al.* (2009). Large-scale analysis of DNA methylation in chronic lymphocytic leukemia. *Epigenomics*. 1, 39

Ramanamurthy, B., Ng, K.K.J., Shah, E.S., Balasubramaniam, N., and Liu, W.T. (2008). Silicon nanopillars substrate for enhancing signal intensity in DNA microarrays. *Biosensors and Bioelectronics*. 24, 723

Roessler, S., Jia, H.L., Budhu, A., Forgues, M., Ye, Q.H., Lee, J.S., Thorgeirsson, S.S., Sun, Z., Tang, Z.Y., Qin, L.X. & Wang, X.W. (2010). A Unique Metastasis Gene Signature Enables Prediction of Tumor Relapse in Early-Stage Hepatocellular Carcinoma Patients *Cancer Res* 70, 10202-10212.

Schena, M., Shalon, D., Davis, R.W. & Brown, P.O. (1995). Quantitative monitoring of gene expression patterns with a complementary DNA microarray. *Science* 270, 467-470.

Stimpson, D.I., Knepper, S.M., Shida, M., Obata, K. & Tajima, H. (2004). Three-dimensional microarray platform applied to single nucleotide polymorphism analysis. *Biotechnol Bioeng* 87, 99-103.

Taylor, J.D., Briley, D., Nguyen, Q., Long, K., Iannone, M.A., Li, M.S., Ye, F., Afshari, A., Lai, E., Wagner, M., Chen, J. & Weiner, M.P. (2001). Flow cytometric platform for high-throughput single nucleotide polymorphism analysis. *Biotechniques* 30, 661-666, 668-669.

Thaitrong N, Toriello NM, Del Bueno N, Mathies RA. (2009). Polymerase chain reaction-capillary electrophoresis genetic analysis microdevice with in-line affinity capture sample injection. *Anal Chem.* 81, 1371-7

Tojo, Y., Asahina, J., Miyashita, Y., Takahashi, M., Matsumoto, N., Hasegawa, S., Yohda, M. & Tajima, H. (2005). Development of an automation system for single nucleotide polymorphisms genotyping using bio-strand, a new three-dimensional microarray. *J Biosci Bioeng* 99, 120-124 .

Wang, D.G., Fan, J.B., Siao, C.J., Berno, A., & Young, P. *et al.* (1998). Large-scale identification, mapping, and genotyping of single-nucleotide polymorphisms in the human genome. *Science* 280, 1077-1082.

Wang, W., Kham, S.K., Yeo, G.H., Quah, T.C. & Chong, S.S. (2003). Multiplex minisequencing screen for common Southeast Asian and Indian beta-thalassemia mutations. Clin Chem. 49, 209-218.

Xu, H., Sha, M.Y., Wong, E.Y., Uphoff, J., Xu, Y., Treadway, J.A., Truong, A., O'Brien, E., Asquith, S., Stubbins, M., Spurr, N.K., Lai, E.H. & Mahoney, W. (2003). Multiplexed SNP genotyping using the Qbead system: a quantum dot-encoded microsphere-based assay. *Nucleic Acids Res* 31, e43.

11

Quartz Crystal Microbalance in Clinical Application

Ming-Hui Yang[1], Shiang-Bin Jong[2,3], Tze-Wen Chung[1],
Ying-Fong Huang[2,3] and Yu-Chang Tyan[2,4,5]
[1]*Department of Chemical and Material Engineering, National Yulin University of Science and Technology*
[2]*Department of Medical Imaging and Radiological Sciences, Kaohsiung Medical University*
[3]*Department of Nuclear Medicine, Kaohsiung Medical University Chung-Ho Memorial Hospital*
[4]*National Sun Yat-Sen University - Kaohsiung Medical University Joint Research Center*
[5]*Center for Resources, Research and Development, Kaohsiung Medical University*
Taiwan

1. Introduction

Human serum albumin (HSA), with a molecular weight of approximately 67 kDa, is a negative acute-phase protein and is the most abundant and characteristic globular unglycosylated serum protein. It is predominantly synthesized in the liver and mainly plays a role in mediating blood volume and regulated by the colloid osmotic pressure (COP) of interstitial fluid bathing the hepatocyte (West, 1990; Peters, 1996). HSA plays an important physiological role as a transporter for various substances. It has a good binding capacity for water, metals (Ca^{2+}, Na^{+}, K^{+}), fatty acids, hormones, bilirubin, ligands, therapeutic drugs and metabolites (Prinsen & de Sain-van der Velden, 2004). In plasma, albumin was comprised about 50% of total plasma protein. This implies that 10-15 g of albumin is produced per day in healthy subjects, which is about 0.4 mg albumin per gram liver per hour. The high steady-state concentration in plasma is 30 to 50 mg/mL (Ballmer et al., 1990). The albumin is minimal urinary loss in healthy subjects. Around 70 kg of albumin that passes through the kidneys each day, only a few grams pass through the glomerular membrane. Nearly all of this is reabsorbed, and urinary loss is usually no more than 10–20 mg per day. Therefore, HSA level in plasma is confirmed to be as a reliable indicator for the prognosis and severity of several diseases, such as liver disease, renal function, infectious disease, and cancer. Hypoalbuminemia, lack of albumin, results from liver disease, over excretion from kidney, excess loss in gastrointestinal system, burns, acute disease, drug effect or malnutrition. Hyperalbuminemia is a sign of serve dehydration or maybe result from the retinol deficiency that all-trans retinoic acid moderate HSA (Rothschild et al., 1988; Moshage et al., 1987; Mariani et al., 1976; Chlebowski et al., 1989; Phillips et al., 1989; Gross et al., 2005).

Self-assembled monolayers (SAMs) have received a great deal of attention for their fascinating potential technical applications such as nonlinear optics and device patterning (Horne & Blanchard, 1998; Morhard et al., 1997; Bierbaum et al., 1995). They also have been used as an ideal model to investigate the effects of intermolecular interactions in the molecular assembly systems (Schertel et al., 1995; Yan et al., 2000; Himmel et al., 1997; Jung et al., 1998). SAMs have been traditionally prepared by immersing a substrate into a solution containing a ligand that is reactive to the substrate surface or by exposing the substrate to the vapor of the reactive species. The most common utilization of the SAMs system is the application of alkanethiolates (AT) on gold (Au), rather than other metals such as platinum, copper, or silver, because gold does not have stable oxide compounds and easily forms a bond with sulfur. The AT SAMs not only provides an excellent model system to study fundamental aspects of surface properties such as wetting (Laibinis et al., 1992) and tribology (Joyce et al., 1992), but also is a promising candidate for potential applications in the fields of biosensors (Gooding &Hibbert, 1999), biomimetics (Erdelen et al., 1994) and corrosion inhibition (Laibinis & Whitesides, 1992).

The quartz crystal microbalance (QCM) with an A-T cut quartz slide equipped with electrodes has been used in various fields, such as environmental protection, chemical technology, medicine, food analysis, and biotechnology (King, 1964; Guilbault, 1983; Guilbault et al., 1988; Guilbault & Luong, 1988; Guilbault et al., 1992; Fawcett et al., 1988). It has been widely used for substance measurement in liquid environments. Previously, research has revealed that measurements in liquid environments are very complicated. Several variations in liquid environments, such as characteristics of crystals and factors of surface interactions, should be controlled and calibrated with accurate and precise machines and mathematical formulas (Attli & Suleman, 1996; Nie et al., 1992; Muramatsu et al., 1988; Voinova et al., 2002). Besides, the amount of sample used in aqueous environments often requires more than can be acquired for analysis from the human body and may be a limitation for use as a clinical immunosensor. The detection theory for QCM can be explained by the Sauerbrey equation, which calculates that the mass change is proportional to the oscillation frequency shift of the piezoelectric quartz crystal (O'Sullivan & Guilbault, 1999). Equation 1 shows the Sauerbrey equation in gas phase. ΔF: the frequency shift (Hz); F: basic oscillation frequency of piezoelectric quartz (Hz); A: the active area of QCM (cm^2); ΔM: the mass change on QCM (g).

$$\Delta F = -2.3 \times 10^{-6} \frac{F^2 \Delta M}{A} \tag{1}$$

This experiment completes a study for a potential biomedical application of functionalized SAMs with the immobilized anti-HSA monoclonal antibody, and a QCM system using the SAMs chip for HSA quantification. The attachment of anti-HSA monoclonal antibody to a SAMs surface was achieved using water soluble N-ethyl-N'-(3-dimethylaminopropyl) carbodiimide hydrochloride (EDC) and *N*-hydroxysuccinimide (NHS) as coupling agents. Surface analyses were utilized by Atomic force microscopy (AFM), X-ray photoelectron spectroscopy (XPS) and Fourier-transformed infrared reflection-reflectance absorbance spectroscopes (FTIR-RAS). The quantization of immobilized antibody was characterized by the frequency shift of QCM and the radioactivity change of ^{125}I labeled antibody. In summary, the limit of detection (LOD) and linear range of the calibration curve of the QCM method were 10 ng/ml and 10 to 1000 ng/ml. The correlation coefficients of HSA concentration between QCM and ELISA were 0.9913 and 0.9864 for the standards and serum samples, respectively. This report illustrates an investigation of SAMs for the preparation of covalently immobilized antibody biosensors.

2. Surface formation, modification and characterization

QCM chips (16MHz, diameter of quartz: 0.8 cm, diameter of Au: 0.5 cm, Yu-kuei, Taiwan) were cleaned by the soxhlet extraction process using a solution (methanol and acetone 1:1) for 24 hrs. Then, the QCM chips were cleaned with ultra pure ethanol (RDH 32205, Riedel-deHaën), and dried with nitrogen. The QCM chips were immersed into a 0.5 mM 11-mercaptoundecanoic acid (11-MUA, $C_{11}H_{22}O_2S$, 450561, Aldrich) ethanol solution for 8 hours and rinsed with pure ethanol twice. The alkanethiols adsorbed spontaneously from solution onto the Au surface. The functionalized thiol groups were chemisorbed onto the Au surface via the formation of thiolate bonds. After being dried by nitrogen, the surface analysis was performed by X-ray photoelectric spectroscopy (XPS) and Fourier-transformed infrared spectroscopy (FTIR).

2.1 Atomic force microscopy image of QCM ship surface

The QCM chip surface was analyzed by the Atomic force microscopy (AFM). The AFM image was acquired with a Slover PRO (NT-MDT, Russia) atomic force microscopy in ambient pressure. The semi-contact mode was used with a frequency of 0.5 μm/s to scan an area of 10×10 μm^2. The AFM probe was a golden silicon probe (NSG11, NT-MDT, Russia) with the length, width, thickness, resonant frequency and force constant as 100 mm, 35 μm, 2.0 μm, 255 kHz and 11.5 N/m^2, respectively.

A rough chip exterior may cause an uneven SAMs surface. To investigate the topology characteristics of the surface, AFM was used to observe the QCM chip surface. In Figure 1, the image of the topographical map taken in the semi-contact mode of a 10×10 μm^2 zone is shown. Figure 1(a) is a surface image of the QCM chip, and Figure 1(b) shows the three-dimensional structure. This impressive image in Figure 1(b) shows a very clear set of surface roughness with a mean depth of about 1.2 μm. A rough surface may provide the opportunity to increase the reaction surface and the effectiveness antibody immobilization. Most SAMs studies were established on the ideal, well-ordered and smooth single-crystal silicon (100 or 111) wafers primed with a metal adhesion layer (Weng et al., 2004, 2006). On the single-crystal silicon wafers, theoretically, all alkanethiols should be bound onto the SAMs surface as an Au-S-C- structure. Unlike the surface of ideal single-crystal silicon wafers, the rough QCM chip surface may be composed of three types of SAMs structures: alkanethiol bound, attachment by adhesion, and sulfonite-Au bonding. The XPS (S 2p, dialkylsulfide and sulfonite species) indicated that the SAMs deposited onto the QCM surface was non-regular.

2.2 Contact angle measurement

The contact angles (θ) were measured in air using a goniometer (Krüss apparatus). A Milli-Q grade water (Millipore Co., Inc.) was used to contact with the sampling dimension by the sessile drop method. For this measurement, 1 μl droplet was placed slightly on the specimen with the needle of a syringe. The value of θ was determined as the volume of the droplet was slowly increased

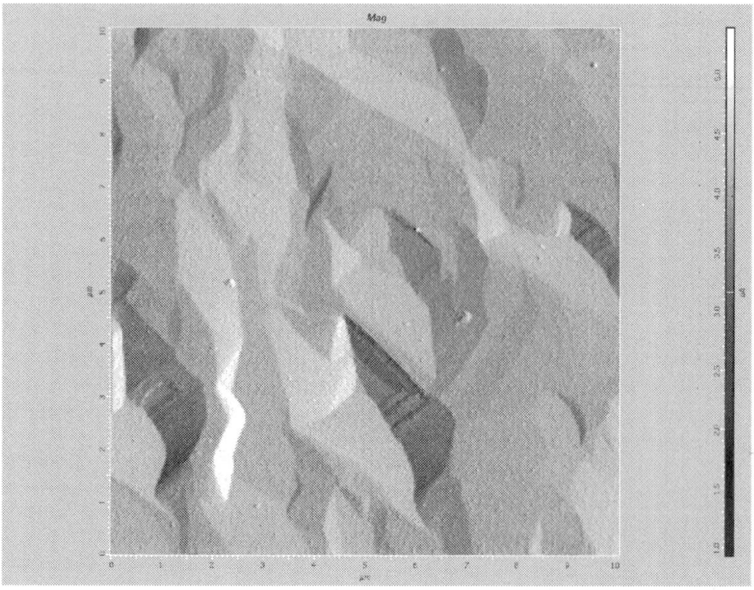

(a)

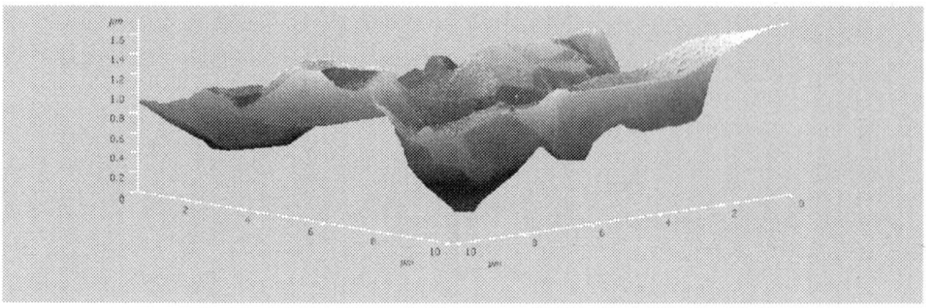

(b)

Fig. 1. AFM images of the Au-covered QCM chip. (a) blank, 10×10 μm, (b) blank, 3D structure. AFM measurements could also be used for measuring the surface roughness of the QCM chip. The mean surface roughness was 1.2 nm.

QCM chip surface	Contact angles (deg)
Au chip	64.1± 2.3
11MUA/Au chip	12.3± 1.6

Table 1. Water Contact Angles Measurement of the SAMs on QCM chip

Contact angles for 11MUA/Au chip using water as probe liquid give advancing contact angles of less than 15°, consistent as a high free energy surface. The SAMs surface with the hydroxyl tail group was hydrophilic. The contact angles agreed well with previous studies (Smith et al., 1992; Lestelius et al., 1997; Laibinis et al. 1991). The above measurements were found unaffected by extending immersion time in the thiol-containing solutions.

2.3 Fourier-transformed infrared reflection-absorption spectroscopy

The infrared (IR) spectroscopy optical benches were acquired with a conventional Fourier-transformed (FT) spectrometer (FTS-175C, Bio-Rad) equipped with a KBr beam splitter and a high-temperature ceramic source. Win-IR, Win-IR Pro (Bio-Rad) and Origin 6.0 (Microcal Software, Inc.) were used for the data acquisition and analysis. The IR spectra were obtained using p-polarized beam incident at a grazing angle of around 80° with respect to the surface normal. The spectra were measured by a liquid-nitrogen cooled, narrow band MCT detector. The spectra were recorded with a resolution of 4 cm^{-1} using about 500 scans and an optical modulation of 15 kHz filter.

The monolayer assembly was routinely characterized with FTIR-RAS upon preparation. Figure 2 shows the FTIR-RAS spectra at 3000~2800 cm^{-1} and 2000~1400 cm^{-1} of the SAMs of carboxylic acid. The peak positions of CH_3 stretching modes were consistent with the presence of a dense crystalline-like phase: r^+, $\upsilon_s(CH_3)$ at 2876 cm^{-1}; FR, $\upsilon_s(CH_3)$ at 2935 cm^{-1}; r^-, $\upsilon_{as}(CH_3)$ at 2963 cm^{-1}. In the spectrum of the SAMs, two absorption peaks at 2920 and 2850 cm^{-1} were assigned to asymmetric (d^-, $\upsilon_{as}(CH_2)$) and symmetric (d^+, $\upsilon_s(CH_2)$) C-H stretching peaks of the methylene groups [1], respectively (Laibinis et al. 1991). The peak positions of 11-MUA/Au indicated that the frequencies at 1705 cm^{-1} was assigned to residual carboxylic acid stretch, υ(C=O) and symmetric carboxylate stretch, $\upsilon_s(COO^-)$ (Frey & Corn, 1996).

2.4 X-ray photoelectron spectroscopy measurement

XPS spectra were acquired with a Physical Electronics PHI 1600 ESCA photoelectron spectrometer with a magnesium anode at 400 W and 15 kV-27 mA (Mg Kα 1253.6 eV, type 10-360 hemispherical analyzer). The specimens were analyzed at an electron take-off angle of 70°, measured with respect to the surface plane. The operating conditions were as follows: pass energy 23.4 eV, base pressure in the chamber below 2×10^{-8} Pa, step size 0.05, total scan number 20, scan range 10 eV (for multiplex scan). The peaks were quantified from high-resolution spectra using a monochromatic Mg X-ray source. Elemental compositions at the surface using C 1s, O 1s and S 2p core level spectra were measured and calculated from XPS peak areas with correction algorithms for atomic sensitivity. The XPS spectra were fitted using Voigt peak profiles and a Shirley background.

The binding structure of the SAMs on the metal surface was monitored by XPS. In the XPS measurements, the variations of O 1s and S 2p with respect to C 1s signal ratios were correlated with the significant presence of chemical species at the SAMs surfaces. The C 1s, O 1s, and S 2p spectra showed the existence of 11-MUA onto the gold-coated QCM chips. The XPS spectra of 11-MUA onto the gold electrode are shown in Figure 3.

In the XPS C 1s spectrum, the peaks of binding energies of core levels at 285.0 eV, 286.9 eV, and 288.8 eV were assigned to the -C-C-, -C-S-, and O=C-O structures, respectively. The C 1s

[1] $\upsilon_{s/as}$: symmetric/asymmetric-stretching modes; FR: Fermi resonance.

core-level spectrum of the peak at 286.9 eV and the S 2p spectrum of the peak in 162.0 eV confirmed the Au-S-$(CH_2)_n$- existence. The C 1s core-level spectrum of the peak at 288.8 eV and the O 1s spectrum of the peaks at 532.0 eV and 533.2 eV provided evidence that the terminal groups of SAMs on the QCM chips were the carboxylic acid groups.
In the O 1s spectrum, the peaks of binding energies of O 1s core levels at 532.0 eV and 533.2 eV were assigned to the carboxylic acid group (O*=C-O and O=C-O* for the * marked O, respectively) structure, which was the characteristic group of 11-MUA.

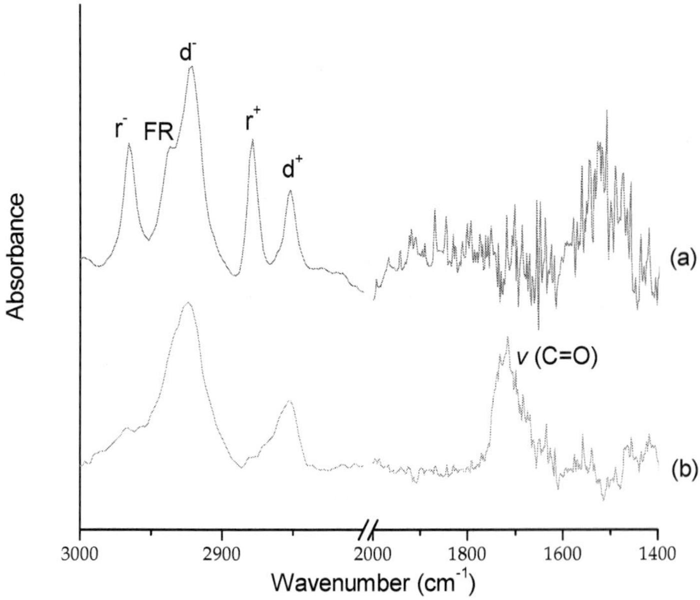

Fig. 2. FTIR-RAS spectra show the frequency regions: 3000 - 2800 and 2000 - 1400 cm^{-1} of the SAMs on the QCM chip. (a) 1-Dodecanethiol (Reference SAMs surface), (b) 11-mercaptoundecanoic acid.

In the S 2p spectrum, the peaks of binding energies of core levels at 162.0 eV, 163.2 eV, and 169.3 eV were assigned to the Au-S-C-, dialkylsulfide, and SO_3^-, respectively. The S 2p spectrum inculcated a doublet structure due to the presence of the S $2p_{3/2}$ and S $2p_{1/2}$ peaks using a 2:1 peak area ratio with a 1.2 eV splitting as shown in Figure 3. The peak at 162.0 eV was assigned to sulfur atoms bound to the gold surface as a thiolate species (Castner et al., 1996). The S 2p spectrum of peak at 163.2 eV was assigned to dialkylsulfide as unbound thiol, which may be due to alkanethiols physisorbed as a double layer or adhesion of alkanethiols (Collinson et al., 1992). The S 2p spectrum of peak at 168.5 eV can be attributed to a sulfonite species (SO_3^-). The sulfonite species formation was from the rapid oxidation of sulfur on the 11-MUA modified QCM chip surface. Since the sulfur atom was at the bottom of the 11-MUA chains, the XPS signal in detecting S-O was much weaker then that of C with O, which was on the top of the chain. Thus, it was not feasible to fit the S-O peak in the O 1s spectrum. Although the SAMs structure on the QCM chip was not ideal, it did not affect the antibody immobilization onto the tail group because the EDC and NHS only functioned on the carboxylic acid group.

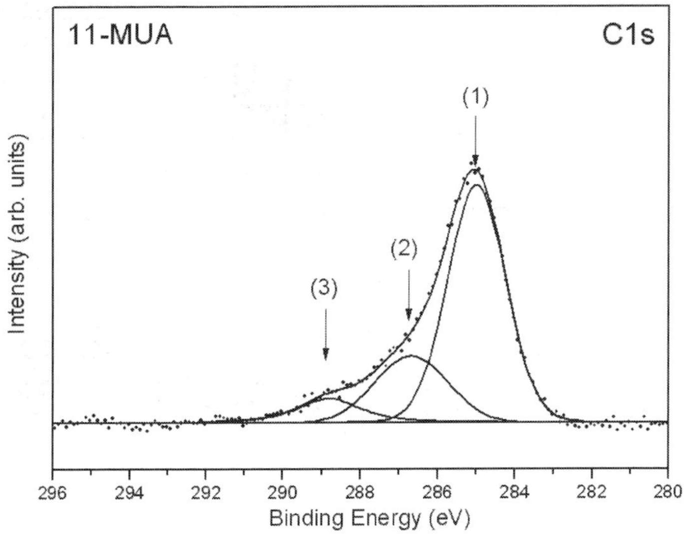

(a)

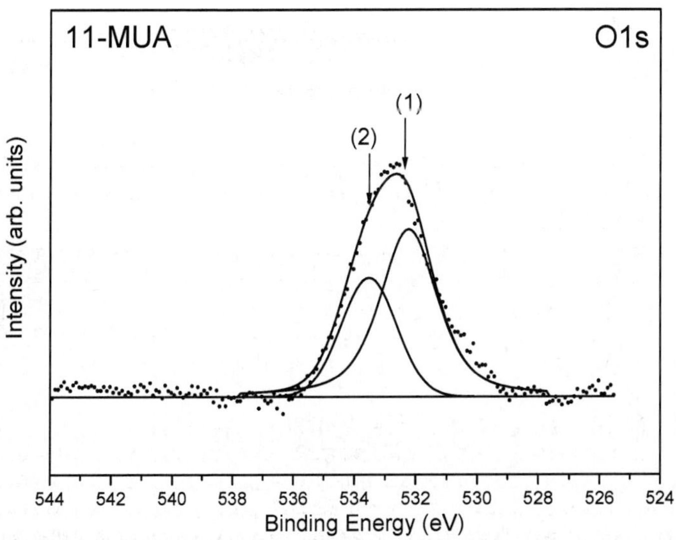

(b)

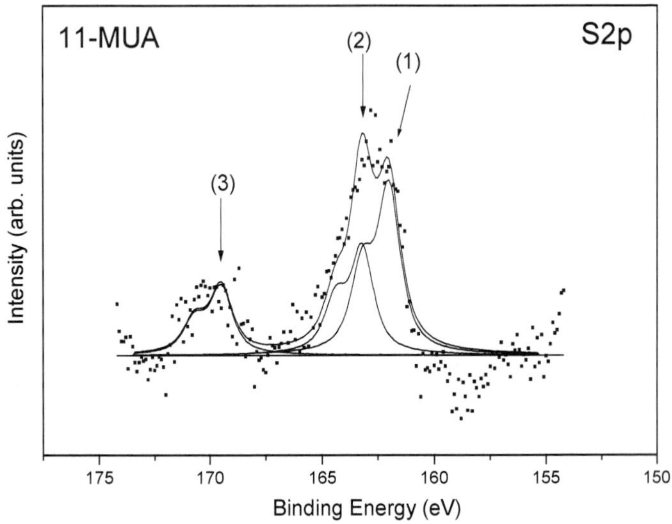

(c)

Fig. 3. XPS spectra of the 11-MUA modified SAMs surface. (a) C 1s, the binding energy at (1) 285.0 eV, (2) 286.9 eV, and (3) 288.8 eV were assigned to the -C-C-, -C-S-, and O=C-O, (b) O 1s, the binding energy at (1) 532.0 eV and (2) 533.2 eV were assigned to the carboxylic acid group, (c) S 2p, the binding energy at (1) 162.0 eV, (2) 163.2 eV, and (3) 169.3 eV were assigned to the Au-S-C-, dialkylsulfide, and SO_3^-, respectively.

2.5 Immobilization of anti-HSA

The labeling procedure was adapted from Chloramine T method. The 2.5 µg anti-HSA was added into sodium phosphate buffer (25 µl, pH= 7.5) with $Na^{125}I$ (0.1 mCi, 2.5 µg/µl). After one minute at room temperature, the reaction was stopped by 25 µl sodium metabisulphite (2.5 µg/µl). The Bio-gel p-60 column was conditioned by sodium phosphate buffer (0.01 M) and NaCl solution (0.15 M, contain 2% BSA) for isolating free iodine from ^{125}I labeled anti-HSA.

In order to immobilize ^{125}I anti-HSA monoclonal antibody, the 11-mercaptoundecanoic acid/Au surface was immersed in the solution containing coupling agents: 75 mM N-ethyl-N'-(3-dimethylaminopropyl) carbodiimide hydrochloride (EDC, E-6383, Sigma) and 15 mM *N*-hydroxysuccinimide (NHS, H-7377, Sigma) at 4 °C for 30 min (van Delden et al., 1997; Kuijpers et al., 2000). Water-soluble EDC and NHS were used to activate O=C-OH (Kang et al., 1993; Tyan et al., 2002) and then the EDC-NHS solution was replaced by a phosphate buffered saline (PBS, URPBS001, UniRegion Bio-Tech), containing 0.2 µg/mL HSA-antibody at 4 °C for 24 hrs. The SAMs chips were thereafter washed by D.I. water and freeze-dried. During the reactions, EDC converted the carboxylic acid group into a reactive intermediate, which was attacked by amines. The radioactivity of each ^{125}I anti-HSA monoclonal antibody immobilized QCM chip was measured by the Scaler cobra II series auto-gamma counting system (Packard, USA, Energy window: 15~75 keV, detection efficiency > 75%, resolution < 34%, detector background <25 cpm).

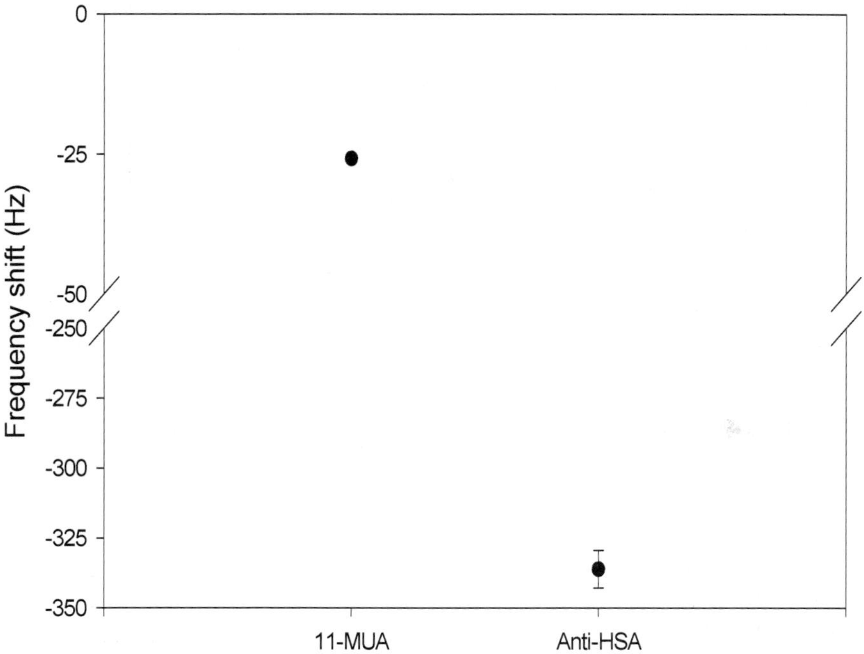

Fig. 4. The oscillation frequency shift of SAMs-QCM chips after 11-MUA and anti-HSA monoclonal antibody immobilization.

The QCM frequency variation after SAMs formation was lowered to around -25.82±4.25 Hz (Figure 4). In this experiment, water-soluble EDC and NHS were used to convert the carboxylic acid of the 11-MUA monolayer to a NHS ester. This reaction activated the 11-MUA-NHS ester monolayer with an aqueous solution of an amine or ammonia, which formed an amide bond with the surface. For the QCM and radioimmunoassay measurements, the frequency variations and count rates were correlated with the data from ^{125}I anti-HSA monoclonal antibody-immobilized SAMs-QCM surface. The QCM frequency decreased after the immobilization of ^{125}I anti-HSA monoclonal antibody (Figure 4). Its average and the coefficient of variations were -336.13±41.50 Hz. The count rate of the radioimmunoassay of ^{125}I anti-HSA monoclonal antibody was 167±18.4 cpm (counts per minute). Thus, the poly-complex between ^{125}I anti-HSA monoclonal antibody and 11-MUA was formed; amino groups in ^{125}I anti-HSA monoclonal antibodies formed complexes with carboxyl groups of 11-MUA. In the QCM measurements, the variations of QCM frequency shift were correlated with the changes of count rates of the radioimmunoassay on the ^{125}I anti-HSA monoclonal antibody immobilized QCM surface. The amount of the ^{125}I anti-HSA monoclonal antibody immobilized onto QCM chips was 59.62±0.47 ng/cm^2. In this study, the surface modification of QCM was analyzed, and the formation of SAMs structure and antibody adsorption were also confirmed.

3. Quantitation of HSA

There are lots of methods for analysis of HSA as Lowry method (Lowry et al., 1951), CBBG-250 (Flores, 1978), enzymatic method (Javed & Waqar, 2001), dye-binding and shift in color method (Gomes et al., 1998), Chemiluminescence technique (Wei et al., 2008), and radioimmunoassay (Catt & Tregear, 1967). The drawbacks of these methods are low sensitivity, narrow linear range, costly, tedious, or protection problem. This experiment of utilizing quartz crystal microbalance provides an alternative method to determine microelement with less test sample and increase the sensitivity. Immumosensors, having the specificity of antibody-antigen (Ab-Ag) affinities and the high sensitivities of various physical transducers, have gained attention for clinical diagnosis (Morgan et al., 1996). Our study combined both techniques of SAMs and QCM for the immumosensor, where a decrease of the resonance frequency is correlated with the mass accumulated on its surface. In this study, the ELISA method was also used for HSA concentration analysis. The feasibility of SAMs-QCM chips can be proofed by the correlation of HSA concentrations measured by the ELISA and QCM methods.

3.1 QCM frequency measurement

The frequency shift of QCM chips was measured by a muti-channel piezoelectric frequency counter with computer signal analysis software (PZ-1001 Immuno-Biosensor System, Universal Sensors Inc., Metairie, LA, U.S.A). For the HSA standard curve and LOD of QCM frequency measurement, the standard solutions with difference concentrations were prepared by dissolving HSA in normal saline and ranged from 5 - 1200 ng/mL. In the QCM frequency measurement of HSA, 10 μL of the HSA standard solutions or serum samples were deposited on the anti-HSA monoclonal antibody immobilized chip. The chips were agitated slowly at room temperature for 10 min, rinsed by D.I. water, and then air-dried.

The QCM instrument was operated in a humidity-controlled cabinet and the humidity was under 50% RH to prevent the moisture interference. The preparation of chips and the tests of serum samples were done under humidity controlled conditions because the high humidity will increase the frequency shift and bias the results. Each concentration was examined six times per chip in a total of six chips. The same procedures were used for the measurement of serum samples. The frequency of the blank was used as a baseline. The frequency of the QCM chip was linearly decreased with the elevation of the HSA concentration. Thus, the amount of negative oscillation frequency shift ($-\triangle F$) was elevated.

The LOD was described as the smallest detectable amount of HSA adsorbed onto the QCM sensor. It used the peak-to-peak value of the noise range (S/N ratio) in the QCM frequency shifts. In this study, the average of S/N ratios of the QCM frequency shift after antibody immobilization were around 1.39, which was over three times of the standard deviation of the background noise (13.72 Hz). Under these criteria, the LOD of this QCM system for HSA detection was around 10 ng/mL and the linear range of the calibration curve of the QCM method was 10 to 1000 ng/ml.

Figure 5 shows the analytic results of the calibration curve, which was plotted with the QCM frequency shift against the actual HSA concentrations. Compared to the actual HSA concentrations, the QCM data was linearized and generated a regression equation as follows: $y=1.3083x-3.4439$ (x-axis, HSA concentration; y-axis, frequency shift; $R^2=0.9913$). It corresponds to the Sauerbrey equation where the frequency shift solely depends on the mass change. In other words, compounds with larger masses will cause more frequency shift than those of smaller masses. In theory, the correlation between the difference of oscillation frequency ($-\triangle F$) and the HSA concentration should be noted as: $C_{(HSA)} = k\cdot(-$

$\triangle$F)+b and b=0. However, the background noise amplitude of the blank chip also existed. In this study, the b value in the equation was -3.4439. Although the QCM chip was freeze-dried, the background noise amplitude may be due to the process of antibody immobilization through wet graft and thus increase the amplitude of oscillation of the QCM. In our previously study, three types of SAMs linkage materials, 11-MUA, cystamine dihydrochloride and cystamine/glutaraldehyde, were compared through the measurements of frequency change and radioactivity decay to determent the optimal linkage material and conditions for antibody immobilization (Jong et al., 2009). The method sensitivity is the slope of the calibration curve that is obtained by plotting the response against the analyte concentration or mass (Figure 6). Thus, in this study, 11-MUA was selected to prepare the HSA biosensors.

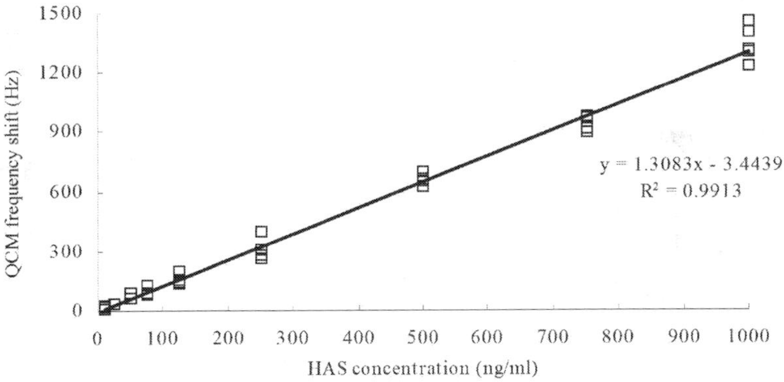

Fig. 5. The calibration curve for HSA standards using anti-HSA monoclonal antibody immobilized QCM chips. The linearity and correlation coefficient were obtained as y=1.3083x-3.4439 and R^2=0.9913.

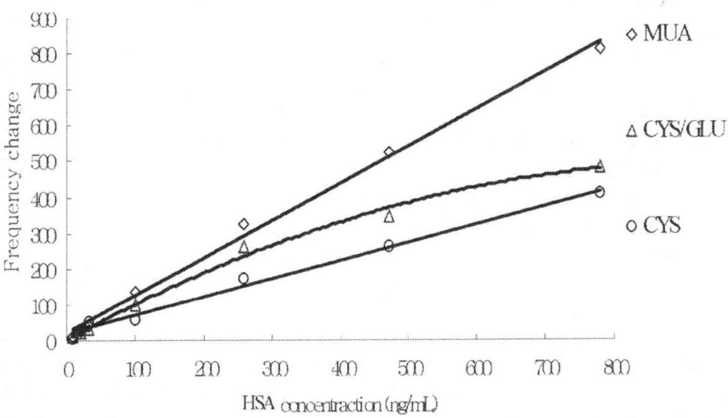

Fig. 6. The slopes of the calibration curve for three types of SAMs linkage materials. The calibration curve of CYS/GLU was a non-linear curve.

3.2 ELISA and QCM measurements of HSA

The HSA concentrations were measured by human albumin ELISA kit (EA2201-1, AssayMax Human Albumin ELISA kit, Assaypro, USA). The HSA standards and serum samples were duplicate counted by the auto-ELISA reader system (Multiskan EX Microplate Photometer, *Thermo* Scientific, USA). The absorbance of the microplate reader was set at a wavelength of 450 nm.

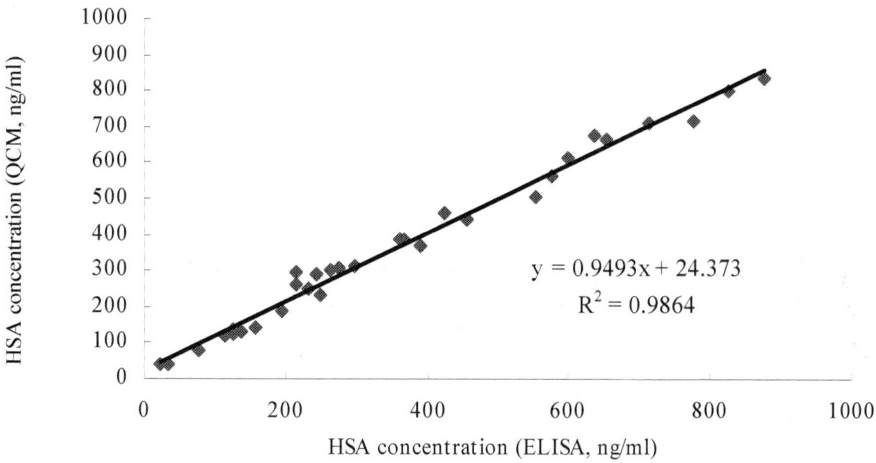

Fig. 7. Detection of HSA in serum samples using QCM chips and ELISA test. The correlation coefficient between the two methods was 0.9864.

The HSA concentrations in serum samples were calculated using the interpolation of the calibration curve and ELISA methods, respectively. Figure 7 shows the correlation of HSA concentrations measured by the QCM and ELISA methods. The linear regression equation for these data is as follows: $y=0.9493x+24.373$ (x-axis, the concentration measured by ELISA, y-axis, the concentrations obtained by QCM, $R^2=0.9864$). The variations between the results of QCM frequency shifts and ELISA measurements were acceptable. The experimental results showed an excellent correlation between ELISA and QCM methods for HSA detection. The materials for SAMs-QCM are easy to obtain, and this technique is simple and easy to apply on surface-based diagnostics or biosensors. Thus, the QCM method may provide a reference method for measuring serum HSA in a laboratory and may be more feasible for clinical applications than the standard methods.

4. Conclusions

This study provides an example of the 11-MUA self-assembled monolayer applications of the QCM chip. SAMs formation provides an easy technique to prepare the structure that can be further functionalized with biomolecules to yield bio-recognition surfaces for medical devices. The carboxyl functional thiol monolayer offers an excellent approach to immobilize antibodies for selected sensing of different analytes. The application of SAMs for the immobilization of antibodies onto Au surfaces has a considerable potential in application of reproducible and reliable biosensors. In this study, the quantization of immobilized antibodies was measured by the shift of QCM frequency and the radioactivity change of ^{125}I labeled antibodies. The LOD of QCM was 10 ng/ml, and the linear range of the calibration curve of QCM method was 10 to 1000 ng/ml. The correlation coefficients between QCM and ELISA were 0.9913 and 0.9864 for HSA in the standards and serum samples, respectively. Compared with ELISA methods, the QCM method was simple and rapid without multiple labeling and purification steps. Our system is different from the conventional approaches in that it operates in the gas phase, not the liquid phase. As a result, there is no waiting time for the frequency to reach stability. In summary, we have presented the modification of the Au interface via 11-MUA SAMs and have proved that the SAMs on Au can be a valid bio-detection chip for HSA concentration analysis by QCM. This assay design of the sensor may develop a potential reference procedure for HSA measurement and has wide applicability in the clinical setting.

5. Acknowledgements

We are thankful to S. Sheldon (ASCP) of the Edmond Medical Center Laboratory (USA) for fruitful discussions. This work was supported by research grants, Q097004 from the Kaohsiung Medical University Research Foundation, NSC96-2321-B-037-006 and NSC97-2320-B-037-012-MY3 from the National Science Council, Taiwan, R.O.C.

6. References

Attli, B.S., Suleman, A.A. (1996). A Piezoelectric Immunosensor for the Detection of Cocaine. *Microchemical Journal*, Vol. 54, No. 2, (August 1996), pp. 174-179, ISSN *0026-265X*.

Ballmer, P.E., McNurlan, M.A., Milne, E., Heys, S.D., Buchan, V., Calder, A.G., Garlick, P.J. (1990). Measurement of albumin synthesis in humans: a new approach employing stable isotopes. *Am J Physiol*, Vol. 259, No. 6, (December 1990), pp. E797-803, ISSN 0193-1849.

Bierbaum, K., Grunze, M., Baski, A.A., Chi, L.F., Schrepp, W., Fuchs, H. (1995). Growth of self-assembled n-alkyltrichlorosilane films on Si(100) investigated by atomic force microscopy. *Langmuir*, Vol. 11, No. 6, (June 1995), pp. 2143-2150, ISSN 0743-7463.

Castner, D.G., Hinds, K., Grainger, D.W. (1996). X-ray Photoelectron Spectroscopy Sulfur 2p Study of Organic Thiol and Disulfide Interactions with Gold Surfaces. *Langmuir*,Vol. 12, No. 2, (October 1996), pp. 5083-5086, ISSN 0743-7463.

Catt, K., Tregear, G.W. (1976). Solid-phase radioimmunoassay in antibody-coated tubes. *Science*, Vol. 158, No. 2, (December 1967), pp. 1570-1572, ISSN 0036-8075.

Chlebowski, R.T., Grosvenor, M.B., Bernhard, N.H., Morales, L.S., Bulcavage, L.M. (1989). Nutritional status, gastrointestinal dysfunction, and survival in patients with AIDS. *Am J Gastroenterol*, Vol. 84, No. 10, (October 1989), pp. 1288-1293, ISSN 0002-9270.

Collinson, M., Bowden, E.F., Tarlov, M.J. (1992). Voltammetry of covalently immobilized cytochrome C on self-assembled monolayer electrodes. *Langmuir*, Vol. 8, No. 2, (May 1992), pp. 1247-1250, ISSN 0743-7463.

Erdelen, C., Haeussling, L., Naumann, R., Ringsdorf, H., Wolf, H., Yang, J., Liley, M., Spinke, J., Knoll, W. (1994). Self-assembled disulfide-functionalized amphiphilic copolymers on gold. *Langmuir*, Vol. 10, No. 4, (April 1994), pp. 1246-1250, ISSN 0743-7463.

Fawcett, N.C., Evans, J.A., Chien, L.C., Flowers, N. (1988). Nucleic acid hybridization setected by Piezoelectric resonance. *Anal Lett*, Vol. 21, No. 7, (July 1988), pp. 1099-1114, ISSN 0003-2719.

Flores, R. (1978). A rapid and reproducible assay for quantitative estimation of proteins using Bromophenol Blue. *Anal Biochem*, Vol. 88, No. 2, (August 1978), pp. 605-611, ISSN 0003-2697.

Frey, B.L., Corn, R.M. (1996). Covalent attachment and derivatization of poly(L-lysine) monolayers on gold surfaces as characterized by polarization-modulation FT-IR spectroscopy. *Anal Chem*, Vol. 68, No. 2, (September 1996), pp. 3187-3193, ISSN *0003-2700.*

Gomes, M.B., Dimetz, T., Luchetti, M.R., Goncalves, M.F., Gazzola, H., Matos, H. (1998). Albumin concentration is underestimated in frozen urine. *Ann Clin Biochem*, Vol. 35, No. 2, (May 1998), pp. 434-435, ISSN 0004-5632.

Gooding, J.J., Hibbert, D.B. (1999). The application of alkanethiol self assembled monolayers to enzyme electrodes. *Trends Anal Chem*, Vol. 18, No. 8, (August 1999), pp. 525-532, ISSN 0165-9936.

Gross, J.L., de Azevedo, M.J., Silveiro, S.P., Canani, L.H., Caramori, M.L., Zelmanovitz, T. (2005). Diabetic nephropathy: diagnosis, prevention, and treatment. *Diabetes Care* , Vol. 28, No. 1, (January 2005), pp. 164-176, ISSN 0149-5992.

Guilbault, G.G. (1983). Determination of formaldehyde with an enzyme-coated piezoelectric crystal detector. *Anal Chem*, Vol. 55, No. 11, (September 1983), pp. 1682-1684, ISSN *0003-2700.*

Guilbault, G.G., Hock, B., Schmid, R.A. (1992). A piezoelectric immunobiosensor for atrazine in drinking water. *Biosensors Bioelectron*, Vol. 7, No. 6, (July 1992), pp. 411-419, ISSN 0956-5663.

Guilbault, G.G., Jordan, J.M., Scheide, E. (1988). Analytical uses of piezoelectric crystals. *Critical Reviews in Analytical Chemistry*, Vol. 19, No. 1, (March 1988), pp. 1-28, ISSN 1040-8347.

Guilbault, G.G., Luong, J.H. (1988). Gas phase biosensors. *J Biotechnol*, Vol. 9, No. 1, (December 1988), pp. 1-9, ISSN 0168-1656.

Himmel, H.J., Weiss, K., Jäger, B., Dannenberger, O., Grunze, M., Woell, C. (1997). Ultrahigh vacuum study on the reactivity of organic surfaces terminated by -OH and -COOH groups prepared by self-assembly of functionalized alkanethiols on Au substrates. *Langmuir*, Vol. 13, No. 19, (September 1997), pp. 4943-4947, ISSN 0743-7463.

Horne, J.C. & Blanchard, G.J. (1998). The role of substrate identity in determining monolayer motional relaxation dynamics. *J Am Chem Soc*, Vol. 120, No. 25, (June 1998), pp. 6336-6344, ISSN 0002-7863.

Javed, M. U., Waqar, S.N. (2001). An enzymatic method for the detection of human serum albumin, *Exp Mol Med*, Vol. 33, No. 2, (June 2001), pp. 103-105, ISSN 1226-3613.

Jong, S.B., Huang, S.L., Lin, C.S., Yang, M.H., Chen, Y.L., Huang, Y.F., Shiea, J.T., Wang, M.C., Tyan, Y.C. (2009). Evaluation the effectiveness of ^{125}I anti-AFP monoclonal antibody on QCM utilizing radioactive measurement. *Chemistry*, Vol. 67, No. 3, (September 2009), pp. 299-307, ISSN 0441-3768.

Joyce, S.A., Thomas, R.C., Houston, J.E., Michalske, T.A., Crooks, R.M. (1992). Mechanical relaxation of organic monolayer films measured by force microscopy. *Phys Rev Let*, Vol. 68, No. 18, (May 1992), pp. 2790-2793, ISSN 0031-9007.

Jung, C., Dannenberger, O., Xu, Y., Buck, M., Grunze, M. (1998). Self-assembled monolayers from organosulfur compounds: A comparison between sulfides, disulfides, and thiols. *Langmuir*, Vol. 14, No. 5, (February 1998), pp. 1103-1107, ISSN 0743-7463.

Kang, I.K., Kwon, B.K., Lee, J.H., Lee, H.B. (1993). Immobilization of proteins on poly(methyl methacrylate) films. *Biomaterials*, Vol. 14, No. 2, (August 1993), pp. 787-792, ISSN 0142-9612.

King, W.H. (1964). Piezoelectric sorption detector. *Anal Chem*, Vol. 36, No. 9, (August 1964), pp. 1735-1739, ISSN *0003-2700*.

Kuijpers, A.J., van Wachem, P.B., van Luyn, M.J., Brouwer, L.A., Engbers, G.H., Krijgsveld, J., Zaat, S.A., Dankert, J., Feijen, J. (2000). In vitro and in vivo evaluation of gelatin-chondroitin sulphate hydrogels for controlled release of antibacterial proteins. *Biomaterials*, Vol. 21, No. 2, (September 2000), pp. 1763-1772, ISSN 0142-9612.

Laibinis, P.E., Nuzzo, R.G., Whitesides, G.M. (1992). The structure of monolayers formed by coadsorption of two n-alkanethiols of different chain lengths on gold and its relation to wetting. *J Phys Chem*, Vol. 96, No. 12, (June 1992), pp. 5097-5105, ISSN 0022-3654.

Laibinis, P.E., Whitesides, G.M. (1992). Self-assembled monolayers of n-alkanethiolates on copper are barrier films that protect the metal against oxidation by air. *J Am Chem Soc*. Vol. 114, No. 23, (November 1992), pp. 9022-9028, ISSN *0002-7863*.

Laibinis, P.E., Whitesides, G.M., Allara, D.L., Tao, Y.T., Parikh, A.N., Nuzzo, R.G. (1991). Comparison of the structures and wetting properties of self-assembled monolayers of n-alkanethiols on the coinage metal surfaces, copper, silver, and gold. *J Am Chem Soc*, Vol. 113, No. 2, (September 1991), pp. 7152-7167, ISSN 0002-7863.

Lestelius, M., Liedberg, B., Tengvall, P. (1997). *In vitro* plasma protein adsorption on ω - functionalized alkanethiolate self-assembled monolayers. *Langmuir*, Vol. 13, No. 2, (October 1997), pp. 5900-5908, ISSN 0743-7463.

Lowry, O.H., Rosebrough, N.J., Farr, A.L., Randall, R.J. (1951). Protein measurement with the Folin phenol reagent. *J Biol Chem*, Vol. 193, No. 2, (November 1951), pp. 265-275, ISSN 0021-9258.

Mariani, G., Strober, W., Keiser, H., Waldmann, T.A. (1976). Pathophysiology of hypoalbuminemia associated with carcinoid tumor. *Cancer*, Vol. 38, No. 2, (August 1976), pp. 854-860, ISSN 1097-0142.

Morgan, C.L., Newman, D.J., Price, C.P. (1996). Immunosensors: technology and opportunities in laboratory medicine. *Clin Chem*, Vol. 42, No. 2, (February 1996), pp. 193-209, ISSN 0009-9147.

Morhard, F., Schumacher, J., Lenenbach, A., Wilhelm, T., Dahint, R., Grunze, M., Everhart, D.S. (1997). Optical diffraction - a new concept for rapid on-line detection of chemical and biochemical analytes. *Proc Electrochem Soc*, Vol. 97, No. 19, (August 1997), pp. 1058-1065, ISSN 0161-6374.

Moshage, H.J., Janssen, J.A., Franssen, J.H., Hafkenscheid, J.C., Yap, S.H. (1987). Study of the molecular mechanism of decreased liver synthesis of albumin in inflammation. *J Clin Invest*, Vol. 79, No. 6, (June 1987), pp. 1635-1641, ISSN 0021-9738.

Muramatsu, H., Tamiya, E., Karube, I. (1988). Computation of equivalent circuit parameters of quartz crystals in contact with liquids and study of liquid properties. *Anal Chem*, Vol. 60, No. 2, (October 1988), pp. 2142-2146, ISSN *0003-2700*.

Nie, L.H., Zhang, X.T., Yao, S.Z. (1992). Determination of quinine in some pharmaceutical preparations using a ring-coated piezoelectric sensor. *J Pharm Biomed Anal*, Vol. 10, No. 2, (July 1992), pp. 529-533, ISSN 0731-7085.

O'Sullivan, C.K., Guilbault, G.G. (1999). Commercial quartz crystal microbalances - theory and applications. *Biosens Bioelectron,* Vol. 14, No. 2, (December 1999), pp. 663-670, ISSN 0956-5663.

Peters, T.J. (1996). *All About Albumin: Biochemistry, Genetics, and Medical Applications.* Academic Press, ISBN 978-0125521109, San Diego, CA, USA.

Phillips, A., Shaper, A.G., Whincup, P.H. (1989). Association between serum albumin and mortality from cardiovascular disease, cancer, and other causes. *Lancet,* Vol. 16, No. 2, (December 1989), pp. 1434-1436, ISSN 0140-6736.

Prinsen, B.H. & de Sain-van der Velden, M.G. (2004). Albumin turnover: experimental approach and its application in health and renal diseases. *Clinica Chimica Acta,* Vol. 347, No. 1-2, (September 2004), pp. 1-14, ISSN 0009-8981.

Rothschild, M.A., Oratz, M., Schreiber, S.S. (1998). Serum albumin. Hepatology, Vol. 8, No. 2, (March 1988), pp. 385-401, ISSN 1665-2681.

Schertel, A., Wöll, C., Grunze, M. (1997). Identification of mono- and bidentate carboxylate surface species on Cu(111) using x-ray absorption spectroscopy. *J Phys IV,* Vol. 7, No. C2, (April 1976), pp. 537-538, ISSN 1155-4339.

Smith, E.L., Alves, C.A., Anderegg, J.W., Porter, M.D., Siperko, L.M. (1992). Deposition of metal overlayers at end-group-functionalized thiolate monolayers adsorbed at gold. 1. Surface and interfacial chemical characterization of deposited copper overlayers at carboxylic acid-terminated structures. *Langmuir,* Vol. 8, No. 2, (November 1992), pp. 2707-2714, ISSN 0743-7463.

Tyan, Y.C., Liao, J.D., Klauser, R., Wu, I.D., Weng, C.C. (2002). Assessment and characterization of degradation effect for the varied degrees of ultra-violet radiation onto the collagen-bonded polypropylene non-woven fabric surfaces. *Biomaterials,* Vol. 23, No. 2, (January 2002), pp. 65-76, ISSN 0142-9612.

van Delden, C.J., Lens, J.P., Kooyman, R.P., Engbers, G.E., Feijen, J. (1997). Heparinization of gas plasma-modified polystyrene surfaces and the interactions of these surfaces with proteins studied with surface plasmon resonance. *Biomaterials,* Vol. 18, No. 2, (June 1997), pp. 845-852, ISSN 0142-9612.

Voinova, M.V., Jonson, M., Kasemo, B. (2002). Missing mass effect in biosensor's QCM applications. *Biosens Bioelectron,* Vol. 17, No. 2, (October 2002), pp. 835-841, ISSN 0956-5663.

Wei, X., Wei, Y., Xing, D., Chen, Q. (2008). A novel chemiluminescence technique for quantitative measurement of low concentration human serum albumin. *Analytical Science,* Vol. 24, No. 2, (January 2008), pp. 115-119, ISSN 1394-2506.

Weng, C.C., Liao, J.D., Wu, Y.T., Wang, M.C., Klauser, R., Grunze, M., Zharnikov, M. (2004). Modification of aliphatic self-assembled monolayers by free-radical-dominant plasma: The role of the plasma composition. *Langmuir,* Vol. 20, No. 2, (October 2004), pp. 10093-10099, ISSN 0743-7463.

Weng, C.C., Liao, J.D., Wu, Y.T., Wang, M.C., Klauser, R., Zharnikov, M. (2006). Modification of monomolecular self-assembled films by nitrogen-oxygen plasma. *J Phys Chem B,* Vol. 110, No. 2, (June 2006), pp. 12523-12529, ISSN 1089-5647.

West, J.B. (1990). *Physiological Basis of Medical Practice.* Williams & Wilkins, ISBN 978-0683089479, Baltimore, MD, USA.

Yan, C., Zharnikov, M., Gölzhäuser, A., Grunze, M. (2000). Preparation and characterization of self-assembled monolayers on indium tin oxide. *Langmuir,* Vol. 16, No. 15, (June 2000), pp. 6208-6215, ISSN 0743-7463.

12

Using the Brain as a Biosensor to Detect Hypoglycaemia

Rasmus Elsborg, Line Sofie Remvig,
Henning Beck-Nielsen and Claus Bogh Juhl
Hypo-Safe A/S, Odense University Hospital, Sydvestjysk Sygehus Esbjerg
Denmark

1. Introduction

1.1 Definition of hypoglycaemia and its clinical importance

Hypoglycaemia can be defined as an abnormally low blood glucose concentration. This rather open definition implies that a strict biochemical definition may be easy and convenient but insufficient. In biochemical terms, blood glucose lower than 3.5 mmol/l will often be considered low in diabetes patients treated with insulin or oral hypoglycaemia agents. Both in diabetes patients and in healthy persons, however, spontaneous blood glucose values lower than this threshold may frequently be measured. Blood glucose values down to 2.7 mmol/l or even lower with limited or no symptoms can be measured following long term fasting in healthy humans (Hojlund et al., 2001). Diabetes patients with tight glucose control and recurrent episodes of hypoglycaemia may lack symptoms of hypoglycaemia even at very low glucose levels down to 1 mmol/l. Consequently, many different definitions of biochemical hypoglycaemia can be found in the literature regarding hypoglycaemia in diabetes.

In clinical terms, hypoglycaemia can be differentiated into mild, moderate or severe events. Mild hypoglycaemia is present when a diabetes patient experiences symptoms of hypoglycaemia such as sweating, shivering or palpitations. The patient is able to react appropriately by eating or drinking and thereby re-establish a normal blood glucose level, avoiding progression into severe hypoglycaemia. Moderate hypoglycaemia is present when the patient may or may not experience hypoglycaemia symptoms but may require help to take action. This could entail simply guiding the patient to eat or drink or a more active approach of giving the patient the food or drink. Severe hypoglycaemia is present when the patient loses consciousness and an active medical approach is needed such as glucose infusion or glucagon injection. The correlation between biochemical and clinical hypoglycaemia is very poor in type 1 diabetes patients (Pramming et al., 1990).

Events of mild hypoglycaemia are not dangerous per se. Diabetes patients often expect this to be a consequence of a strict insulin treatment regime. The problem, however, is that frequent events of mild hypoglycaemia reduce the patient's awareness of hypoglycaemia, initiating a vicious cycle of recurrent events and thereby increasing the risk of severe hypoglycaemic events. Episodes of severe hypoglycaemia are associated with both risk and fear of recurrent episodes, which may result in the patient striving for a higher glucose target, and thereby, increased risk of late diabetes complications. In addition, hypoglycaemia related visits to the emergency room and hospitalization constitute a heavy economic burden (Hammer et al., 2009; Lammert et al., 2009). Clearly, there are several reasons to consider alternative methods of reducing this risk of hypoglycaemia events.

1.2 Sympato-adrenal warning symptoms and hormonal counter regulation

Healthy humans have two major supplementary mechanisms to avoid severe hypoglycaemia. The first line of defence is the hormonal counterregulation. When blood glucose falls below 3.5 mmol/l, insulin release will be suppressed and the pancreatic alpha cells will release glucagon. This results in an increased glucose release from the hepatic store. Also adrenalin, cortisol and human growth hormone are released as a consequence of hypoglycaemia and contribute to re-establish euglycaemia. The second line of defence arises from an activation of the sympathetic nervous system resulting in the hypoglycaemic symptoms described above. Awareness of these symptoms alerts the patient and enables an appropriate reaction.

1.3 Hypoglycaemia unawareness

In newly diagnosed diabetes, hormonal counterregulation resembles that of a healthy person despite the fact, of course, that insulin release cannot be suppressed since this is externally delivered. With increased duration of diabetes, hormonal counterregulation may fail. Within five years of diabetes onset, most patients have lost their ability to release glucagon upon hypoglycaemia. Although the release of human growth hormone and cortisol may persist, these hormones are less effective and slower acting and do not prevent the development of severe hypoglycaemia.

With increased diabetes duration the sympato-adrenal activation may likewise fail resulting in impaired awareness of hypoglycaemia and ultimately, hypoglycaemia unawareness (Howorka et al., 2000). This is defined by a severe cognitive impairment occurring without subjective symptoms of hypoglycaemia.

A number of factors contribute to deterioration of the hypoglycaemic defences: Recent hypoglycaemic events, tight glycaemic control, sleep, a supine position and alcohol consumption all tend to reduce the hypoglycaemic defences due to the mechanisms described above, thereby increasing the risk of severe hypoglycaemia (Amiel et al., 1991; Geddes et al., 2008; Howorka et al., 2000). Approximately 25% of all type 1 diabetes patients suffer from hypoglycaemia unawareness and most events of severe hypoglycaemia take place within this group of patients (Pedersen-Bjergaard et al., 2004). The risk of severe hypoglycaemia is estimated to be five to ten times higher in patients suffering from hypoglycaemia unawareness (Geddes et al., 2008; Gold et al., 1994; Pedersen-Bjergaard et al., 2004). The term hypoglycaemia associated autonomic failure (HAAF) has been proposed for the concomitant lack of counterregulatory hormonal release and the lack of sympatoadrenal symptoms (Cryer, 2005).

1.4 How to reduce the risk of severe hypoglycaemia

Assuming that the risk and fear of hypoglycaemia is a major hindrance in achieving an optimal glucose control, all possible efforts should be done to reduce them. The first priority must be to optimize the insulin regime. Often a thorough interview with the patient including a review of blood glucose measurements can uncover risk factors for severe hypoglycaemic events in the individual patient. Adjustment of the insulin dose and timing may consequently reduce the risk. Switching from one insulin type to another may ensure a better convergence between insulin concentration and insulin need. The long acting insulin analogues insulin glargine and insulin detemir reduce the risk of hypoglycaemia particularly at night-time (Monami et al., 2009). Use of continuous insulin infusion (insulin pump therapy) rather than multiple injection therapy has been shown to enable a more strict diabetes regulation and also a significant reduction in the risk of severe hypoglycaemia (Pickup et al., 2008). However, severe hypoglycaemia is still a common and feared complication in type 1 diabetes (Anderbro et al., 2010).

Much effort has been put into the development of continuous glucose monitoring (CGM) systems. Ideally, CGM will provide a better protection against severe hypoglycaemia by frequent glucose measurements in the interstitial tissue and alarms based on actual glucose measurements or prediction algorithms. Large clinical studies have shown that the use of CGM enables a more tight glucose control without increased risk of hypoglycaemia, but so far CGM has not been shown to reduce the risk of severe hypoglycaemic events (The Diabetes Control and Complication Trial, 2009; Bergenstal et al., 2010; Tamborlane et al., 2008). Still, CGM studies have taught us that hypoglycaemia is much more common than previously thought and is likely to be significantly underreported (JDRF CGM Study Group, 2010). One shortcoming of CGM is that adherence to therapy seems to decline with long term use, so use of the device calculated as hours per week was reduced to 35-70% depending on age group already after six months of use in clinical trials (JDRF CGM Study Group, 2008).

2. EEG for hypoglycaemia detection

2.1 The concept of an EEG based biosensor as a hypoglycaemia alarm

While hormonal counterregulation and sympatoadrenal symptoms often diminish or disappear with long term diabetes, the devastating effect of low blood glucose on organ function persists. The most important dysfunctions arise from the glycopenic effects on the brain and the heart. Neuroglycopenia results in a gradual loss of cognitive functions. In the early stage, this may only be apparent during systematic cognitive testing. As the glucose concentration falls, the cognitive function continues to decline resulting in slower speed of reaction, blurred speech, loss of consciousness, seizures and ultimately death. The effect of hypoglycaemia on the heart is less well described but comprises prolongation of the QT-interval which is a known cause of cardiac arrhythmia. In fact death among younger patients with insulin treated diabetes is assumed often to be related to malignant cardiac arrhythmia.

The blood glucose threshold at which the organ function is affected varies both between and within diabetes patients. Diabetes patients with tightly controlled blood glucose and frequent hypoglycaemic events may not be severely affected despite a blood glucose level as low as 1.5 mmol/l or even lower. This means, however, that just a slight further reduction in the glucose concentration will result in the serious effects of severe hypoglycaemia.

The concept of a hypoglycaemia alarm based on biosensing involves continuous monitoring of organ function, a real-time signal processing and an alarm device. Preferably, such a biosensor should be able to sense subtle change in brain function (e.g. electroencephalography), cardiac function (e.g. electrocardiography) or any other organ changes preceding cognitive dysfunction which will preclude the patient from taking action and thereby avoid severe hypoglycaemia.

This chapter focuses on the possibility to construct a hypoglycaemia alarm system based on continuous EEG monitoring and real-time data processing by means of a multi-parameter algorithm. Such a device may comprise an alternative to self-glucose testing or continuous glucose monitoring as a guard against severe hypoglycaemia. Analysis of EEG changes as a predictor of severe hypoglycaemia was already proposed by Regan et. al. in 1956 (Reagan et al., 1956). Iaione published the development of an automated algorithm using digital signal processing and artificial neural networks with the aim of developing a hypoglycaemia detector system, and achieved a fair sensitivity and specificity in the detection of hypoglycaemia (Iaione et al., 2005). Our aim is to develop this further to a portable real-time hypoglycaemia alarm device, which can be used by type 1 diabetes patients with hypoglycaemia unawareness. For such a device to be suitable for clinical use, it must fulfil a number of criteria: It must have a high sensitivity with low occurrence of false positive alarms, preferably it should require little or no calibration, and it must be suitable for use over long periods with minimal discomfort for the patient.

2.2 Hypoglycaemia related EEG changes

The electroencephalogram (EEG) is usually measured on the scalp, using surface electrodes that are glued to the scalp with conducting gels. The surface EEG represents the electrical activity taking place inside the brain and originates from the firing neurons, mainly in the superficial part of the brain. When a neuron fires, a very small electrical charge is released, which in itself cannot be measured on the scalp. But the macro pattern that appears when many neurons fire in a synchronized manner, builds up larger electrical signals, which can be measured on the scalp. When measuring the EEG, all the micro changes in the firing pattern disappear due to the averaging effect through the scalp, and only the macro changes remain. The EEG, which is measured outside the scalp, can therefore be used to detect macro changes in the electrical behaviour of the brain. In general, during daytime, the healthy brain is less synchronized than during sleep, and only few daytime phenomena can be characterized and detected. During sleep, the brain is more synchronised and emits many characteristic wave patterns that reflect the different sleep phases (Iber et al., 2007). Many brain related diseases, like e.g. epilepsy, do result in synchronization of the brain waves, which can be seen in the EEG patterns. This is also the case for patients experiencing hypoglycaemia.

Glucose is an essential substrate for brain metabolism. Accordingly, low blood glucose resulting in neuroglycopenia can be assumed to result in EEG changes. In the 1950's, the first studies of hypoglycaemia related EEG changes (HREC) were published (Ross et al., 1951; Regan et al., 1956) and already by then, it was proposed that EEG might add information on whether a patient's blood glucose concentration falls below a critical threshold (Regan et al., 1956). Pramming et al studied EEG changes during insulin induced hypoglycaemia in type 1 diabetes patients (Pramming et al., 1988). They found that the EEG was unaffected when the blood glucose concentration was above 3 mmol/l. Following a gradual decline in blood glucose the EEG changes became apparent in all the patients. At a median blood glucose concentration of 2.0 mmol/l the alpha activity (8-12 Hz) decreased while theta activity (4-8 Hz) increased, reflecting a cortical dysfunction. Importantly, HREC disappeared when the blood glucose was normalized and a normal EEG was re-established when the blood glucose concentration exceeded a level of 2.0 mmol/l. It was concluded that "changes in electroencephalograms during hypoglycaemia appear and disappear at such a narrow range of blood glucose concentrations that the term threshold blood glucose concentration for the onset of such changes seems justified".

A number of studies have further characterized the EEG-changes associated with hypoglycaemia (Bedtsson et al., 1991; Bjorgaas et al., 1998; Hyllienmark et al., (2005); Juhl et al., (2010); Tamburrano et al., 1988; Tribl et al., 1996). Although some discrepancy exists with respect to the spatial location of the EEG changes (see section 2.4) and the persistence of these changes after restoration of euglycaemia, it is well established that hypoglycaemia is associated with an increased power in the low frequency bands. Figure 1 shows an example of a single channel EEG recorded during euglycaemia and hypoglycaemia during daytime. Comparing the two signals, it is evident that the hypoglycaemic EEG originates from a process of lower frequency, which is more synchronized, leading to EEG of higher amplitude.

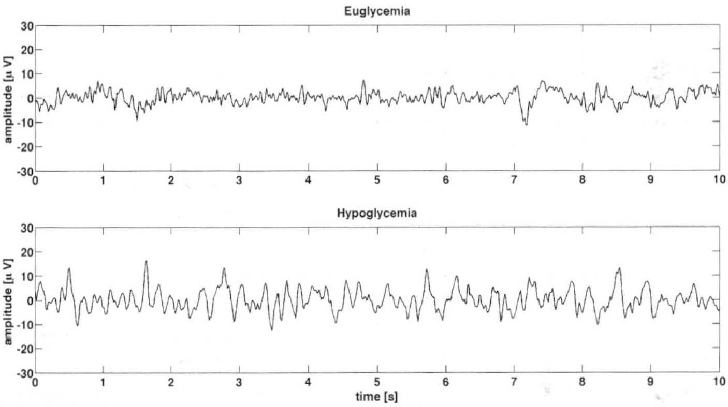

Fig. 1. Representative examples of single channel EEG recorded during euglycaemia and hypoglycaemia in the same person.

Bendtson et al. studied type 1 diabetes patients during sleep and found widespread occurrence of low frequency waves which could be differentiated from the delta and theta-band by the frequency (Bentson et al., 1991). These changes were only detectable in patients with lack of glucagon response. This observation has been challenged by our research team which found EEG changes irrespective of glucagon response (Juhl et al., 2010).

Though the two signals in Figure 1 are very easy to distinguish and the HREC paradigm is relatively well established, the HREC detection problem is not as trivial as it seems. The illustrated signals constitute textbook examples, and the exact signal characteristics vary considerably between subjects - both during euglycaemia and hypoglycaemia. In addition, many everyday activities induce EEG activity in the same frequency band as the HREC paradigm. Examples of this are low-frequency deep sleep patterns and broadband noise signals.

2.3 Long-term EEG recording: scalp vs. subcutaneous EEG

Using the brain as a biosensor for hypoglycaemia detection throughout the day requires a stable long-term EEG recording system. The usual 10/20 EEG system (Crespel et al., 2005) with surface electrodes glued to the scalp is not an option, since surface electrodes are highly exposed to movement artefact. Therefore, in our setting, the EEG is measured by electrodes placed in the subcutaneous layer, a few millimetres below the skin, thereby giving the advantage of being more robust to noise and artefact signals. The subcutaneous measurements were tested compared to scalp electrodes and were found to be very similar, showing very high correlation.

In the initial experiments, four single subcutaneous electrodes were placed, while in the sleep studies a single electrode with three measuring points were inserted in the temporal area and connected to an EEG device.

2.4 Spatial considerations

In general, EEG patterns have different characteristics depending on the spatial location of the measurement. While some EEG changes are generalized and apparent on the entire surface of the brain, some paradigms are only present in smaller areas, which make detailed measurements in certain locations necessary.

Regarding the spatial distribution of the HREC, some discrepancy exists. The topographic maximum has been demonstrated to be located in the lateral frontal region during mild hypoglycaemia. This shifts towards the centroparietal and parieto-occipital region in deeper hypoglycaemia (Tribl et al., 1996). Hyllienmark et al on the other hand studied type 1 diabetes patients with a history of recurrent hypoglycaemia, and the EEG recording was conducted during a period of normal blood glucose. They found similar HREC characteristics as previously described, however predominantly in the frontal region. (Hyllienmark et al., 2005). In addition, this could indicate that EEG changes in some cases may become permanent.

In order to be able to detect HREC with a single or a few electrodes we investigated the spatial distribution of the changes. The hypoglycaemia changes are generally present on most of the scalp area. The spatial distribution of the artefacts particularly derived from muscle activity during facial mimicking, eating, eye movement and sleep related movements, should be taken into account when the optimal electrode placement is to be defined. In contrast to the HREC, these artefacts are more localized, making the location important. Artefact related to electrode movements and the mechanics of the electrode contact are not dependent on the spatial location. The ability to detect the HREC when artefact signals are present is illustrated in Figure 2, where the HREC signal is detected from a single electrode channel on five diabetes patients.

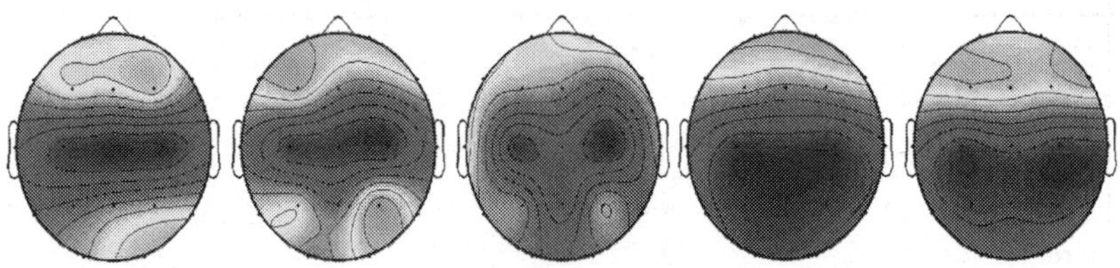

Fig. 2. Illustration of the spatial influence on the ability to detect the HREC paradigm. The red areas in the figure indicate that the HREC paradigm detection performance is high, whereas green areas indicate low performance.

Taking into consideration the spatial influence and the electrode type we have chosen the final measurement location shown in Figure 3.

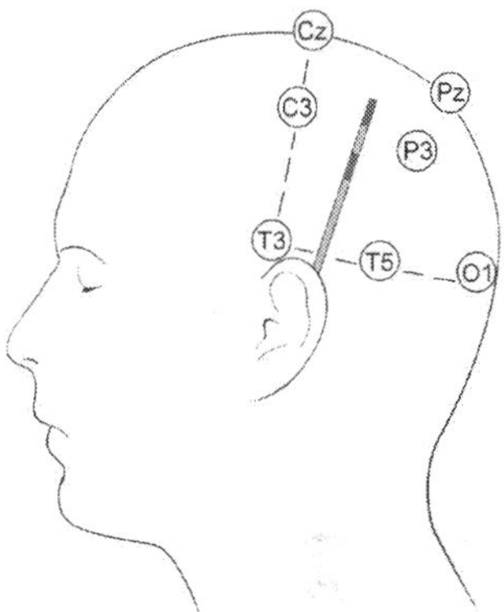

Fig. 3. Location of the subcutaneous EEG electrode. The subcutaneous electrode is inserted in a location behind the ear towards vertex cranii between Cz and Pz. The measurement points are shown in red, giving one differential channel.

3. The development of the algorithm

In the following paragraphs we describe in detail the development of the algorithm, which distinguishes HREC from normal daytime and sleep EEG. This process required a series of insulin-induced hypoglycaemia experiments with continuous improvements of the algorithm and repetitive testing. The series of clinical trials from which the data were obtained are outlined in Figure 4.

The measurement system used to acquire EEG data, samples the EEG at a sampling frequency of 512 Hz. The EEG is filtered so that all the frequency components above 32 Hz are removed, leaving us with a signal bandwidth of 32 Hz and a sampling frequency of 64 Hz for the HREC detection algorithm. The dynamic range of the measured signal is ± 512μV with a signal resolution (1 LSB) of 1μV. The internal noise level in the analogue data acquisition system is 1.3μV RMS.

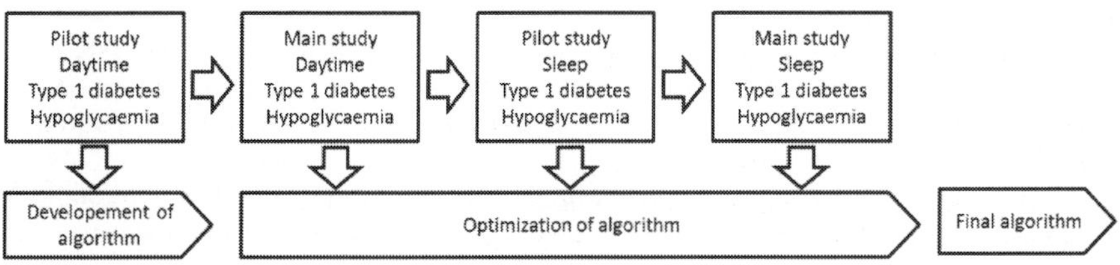

Fig. 4. Illustration of the flow of clinical studies leading to the development of the algorithm. Continuous optimizations were conducted on the basis of consecutive daytime and sleep experiments.

The HREC can be detected by visual inspection by a neurophysiologist, who inspects the waveforms of the EEG. However, if the EEG of the diabetes patients is to be analysed in real-time throughout the day this must be done automatically using an algorithm. The algorithm structure for hypoglycaemia detection is shown in Figure 5.

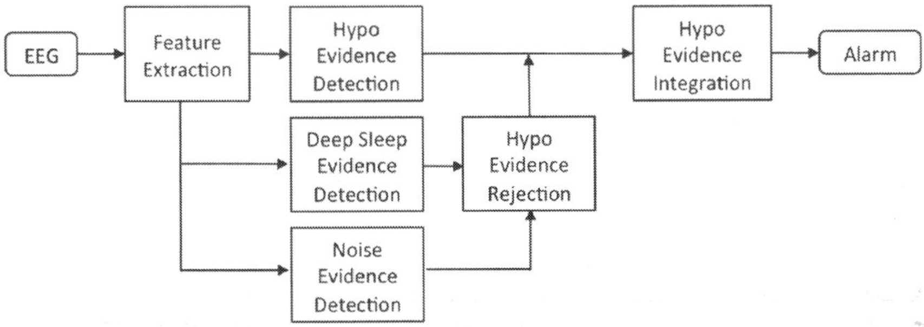

Fig. 5. Structure of the hypoglycaemia detection algorithm.

Overall, the algorithm works in four sequential levels that process the EEG signal and determines whether sufficient evidence of hypoglycaemia is present for an alarm to be triggered. At the first level, the feature extraction process maps the raw EEG into an appropriate feature space in which it is possible to distinguish HREC from normal EEG. The second level consists of three blocks, each of which analyses the features to determine if there is evidence of impending hypoglycaemia, deep sleep patterns, or noise contamination, respectively. At the third level, hypoglycaemia evidence is rejected when deep sleep patterns and/or noise are present. Lastly, taking the recent history into account it is determined whether or not a sufficient amount of hypoglycaemia evidence is present to constitute an alarm. Each of the algorithm blocks will be described in the following sections.

3.1 Feature extraction

The raw EEG signal waveform can easily be analysed by the trained human eye, which interprets the shape of the waves and draws a conclusion based on this. However, the raw waveform representation is not directly interpretable for a machine decision network, which needs the EEG in a different presentation. The feature extraction part of the algorithm maps the raw EEG into another form that represents the distribution of different kinds of waveforms. Since the hypoglycaemia paradigm in EEG is characterized by the existence of waveforms of specific frequency content, the features calculated are designed to reflect this.
The EEG waveforms are transformed to features by sending the EEG through an IIR filter bank, taking the 1-norm of the filtered signals, integrating the values in another filter, and by finally subsampling the integrated signal.
When analysing EEG, the signal is traditionally split into 5 frequency bands (delta, theta, alpha, beta, and gamma). However, this frequency resolution is not sufficient for an optimal performance of the hypoglycaemia detection system.
Our IIR filter bank consists of 32 filters where each filter has a bandwidth of 1Hz and a sub-band attenuation of 30 dB or more. In Figure 6, a 20-minute sample of EEG is represented in feature space.

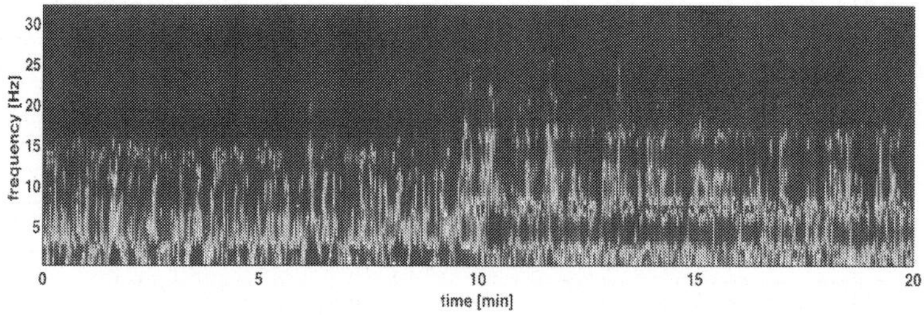

Fig. 6. Feature space representation of an EEG signal during a transition from euglycaemia (first 10 min) to hypoglycaemia (last 10 min), where HREC's are present. It is evident that a strong 7-8 Hz activity is present during hypoglycaemia in this sample.

We will see later (Figure 9) that many of the filter bands are irrelevant for the overall performance of the algorithm, but all bands have been included here to give a better understanding of the importance of each band. It should be noted that the fast Fourier transform (FFT) algorithm could easily substitute the IIR filter bank, if the process memory requirements are of no concern. Each filter in the filter bank consists of four sequential direct form-2 transpose 2nd order filter sections (Van den Enden et al., 1989). The direct form-2 transpose filters maintain the dynamic range of the signal in the fixed-point filter structure that we have chosen.

The output of the filters are normalized by the 1-norm and then integrated over a certain amount of time to get an estimate of the signal energy during this time period. We have used an IIR filter to facilitate the integration, which is a processing-wise cheap way of carrying this out. The integrator remembers the history approximately one second back in time. The integrator output is finally subsampled into a 1 Hz feature interval to eliminate redundant information. In this manner, feature vectors representing 1-second epochs are fed into the classifier.

3.2 Classifying evidence of hypoglycaemia

An important part of the algorithm is the classifier, which determines if there is evidence of hypoglycaemia in a small part of the EEG signal. The classifier bases its judgment on the extracted features, which represent the statistical properties of the EEG during 1-second epochs. The classifier combines the input statistics in a mathematical expression that results in either a "1" if the EEG has a hypoglycaemia pattern or a "0" otherwise.

There are many ways of setting up the mathematical classifier expression, and depending on this expression, the ability to classify the hypoglycaemia pattern varies. We have experimented with different kinds of classifier methods and found that the performance variation between them is small. The more advanced non-linear classifiers like support vector machines (SVM) (Joakims, 2002) and artificial neural networks (ANN) do however have small performance advantages over the more simple classifiers such as linear classifiers or the Bayes classifier with a Gaussian kernel (Bishop, 1998).

Based on our results, we have chosen to use a two-layer feed-forward ANN classifier structure to do all classification tasks in the hypoglycaemia alarm system. The ANN has a number of hidden units and uses the tanh sigmoid function for non-linear mappings.

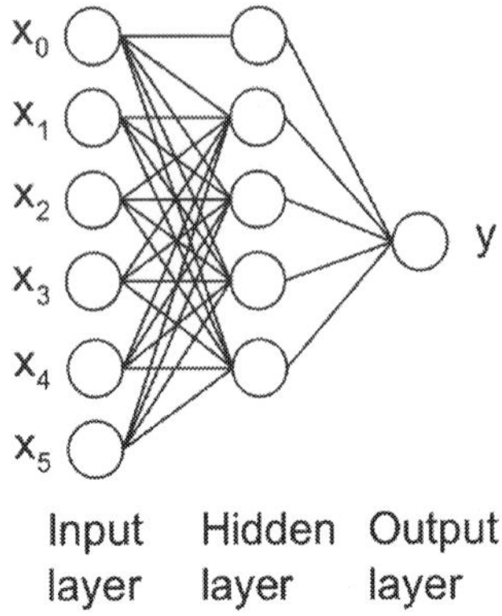

Fig. 7. Structure of the artificial neural network that detects HREC. It consists of a number of inputs and hidden layers, but only one final output determining whether or not the input epoch contains HREC.

The input layer values (x_0 - x_5) contain the feature values, where x_0 is a bias. The ANN classifier expression is shown in equation (1),

$$y_n = a\left(\sum_{h=0}^{N_h} z_h g\left(\sum_{i=0}^{N_i} w_{h,i} x_{n,i}\right)\right) \quad (1)$$

where $x_{n,i}$ is the input feature number i at time *n*, $w_{h,i}$ is the input feature weight for the mapping to the hidden unit h, N_h is the number of input features, g is the nonlinear mapping function (tanh), z_h is the output weight for the hidden unit h, N_h is the number of hidden units, a is the output activation function and y_n is the classifier output at time *n*. In our setting, the output activation function is simply a logic expression that determines whether or not the contained value has exceeded a threshold. The output y_n is shown as "1" if a HREC is detected, or otherwise, as "0".

3.3 Classifier training

The optimal parameters of the classifier ($w_{h,i}$ and z_h) can be estimated by using the back-propagation method (Bishop, 1998), based on a training set of labelled data points. We have used a neural network toolbox that applies a maximum a posteriori approach when finding the optimal weights (Sigurdsson et al., 2002). The precise classifier parameter optimization approach is of little importance in this application. Instead, the data labelling method impacts the classifier performance more. We have experimented with two data labelling approaches, where the first approach is based on expert labelling of experiment data, and the second approach is a flexible automatic labelling based on standard experiment parameters.

In the first data labelling approach, a neurophysiologist labelled a training set of EEG data, based on visual inspection of the raw EEG. The visual inspection is rather time consuming and is not feasible when larger amounts of data are used for training of the classifier. During the process of marking the data, the neurophysiologist was blinded to the timeline and associated blood glucose sample values that had been measured while sampling the EEG. The neurophysiologist only knew that the EEG originated from a diabetes patient where both euglycaemia and hypoglycaemia situations were present in each experiment EEG dataset.

The second approach to data labelling is automatic and based on parameters that are associated with the experiment timeline and glucose values measured during the experiment. One direct advantage of using this approach is that all data can be used for modelling, and not just the data marked by the neurophysiologist. This allows for better modelling of the inter-subject variability. When using the second approach, the labelling is not predefined. Instead, time intervals with different reward functions are defined. Within such a time interval, the number of positive and negative labels rather than the exact timestamp of the label is used to determine the cost function of the classifier model. The time segments with different reward functions are shown in Figure 8, where β is the glucose threshold of 3.5 mmol/l that determines when an alarm may, but not necessarily will, be set off. T_0 is the point in time when cognition has deteriorated too much for the subject to be able to react to an alarm, $T_{0-\tau}$ is 10 minutes prior to T_0 and $T_{GL<\beta}$ are the times where the glucose level passes the threshold of 3.5 mmol/l.

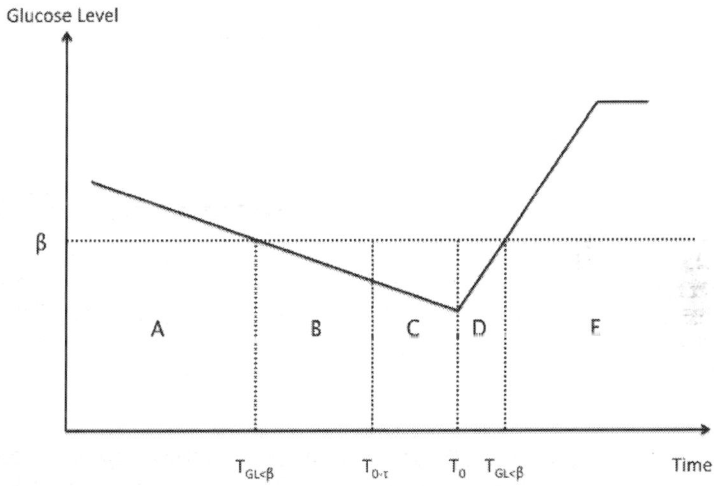

Fig. 8. Reward function time segments used to train the classifier.

In segment A and E, the classifier cost function is punished for detecting HREC, while rewarded in segment B and C. In segment D, the classifier is neither rewarded nor punished for its behaviour. The exact expression for the cost function is given in equation (2).

$$C = -\left(\sum_A y_n\right) + \left(\sum_B y_n\right) + \left(2\sum_C y_n\right) - \left(\sum_E y_n\right) \tag{2}$$

When the cost function expression is applied to a linear classifier with a single hidden unit, and optimized, we get the basic influences of the features. The classifier input weights $w_{h,i}$

show the importance of each feature. In Figure 9 the weights are shown for the linear classifier.

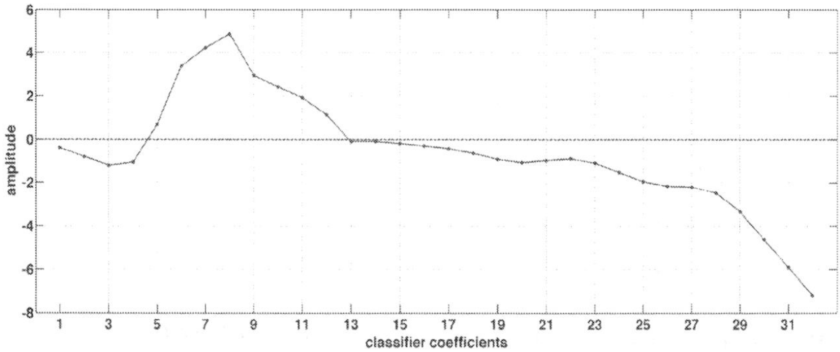

Fig. 9. Coefficients of a linear HREC classifier.

Many of the coefficients have small values and could be disregarded and many features could be joined since they have similar influence on the classifier output. It is evident that the HREC paradigm is characterized by high 6-8 Hz activity and some alpha activity.

3.4 Integration of evidence

Single events detected by the classifier do not make up sufficient evidence to trigger an alarm. The brainwaves are contaminated with noise and artefacts, leading to false detections. Furthermore, brainwaves similar to those seen during hypoglycaemia also appear sporadically during euglycaemia. It is therefore necessary to take the history of detected events into account before giving a hypoglycaemia alarm. We used the history by integrating the events that were detected during the past 10 minutes. The integrator is implemented as an IIR filter which makes it computationally cheap while only consuming little memory. The integration structure is shown in Figure 10.

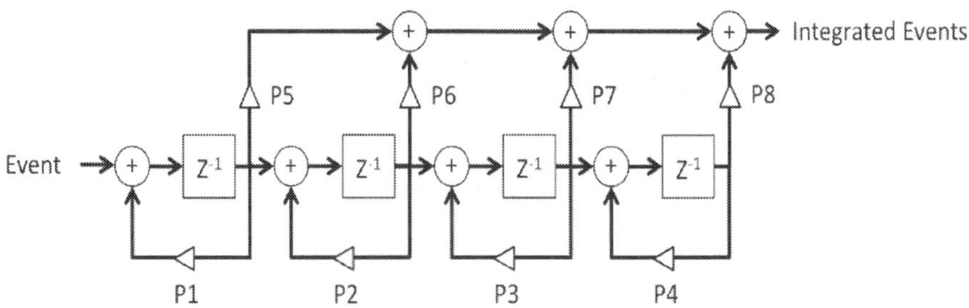

Fig. 10. Filter structure used for integration of evidence.

The coefficients P1-P8 are set to make the resulting time-function resemble a 5-minute square window. The shape of the integrator can easily be changed to have different weight and time perspectives, by changing the coefficients.

An example of the integrator output is shown in Figure 11, where a diabetes patient undergoes hypoglycaemia and recovers from the situation.

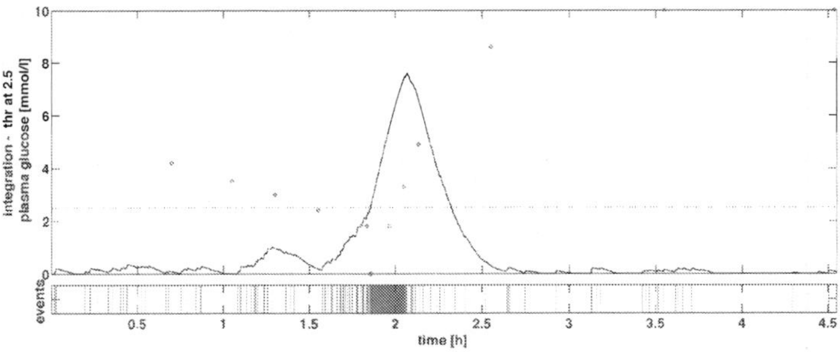

Fig. 11. Example of integrated evidence of the HREC. The red dots are blood glucose sample values sampled during the experiment. The solid line shows the value of the integration function, which alarms the subject when exceeding the predefined threshold of 2.5. The lower graph displays the events. One red vertical line represents an epoch in which HREC is detected.

3.5 Deep sleep algorithm

Initially, the hypoglycaemia algorithm was based on EEG from daytime experiments only. Figure 12 shows the output when it is applied on EEG recorded during sleep. The result is repeated detections of EEG changes compatible with hypoglycaemia during the night.

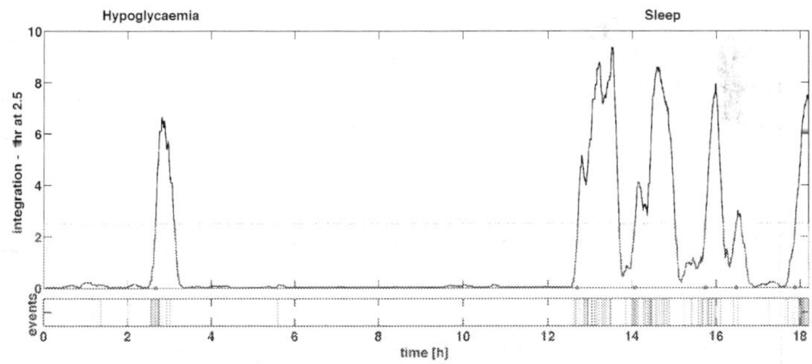

Fig. 12. Integrated events of EEG changes compatible with hypoglycaemia in a diabetes patient exposed to hypoglycaemia during the daytime and continued EEG recorded during sleep. The algorithm clearly detected repeated episodes during sleep as being consistent with hypoglycaemia.

Nocturnal hypoglycaemia thus encompasses a distinctive challenge with respect to a hypoglycaemia alarm. Not only do approximately half of all hypoglycaemic events take place during sleep (Woodward et al., 2009), but also the nocturnal EEG is distinctly different from the daytime EEG. During stages of deep sleep, the EEG pattern is characterized by slow wave patterns much like the hypoglycaemia EEG. It is therefore a challenge to distinguish deep sleep EEG patterns from HREC. In order to suppress falsely detected hypoglycaemia events, we used a learning process that is similar to learning the HREC to construct a classifier that can detect when deep sleep patterns are contaminating the EEG signal. It should be noted that during the 27 insulin-induced hypoglycaemia night experiments that we have conducted so far, no deep sleep patterns have been present simultaneously with HREC.

3.6 Noise and artefact suppression

In an everyday life environment, the presence of noise and artefacts is substantial. Some of these operate in the same frequency band as the HREC, potentially leading to false alarms. Figure 13 shows an example of a false alarm detected during euglycaemia and normal daytime activities. The false alarm is caused by muscle activity when chewing. Many other daytime activities also come close to setting off false alarms.

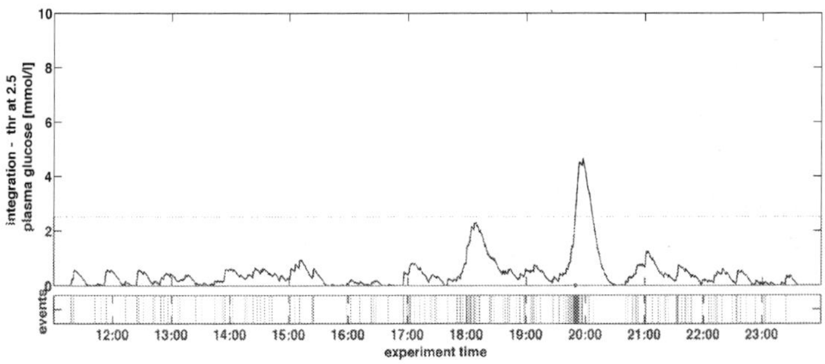

Fig. 13. Integrated HREC evidence during normal everyday activity. A false alarm is declared just before 20:00.

In order to suppress falsely detected hypoglycaemia events due to noises and artefact, we have constructed a classifier that can detect when noise and artefacts are contaminating the EEG signal using a learning process similar to learning the HREC. When this noise/artefact detection system is applied to the algorithm, the false alarm in Figure 13 is removed, and other false events are handled. The result is displayed in Figure 14. The integrated evidence is now generally lower during the normal situation, allowing us to make the HREC classifier more sensitive.

4. Clinical results

The following paragraph will focus on the clinical studies we have conducted. The focus of these studies has been the development of the algorithm for an EEG-based hypoglycaemia alarm device. The results we have achieved give an indication of the clinical applicability of the device. Here we will briefly summarize the results from the clinician's point of view.
Altogether, we have studied more than 50 patients. An important observation is that *all* patients studied so far have developed EEG changes compatible with previously described hypoglycaemia associated changes. This has allowed us to develop a general algorithm for EEG analysis, which can be applied to all diabetes patients.

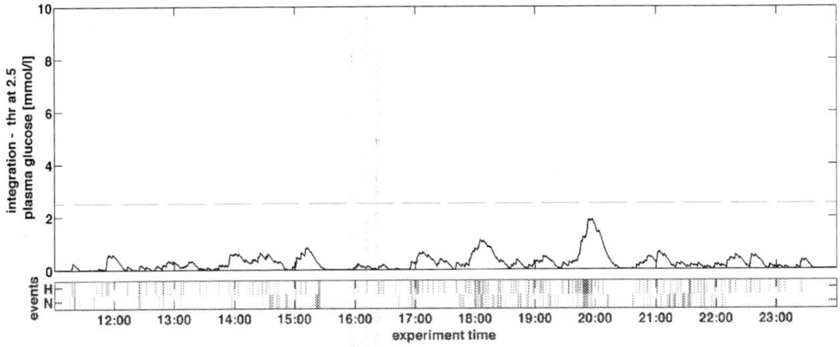

Fig. 14. Integrated HREC evidence after suppression of noise and artefacts. The vertical lines in the lower graph display the detected hypoglycaemia (red) and noise (green) events.

Initially, continuous EEG was recorded during insulin-induced hypoglycaemia experiments in 15 type 1 diabetes patients during daytime. Four subcutaneous electrodes located in the temporal region were applied along with a standard scalp 10/20 system recording. The cognitive function was evaluated by repeated cognitive testing (a backward counting test and a minus-seven test). Insulin infusion was terminated when plasma glucose reached 1.8 mmol/l or when the subjects showed obvious signs of cognitive dysfunction such as severely reduced speech velocity or heavy sweating. EEG was analysed post hoc by the automated mathematical algorithm. HREC were detected in all 15 subjects. Plasma glucose at the time of EEG changes above the threshold value indicating hypoglycaemia, ranged from 2.0 to 3.4 mmol/l and occurred 29±28 minutes (mean±SD)(range 3 - 113 minutes) before termination of insulin infusion. In this study, patients did not receive a real-time alarm, and therefore, it is not possible to state if they would have been able to react following an alarm. In 12 of 15 patients, however, EEG changes occurred before severe neuroglycopenia was apparent as evaluated by the cognitive testing. In three cases, the patients were moderately cognitively impaired at the time of EEG changes, they were, however, still awake. The presence and the time of alarm were independent of age, diabetes duration and glucose regulation (Juhl et al., 2010). Although this study did not prove that an alarm could be given in time for the patient to react, it indicated that it would in most cases.
Due to the characteristic EEG pattern during sleep, occasionally resembling HREC, it is essential to study the applicability of the algorithm during sleep. Initially, we performed a number of pilot experiments in type 1 diabetes patients exposed to insulin-induced hypoglycaemia during sleep. The original algorithm was trained on these data, and the algorithm was optimized to distinguish hypoglycaemia from deep sleep. Ten type 1 diabetes patients (mean age 47 years, diabetes duration 23.7 years, HbA1c 7.5%) all suffering from hypoglycaemia unawareness, were subsequently subjected to induced hypoglycaemia by graded insulin infusion both during daytime and during sleep at night-time. EEG was recorded from a single electrode with three measurement points placed subcutaneously in the temporal region and was analysed real-time. The patient received an auditory alarm when EEG-changes met a predefined threshold. The patients were instructed beforehand to consume a sandwich and a juice at the time of alarm. Figure 15 illustrates the procedure of a night experiment.

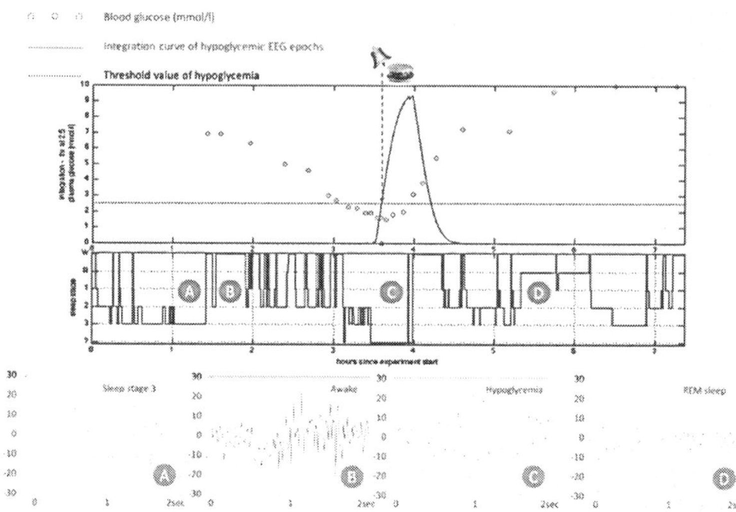

Fig. 15. Representative example of a night-time experiment. The upper panel shows the blood glucose profile (red circles) and the curve for integrated EEG-events of hypoglycaemia (black line). The integration curve rose steeply following hypoglycaemia. The patient received an alarm at blood glucose 1.8 mmol/l, where the integration curve crossed the threshold (blue dotted line). Blood glucose increased following ingestion of the meal, and the integration curve normalized accordingly. The middle panel shows the sleep stage according to AASM scoring. The patient clearly went through all stages of sleep during the night. After a short awake period following the hypoglycaemia event, the patient went back to sleep. The lower panels show two-second epochs of EEG while awake (B), REM sleep (D), stage three sleep (A) and hypoglycaemia (C).

If blood glucose fell to 1.7 mmol/l without triggering the alarm or if the patient was not able to react at the time of the alarm, hypoglycaemia was ceased by glucose infusion. The alarm was triggered for seven out of nine patients during daytime (mean blood glucose (BG) 2.7 mmol/l). Six of these seven patients were able to reverse hypoglycaemia by carbohydrate ingestion. During sleep, the alarm was triggered in nine out of ten subjects (mean BG 2.0 mmol/l) and eight awoke due to the alarm. Four corrected hypoglycaemia by food ingestion (mean BG 2.2 mmol/l) while the remaining four (mean BG 1.9 mmol/l) were supplemented with glucose due to cognitive impairment. Two events of false alarm were observed. EEG was also recorded from surface electrodes placed according to the 10/20 system and analysed by the American Academy of Sleep scoring manual to determine sleep stages (Iber et al., 2007). HREC occurred irrespective of the sleep stages and seemed to overrule physiological sleep related patterns.

By post hoc improvements of the algorithm (e.g. inclusion of hypoglycaemia evidence rejection due to deep sleep patterns and/or noise artefacts) it was possible to detect hypoglycaemia in all patients, while eliminating the false alarms. In addition, hypoglycaemia could be detected on average three (daytime experiments) and six (sleep experiments) minutes earlier than with the original algorithm, improving the sensitivity of the alarm.

Overall, it seems possible to detect hypoglycaemia in diabetes patients irrespective of the time of the day, duration of diabetes, awareness status and hormonal counter-regulation. The core question is whether this detection precedes serious cognitive impairment, allowing the patient to react. This is currently being tested in clinical trials.

5. An EEG based hypoglycaemia device for permanent use

The EEG based hypoglycaemia alarm system consists of two main parts: An implanted device that captures the EEG signal, and a non-implanted device, which stores and processes the EEG signal. This is illustrated in Figure 16.

The inner device is implanted subcutaneously, with the main part behind the ear and the electrode pointing towards the top of the head. The electrode has three measurement points, a length of 8 cm and a diameter of 1.1 mm.

Data is transmitted from the inner device to the outer device through a near field communication link. Therefore, the two devices have to be closely aligned for the system to function. The outer device is designed as an ear hanger, illustrated on the right panel of Figure 16. It is therefore easy to wear with a minimum of discomfort for the user. The outer device contains a sound generator and a light indicator to inform the user of critical events, e.g. impending hypoglycaemia.

The outer device contains a power source. When the outer device is placed behind the ear, the power source is shared with the inner device through the communication link. When the power source in the outer device is depleted, it must be recharged in a charging station. A full recharge allows for approximately 18 hours of use.

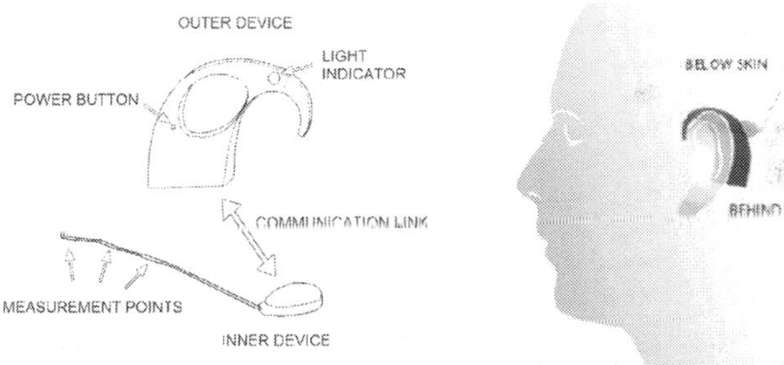

Fig. 16. The EEG based hypoglycaemia alarm system consisting of an inner and an outer device.

The implantation procedure is simple and takes approximately 15 minutes. The implanted device must be replaced only after two years of use.

6. Conclusion

Type 1 diabetes patients suffering from hypoglycaemia unawareness are significantly disposed to episodes of severe hypoglycaemia. This is associated with a risk of glucose metabolic dysregulation and a reduced quality of life (Anderbro et al., 2010; Barnard et al., 2010; Frier, 2008). Despite self-monitoring of blood glucose, the use of insulin analogues and increased knowledge of the mechanisms of unawareness, the risk of hypoglycaemia remains a major barrier to optimized glucose control. If just one of the two components of hypoglycaemia associated autonomic failure (Cryer, 2005) (i.e. hypoglycaemia unawareness or reduced hormonal counter-regulation) could be re-established, these patients would be much less prone to severe hypoglycaemia.

The initial clinical studies of continuous EEG recording and real-time data processing during insulin-induced hypoglycaemia in type 1 diabetes patients indicate that it will be possible to predict incidents of severe hypoglycaemia before the patients are severely cognitive impaired both during daytime and sleep. The studies conducted so far, though, have taken place in clinical research units. We are now testing the hypoglycaemia alarm in an out-patient setting.

It is of utmost importance that an alarm device has a high sensitivity and specificity. False alarms may be annoying to the patients yet they are not dangerous. Missed alarms, on the other hand, may render the patient with a false feeling of security. On the other hand, a sensitive and reliable alarm device will allow the patient to achieve a better glucose control with less fear of hypoglycaemia events. The studies conducted so far hold promises that an EEG based device might fulfil these goals.

7. Acknowledgement

First of all, we would like to thank the patients who volunteered to participate in the clinical trials. Conducting these studies was essential in the development of the algorithm. Thanks to Marianne Bötcher, Lone Jensen, and Charlotte Olsen for excellent technical assistance during the conduction of the hypoglycaemia studies. Thanks to Poul Jennum and Michaela Gjerstadt for analyses of and advice regarding the recording and analysis of sleep EEG.

8. References

Amiel, SA.; Pottinger, RC.; Archibald, HR.; Chusney, G.; Cunnah, DT.; Prior, PF. & Gale, EA. (1991). Effect of antecedent glucose control on cerebral function during hypoglycemia. *Diabetes Care*, Vol.14, No.2, pp. 109-118.

Anderbro, T.; Amsberg, S.; Adamson, U.; Bolinder, J.; Lins, PE.; Wredling, R.; Moberg, E.; Lisspers, J. & Johansson UB. (2010). Fear of hypoglycaemia in adults with Type 1 diabetes. *Diabet Med*, Vol.27, No.10, pp. 1151-1158.

Barnard, K.; Thomas, S.; Royle, P.; Noyes, K. & Waugh, N. (2010). Fear of hypoglycaemia in parents of young children with type 1 diabetes: a systematic review. BMC Pediatr, 10:50.

Bendtson, I.; Gade, J.; Rosenfalck, AM.; Thomsen, CE.; Wildschiodtz, G & Binder, C. (1991). Nocturnal electroencephalogram registrations in type 1 (insulin-dependent) diabetic patients with hypoglycaemia. *Diabetologia*, Vol. 34, No.10, pp. 750-756.

Bergenstal, RM.; Tamborlane, WV.; Ahmann, A.; Buse, JB.; Dailey, G.; Davis, SN.; Joyce, C.; Peoples, T.; Perkins, BA.; Welsh, JB.; Willi, SM. & Wood, MA. (2010). Effectiveness of sensor-augmented insulin-pump therapy in type 1 diabetes. *N Engl J Med*, Vol.363, No.4, pp.311-320.

Bjorgaas, M.; Sand, T.; Vik, T. & Jorde, R. (1998). Quantitative EEG during controlled hypoglycaemia in diabetic and non-diabetic children. *Diabet Med*, Vol. 15, No.1, pp. 30-37.

Bishop, CM. (1998). *Neural Networks for Pattern Recognition*. 1st ed. Oxford University Press, New York, USA.

Crespel, A. & Gélisse, P. (2005). *Altas of Electroencephalography*. 1st ed. John Libbey Eurotext, Montrouge, France.

Cryer, PE. (2005). Mechanisms of hypoglycemia-associated autonomic failure and its component syndromes in diabetes. *Diabetes*, Vol.54, No.12. pp. 3592-3601.

Frier BM. (2008). How hypoglycaemia can affect the life of a person with diabetes. Diabetes Metab Res Rev 2008 Vol. 24, No.2, pp. 87-92.

Geddes, J.; Schopman, JE.; Zammitt, NN. & Frier, BM. (2008). Prevalence of impaired awareness of hypoglycaemia in adults with Type 1 diabetes. *Diabet Med*, Vol.25, No.4, pp. 501-504.

Gold, AE.; MacLeod, KM. & Frier, BM. (1994). Frequency of severe hypoglycemia in patients with type I diabetes with impaired awareness of hypoglycemia. *Diabetes Care*, Vol.17, No.7, pp. 697-703.

Hammer, M.; Lammert, M.; Mejias, SM.; Kern, W. & Frier, BM. (2009). Costs of managing severe hypoglycaemia in three European countries. *J Med Econ*, Vol. 12, No.4, pp. 281-290.

Hojlund, K.; Wildner-Christensen, M.; Eshoj, O.; Skjaerbaek, C.; Holst, JJ.; Koldkjaer, O.; Møller Jensen, D. & Beck-Nielsen, H. (2001). Reference intervals for glucose, beta-cell polypeptides, and counterregulatory factors during prolonged fasting. *Am J Physiol Endocrinol Metab*, Vol.280, No.1, pp. E50-E58.

Howorka, K.; Pumprla, J.; Saletu, B.; Anderer, P.; Krieger, M. & Schabmann, A. (2000). Decrease of vigilance assessed by EEG-mapping in type I diabetic patients with history of recurrent severe hypoglycaemia. *Psychoneuroendocrinology*, Vol. 25, No.1, pp. 85-105.

Hyllienmark, L.; Maltez, J.; Dandenell, A.; Ludvigsson, J. & Brismar T. (2005). EEG abnormalities with and without relation to severe hypoglycaemia in adolescents with type 1 diabetes. *Diabetologia*, Vol.48, No.3, pp. 412-419.

Iaione, F. & Marques, JL. (2005). Methodology for hypoglycaemia detection based on the processing.; analysis and classification of the electroencephalogram. *Med Biol Eng Comput*, Vol.43, No.4, pp. 501-507.

Iber, C.; Ancoli-Isreal, S.; Chesson, A.; & Quan, SF. (2007). The AASM Manual for the Scoring of Sleep and Associated Events, Rules, Terminology and Technical Specifications. 1st ed. American Academy of Sleep Medicine, Westchester, Illinois.

JDRF CGM Study Group. (2010). Prolonged nocturnal hypoglycemia is common during 12 months of continuous glucose monitoring in children and adults with type 1 diabetes. *Diabetes Care*, Vol. 33, No.5. pp. 1004-1008.

JDRF CGM Study Group. (2008). Continuous glucose monitoring and intensive treatment of type 1 diabetes. N *Engl J Med*, Vol. 359, pp. 1464–1476.

Joakims, T. (2002). *Leaning to Classify test using Support Vector Machines*. 1st ed. Kluwer Academic Publishers. Boston, USA.

Juhl, CB.; Hojlund, K.; Elsborg, R.; Poulsen, MK.; Selmar, PE.; Holst, JJ.; Christiansen, C & Beck-Nielsen, H. (2010). Automated detection of hypoglycemia-induced EEG changes recorded by subcutaneous electrodes in subjects with type 1 diabetes-The brain as a biosensor. *Diabetes Res Clin Pract*, Vol.88, No.1, pp. 22-28.

Lammert, M.; Hammer, M. & Frier, BM. (2009). Management of severe hypoglycaemia: cultural similarities.; differences and resource consumption in three European countries. *J Med Econ*, Vol.12, No.4, pp. 269-280.

Monami, M.; Marchionni, N. & Mannucci, E. (2009). Long-acting insulin analogues vs. NPH human insulin in type 1 diabetes. A meta-analysis. *Diabetes Obes Metab*, Vol. 11, No.4, pp. 372-378.

Pedersen-Bjergaard, U.; Pramming, S.; Heller, SR.; Wallace, TM.; Rasmussen, AK.; Jorgensen, HV.; Matthews, DR.; Hougaard, P & Thorsteinsson, B. (2004). Severe hypoglycaemia in 1076 adult patients with type 1 diabetes: influence of risk markers and selection. *Diabetes Metab Res Rev*, Vol.20, No.6, pp. 479-486.

Pickup, JC. & Sutton, AJ. (2008). Severe hypoglycaemia and glycaemic control in Type 1 diabetes: meta-analysis of multiple daily insulin injections compared with continuous subcutaneous insulin infusion. *Diabet Med*, Vol.25, No.7, pp. 765-774.

Pramming, S.; Thorsteinsson, B.; Stigsby, B. & Binder, C. (1988). Glycaemic threshold for changes in electroencephalograms during hypoglycaemia in patients with insulin dependent diabetes. *Br Med J (Clin Res Ed)* Vol.296, No.6623, pp.665-677.

Pramming, S.; Thorsteinsson, B.; Bendtson, I.; & Binder, C. (1990). The relationship between symptomatic and biochemical hypoglycaemia in insulin-dependent diabetic patients. *J Intern Med*, Vol.228, No.6, pp. 641-646.

Regan, PF. & Browne-Mayers, AN. (1956). Electroencephalography, frequency analysis and consciousness, a correlation during insulin-induced hypoglycemia. *J Nerv Ment Dis*, Vol.124, No.2, pp.142-147.

Ross, IS. & Loeser, LH. (1951). Electroencephalographic findings in essential hypoglycemia. *Electroencephalogr Clin Neurophysiol*, Vol.3, No.2, pp. 141-148.

Sigurdsson, S.; Larsen J.; Hansen LK.; Philipsen PA. & Wulf, HC. (2002). Outlier estimation and detection: Application to Skin Lesion Classification. *Proceedings of IEEE International conference on acoustics.; speech and signal processing.*

Tamborlane, WV.; Beck, RW.; Bode, BW.; Buckingham, B.; Chase, HP.; Clemons, R.; Fiallo-Scharer, R.; Fox,LA.; Gilliam,LK.; Hirsch, IB.; Huang, ES.; Kollman, C.; Kowalski, AJ.; Laffel, L.; Lawrence, JM.; Lee, J.; Mauras, N.; O'Grady, M.; Ruedy, KJ.; Tansey, M.; Tsalikian, E.; Weinzimer, S.; Wilson, DM.; Wolpert, H.; Wysocki, T. & Xing, Dl. (2008). Continuous glucose monitoring and intensive treatment of type 1 diabetes. *N Engl J Med*, Vol.359, No.14, pp.1464-1476.

Tamburrano, G.; Lala, A.; Locuratolo, N.; Leonetti, F.; Sbraccia, P.; Giaccari, A.; Busco, S. & Porcu, S. (1988). Electroencephalography and visually evoked potentials during moderate hypoglycemia. *J Clin Endocrinol Metab*, Vol.66, No.6, pp. 1301-1306.

The Diabetes Control and Complications Trial Research Group. (2009). The effect of continuous glucose monitoring in well-controlled type 1 diabetes. *Diabetes Care*, Vol.32, No.8, pp. 1378-83.

Tribl, G.; Howorka, K.; Heger, G.; Anderer, P.; Thoma, H. & Zeitlhofer, J. (1996). EEG topography during insulin-induced hypoglycemia in patients with insulin-dependent diabetes mellitus. *Eur Neurol*, Vol.36, No.5, pp. 303-309.

Van Den Enden, AWM. & Verhoeckx, NAM. (1989). Discrete-time signal processing. Prentice Hall. Hertfordshire, UK.

Woodward, A.; Weston, P.; Casson, IF. & Gill, GV. (2009). Nocturnal hypoglycaemia in type 1 diabetes-frequency and predictive factors. QJM, Vol.102, No.9, pp. 603-607.

13

Electrochemical Biosensor for Glycated Hemoglobin (HbA1c)

Mohammadali Sheikholeslam, Mark D. Pritzker and Pu Chen
University of Waterloo
Canada

1. Introduction

Diabetes is recognized as a group of heterogeneous disorders with the common elements of hyperglycaemia and glucose intolerance due to insulin deficiency, impaired effectiveness of insulin action or both (Harris & Zimmet, 1997). If left untreated or improperly managed, diabetes can result in a variety of complications, including heart disease, kidney disease, eye disease, impotence and nerve damage. Diagnosis and management of the disease require a tight monitoring of blood glucose levels that serves a number of purposes:

- provides a quick measurement of blood glucose level at a given time.
- determines if a diabetic person has a high or low blood glucose level at a given time.
- demonstrates the link between lifestyle, medication and blood glucose levels.
- helps diabetics and diabetes health-care teams make changes to lifestyle and medication that will improve blood glucose levels.

Electrochemical biosensors for glucose (glucose meters) play a leading role for this purpose. For the purpose of measuring daily glucose levels to control food intake and insulin usage, these glucose meters work although some difficulties exist. For example, blood glucose level measurements are recommended three to four times per day. Due to the large fluctuations in glucose levels that naturally occur over the course of a day, measurements on an empty stomach and within 2 h of eating are required for comparison purposes. These problems are more prominent for the diagnosis of diabetes and determining the link between lifestyle and medication once a patient has been diagnosed with this disease.

Historically, measurement of glucose levels has been the method universally used to diagnose diabetes. Laboratory methods such as fasting plasma glucose (FPG) or 2-h plasma glucose (2HPG) level have been used for this purpose. However, this approach still suffers from the same problems and difficulties associated with glucose biosensors such as the need for fasting, biological variability and the effects of acute perturbations (e.g., stress- or illness-related) on glucose levels. It has recently been concluded that the best marker for long term glycaemic control is whole blood glycated hemoglobin (i.e., hemoglobin A1c denoted as HbA1c) since its levels respond to the long-term progression of diabetes without the short-term fluctuations characteristic of glucose (Berg & Sacks, 2008). Also, the use of this approach solves many of the problems associated with FPG or 2HPG methods based on glucose measurements such as no need for fasting, substantially less biological variability and relative insensitivity of HbA1c levels to acute perturbations. On the other hand with advances in instrumentation and standardization, the accuracy and precision of A1C assays at least match those of glucose assays. Consequently, the decision was made by the International Expert Committee (with members appointed by the American Diabetes Association, the European Association for the Study of Diabetes, and the International Diabetes Federation) that the A1c assay should be considered as the primary method for the diagnosis of diabetes (Nathan, 2009).

HbA1c is a stable glycated hemoglobin derivative formed by the non-enzymatic reaction of glucose with the N-terminal valine of the β-chain of normal adult Hb (HbA). Since it reflects the average blood glucose level over the preceding 2-3 months and is not affected by the daily fluctuation of the glucose level, the HbA1c level provides a more accurate index for diagnosis and long term control of the disease. Traditionally, clinical laboratory assays for HbA1c have been obtained by ion-exchange chromatography, immunochemical methods, electrophoresis and boronate affinity chromatography. However, these methods are time-consuming, require trained personnel and expensive equipment and have limited availability in many areas of the world. So point-of-care (POC) devices are needed for diabetes diagnosis and management. Point-of-care testing (POCT) is defined as diagnostic testing at or near the site of patient care (Kost, 2002). The driving notion behind POCT is to bring the test conveniently and immediately to the patient. This increases the likelihood that the patient will receive the results in a timely manner. Such devices would allow for immediate availability of A1C measurements and greatly enhance diabetes care. Currently, eight HbA1c POC devices are available commercially with generally accepted performance criteria for HbA1c, but only one of them has met the acceptance criteria of NGSP[1] with two different reagent lots. Also, the reproducibility of production of the different reagent lots of the POC instruments investigated appears inadequate at this moment for optimal clinical use (Lenters-Westra & Slingerland, 2010). As a result, the American Diabetes Association (ADA) recently decided to exclude POC methods from their list of recommended methods for HbA1c diagnosis, stating that they are not yet accurate enough (NGSP, 2010). Also, among these POC instruments, only one is designed for patient use at home, whereas the others are suitable only for clinics and physician offices due to their high price ($1000-$3000) and complicated operation. Consequently, considerable work is still needed for the development of accurate, simple and cheap HbA1c biosensors. Although an HbA1c measurement is recommended quarterly and not as frequently as in the case of glucose, its role in prevention, diagnosis and management of diabetes is critical.

2. Electrochemical biosensors

A biochemical sensor is a small device consisting of a transducer covered by a biological recognition layer which interacts with the target analyte. The chemical changes resulting from this interaction are converted by the transducer into electrical signals. Electrochemical biosensors combine the analytical power of electrochemical techniques with the specificity of biological recognition processes to produce an electrical signal that is related to the concentration of an analyte (Wang, Analytical Electrochemistry, 2006). In electrochemical biosensors, the transducer is an electrode. Based on the nature of the biological recognition process, two general categories of electrochemical biosensors can be defined: biocatalytic devices (utilizing enzymes, cells or tissues as immobilized biocomponents) and affinity

[1] National Glycohemoglobin Standardization Program

sensors (based on antibodies, membrane receptors or nucleic acids) (Wang, Analytical Electrochemistry, 2006). Electrochemical biosensors can be further divided into the sub-categories of potentiometric, amperometric and impedimetric biosensors depending on their mode of operation (Pohanka & Skládal, 2008). Electrochemical biosensors are widely used in the medical field. One of the most important applications of such devices is for the diagnosis and management of diabetes, a topic which has received a great deal of interest due to its urgent need and as a model system for sensor development.

2.1 Glucose biosensors

Glucose biosensors are one of the key elements in treating and management of diabetes. Many diabetics use these devices to measure their blood glucose level every day. In fact, glucose biosensors occupy 85% of the entire biosensor market. Such huge market size has made diabetes a model disease for developing new biosensing concepts (Wang, Electrochemical Glucose Biosensors, 2008). It is has been about 36 years since the first commercial glucose biosensor was introduced into the commercial market (Pohanka & Skládal, 2008). From that date, different approaches have been explored and many devices have been designed for individual diabetes control. In spite of the huge development in glucose biosensors, diabetes control still has problems and so efforts are still being made to further improve their use. Issues such as *in vivo* glucose measurement and insulin delivery and long-term glucose level measurement are some areas of interest. As mentioned previously, the problems associated with the measurement of long-term blood glucose levels are leading to the development of HbA1c biosensors. HbA1c biosensors integrated with personal glucose biosensors can greatly improve management and treatment of diabetes.

3. HbA1c biosensors

3.1 Biosensors based on Fructosyl Valine (FV)

As mentioned previously, the problems associated with the measurement of long-term blood glucose levels are leading to the development of HbA1c biosensors. HbA1c biosensors integrated with personal glucose biosensors can greatly improve management and treatment of diabetes. As mentioned previously, HbA1c is formed through the non-enzymatic glycation of the terminal valine of beta sheets in hemoglobin. This HbA1c can be digested to small glycated peptide fructosyl valine (FV) that can be further oxidized by the enzyme fructosylamine oxidase (FAO). Enzymatic assay of HbA1c is based on the oxidation of FV (as a model compound).

In one of the first studies on FV enzyme sensors, Sode et. al. used an isolated fructosyl amine oxidase from marine yeast (Tsugawa, Ishimura, Ogawa, & Sode, 2000). They fabricated 2 types of sensors: a mediator-type enzyme sensor (using carbon paste electrode) and a hydrogen peroxidise-based enzyme electrode. Although lower potentials (150 mV vs. Ag/AgCl) were applied for the mediator-type probe than for the other one (600 mV vs. Ag/AgCl), the sensitivity of the hydrogen peroxidise sensor was found to be higher (0.42 $\mu A\ mM^{-1}\ cm^{-2}$). Consequently, further optimization of the operating conditions was needed as well as the sensor design. In a subsequent study, this group developed an FAO-peroxidase-ferrocene sensor and a Prussian blue-based FAO sensor (Tsugawa, Ogawa, Ishimura, & Sode, 2001). The sensitivities of these probes were found to be similar to that of the earlier hydrogen peroxidise sensor but the applied potentials were lowered dramatically

(-250 mV and -50 mV for FAO-peroxidase-ferrocene sensor and Prussian blue-based FAO sensor, respectively). However the linear range of the current-concentration calibration curves for both sensors was narrower and the response times were longer than in the case of the hydrogen peroxidase sensor.

Molecular imprinting is a technique to create template-shaped cavities in polymer matrices with memory for the template molecules to be used in molecular recognition (Alexander, et al., 2006). Sode et. al. employed a synthetic polymer (polyvinylimidazole denoted as PVI) as a catalyst for fabrication of an amperometric FV sensor (Sode, Takahashi, Ohta, Tsugawa, & Yamazaki, 2001). They combined this catalytic center with molecular imprinting for oxidative cleavage of FV. In their method, a mixture of carbon paste and PVI was applied on the electrode. The constructed electrode was then immersed in the phosphate buffer electrolyte containing m-PMS as mediator (Fig. 1). The current for the anodic oxidation of the reduced mediator (resulting from oxidation of FV) was monitored after applying an electrode potential of +100mV vs. Ag/AgCl. This system showed a linear relation between the current and the fructosylvaline concentration over the range from 50µM to 10mM in the presence of 5mg/ml PVI. Fig. 2 shows an excellent linear response of the current over a FV concentration range from 20µM to 0.7mM. Although the electrode sensitivity was not reported, they reported a detection limit for the sensor of about 20µM, which is acceptable for diabetes diagnosis, and measurement reproducibility within 10%. Also, the current response of a bare carbon electrode was found to be about 15% of that obtained in the presence of the PVI catalyst.

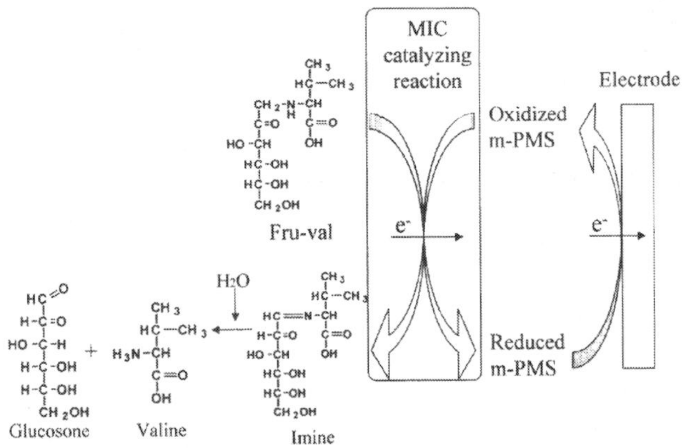

Fig. 1. Oxidative fructosylamine cleavage reaction and detection on MIC-employing electrode (Sode, Ohta, Yanai, & Yamazaki, 2003).

Since FV is an expensive reagent, it is the limiting factor for its utilization as the template for sensor fabrication. Proteolytic digestion of HbA1c for production of FV also leads to the formation of another fructosylamine compound (fructosyl lysine denoted as Fru-ε-lys) which is the proteolytic product of digestion of glycated albumin in the blood and can interfere with the detection of FV. So Sode and coworkers developed a sensor for better selectivity for FV over fructosyl lysine and used methyl valine (m-val) which is a cheaper analogue of expensive FV as the template (Sode, Ohta, Yanai, & Yamazaki, 2003). Also, they used the positively charged functional monomer allylamine to improve the selectivity of the

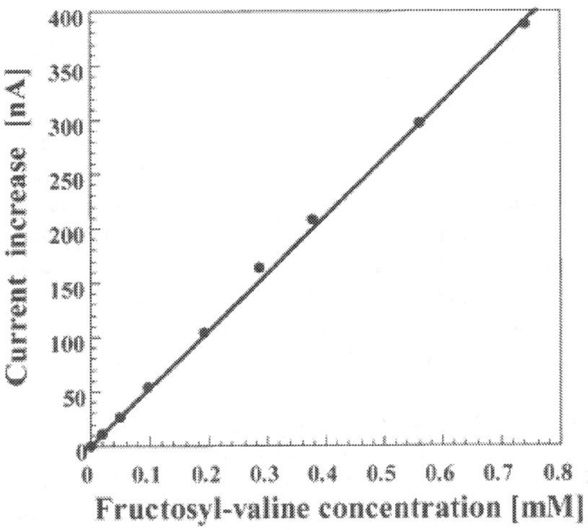

Fig. 2. Calibration curve for amperometric fructosylamine sensor employing PVI as the catalyst. The measurements were carried out in 10mM potassium phosphate buffer (pH 7.0) containing 1mM m-PMS at 50◦C (Sode, Takahashi, Ohta, Tsugawa, & Yamazaki, 2001).

sensor toward FV. Both the sensitivity and selectivity (FV/Fru-ε-lys) decreased from 135nA/mM to 95nA/mM and 1.8 to 1.6, respectively, after replacing the FV template with m-val. However, with the introduction of allylamine as the functional monomer, the selectivity increased to 1.9, while a sensitivity of 95nA/mM could be maintained. Thus, with these two modifications, selectivity increased slightly, while the sensitivity decreased in exchange for a more inexpensive template (m-val). Table 1 shows a comparison of the sensitivities and selectivities achieved by the use of different polymers in their study.

Polymer	Template	Allylamine	Sensitivity (nA/mM)		Selectivity (Fru-val/Fru-ε-lys)
			Fru-val	Fru-ε-lys	
P1	—	—	79 (R^2 > 0.984)	70 (R^2 > 0.988)	1.1
P2	Fru-val	—	135 (R^2 > 0.992)	75 (R^2 > 0.982)	1.8
P3	m-val	—	95 (R^2 > 0.984)	60 (R^2 > 0.968)	1.6
P4	m-ε-lys	—	84 (R^2 > 0.980)	101 (R^2 > 0.976)	0.8
P5	—	+	91 (R^2 > 0.996)	54 (R^2 > 0.998)	1.7
P6	m-val	+	95 (R^2 > 0.992)	50 (R^2 > 0.980	1.9

Table 1. Sensitivity and selectivity of polymers for fructosylamine compounds (Sode, Ohta, Yanai, & Yamazaki, 2003).

Fang and his coworkers developed a single-use, disposable fructosyl valine amperometric biosensor. Since HbA1c measurement is vital for long-term management of diabetes in patients, a cheap single-use disposable HbA1c sensor could be very useful in this regard. They used screen-printed electrodes for sensor fabrication and incorporated iridium into the electrodes as a catalyst (Fig. 3). Both the working and counter electrodes were iridium-modified carbon, while the reference electrode was Ag/AgCl. Fructosyl amine oxidase

(FAO) was immobilized on the working electrode for detection of H_2O_2 produced enzymatically from FV in a 3μL sample. Amperometric measurements were done in a medium containing PBS, FV and potassium chloride as the supporting electrolyte at pH 7.0 and room temperature for 120 seconds after applying an electrode potential of +0.25 V at HbA1c concentrations from 0 to 2 mM that correspond to the range relevant to physiological conditions. The results are shown in Fig. 4 and Fig. 5. Fang et al claimed a sensitivity of 21.5 μA mM^{-1} cm^{-2} for their sensor which is several orders of magnitude larger than the value reported in the physiological range. At the same time, their applied potential of +0.25 V was lower than that used in most previous studies on this type of sensor. However their FV samples were synthesized using L-valine and glucose and so should not have experienced the potential interferences due to the presence of the proteolytic products of HbA1c other than FV.

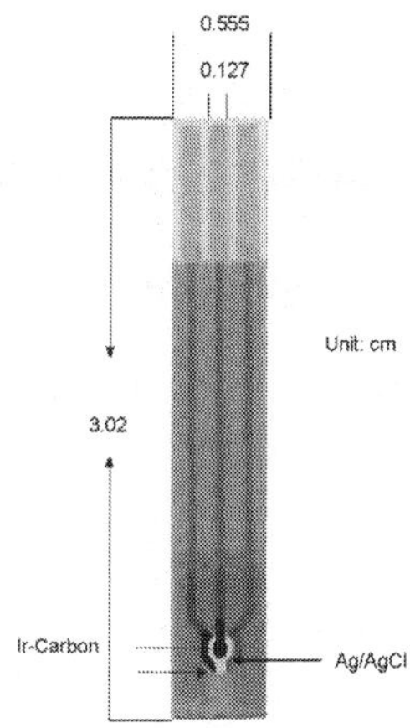

Fig. 3. The configuration of the thick-film sensor (Fang, Li, Zhou, & Liu, 2009).

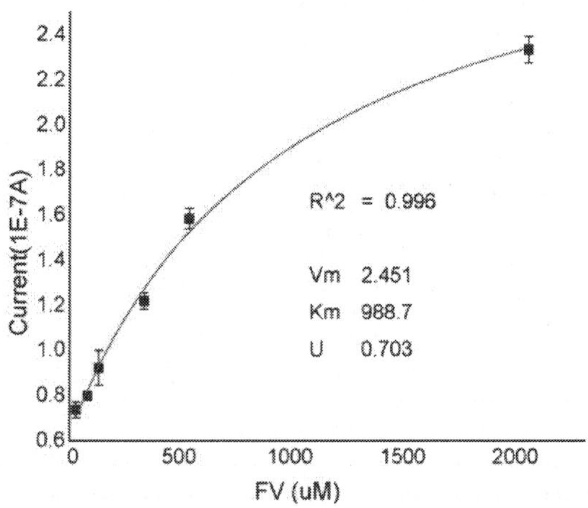

Fig. 4. Calibration curve for the FV biosensor (Fang, Li, Zhou, & Liu, 2009).

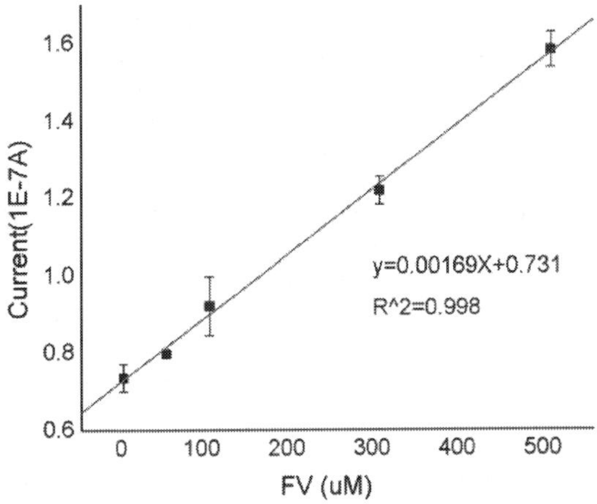

Fig. 5. Calibration curve for the FV biosensor at concentrations below 1mM FV (Fang, Li, Zhou, & Liu, 2009).

In another study, Chuang et. al. used the same technique of molecular imprinting to fabricate a potentiometric FV biosensor (Chuang, Rick, & Chou, 2009). They made molecular imprints of FV in a poly-aminophenylboronic acid (p-APBA) polymer on conductive indium-doped tin oxide (ITO) electrodes. Electrochemical characterization of the fabricated biosensor was carried out by comparing the open circuit potential (E_{oc}) of the ITO carrying the molecular imprinted polymer (MIP) with that measured on a non-imprinted control in 10mL phosphate buffer (pH 7.0) with a standard Ag/AgCl reference electrode to assess the affinity of the FV imprints for FV, D-fructose, D-glucose and L-valine. The ΔE_{oc} values obtained when the imprinted electrode was introduced into solutions containing 10 mM FV, 10 mM D-fructose, 10 m D-glucose and 10 mM L-valine were found to be ~5.0×10^{-3} V , ~2.9×10^{-3} V, ~4.0×10^{-4} V and less than 1.0×10^{-5} V, respectively. The higher ΔE_{oc} values measured in the presence of D fructose than D glucose indicates that the electrode recognises the limited structural similarity between D-fructose and D-glucose. Also, it is apparent that the affinity of the imprinted electrode for FV is higher than for the others. The suggestion was made that this may be due to both shape complementarity (as evident in the case of D-fructose and D-glucose) and charge effects. The p-APBA polymer has a net positive charge in pH 7.0 buffer while FV is negatively charged. Selectivity through shape recognition was attributed mainly to the imprinting of the carbohydrate component of FV, as suggested from a comparison of the ΔE_{oc} values for fructose, glucose and valine.

Electrochemical oxidation of FV on a bare glassy carbon paste electrode (GCPE) in the absence of an enzyme was reported by Chien et. al (Chien & Chou, 2010). The electrode was prepared by applying a glassy carbon microparticle paste on the ITO substrate using a baking process. This GCPE was characterized and reported to have higher sensitivity on FV and lower background current compared with conventional glassy carbon electrodes. After studying the polarization behaviour of FV to determine an appropriate applied potential that would yield higher sensitivity and signal-to-noise ratio (+0.1 V), the current response of the GCPE to successive additions of FV (0 to 1mM) was collected by chronoamperometric measurement in a phosphate buffer (pH 7.4) (Fig. 6). The average response time and stabilization time between each addition was found to be 40 and 100 seconds, respectively. According to the data (correlation between FV concentration and the response current in phosphate buffer) shown in the inset of Fig.6, the response current increased from 0.27 μA to 5.52 μA as the FV concentration increased from 0 to 1.0 mM. These data also show a good linearity with an R^2 value of 0.999. The sensitivity of the biosensor was found to be 5.26 μAmM^{-1} and the minimum detection limit less than 0.1 mM. Chien et al. also showed that an increase in pH leads to a rise in the oxidation current. Moreover, the biosensor exhibited a high selectivity for FV as D-glucose, D-fructose and L-valine had no interference on the current response. However, it should be acknowledged that their FV samples were synthesized using L-valine and glucose so the use of a high applied potential may cause interference and necessitate the inclusion of a mediator in future applications.

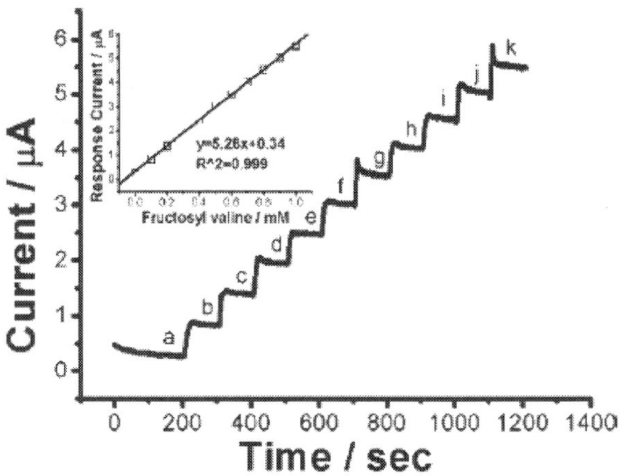

Fig. 6. Chronoamperometric response at GCPE (glassy carbon microparticles/mineral oil 50/50 (w/w) %). FV concentrations, increasing in mM L^{-1} increments, are shown as: (a) 0, (b) 0.1, (c) 0.2, (d) 0.3, (e) 0.4, (f) 0.5, (g) 0.6, (h) 0.7, (i) 0.8, (j) 0.9, (k) 1. The current readings were observed to stabilize for approximately 100s. The supporting electrolyte was phosphate buffer (pH 7.4), the operating potential was +1.0 V (vs. Ag/AgCl) with the measurements being made at ambient temperature. Inset: Calibration curve obtained for different concentrations of FV (Chien & Chou, 2010).

3.2 Biosensors based on HbA1c

Other types of HbA1c biosensors detect HbA1c directly. Different methods and techniques have been applied for these types of HbA1c biosensor. One of their potential advantages is that there is no need for two time-consuming preliminary steps to release fructosyl valine from HbA1c by a protease (one of the main drawbacks with FV POC instruments).

Stöllner et al. developed an immunoenzymometric assay (IEMA) in which a glycated pentapeptide (with an amino acid sequence corresponding to the first 5 amino acids of the N-terminal hemoglobin sequence of the beta-chain) was used as an HbA1c analogue on the surface of either a microtiter plate or an amino-modified cellulose membrane (Stöllner, Warsinke, Stöcklein, Dölling, & Scheller, 2001). In this sensor, this glycated peptide competes with HbA1c in the sample for antigen binding sites of anti-HbA1c. After a washing step, a glucose oxidase-conjugated antibody is applied to indicate the previously bound antibodies to the glycated peptide. Then the bound enzyme conjugates are measured optically. This procedure yielded the relation between signal intensity and HbA1c concentration shown in Fig. 7. At a total hemoglobin concentration of 30 µg ml^{-1} (456 nM), a reasonably linear dependence of absorbance on concentration is obtained in the range of 5-50% HbA1c. Furthermore, the authors reported no decrease in binding affinity of the glycated pentapeptide modified substrate to the anti-HbA1c antibodies even after being subjected to more than 20 repeated regeneration cycles. The authors did not present a similar diagram for their biosensor based on a cellulose membrane.

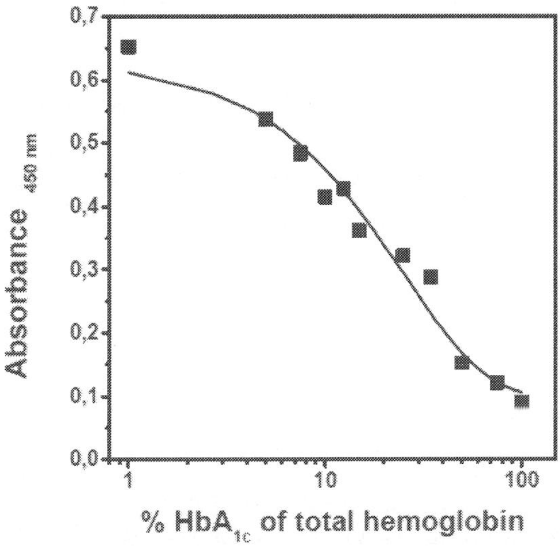

Fig. 7. Calibration curve for HbA1c measured with the Hemoglobin-A1c-ELISA at a final concentration of total hemoglobin of 30 mg ml-1 (465 nM) (Stöllner, Warsinke, Stöcklein, Dölling, & Scheller, 2001).

In a subsequent study, Stöllner et al and co-workers modified this biosensor for use as an amperometric immunosensor (Stöllner, Stöcklein, Scheller, & Warsinke, 2002). Their system works in 2 steps: selective enrichment of total hemoglobin on the surface of an affinity matrix followed by specific detection of immobilized HbA1c using a GOx-conjugated anti-HbA1c antibody. The affinity matrix consists of a cellulose membrane (fixed to a platinum surface) covalently immobilized by either haptoglobin (strong hemoglobin-binding protein) or anti-hemoglobin antibody. In this way, the surface of the biosensor becomes saturated with a variety of hemoglobin and HbA1c-type compounds that can be detected by amperometric (or optical) measurement of enzymatically produced H_2O_2 from GOx labels (Fig. 8). Electrochemical measurement was done in a PBS electrolyte after allowing the system to reach equilibrium after a potential of +600 mV vs. Ag/AgCl was applied. By preparing HbA1c samples with known concentrations in 3%BSA/PBS (blocking buffer), they did not have to determine the total hemoglobin concentration.

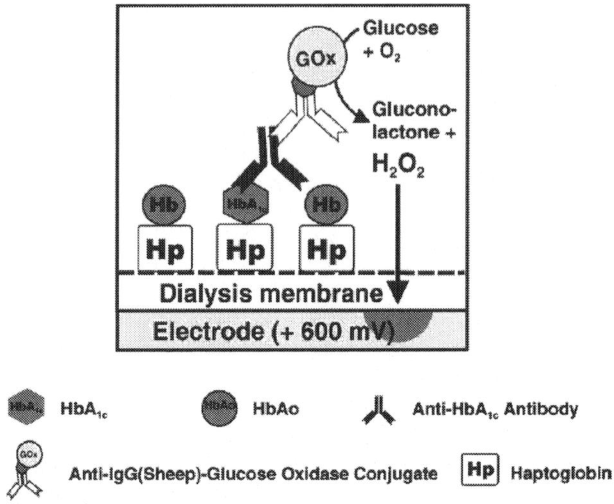

Fig. 8. Principle of the electrochemical HbA1c immunosensor (Stöllner, Stöcklein, Scheller, & Warsinke, 2002).

Their ELISA analysis showed a better reproducibility, higher sensitivity and signal-to-background ratio for the haptoglobin-based sensor than the one based on the anti-hemoglobin antibody. These researchers mentioned that this may be due to the more accessible glycated N-terminus of the β-chain of hemoglobin as a result of hemoglobin unfolding prior to the formation of a complex with haptoglobin. On the other hand, in the case of anti-hemoglobin antibody, the glycated N-terminal of the β-chain might be sterically hindered and less accessible for the anti-HbA1c antibody due to random orientation of hemoglobin molecules and a slight denaturation, As shown in Figs. 9 and 10, both ELISA and electrochemical analysis of HbA1c showed a linear correlation between %HbA1c of total hemoglobin and the signal (either absorbance or current) in the clinically relevant range of 5-20% HbA1c. The signal at 0% HbA1c corresponds to background effects. As can be seen, this background signal is relatively low in the case of the ELISA method, but comparable to the measurement obtained at 5% HbA1c using the electrochemical method. This background effect may be due to non-specific binding of the anti-HbA1c-GOx conjugate. The other problem with the electrochemical method is a standard deviation of 5-15% due to the use of one haptoglobin-modified membrane per sample in comparison to parallel screening with the ELISA method. Also, separate immunochemical reaction and indication steps of the bound GOx are required because of unspecific binding of the involved proteins to the plastic wall of the electrochemical cell. The time needed for HbA1c measurement in this work is approximately 3h due to non-optimized incubation times.

More recently, the same group published another study on an HbA1c biosensor based on electrochemical detection of ferroceneboronic acid (FcBA)-bound HbA1c (Liu, Wollenberger, Katterle, & Scheller, 2006). They introduced more electrochemical techniques in this approach. A zirconium dioxide nanoparticle-modified pyrolytic graphite electrode (PGE) was used in the presence of didodecyldimethylammonium bromide (DDAB) for total hemoglobin immobilization rather than a haptoglobin-modified cellulose membrane on a

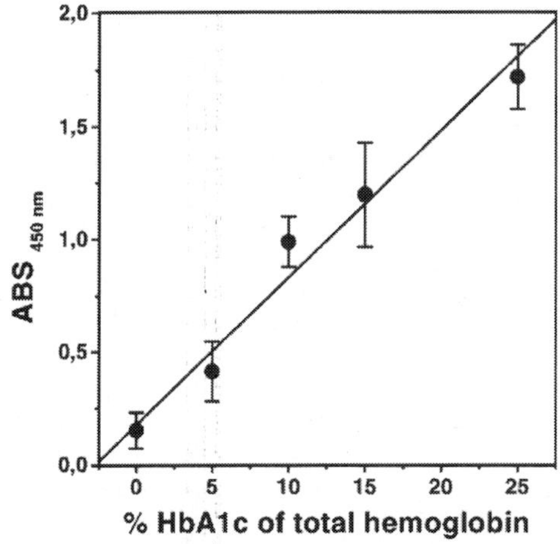

Fig. 9. Calibration curve for HbA1c measured with the sandwich immunoassay carried out on haptoglobin-modified cellulose membranes. The enzyme label GOx was detected optically (Stöllner, Stöcklein, Scheller, & Warsinke, 2002).

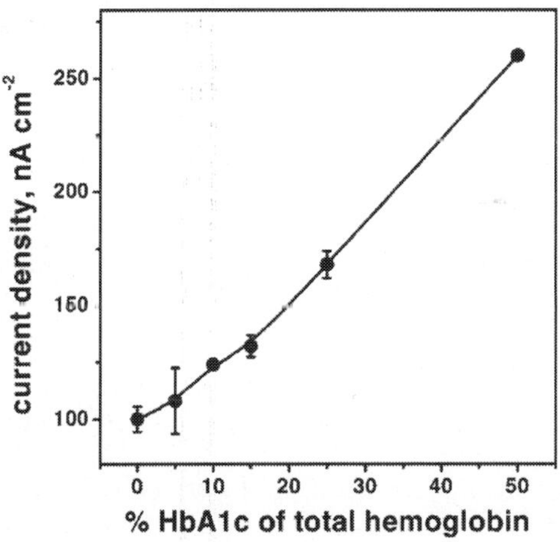

Fig. 10. Calibration curve for HbA1c using amperometric indication of the produced H_2O_2. The haptoglobin-modified cellulose membranes were fixed onto a Clark-type electrode (Stöllner, Stöcklein, Scheller, & Warsinke, 2002).

platinum electrode. Also, electrochemical measurement of HbA1c involved the use of FcBA instead of an anti-HbA1c-GOx conjugate. The PGE is used for protein (total hemoglobin) immobilization and DDAB accelerates electron transfer between hemoglobin and the electrode. Purified hemolysed erythrocytes from real human blood sample were mixed with the suspension of ZrO_2 nanoparticles in the DDAB solution and then applied to the electrode surface for total hemoglobin immobilization. Afterward, the electrode with immobilized hemoglobin was incubated in FcBA solution for 30 min. The aromatic derivatives of boronic acid can react with 1,2- or 1,3-cis-diols to form reversible cyclic boronic esters in aqueous solutions under mild and easily controllable reaction conditions (Fig. 11). Consequently, FcBA serves 2 functions: selective binding to HbA1c over the other immobilized hemoglobins (using boronic acid part) and participation in the electrochemical reaction for HbA1c measurement through its ferrocene part. The total immobilized hemoglobin content was determined using cyclic voltammetry (CV) in pH 8.0 PBS solution, while the bound FcBA was detected using square wave voltammetry (SWV). SWV was used instead of CV since the chemically modified sensor with bound hemoglobin exhibited a relatively large charging current and higher sensitivity for the Fc label. The cyclic voltammogram obtained in the presence of hemoglobin-immobilized PEG showed 2 peaks related to the Fe(II)-Fe(III)-couple of the heme groups in hemoglobin. The hemoglobin concentration was obtained by integration of the reduction peak. Fig. 12 shows square wave voltammograms for a hemoglobin sensor obtained in solutions containing 2 different HbA1c concentrations before and after incubation in the presence of FcBA. The peak current increases significantly after incubation in the presence of FcBA and with increasing HbA1c percentage in total hemoglobin. Calibration curves for determination of %HbA1c at various total hemoglobin concentrations are presented in Fig. 13. From the point of view of sensitivity, the optimal total hemoglobin concentration is between 20-50μM. Measurement reproducibility of the fabricated sensor reported for 10.2% HbA1c samples at the different total hemoglobin concentrations was found to be 12.7% on average. Deviation of the HbA1c% measurements from the values obtained using the HPLC-based standard reference method was found to be quite high and vary from -10.7% to 31% for the 20 samples analyzed. The requirement for the separate determination of the total hemoglobin content also makes this an inconvenient aspect of this method.

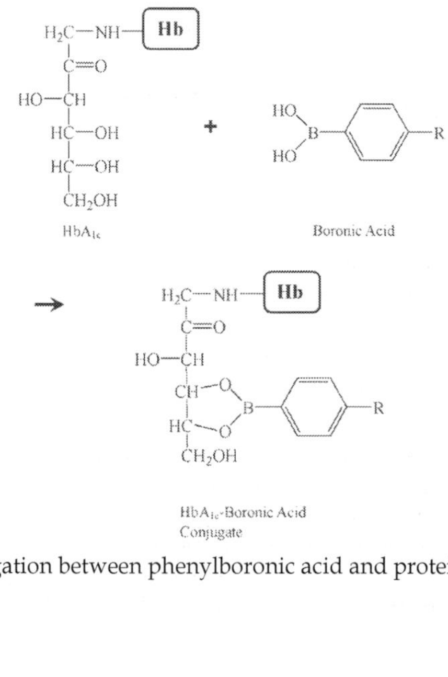

Fig. 11. Mode of conjugation between phenylboronic acid and protein HbA1c (Song & Yoon, 2009).

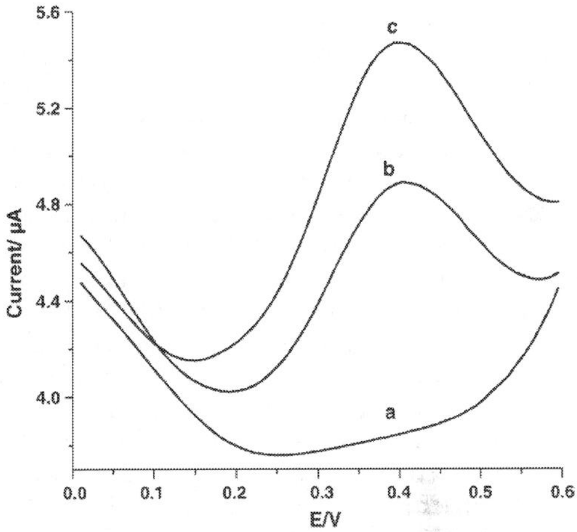

Fig. 12. Square wave voltammograms of a sensor containing 6.8% glycated hemoglobin before (a) and after incubation in FcBA (b) and Hb containing 14% glycated hemoglobin after incubation in FcBA (c) (Liu, Wollenberger, Katterle, & Scheller, 2006).

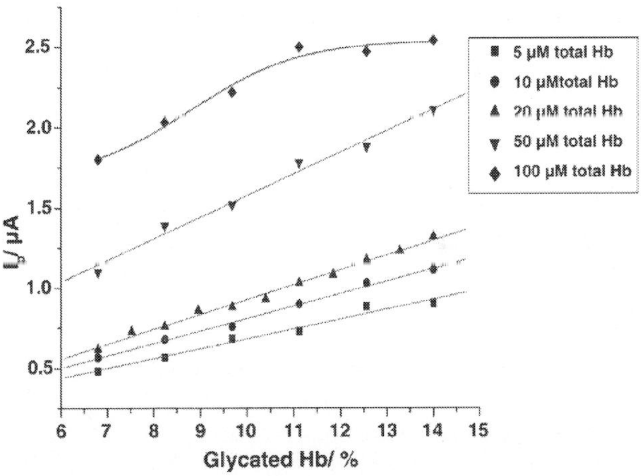

Fig. 13. Calibration curve for glycated hemoglobin determination for 3 µl 5µM total Hb (■), 10µM total Hb (•), 20µM total Hb (▲), 50µM total Hb (▼) and 100µM total Hb (♦) (Liu, Wollenberger, Katterle, & Scheller, 2006).

More recently, Scheller et. al. further modified their previous amperometric HbA1c sensor into an electrochemical piezoelectric sensor (Halámek J. , Wollenberger, Stöcklein, & Scheller, 2007). The total hemoglobin content was determined using a mass-sensitive quartz crystal modified with a surfactant, while the FcBA-bound HbA1c on the surface was measured using square wave voltammetry. A piezoelectric quartz crystal was coated with gold and covalently modified with the surfactants. Of the four surfactants evaluated, deoxycholate (DOCA) was found to be optimal with regard to hemoglobin surface loading, regeneration and direct reduction of the bound hemoglobin. Unlike their previous work, blood samples were first incubated with FcBA and then applied on the modified surface. The boronic acid/diol interaction is much faster in alkaline conditions; on the other hand, hemoglobin has lower stability at these pHs. Consequently, the optimum pH for incubation was found to be 8.0. Denaturation of hemoglobin before incubation with FcBA (by heat treating at 75 °C for 300s) is required for detection of HbA1c and the electrochemical response of the heme groups and also increases binding with DOCA-modified surface. The amount of the total hemoglobin bound to the surface is monitored by a quartz crystal nanobalance (QCN). Upon immobilization of hemoglobin on the electrode surface, the oscillation frequency of the quartz crystal decreases. The decrease in the frequency is proportional to the amount of adsorbed total hemoglobin. Fig. 14 shows a typical response of the QCN upon hemoglobin binding and regeneration of the DOCA-modified piezosensor. The oscillation frequency decreases after hemoglobin binding, but increases again after washing loosely bound hemoglobin and returns back to the baseline after regeneration and removal of bound hemoglobin. More than 30 binding-regeneration cycles were possible without loss of sensitivity.

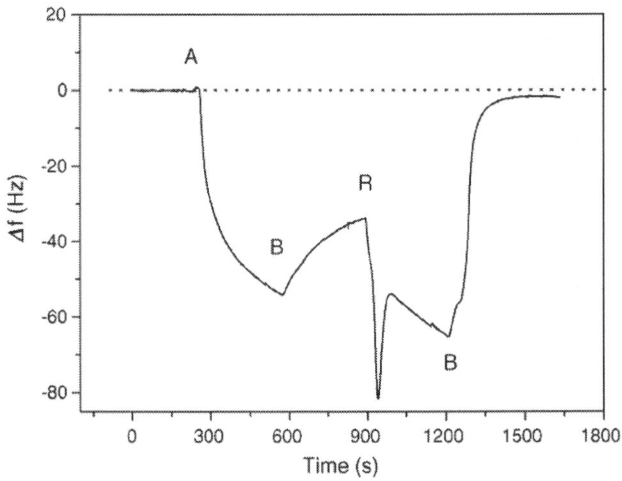

Fig. 14. Typical QCN response after Hb-binding to the DOCA-modified piezosensor. (A) Injection of Hb (7.75μM) is followed by (B) washing with buffer (Sörensen phosphate buffer pH 7.5) and (R) 5 min regeneration using pepsin solution. The dotted line represents the baseline of the piezoelectric quartz crystal. Before measurement, Hb was incubated at 75 °C for 300 s (Halámek J. , Wollenberger, Stöcklein, & Scheller, 2007).

These researchers used the same method of square wave voltammetry used in their earlier work for measurement of the FcBA-bound HbA1c (Fig. 15). To ensure that all HbA1c molecules are bound to FcBA, they added a 12-fold excess of FcBA to total hemoglobin. Fig. 16 shows the dependence of the current peak height of the SWV on %HbA1c. The standard deviation of this calibration curve obtained from 5 measurements of each sample is relatively high. This was partly attributed to the fact that the data were obtained in experiments performed over a period of 5 days. Further optimization of the technique to reduce the measurement variability and attain a detection limit below 5% HbA1c is needed.

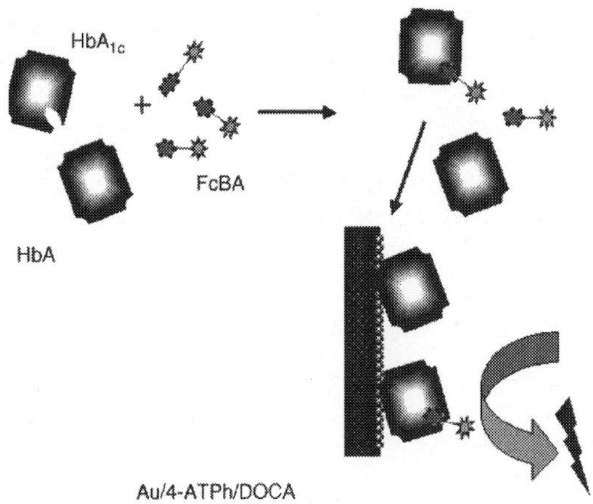

Fig. 15. Scheme of the electrochemical HbA1c sensor based on binding of FcBA-labelled HbA1c to the surface of the DOCA-modified piezoelectric quartz crystal and voltammetric read out of the label (Halámek J. , Wollenberger, Stöcklein, & Scheller, 2007).

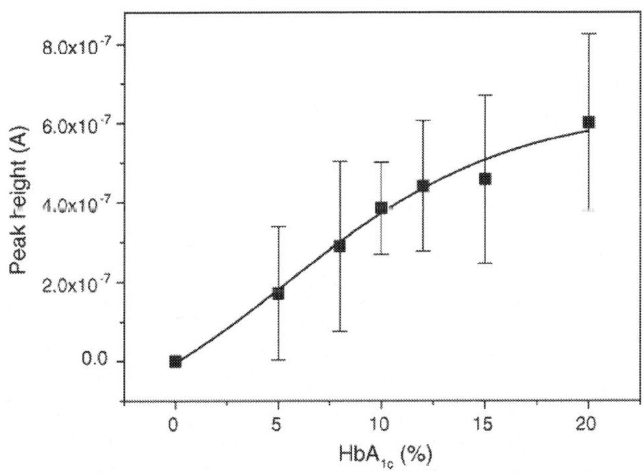

Fig. 16. Dependence of peak height of the SWV at +200mV vs. Ag/AgCl (1M KCl) on HbA1c content in Hb sample. Hb samples (7.75μM solution in Sörensen phosphate buffer pH 8.0) were preincubated with 1mMFcBAsolution at 75 °C for 300 s (number of measurements per sample n = 5) (Halámek J. , Wollenberger, Stöcklein, & Scheller, 2007).

The same sensor was modified to enhance the signal by *in situ* tagging of an anti-HbA1c antibody with FcBA (Halámek J. , Wollenberger, Stöcklein, Warsinke, & Scheller, 2007). Measurement of the total immobilized hemoglobin was done by QCN as before, but an additional step of incubating the anti-HbA1c antibody for 300s was done before introducing FcBA to the system. This antibody selectively binds to the glycated N-terminus of the β-chains of HbA1c. According to its structure, at least 5-6 terminal glycated residues contain vicinal cis-diol groups compared with 1-2 terminal sugar residues of the β-chains of HbA1c. Therefore, more FcBA per HbA1c molecule can bind to the surface and produce a higher SWV peak current and thereby increase the electrochemical signal. A comparison of this approach with that of direct tagging of HbA1c with FcBA described previously shows a 3.6-fold increase in sensitivity (Fig. 17). Although all the experiments were conducted in a single day, the standard deviations based on 3 measurements per sample were still high and accurate detection of HbA1c levels below 5% was still a problem.

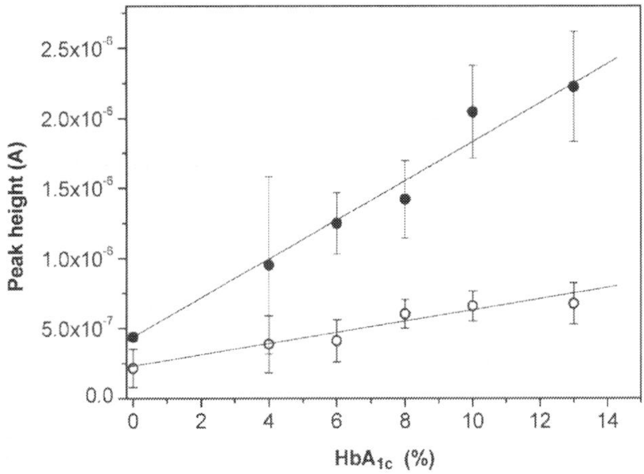

Fig. 17. Dependence of peak height of the SWV at +300 mV versus Ag/AgCl (1M KCl) on the HbA1c content in the Hb sample (total Hb 7.75 µM in Sörensen buffer pH 8.0, preincubated at 75°C). After immobilization of Hb onto the DOCA sensor, either FcBA (○) or anti-HbA1c Ab and then FcBA (•) was injected. SWV were then measured in stopped flow (Halámek J. , Wollenberger, Stöcklein, Warsinke, & Scheller, 2007).

Son et al fabricated a disposable biochip for electrochemical HbA1c measurement (Son, Seo, Choi, & Lee, 2006). They used ferricyanide ($K_3Fe(CN)_6$) as mediator so that the electrons released from the oxidation of Fe^{2+} in hemoglobin were transferred to the electrode by the ferricyanide/ferrocyanide couple. A schematic view of their %HbA1c measurement procedure is shown in Fig. 18. The components integrated in the system are a pair of interdigitated array (IDA) electrodes, HbA1c binding chamber, blood lysis chamber, filter, micro-pump and microchannel. After plasma separation (1) and red blood cell (RBC) lysis (2), the total hemoglobin stream branches off into two separate streams: in the lower stream HbA1c is immobilized on a packed agarose bead containing m-amino-phenylboronic acid (m-APBA) in the binding chamber and releases hemoglobin, while total hemoglobin flows in the upper stream (3). The ratio of the resulting electrochemical signals from the lower and upper streams after passing through the IDA electrodes yields the %HbA1c. Due to the non-homogeneous distribution of hemoglobin, the instantaneous current varies as a sample flows through the IDA electrodes. Consequently, the integral of the current over time was used for measurement. Unfortunately, no information on the performance of this biosensor was provided in the article.

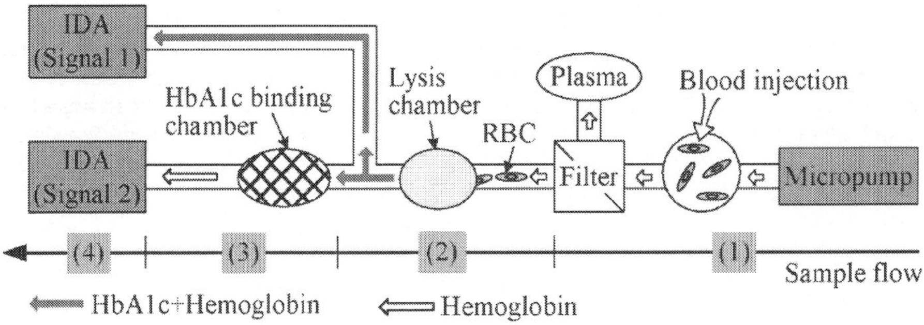

Fig. 18. Schematic of the %HbA1c measurement process (Son, Seo, Choi, & Lee, 2006).

In another study, Park et. al. reported an electrochemical HbA1c measurement method based on selective immobilization of HbA1c on a gold electrode covered with a thiophene-3-boronic acid (T3BA) self-assembled monolayer (SAM) and detecting HbA1c by label-free electrochemical impedance spectroscopy (EIS) (Park, Chang, Nam, & Park, 2008). Presumably, these researchers chose to modify the gold electrode with T3BA based on the common use of 3-aminophenylboronic acid to bind to a solid support for HbA1c separation from hemoglobin in boronate affinity chromatography. This species can form a self assembling monolayer (SAM) on a gold surface. The reported binding mechanism is based on bonding between the sulphur atom of the π-stacked thiophene SAM and the gold. The binding of T3BA and formation of a SAM on the gold was confirmed by the use of a quartz crystal microbalance (QCM), atomic force microscopy (AFM) and EIS experiments. Figs. 19 and 20 show the progress of T3BA binding over time as measured by QCM and an AFM image of a HbA1c/T3BA-SAM, respectively.

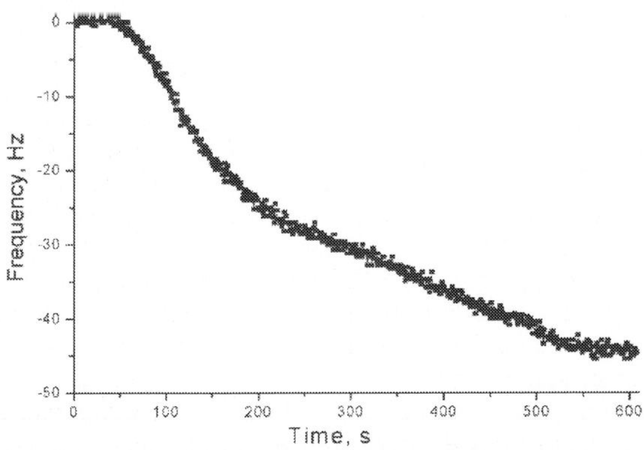

Fig. 19. QCM results for the HbA1c binding upon injection of 100 μL of diluted 11.6% HbA1c solution into 2 mL of the pH 8.5 buffer solution (10 mM 4-ethylmorpholine) (Park, Chang, Nam, & Park, 2008).

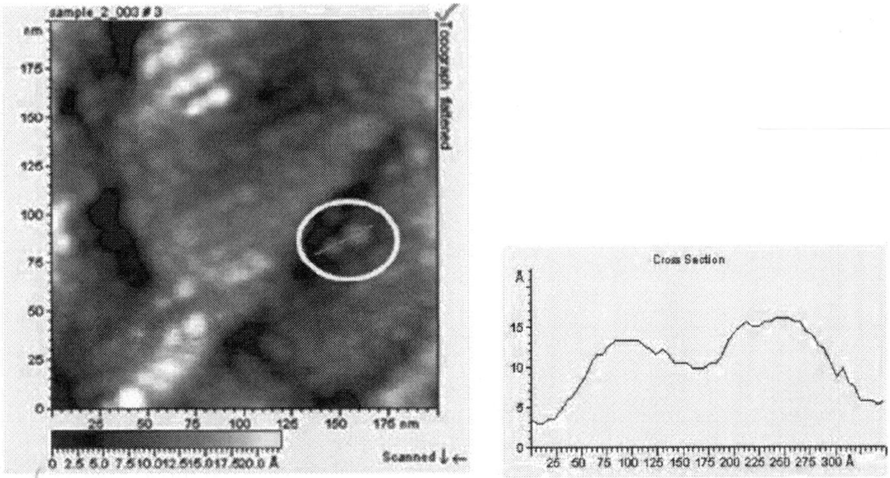

Fig. 20. AFM image the HbA1c/T3BA-SAM immobilized on it (left) along with corresponding cross-sectional profiles of the spots marked by white circles on the images (right) (Park, Chang, Nam, & Park, 2008).

Electrochemical determination of selectively immobilized HbA1c on the T3BA SAM is based on measuring the change in the capability of the gold electrode for electron transfer due to blocking of the electrode surface by HbA1c after immobilization. This is conducted using standard HbA1c solutions diluted with a buffered (pH 8.5) solution containing 10 mM 4-ethylmorpholine in a 3-electrode cell including a gold disk working electrode (0.020 cm^2), Ag/AgCl reference electrode and platinum spiral wire counter electrode. The T3BA SAM has been found to have relatively high electrochemical activity since the charge transfer resistance R_{ct} is small only when it forms on the surface. On the basis of the shape of the EIS Nyquist plot obtained, the SAM appears to cover the electrode surface uniformly with no significant defects. The subsequent addition of HbA1c to the system causes the R_{ct} value to increase significantly. As shown in Fig. 21, the ratio of R_{ct} obtained in the presence of HbA1c to that obtained in its absence increases linearly with HbA1c concentration. Similarly, this ratio varies linearly with %HbA1c in samples with the same total hemoglobin concentration (Fig. 22). Such linear behaviour makes the T3BA-SAM modified electrode a satisfactory platform for a HbA1c sensor. On the other hand, these results indicate that the variation of this signal with HbA1c concentration also depends on total hemoglobin concentration. Consequently, the total hemoglobin concentration must also be determined to obtain the HbA1c content. Electrode regeneration can be carried out by washing with a sodium acetate buffer at pH 5.0. Since this method is not selective for HbA1c over glycated albumin (also present in blood under hyperglycemic conditions), glycated albumin must be separated from RBC by centrifugation.

In another study, Song and Yoon used a boronic acid-modified thin film interface for selective binding of HbA1c followed by electrochemical biosensing using an enzymatic backfilling assay (Song & Yoon, 2009). They used a freshly evaporated gold working electrode for the bottom-up layer formation process (Fig. 23). This procedure began with the formation of an amine-reactive DTSP SAM on the gold which was then transferred to a

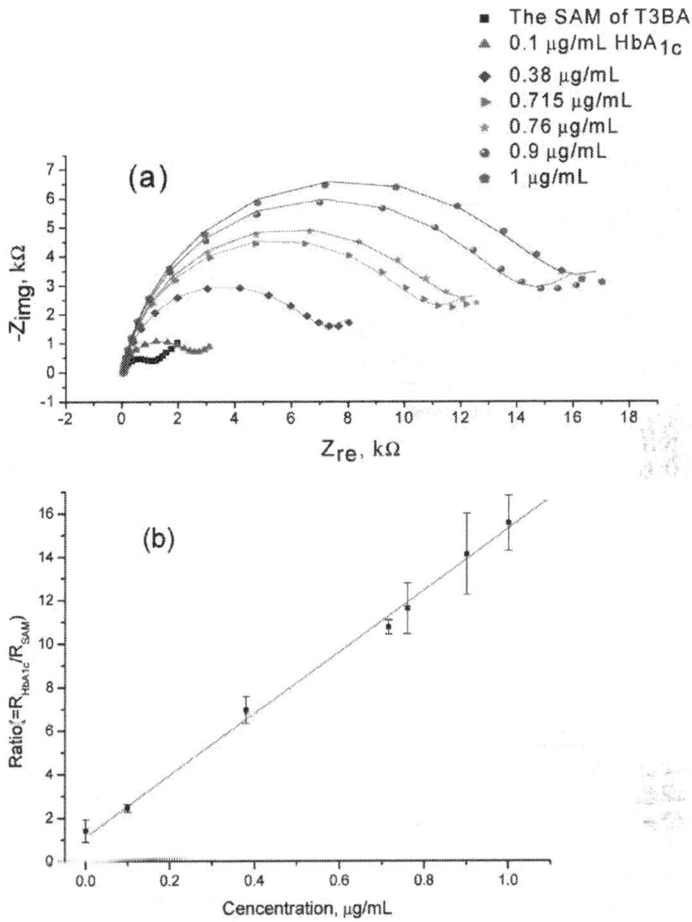

Fig. 21. (a) Impedance data obtained for the T3BA-SAM-covered electrode before and after immersion into various HbA1c concentrations diluted with 10 mM 4-ethylmorpholine buffer (pH 8.5) for 5 min. (b) The ratio of resistances plotted versus HbA1c concentration (μg/mL) (Park, Chang, Nam, & Park, 2008).

poly(amidoamine) G4 dendrimer solution. Then 4-formyl-phenylboronic acid (FPBA) was immobilized on the dendrimer layer selective for HbA1c. FPBA functionalization was confirmed by XPS and cyclic voltammetry. To carry out the backfilling assay, samples with various ratios of HbA1c/HbA0 (with normal adult human hemoglobin concentration i.e. 150 mg/ml) in a pH 9.0 bicarbonate buffer were contacted with the functionalized surface to react with FPBA for 1 hour. After rinsing with buffer and PBS, 1 mg/ml activated GOx in PBS was added in order to bind to the remaining unreacted amine groups on the dendrimer-FPBA layer or 30 minutes. The response of this electrode sensor was assessed by subjecting it to a voltammetric scan from 0 to +500 mV vs. Ag/AgCl at a rate of 5 mV/s in PBS in the presence of 0.1 mM ferrocenemethanol (as mediator) and 10 mM glucose (as substrate). The anodic current measured at +400 mV was chosen as the sensor signal because of stable current at this potential in the voltammogram. Fig. 24(A) shows voltammograms obtained at different HbA1c concentrations. As expected, an increase in the HbA1c concentration leads to a decrease in the resulting current due to less available space for GOx on the electrode. The corresponding calibration curve for the anodic current at +400 mV as a function of HbA1c concentration is shown in Fig. 24(B). Although this sensor has the advantage of signal amplification without the need for pretreatment such as labelling or use of labelled secondary antibody, incubation of the hemoglobin sample and then GOx solution requires 1 hour and 30 minutes, respectively. In addition, the sensitivity at HbA1c levels below 5% is not sufficient.

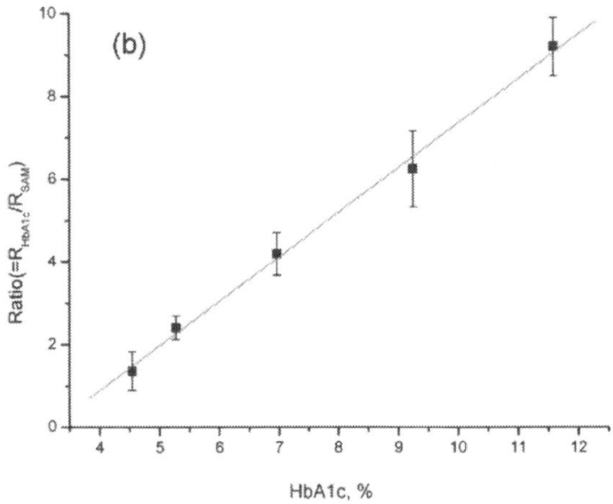

Fig. 22. R_{ct} ratio obtained at five HbA1c concentrations 20 minutes after sample injection (Park, Chang, Nam, & Park, 2008).

Qu and coworkers fabricated a micro-potentiometric Hb/HbA1c immunosensor based on an ion-sensitive field effect transistor (ISFET) using a MEMS fabrication process (Qu, Xia, Bian, Sun, & Han, 2009). Such ISFET biosensors have numerous advantages such as easy miniaturization and mass-production and rapid and label-free detection of a wide range of chemical and biochemical species. The procedure involved modification of the gold working electrode by electropolymerization of a polypyrrole (PPy)-$HAuCl_4$ composite followed by electrochemical synthesis of gold nanoparticles (AuNP) and modification of the gold reference electrode by applying a PPy film. The presence of AuNP on the surface (confirmed by FE-SEM) is reported to enhance antibody immobilization. Also, the PPy-AuNp electrode was electrochemically characterized by cyclic voltammetry and shown to exhibit better redox reaction reversibility than a PPy electrode. For hemoglobin and HbA1c immunosensor fabrication, anti-Hb antibodies and anti-HbA1c antibodies, respectively, were immobilized on the modified working electrodes. The fabricated microelectrode chip was then connected to an ISFET integrated chip. Charge adsorption at the ion/solid interface of the sensing layer leads to a potential drop and influences the gate voltage of the ISFET which is reflected by the change in the threshold voltage of the ISFET. Measurement of the hemoglobin level was done by successive injection of 10 μL of hemoglobin solutions with concentrations of 60-180 µg/ml in PBS (pH 7.4) onto the SU-8 reaction pool of the sensor. Fig. 25 shows the change in differential voltage response (ΔE) upon successive addition of the samples (in comparison with the initial response in PBS). A linear relation between the hemoglobin concentration and voltage response is observed between 60 and 180 µg/ml. The corresponding sensor sensitivity and variation coefficient of ΔE was reported to be 0.205 mV μg^{-1} ml and 21%. A similar experiment on whole blood samples yielded a linear relation between ΔE and hemoglobin concentrations between 125-197 µg/ml with a sensitivity of 0.20 mV μg^{-1} ml.

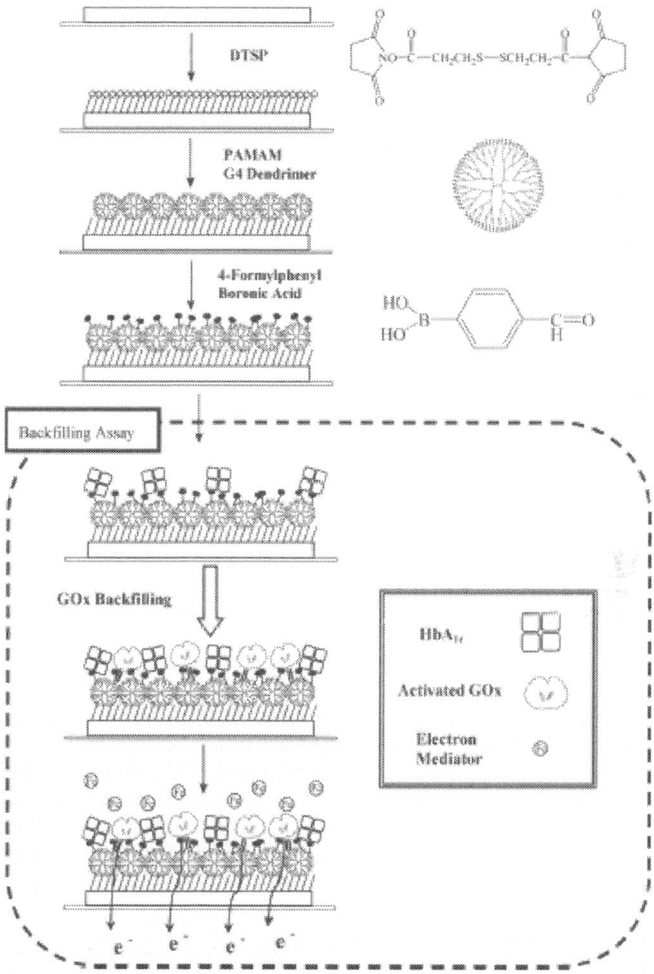

Fig. 23. Schematic diagram of "backfilling assay" between HbA1c and activated GOx. HbA1c binds to boronic acid and activated GOx binds to the remaining amine on the dendrimer monolayer (Song & Yoon, 2009).

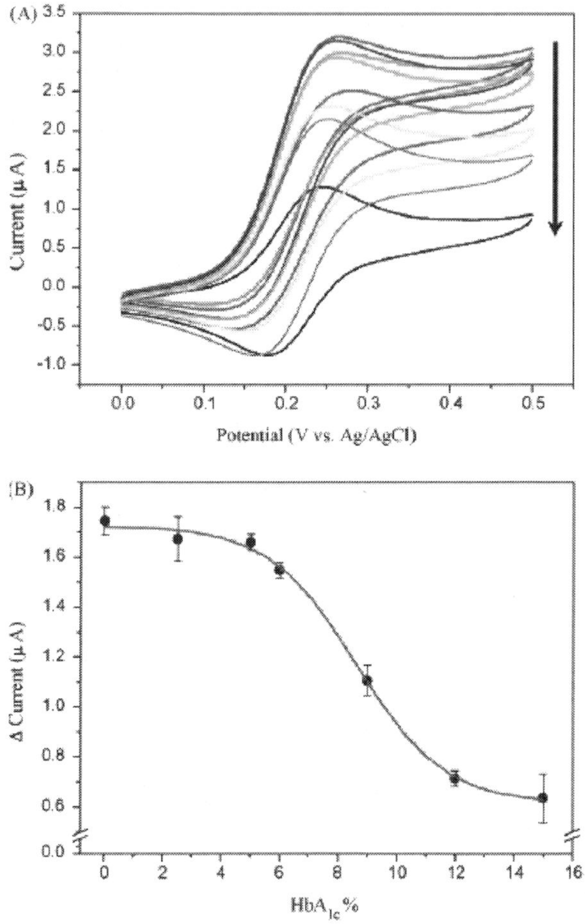

Fig. 24. Electrochemical biosensing of HbA1c by using Dend-FPBA electrodes. (A) Cyclic voltammograms of the backfilling assay between HbA1c and activated GOx at different HbA1c concentrations in the presence of ferrocenemethanol (0.1mM)in electrolyte with glucose (10mM)in 0.1MPBS (pH 7.2) at a 5mV/s sweep rate. A voltammogram before glucose addition is also included for comparison. (B) Calibration curve from the resulting backfilling assay as a function of target HbA1c concentration. Signal current levels were masured at +400mV from the background-subtracted voltammograms for respective analyte concentrations. The mean value from three independent analyses is shown at each concentration with error bar indicating the standard deviation (Song & Yoon, 2009).

The HbA1c concentration was measured using the same procedure on 10 μL solutions containing concentrations of 4-18 μg/ml HbA1c in PBS (pH 7.4) Fig. 26 shows a linear dose-response over this concentration range. Sensor sensitivity and variation coefficient of ΔE was reported to be 1.5087 mV μg^{-1} ml and 24%. The change in response due to the addition of potential interferents such as immunoglobin G (100 µg/ml), α-fetoprotein (2.5 µg/ml) and BSA (1%) was found to be less than 9.2%. It was also found that the ΔE of the hemoglobin sensor decreased about 33.2% after storage at 4°C under dry conditions for 5 days in 100 µg/ml hemoglobin in PBS (pH 7.4). The same trend was observed for a HbA1c sensor which showed a decrease in ΔE by about 35.1% after storage at 4°C under dry conditions for 5 days in 8 µg/ml hemoglobin in PBS (pH 7.4). This change in response was attributed to the slow deactivation of antibodies during storage. Although this sensor has a short response time (less than 1 min) in comparison to other HbA1c biosensors and low fabrication costs (in the case of batch produced electrode chips), its low stability and the relatively high variability of its signal are problems requiring further improvement.

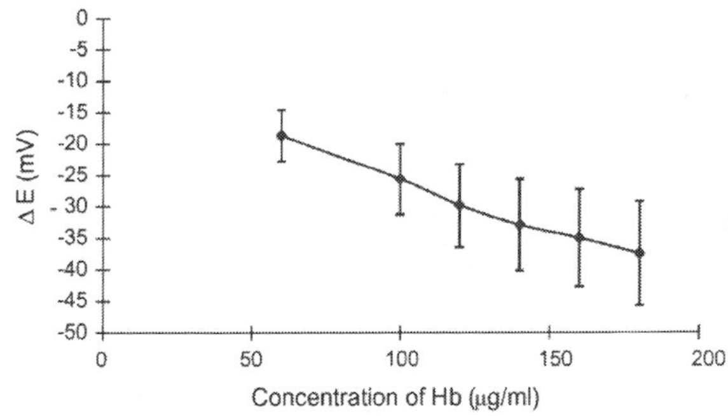

Fig. 25. Differential voltage response of the ISFET hemoglobin immunosensor to successive injections of Hb solutions with concentrations of 60, 100, 120, 140, 160 and 180µg/ml in PBS (pH 7.4). The coefficient of variation of the change of voltage response ΔE was 21% for measurements with three independently prepared electrodes. Voltages were measured 60 s after sample injection (Qu, Xia, Bian, Sun, & Han, 2009).

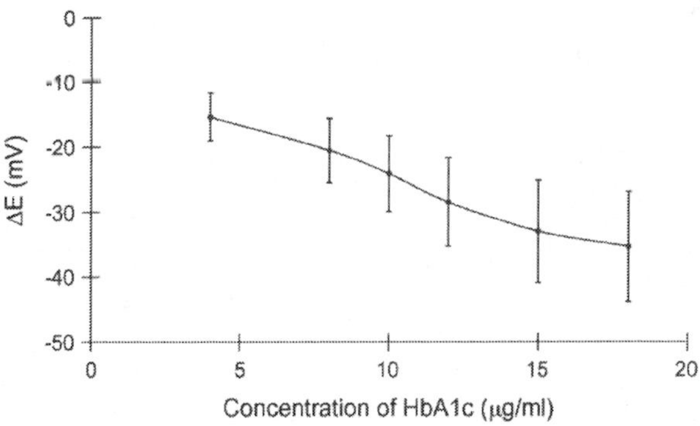

Fig. 26. Differential voltage response of the ISFET hemoglobin-A1c (HbA1c) immunosensor to successive injections of 4, 8, 10, 12 and 15µg/ml HbA1c solution in PBS (pH 7.4). The coefficient of variation for the change of voltage response ΔE was 24% for measurements with three independently prepared electrodes. Reported voltages were taken 60 s after HbA1c injection (Qu, Xia, Bian, Sun, & Han, 2009).

The same group further extended their approach by using SAMs (Xue, Bian, Tong, Sun, Zhang, & Xia, 2011). They designed a micro-potentiometric immunosensor based on mixed SAMs containing an array of gold nanospheres (instead of a PPy-AuNP layer) for HbA1c measurement (Fig. 27). The surfaces of nano-gold particles and a gold electrode were both modified by SAMs. This modification was done to address some of the problems associated with the use of nanoparticles in immunosensor fabrication. It also plays a role as an insulating film which is suitable for a FET, stabilizes covalent immobilization of antibodies and can eliminate the nonspecific sites to prevent noise interferences. The two-layer structure of SAMs with different chain lengths also helps reduce steric hindrance.

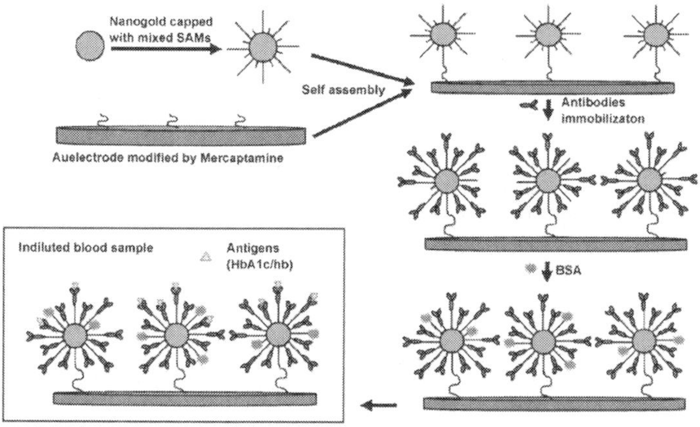

Fig. 27. Schematic diagram of electrode modification process and specific binding in diluted blood sample (Xue, Bian, Tong, Sun, Zhang, & Xia, 2011).

The electrode surface was modified by combining AuNPs with a mixed thiol solution (10 mM of both 16- and 3- mercaptohexadecanoic acid in ethanol) to form a two-layer SAM on AuNP followed by covalent immobilization on a gold electrode already modified with mercaptoethylamine-SAM using NHS and EDC. Antibodies were immobilized on the modified electrode using NHS and EDC as well. SEM images of the modified electrode showed a more uniform distribution of AuNPs which was attributed to the presence of SAMs. Electrochemical characterization of the modified electrode using CV and EIS confirmed that the SAMs had an insulating effect by decreasing the oxidation/reduction current and increasing the interfacial resistance. Also, the presence of AuNP increased the electrode sensitivity about 2-fold by raising the surface area-to-volume ratio of the sensor and making more sites available for antibody immobilization (Fig. 28A).

Measurements of hemoglobin and HbA1c content were conducted on 5 μL samples of simulated blood solution. Hemoglobin with concentrations of 166.67-570 ng/ml and HbA1c with concentrations of 1.67-170.5 ng/ml were analyzed. Figs. 28B and C indicate that linear relations between reagent dose and the electrode response were obtained over the concentration ranges from 166.67 to 570 ng/ml for hemoglobin and from 50 to 170.5 ng/ml for HbA1c. Sensor sensitivity was also reported to be 40.42 μV/(ngmL^{-1}) and 94.73 μV/(ngmL^{-1}) for hemoglobin and HbA1c, respectively. Also, the relative standard deviation of the measurements (RSD) was 5%. The good linearity of the results was attributed to the absence of significant interferences from bovine serum albumin, lysis solution, potassium ions and chloride ions in the simulated blood sample as well as good biocompatibility of the method and a stable combination with antibodies. In comparison with their previous sensors based on mixed SAMs, the use of wrapped AuNP arrays increased the sensor sensitivity from the order of μg/mL to ng/mL and lowered the standard deviation from above 20% to 5%, while reaching a dilution factor of 150,000 times.

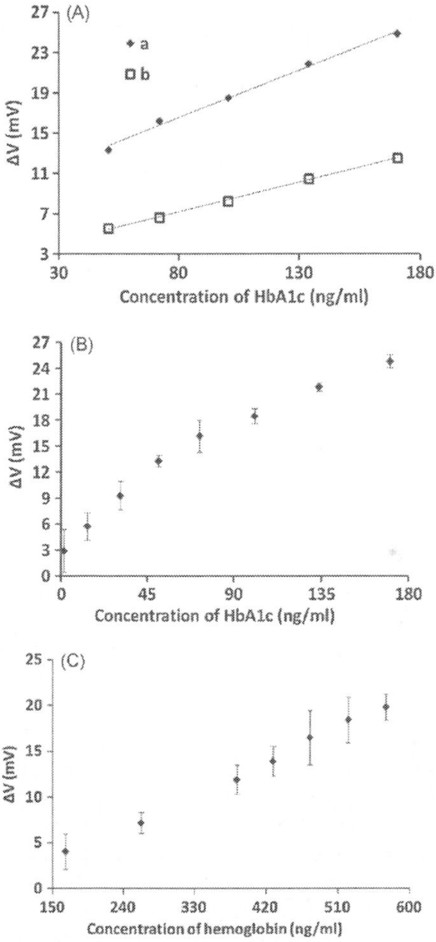

Fig. 28. Potential output of the immunosensor in a phosphate buffer solution of pH7.4 in the presence of simulated blood samples containing different concentrations of HbA1c and hemoglobin: (A) effect of HbA1c using two methods: (a) mixed SAM wrapped nano-spheres method and (b) mixed SAM method); (B) response to HbA1c; (C) response to hemoglobin. The results are the mean values of 3 measurements (Xue, Bian, Tong, Sun, Zhang, & Xia, 2011).

4. Conclusion

HbA1c point-of-care (POC) devices can potentially play an important role in diabetes diagnosis and management. However, they suffer from problems of low accuracy and reproducibility and so are not yet reliable enough to be recommended for clinical use at this time. This chapter reviews the research that has been done in the past decade or so to fabricate and improve the performance of HbA1c biosensors. A variety of approaches has been adopted to fabricate these sensors, making it difficult to compare them. However, based on the research to date, it appears that FV-based sensors require more steps for sample preparation, making their application in POC devices less favourable. Sensors that use label-free methods based on FET are less complicated for the user and require less time for measurement of HbA1c levels, but improvement to their sensitivity and especially reproducibility are needed in order to be accepted by clinicians and be suitable for introduction to the commercial market. Consequently, considerable work is still needed for the development of accurate, simple, reliable and cheap HbA1c biosensors.

5. Acknowledgment

Support for this research has been provided to two of the authors (PC and MP) by the Natural Sciences and Engineering Research Council of Canada (NSERC) and to one of the authors (PC) by the Canadian Foundation for Innovation (CFI) and the Canada Research Chairs (CRC) Program.

6. References

Alexander, C., Andersson, H. S., Andersson, L. I., Ansell, R. J., Kirsch, N., Nicholls, I. A., et al. (2006). Molecular imprinting science and technology: a survey of the literature for the years up to and including 2003. *JOURNAL OF MOLECULAR RECOGNITION* , Vol. 19, pp. 106–180

Berg, A. H., & Sacks, D. B. (2008). Haemoglobin A1c analysis in the management of patients with diabetes: from chaos to harmony. *Journal of Clinical Pathology* , Vol. 61, pp. 983-987

Chien, H.-C., & Chou, T.-C. (2010). Glassy Carbon Paste Electrodes for the Determination of Fructosyl Valine. *Electroanalysis* , Vol. 22, No. 6, pp. 688 - 693

Chuang, S.-W., Rick, J., & Chou, T.-C. (2009). Electrochemical characterisation of a conductive polymer molecularly imprinted with an Amadori compound. *Biosensors and Bioelectronics* , Vol. 24, pp. 3170–3173

Fang, L., Li, W., Zhou, Y., & Liu, C.-C. (2009). A single-use, disposable iridium-modified electrochemical biosensor for fructosyl valine for the glycoslated hemoglobin detection. *Sensors and Actuators B* , Vol. 137, Vol. 235–238

Halámek, J., Wollenberger, U., Stöcklein, W. F., Warsinke, A., & Scheller, F. W. (2007). Signal Amplification in Immunoassays Using Labeling via Boronic Acid Binding to the Sugar Moiety of Immunoglobulin G: Proof of Concept for Glycated Hemoglobin. *Analytical Letters* , Vol. 40, pp. 1434–1444

Halámek, J., Wollenberger, U., Stöcklein, W., & Scheller, F. (2007). Development of a biosensor for glycated hemoglobin. *Electrochimica Acta* , Vol. 53, pp. 1127–1133

Harris, M., & Zimmet, P. (1997). *Classification of diabetes mellitus and other categories of glucose intolerance* (Second Ausg.). (K. Alberti, P. Zimmet, & R. Defronzo, Hrsg.) Chichester: John Wiley and Sons Ltd.

Kost, G. J. (2002). 1. Goals, guidelines and principles for point-of-care testing. In *Principles & practice of point-of-care testing* (S. 3–12). Lippincott Williams & Wilkins.

Lenters-Westra, E., & Slingerland, R. J. (2010). Six of eight hemoglobin A1c point-of-care instruments do not meet the general accepted analytical performance criteria. *Clinical Chemistry* , Vol. 56, pp. 44-52

Liu, S., Wollenberger, U., Katterle, M., & Scheller, F. W. (2006). Ferroceneboronic acid-based amperometric biosensor for glycated hemoglobin. *Sensors and Actuators B* , Vol. 113, pp. 623–629

Nathan, D. M. (2009). International Expert Committee Report on the Role of the A1C Assay in the Diagnosis of Diabetes. *DIABETES CARE* , Vol. 32, No. 7, pp. 1327-1334

NGSP. (June 2010). Abgerufen am 9. 1 2010 von http://www.ngsp.org/CAC2010.asp

Park, J.-Y., Chang, B.-Y., Nam, H., & Park, S.-M. (2008). Selective Electrochemical Sensing of Glycated Hemoglobin (HbA1c) on Thiophene-3-Boronic Acid Self-Assembled Monolayer Covered Gold Electrodes. *Analytical Chemistry* , Vol. 80, pp. 8035–8044

Pohanka, M., & Skládal, P. (2008). Electrochemical biosensors - principles and applications. *Journal of Applied Biomedicine* , Vol. 6, pp. 57–64

Qu, L., Xia, S., Bian, C., Sun, J., & Han, J. (2009). A micro-potentiometric hemoglobin immunosensor based on electropolymerized polypyrrole–gold nanoparticles composite. *Biosensors and Bioelectronics* , vol. 24, pp. 3419–3424

Sode, K., Ohta, S., Yanai, Y., & Yamazaki, T. (2003). Construction of a molecular imprinting catalyst using target analogue template and its application for an amperometric fructosylamine sensor. *Biosensors and Bioelectronics* , Vol. 18, pp. 1485-1490

Sode, K., Takahashi, Y., Ohta, S., Tsugawa, W., & Yamazaki, T. (2001). A new concept for the construction of an artificial dehydrogenase for fructosylamine compounds and its application for an amperometric fructosylamine sensor. *Analytica Chimica Acta* , Vol. 435, 151–156

Son, S. U., Seo, J. H., Choi, Y. H., & Lee, S. S. (2006). Fabrication of a disposable biochip for measuring percent hemoglobin A1c (%HbA1c). *Sensors and Actuators A* , Vol. 130–131, pp. 267–272

Song, S. Y., & Yoon, H. C. (2009). Boronic acid-modified thin film interface for specific binding of glycated hemoglobin (HbA1c) and electrochemical biosensing. *Sensors and Actuators B* , Vol. 140, pp. 233–239

Stöllner, D., Stöcklein, W., Scheller, F., & Warsinke, A. (2002). Membrane-immobilized haptoglobin as affinity matrix for a hemoglobin-A1c immunosensor. *Analytica Chimica Acta* , Vol. 470, pp. 111–119

Stöllner, D., Warsinke, A., Stöcklein, W., Dölling, R., & Scheller, F. (2001). Immunochemical Determination of Hemoglobin-A1c Utilizing a Glycated Peptide as Hemoglobin-A1c Analogon. *BIOSENSOR Simposium.* TÜBINGEN.

Tsugawa, W., Ishimura, F., Ogawa, K., & Sode, K. (2000). Developement of an Enzyme Sensor Utilizing a Novel Fructosyl Amine Oxidase from a Marine Yeast. *Electrochemistry* , Vol 68, No. 11, 869-871

Tsugawa, W., Ogawa, K., Ishimura, F., & Sode, K. (2001). Fructosyl Amine Sensing Based on Prussian Blue Modified Enzyme Electrode. *Electrochemistry* , Vol 69, No. 12, pp. 973-975

Wang, J. (2006). *Analytical Electrochemistry.* United States of America: John Wiley & Sons, Inc.

Wang, J. (2008). Electrochemical Glucose Biosensors. *Chemical Reviews* , Vol. 108, No. 2, pp. 814-825

Xue, Q., Bian, C., Tong, J., Sun, J., Zhang, H., & Xia, S. (2011). A Micro Potentiometric Immunosensor for Hemoglobin-A1c Level Detection Based on Mixed SAMs Wrapped Nano-spheres Array. *Biosensors and Bioelectronics* , Vol. 26, pp. 2689–2693

14

Electrochemical Biosensors for Virus Detection

Adnane Abdelghani
National Institute of Applied Science and Technology, Charguia Cedex
Tunisia

1. Introduction

The rabies constitutes one of the most dangerous viruses causing many death cases every year. Each year approximately 55,000 people die of rabies, with high percentage of children [S et al., 2007; L et al., 2000; FX et al., 1994). High percentages (99%) of the registered cases were in Asia and Africa. In order to fight this dangerous disease, many techniques are usually used for diagnostic but are usually complex, time consuming, expensive, difficult to implement, and this is a necessity for developing new detection process [N et al., 1993; Crepin et al., 1998]. Avian Influenza Virus (AIV) infections are a major cause of mortality and rapid identification of the virus has important clinical, economical and epidemiological implications. The traditional methods for virus diagnostic are Enzyme Linked Immunosorbent Assay (ELISA) and Reverse Transcriptase Polymerase Chain Reaction (RT-PCR) which are time consuming and expensive. Biosensors can play an important role in areas such as diagnostic of diseases, drug detection and food quality control. Biosensors are devices with qualities quoted as rapidity, sensitivity and specificity [G et al., 2002; D et al., 1999). Biacore based on Surface Plamson Resonance technique is effectively a successful biosensor used for antigen-antibody interaction [J et al., 1999]. Others commercialized biosensors such us glucometer was developed for self-monitoring of glucose in blood for diabetes care.

In terms of the transduction techniques used, the three main classes of biosensors are optical, electrochemical and piezoelectric. Out of the three, optical methods appear to be the most sensitive, with surface plasmon resonance and waveguide based devices being the technological spearhead. As for Electrochemical biosensors, they are cheaper than optical ones. They can be amperometric or impedimetric, depending on whether they monitor a current as a function of potential or the resulting sensor impedance as a function of frequency. The advantage of impedimetric methods is that, unlike amperometry, they do not need of enzymatic labels in order to detect. In this work, we use the high sensitive impedance spectroscopy technique for biosensors applications. This technique is very known to characterize the electrical properties of materials and their interfaces exposed to electronically conducting electrodes [A et al., 2004; S et al., 2006; A et al., 2006]. It may be used to investigate the dynamics of bound and mobile charges in the bulk or interfacial regions of any kind of solid or liquid material: ionic semiconducting, mixed electronic-ionic and dielectric. The biosensor is based on the immobilization of specific anti-rabies polyclonal antibodies and specific anti-H_7N_1 antibodies onto a functionalized gold electrode with micrometer size. The affinity interaction of the antibody with the specific antigen can be measured with a good reproductibility with impedance spectroscopy [M et al., 2008; M et al., 2008]. The different steps of biosensor conception were characterized by Electrochemical Impedance Spectroscopy (EIS). The obtained limit detection was better than those obtained with the others traditional methods for clinical use. The non-specific interaction has been tested with the Newcastle antigen virus.

2. Experimental set-up

2.1 Specific rabies antibody preparation

Rabies immunoglobulins were produced by horse immunization. The immunization was carried out using human vaccine "RABIPUR" manufactured by "Chiron Behring Vaccines " in Ankleshwar (Gujarat), India. The horses were exposed to a series of injections to increase vaccine amounts. The immunization period lasted for 105 days (M et al., 2008).

2.2 Specific rabbit antibody (anti-H_7N_1) preparation

Three male rabbits were injected sub-cutaneously with different doses of NobilisTM, INFLUENZA H_7N_1 vaccine in different periods (15 days, 30 days, 45 days, 65 days). For each period, quantity of blood were analysed to study the kinetic of the rabbit vaccine immuno-response. Hyper immuno serums has been collected and specific rabbit-polyclonal antibodies (anti-H7N1) has been purified with affinity chromatography (M et al., 2008).

2.3 Antibody immobilization on gold electrode

The gold electrodes were cleaned with organic solvents (acetone and ethanol) and with piranha solution (1:3 H_2O_2 - concentrated H_2SO_4) for 1 min. After each treatment, the gold substrates were rinsed with ethanol and dried under nitrogen flow. The pretreated electrodes were immersed in 11-mercaptoundecanoic acid 1 mM in ethanol solution for 12 h in order to form a self-assembled monolayer (SAM). The substrates were then rinsed with ethanol in order to remove the unbonded thiols. To convert the terminal carboxylic groups to an active NHS ester, the thiol-modified electrodes were treated with 0.4 mM EDC-0.1 mM NHS for 1 h. After gold electrodes were rinsed with water and dryed under nitrogen, 20 µg/ml of Anti-Rabies IgG (respectively 5 µg/ml of Anti-H7N1) were dropped onto the surface at 37 °C for one hour. The excess antibodies were removed by rinsing with PBS. Then, the antibody-modified electrodes were treated with 0.1% BSA for 30 min, to block the unreacted and non-specific sites. After rinsing with PBS and water, the electrodes were dried under nitrogen (Figure.1).

2.4 Impedance spectroscopy

Many reports show that impedance spectroscopy is a useful tool to characterize self assembled monolayer on surfaces (A et al., 2004). A capacitor is formed between the conducting electrode and the electrolyte. The absolute impedance is related to the frequency by the equation:

$$|Z| = \frac{1}{2\pi fC} \tag{1}$$

where f is the frequency (in Hz) at which Z is measured.

The complex impedance can be presented as a combination of the real impedance (Z_{re}) and imaginary impedance (Z_{im}), Nyquist plot. To fit the measured spectra with the impedance spectra out of ideal elements, the ideal elements have been replaced with the constant phase elements (CPE):

$$Z_{CPE} = K\omega^{-\alpha} \tag{2}$$

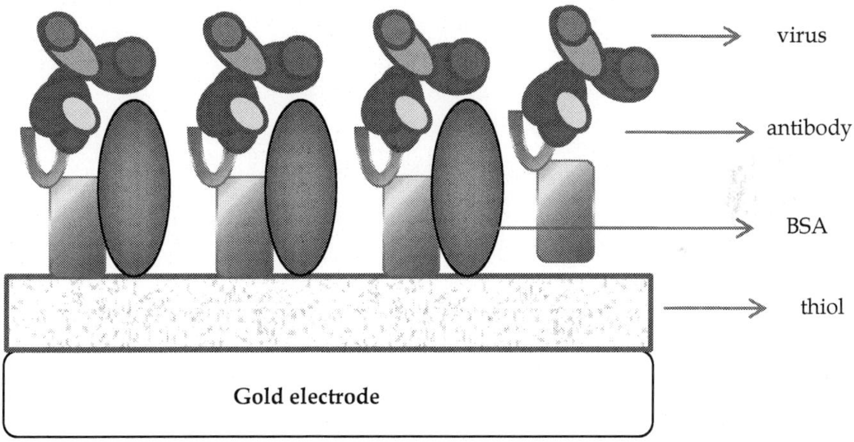

Fig. 1. Biosensor multilayer configuration

The frequency exponent is $\alpha = 1$ and $K = 1/C$ for an ideal capacitance, and $\alpha = 0$ and $K = R$ for an ideal resistance, respectively. The exponent α could be obtained, when the membrane capacitance (or layer capacitance) was replaced by a constant phase element Z_{CPE}. The deviation of the exponent α from the ideal values is attributed to the inhomogeneities of the analyzed layer, like defects or roughness. The measured spectra of the impedance were analyzed in terms of electrical equivalent circuits using a analysis program. The mathematical expressions of the equivalent circuit models were fitted to the data. The electric parameters of the system were calculated with the computer program and the fit error was kept under a maximum of 10%. The impedance analysis was performed with the Voltalab 40 impedance analyser in the frequency range 0.05 Hz - 100 kHz, using a modulation voltage of 10 mV. Three-electrode system was employed with a saturated calomel electrode (SCE), an immunosensor working electrode (0.19 cm^2), and a platinum strip counter electrode (0.385 cm^2). The impedance measurements were performed in the presence of a 5 mM $K_3[Fe(CN)_6]$/ $K_4[Fe(CN)_6]$ (1:1) mixture as redox probe in PBS. The measured spectra of the impedance and phase were analysed in terms of electrical equivalent circuit model using a Zview modelling programme (Scribrer and associates, Charlottesville, VA). All electrochemical measurements were carried out at room temperature and in a faraday cage. More details on electrochemical impedance spectroscopy can be found in reference (A et al., 2004; M et al., 2008).

3. Results and discussions

3.1 Avian influenza virus biosensor

First, we study the variation of the impedance spectra (the real part, it means the charge transfer resistance) of the functionalized gold electrode with different concentration of immobilised antibody. This allows us to know the saturation concentration of the antibody on our gold electrode, which will leads to the high sensitivity detection. Figure.2 shows the impedance spectra of the functionnalized gold electrode after the immobilisation of antibody with different concentration.

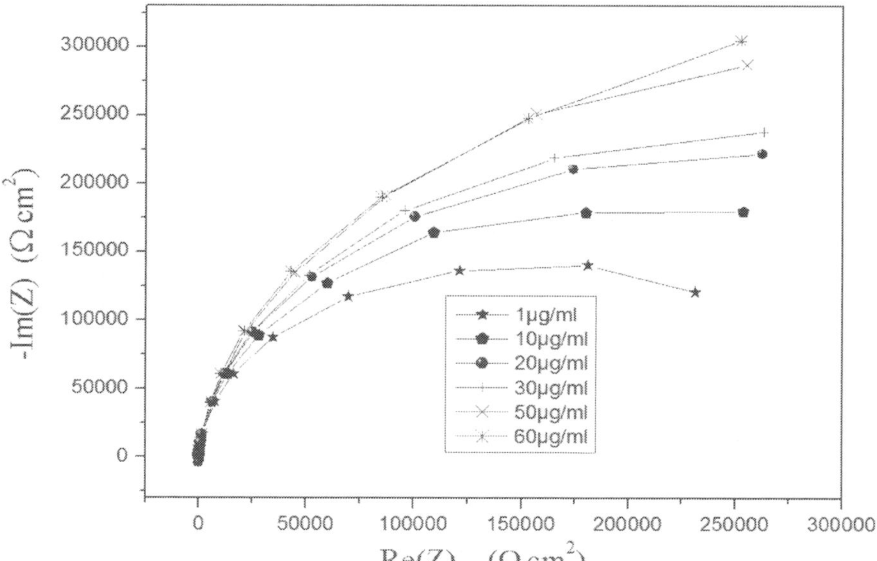

Fig. 2. Impedance spectra of the functionalized gold electrode after the immobilisation of different antibody concentration

The impedance spectra can be fitted with computer simulated program using the electric circuit shown in figure 3. This equivalent circuit includes the ohmic resistance of the electrolyte solution R_0, the constant phase element Z_{CPE} and electron transfer resistance R_1. An excellent fitting between the simulated and experimental spectra was obtained for each antibody concentration. Figure4 shows the variation of the impedance versus the antibody concentration. We can see that the surface saturation can be obtained with 60μg/ml antibody concentration. For specific and non specific antigen detection, we will use this antibody concentration

3.1.1 Virus detection

Figure 5 show the impedance spectra of the functionalized gold electrode recorded at 0 V in PBS buffer at pH=7.2 in the range of 50 mHz to 100 KHz before and after addition of different H_7N_1 antigen concentration.

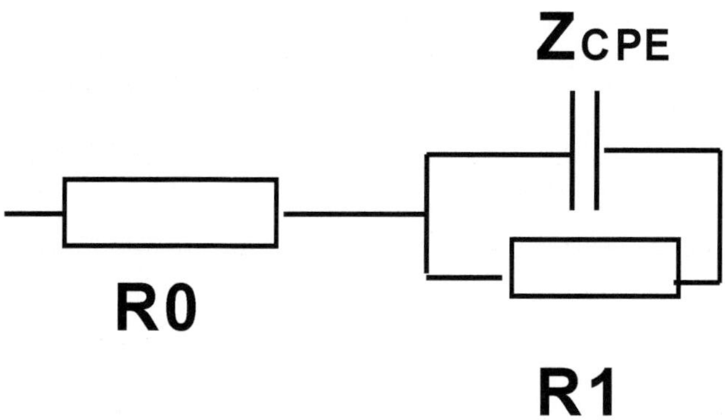

Fig. 3. Electric model

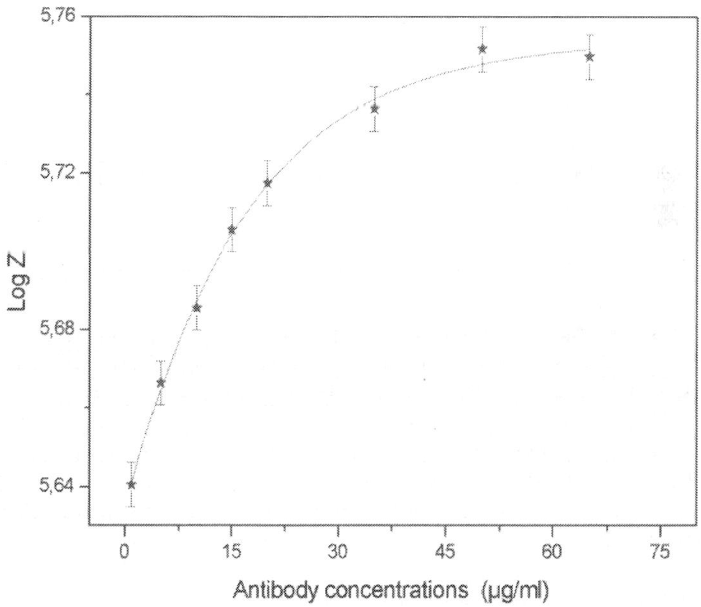

Fig. 4. Impedance spectra of the functionalized gold electrode after the immobilisation of different antibody concentration

The interface can be modelized with the electric model shown in figure3. An excellent fitting between the simulated and experimental spectra was obtained.

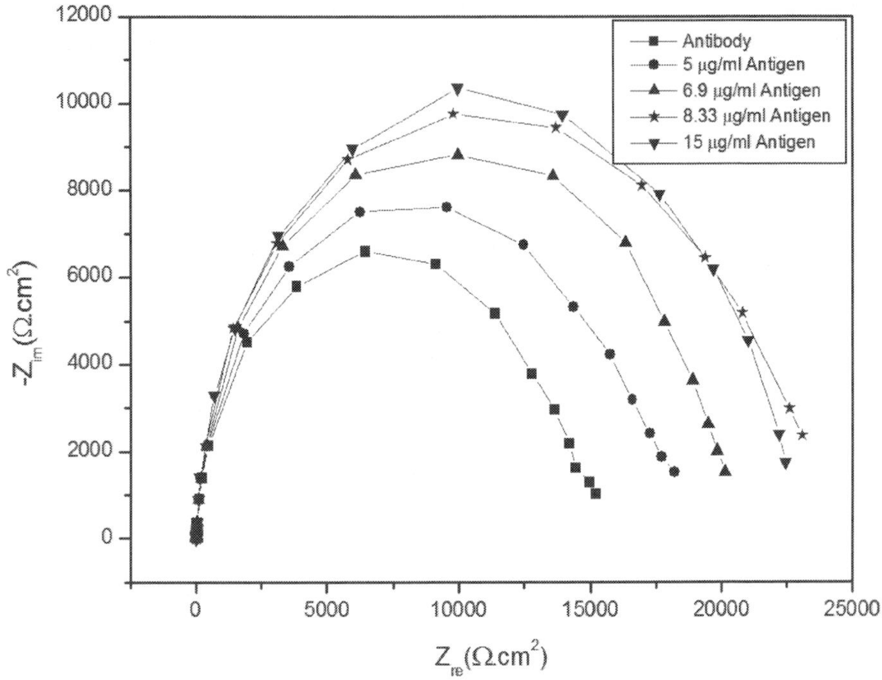

Fig. 5. Impedance spectra of the functionalized gold electrode before and after addition of different H_7N_1 antigen concentration.

The charge transfer resistance increases and reaches a new saturation value that can be determined with the fitting program. This increase could be attributed to a rearrangement in the structure of the antibody and a variation of the dielectric constant. The lowest detection limit that induces a signal variation is equal to 5 µg/ml . This value was lower than the limit detection obtained with ELISA technique.

3.1.2 Calibration and selectivity

In order to obtain the calibration data set, the values of log Z/Z_o versus the antigen H_7N_1 concentration were plotted in figure 6 , where Z is the value of the impedance resistance after antigen binding to antibody, Z_0 is the value of impedance as antibody immobilized on the electrode.

As we can be see in the figure6, the plot is linear and saturate at the higher concentration. To confirm that the above-observed impedance changes generated from the result of specific antibody-antigen interaction, the sensor was exposed to the solution of Newcastle antigen that are expected to bind non-specifically. Figure 6 shows the variation of the impedance versus the non-specific antigen concentration. As we can see, the sensor was not subjected to the non-specific binding and applicable to the selective determination of H_7N_1.

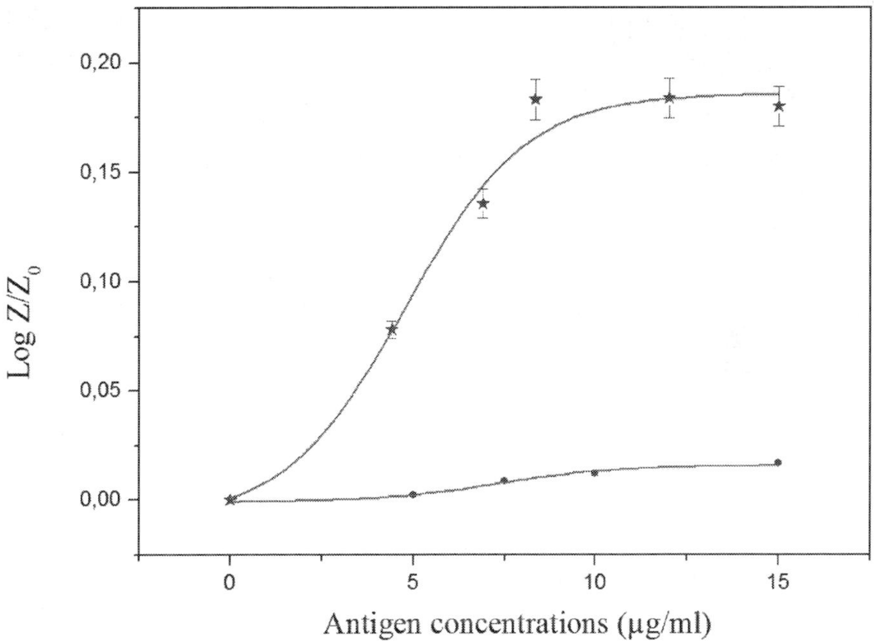

Fig. 6. Calibration curves and selectivity of the developed biosensor.

3.2 Rabbies virus biosensor

We start to characterise the insulating properties of the thiol monolayer on gold surface. The Nyquist diagram of bare gold (fig.7) presents a half-circle, characteristic of a resistance in parallel with a capacity and a linear part which appears at low frequencies and which is assigned to diffusion phenomenon [17]. However, after acid thiol treatment, the diameter of the half-circle of Nyquist diagram increases clearly and the Warburg impedance was not observed. This is shows the high insulating properties of the acid thiol (M et al., 2008).

After, impedance measurements were performed after gold surface activation with EDC/NHS, antibody immobilization and BSA blocking step. After each step, acquisitions of impedance data in PBS were carried out over 5 decades of frequency. Figure 8 presents the Nyquist diagram for the various steps of the biosensor development: SAM layer, antibody layer, blocking with BSA and antigen injection.

We observe that each layer deposition on the gold surface generates an impedance increase. This increase is due to the change of the electric properties of the gold/electrolyte interface.

3.2.1 Calibration and selectivity

For rabbies detection, Figure 9 presents the calibration of the developed biosensors for specific and non-specific detection. It shows a dynamic range between 0.1 µg/ml and 4 μg/ml and a saturation reached at 4 μg/ml. This behaviour can be explained: when the antigen concentration increases in the electrochemical cell, the number of immobilized antibodies, but not complexed, decreases and reaches zero when concentration of antigen is higher than 4 μg/ml. The limit detection of this sensor is about 0.5 μg/ml. This limit detection is better than the limit detection obtained with the others traditional methods for clinical use. In order to prove sensor selectivity, the immunosensor was exposed to a solution containing the Newcastle antigen viruses.

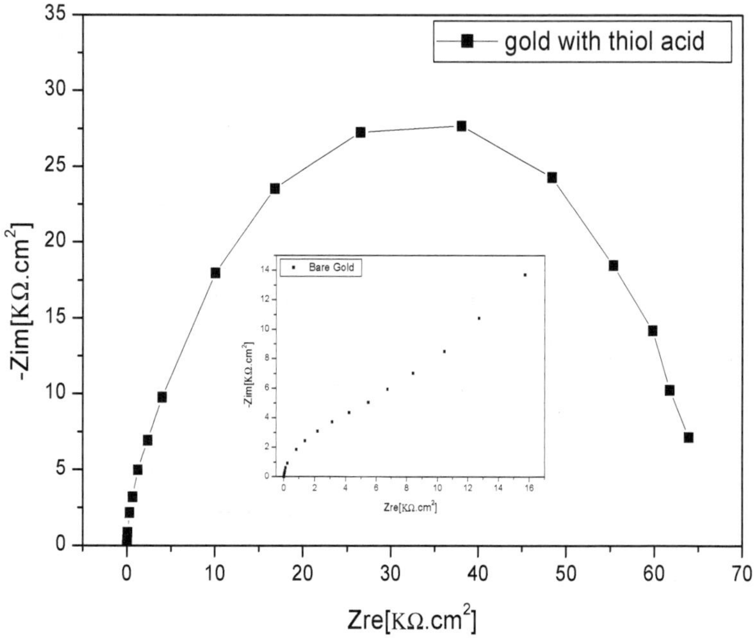

Fig. 7. Nyquist plot for bare gold (small curve) and gold with thiol acid (big curve) in PBS solution with 1 mM redox couple

As shown in figure 9, there is a little variation of impedance after no-specific antigen addition. This little non specific variation can be explained by the use of polyclonal antibodies. In order to avoid non specificity, the use of monoclonal immunoglobulins G (IgGs) is necessary.

4. Conclusion

In this study, we reported the development of biosensor for rabies and for H_7N_1 antigen detection. The affinity interaction of the antibody with specific antigen can be measured with detection limit of 0.5 and 5 μg/ml respectively. The impedance spectroscopy technique is a higher sensitive technique which can be used to measure the high insulating properties of biomembranes. The different steps of biosensor conception were characterized by

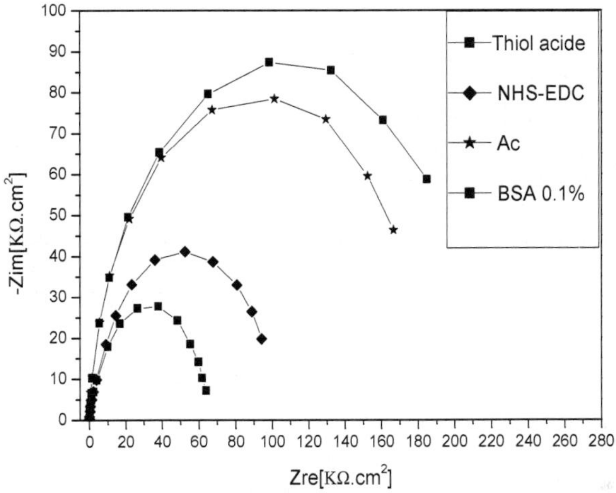

Fig. 8. Nyquist plot of the different layers of the rabies biosensors

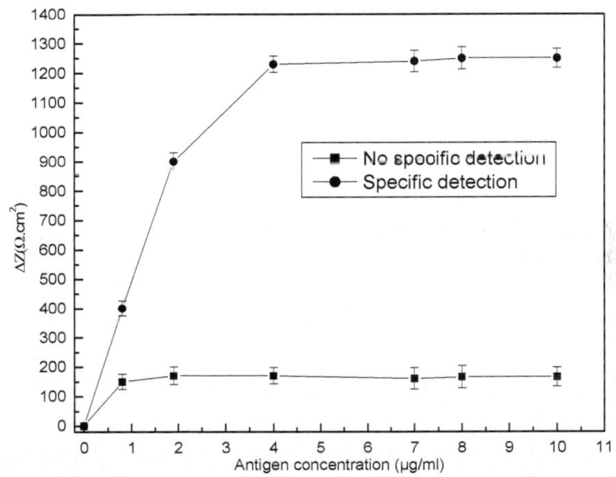

Fig. 9. Selectivity of the developed biosensor.

electrochemical impedance spectroscopy. The sensitivity of miniaturized biosensor prototype will be improved by using interdigitated gold microelectrodes with microfluidic cell for industrial development and clinical use.

5. Acknowledgements

The authors thank the NATO through collaborative Linkage Grant CBP.MD. CLG 982802. and the Alexander Von Humboldt Stiftung (Germany) for the material donation.

6. References

[1] S, E. Sloan.; C, Hanlon.; W. Weldon.; M, Niezgoda.; J, Blanton. (2007). Identification and characterization of a human monoclonal antibody that potently neutralizes a broad panel of rabies virus isolates. Vaccine, Vol.25, pp. 2800-2810.

[2] L, Martinez.; Global infectious disease surveillance.(2000). International Journal Infections Diseases ;Vol. 4, N0. 222, pp. 10-28.

[3] FX, Meslin.; DB, Fishbein. (1994). Rationale and prospects for rabies elimination in developing countries. Current Trop Microbiology Immunology, Vol.187, pp. 1-26.

[4] World Health Organization. (2002). Rabies vaccines Weekly epidemiological record. Vol. 14, N0. 77, pp. 109-11.

[5] N, Kamolvarin.; T. Tirawatnpong.; R, Rattanasiwamoke.; S, Tirawatnpong.; T, Panpanich.; and T. Hemachudha. (1993). Diagnosis of rabies by polymerase chain reaction with nested primers. Journal of Infections Diseases, Vol. 167, pp.207-210.

[6] Crepin, P.; L. Audry.; Y. Rotivel.; A. Gacoin.; C. Caroff.; and H. Bourhy. (1998). Intravitam diagnosis of human rabies by PCR using saliva and cerebrospinal fluid. Journal Clinical Microbiology. Vol, 36, pp. 1117-1121.

[7] Perrin, P.; and P,. Sureau. (1987). A collaborative study of an experimental kit for rapid rabies enzyme immunodiagnosis (RREID). Bull World Health Organization.pp.489-493.

[8] A, Ermine.;. N, Tordo.; and H, Tsiang. (1998). Rapid diagnosis of rabies infection by means of a dot hybridization assay. Molecular Cell Probes, Vol.2, pp. 75-82.

[9] G, A.Rand.; J, Ye.; C.W, Brown.; S.V, Letcher. (2002). Optical biosensors for food pathogen detection. Food Technology, Vol. 56 , pp.32–37.

[10] D, Ivnitski.; I.A, Hamid.; P, Atanasov.; E, Wilkins. (1999). Biosensors for detection of pathogenic bacteria. Biosensors and Bioelectronics, Vol. 14 , pp. 599–624.

[11] J, Homola.; S.S, Yee. ; G, Gauglitz. (1999). Surface plasmon resonance sensors. Sensors and Actuators B, Vol. 54 , pp. 3–15.

[12] A, Tlili.; S, Hleli.; A, Abdelghani.; M.A, Maaref . (2004). Electrical Characterization of a Thiol SAM on Gold as a First Step of the Fabrication of an Immunosensors based on a Quartz Crystal Microbalance. Sensors, Vol.4, pp. 104-114.

[13] S, Hleli.; C, Martelet.; A, Abdelghani.; N, Jaffrezic-Renault. (2006). Atrazine analysis using impedimetric immunosensors based on mixed biotinylated self-assembled monolayer. Sensors and Actuators B, Vol.113 , pp. 711–717.

[14] A, Abdelghani.; K, Cherif.; M, Maaref. (2006). Impedance Spectroscopy on Xerogel Layer for Chemical Sensing. Materials Science and Engineering C, Vol. 26, pp. 542 - 545.

[15] A, Tlili.; A, Abdelghani.; S, Ameur.; N, Jaffrezic-Renault. (2006). Impedance spectroscopy and affinity measurement of specific antibody-antigen interaction. Materials Science and Engineering C, Vol. 26, pp. 546 - 550.

[16] M, Hnaien.; S, Hleli.; M, Diouani.; I, Hafaid.; W, Hassen.; N, Jaffrezic- Renault.; A, Abdelghani. (2008). Immobilisation of Specific Antibody on SAM Functionalized Gold Electrode for Rabies Virus Detection by Electrochemical Impedance Spectroscopy. Biochemical Engineering Journal, Vol. 39, N0. 3, pp. 443-449.

[17] M, .Diouani.; S, Hleli.; I, Hafaid.; A, Snousi.; A,Ghram.; A,Abdelghani. (2008). Immobilisation of Specific Antibody on Functionnalised Gold Microelectrode for Avian Influenza Virus H7N1 Detection. Materials Science and Engineering C, Vol. 28, N0. 5-6 , pp. 580-583.

15

Microfaradaic Electrochemical Biosensors for the Study of Anticancer Action of DNA Intercalating Drug: Epirubicin

Sweety Tiwari and K.S. Pitre
Dr. Harisingh Gour University
India

1. Introduction

In the past two decades chemically modified electrodes (CME) have attracted considerable interest of researchers to exert a direct control over the chemical nature of electrodes. CMEs have found a large number of useful applications in different fields viz. selective electro-organic synthesis, biomedical analysis, electro analyses etc. The ability to manipulate the molecular architecture of bulk matrix of the electrode, particularly its surface has led to a wide range of analytical applications of CMEs and created opportunities for electroanalysts to fabricate useful biosensors

The CMEs have shown remarkable specificity for biological recognition processes which has led to the development of highly selective biosensing devices. The electrochemical biosensors hold a leading position among the bioprobes currently available and hold great promise for the tasks of study of in-vivo mechanism of action of large number of drugs. These electrochemical biosensors consist of two components (1) a biological entity that recognises the target analyte and (2) the electrode transducer that translates the biorecognition event in to a useful electrical signal.

Modern methods of analysis specially designed for drug discovery are mostly high-through put systems. The target samples are either obtained by natural origin generated by combinational chemistry or produced by biochemical methods. Hundreds and thousands of synthetic compounds are available in modern substance libraries, which have to be tested individually for their use as useful drugs. In addition to this, some natural resources including tropical rain forests and marine environments are of great interest for the development of potential new drugs. In the past, a large number of plants and samples obtained from biological sources of these habitats have been used as traditional medicine of native population. Scientific knowledge about these traditional medicines has attracted the attention of scientists working in the field of development of nature derived drugs.

1.1 Biosensors

In the present times most of the screening systems used are enzyme or whole cell based and these biological substances have also been used as biological recognition elements of biosensors. We may consider a biosensor as a device consisting of a biological part and a physical transducer (Figure-1).

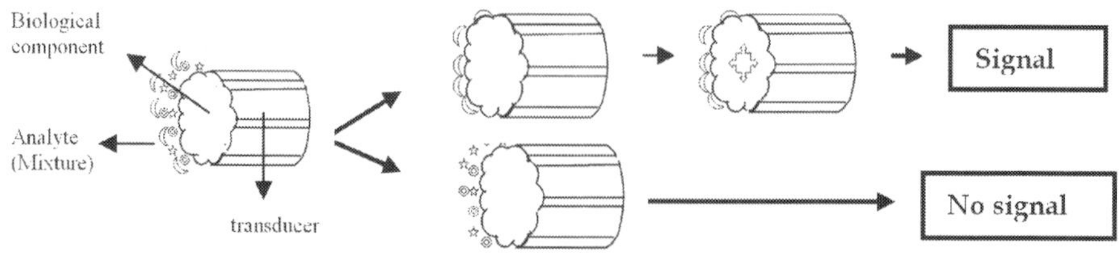

Fig. 1. Typical function of a biosensor. One of the compounds of a mixture of substances interacts with biological part of the biosensor. The biological signal so produced is converted to some physical signal (optical, electric) by the transducer. Compounds which do not interact with biological part do not produce any signal.

According to a recent IUPAC document, a biosensor is defined as a specific type of chemical sensor comprising a biological recognition element and physiochemical transducer. The biological element is capable of recognizing the presence of activity or concentration of specific analyte in solution. The recognition may be either a binding process i.e. affinity ligand based biosensor when the recognition element is an antibody /DNA segment /cell receptor or biocatalytic reaction i.e. enzyme based biosensors.

Both the components of the biosensor are in direct contact and may be used for several measurements. The selectivity of the biosensor depends on integrated biological component. The substances which have a specific tendency interact with the biological part of the biosensor produce optical or electrical signals of the transducers. In addition to cell and enzyme, some other compounds such as DNA, receptor and antibodies have also frequently been used as component of biosensors.

The increasing need to develop specific biosensors for fast routine measurement in several fields of analysis has generated interest of a large number of scientists in the field of biosensor research. As a result, a fairly high number of recently developed specific biosensors are in use for the detection and analysis of hundreds of compounds in analytes of different origin e.g. sugars, amino acids and enzyme co-factor which have utmost biological relevance (Paddle,1996, Meadows,1996, Bousse,1996, Ziegler et al., 1998).

Some electrical devices such as semiconductors and electrodes, some optical components such as fiber optics, quartz microbalances have also been used as transducer part of biosensor. These transducers have been miniaturized in order to obtain chip based sensors.

Though, initially biosensors were developed with an aim of clinical diagnosis e.g. in the determination of blood sugar level but in recent years biosensors have been fabricated for their possible application in food industry for quality control purpose, environmental analysis and biomedical analysis etc.

1.2 Electrochemical biosensor

The first scientifically proposed as well as successfully commercialized biosensors were those based on electrochemical sensors for multiple analysis. More than fifty percent sensors reported in the literature are electrochemical and can be classified as amperometric, potentiometric or conductometric sensors (Meadows,1996).

Electrochemical biosensors have been studied for a long time. They have been the subject of basic as well as applied research for nearly fifty years. Leland C Clark introduced the principle of the first enzyme electrode with immobilized glucose oxidase (Clark et al., 1962).

The first commercially produced biosensor was introduced in the market in 1975. This biosensor was used for the fast glucose assay in blood samples from diabetics. Today there is a large number of proposed and already commercialized devises based on the principle of biosensor including those for the analysis of pathogens and toxins.

1.2.1 Amperometric biosensor

In amperometric sensors, an enzyme is typically immobilized at the surface of an amperometric electrode; this immobilized enzyme reacts with the substrate (e.g. phenolic compounds/sugar) and produces current that depends on the concentration of the analyte (Figure-2).

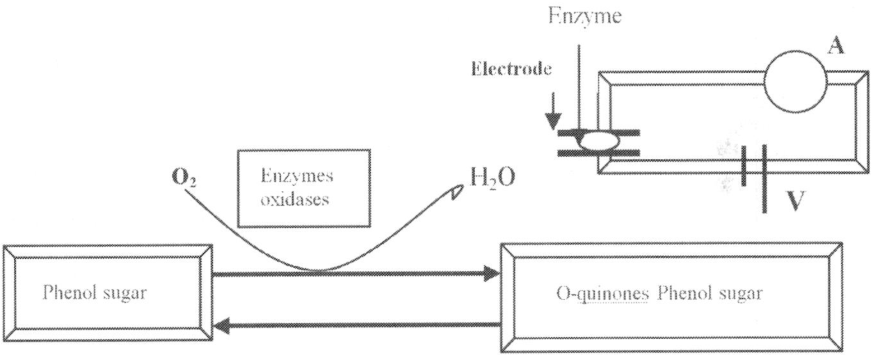

Fig. 2. A typical amperometric sensor for the assay of phenols and sugars: The enzyme is immobilized at the top of electrode, the current between electrodes gives information about the analyte.

In a simple biosensor of above type an oxygen consuming enzyme (phenolase/glucose oxidase) is immobilized on a platinum electrode and the reduction of oxygen at the electrode results in a current that is inversely proportional to the analyte concentration.

1.2.2 Potentiometric biosensor

This type of biosensor is based on the use of ion selective electrodes and ion-sensitive field effect transistors. Possibly the primary out put signal is due to the ions accumulated at the ion-selective membrane interface. The presence of the monitored ion due to reaction at the electrode surface is indicated by change in some physical parameters like pH etc. For example, the enzyme glucose oxidase can be immobilized at the pH electrode surface. The compound glucose has minimal influence on pH in working medium but the formation of gluconate due to its interaction at the enzyme immobilized pH electrode the solution becomes acidic, which can be easily detected. In general a potentiometric biosensor can be represented as under Figure 3.

Some semiconductor based physico-chemical transducers are commonly used for the construction of biosensors. The ion selective field effect transistors (ISFET) and light addressable potentiometric sensors (LAPS) are convenient biosensor materials. The working principle of ISFET is based on the generation of potential by surface ions in a solution

(Yuging et al., 2003, 2005). The generated potential modulates the current flow across silicon semiconductors. A selective membrane fabricated from compounds viz. Si_3N_4 (silicon nitrite), Al_2O_3 (Alumina), ZrO_2 (Zirconium oxide), Ta_2O_5 (Tantalum oxide) is used to cover the transistor gate surface to enable pH measurement. However, the LAPS working are based on semiconductor activation by light emitting diode (LED). Both types of biosensors have proved their applicability for bioassay.

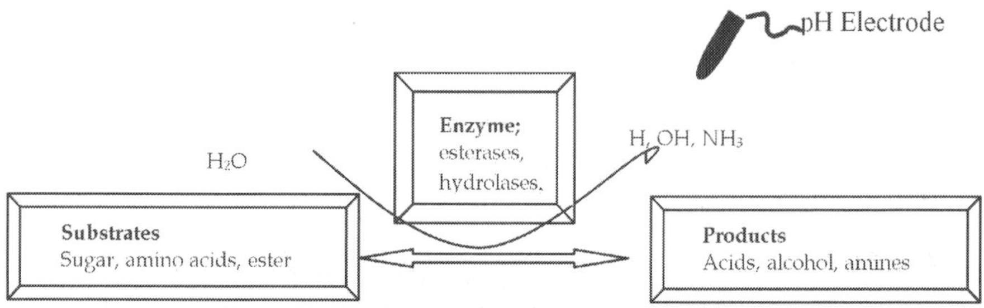

Fig. 3. Principle of working of a potentiometric sensor for the analysis of amino acids, sugars and esters. The enzymes are immobilized at the pH-electrode surface and the change in pH caused due to enzymatic conversion of the substrate is recorded, which is proportional to analyte concentration.

1.2.3 Impedimetric / conductometric biosensors

These types of biosensors measure either impedance or its components resistance/conductance and capacitance. These biosensors have been used for the assay of urea, using urease as biorecognition component. Though, the use of impedimetric biosensor is less frequent as compared to potentiometric and amperometric biosensors but their use in the study of hybridization of DNA fragments previously amplified by a polymerase chain reaction and also in monitoring the microorganism growth due to the production of conductive metabolites (Silley et al., 1996) and some other studies has produced promising results.

1.3 Electrochemical biosensors in biomedical analysis

With increasing demand for the development of low cost analytical techniques for selective and accurate analysis of drugs and other analytes and also for suggesting the mechanism of action of drugs, scientists working in the field of electroanalytical chemistry have designed electrochemical biosensors.

The developed biosensors have been successfully used for pharmaceutical analysis (Gil et al., 2010) and also for biomedical purpose. Since a large variety of biological systems can be used as recognizing agents, as such, it allows the fabrication of specific biosensors for a large variety of analytes and the electrochemical transducers impart high sensitivity to these devices (Lojou et al., 2006). The analyte-bio-recognizing agent interaction is monitored by the transducer and in the case of an electrochemical biosensor the signal detection occurs at the electrode-solution interface, which may be dynamic or static. In case of former methods i.e. voltammetry, amperometric biosensors are used, the interaction involves redox process followed by transfer of electrons. Whereas, in static methods, potentiometric biosensors are used to monitor the concentration of charged species as a function of electrochemical potential (Ravishanker, et al 2001). The correct choice of a biosensor for the study of a particular analyte depends on the selection of the recognizing agent and transducer, both suited to the target molecule.

Thus, the selection of the above biosensors depends on the characteristics of the analyte i.e. while using amperometric biosensors the organic/inorganic species should undergo a redox process at working potentials. Whereas, the static methods (using potentiometric biosensors) involve charged species. In pharmaceutical analysis, the commonly used recognizing agents are enzymes, antibodies, DNA, drug receptors etc. For the fabrication of electrochemical biosensors the main transducing elements in use are some noble metals viz. Pt and Au and also some carbon based electrode materials viz. glassy carbon, carbon paste. These electrodes, after proper modification are being widely used in the field of pharmaceutical and biomedical analysis.

In addition to the above materials the advancement made in the field of materials science and nanotechnology, has led to significant development of many electrochemical transducers like conducting polymers with suitable characteristic for electrochemical sensors, carbon nanotubes, nanomaterials with molecular dimensions (porous and monodispersive particles of clay with high superficial area etc).

Nevertheless, the efficient immobilization of recognizing agents for transducer is still a challenging task in electrochemical biosensor technology. Some immobilization techniques have been reported in the literature (Nakamura et al., 2003).

The field of research and development of biomedical and pharmaceutical analysis embraces comprehensive procedures in a bid to fulfill the requirements of the analysis i.e. accuracy, selectivity, precision, simplicity and low cost. Since, biosensors fulfill the above requirements, their possible use in the field of biomedical, pharmaceutical, food and environment etc analytes is widely being proposed.

1.4 Electrochemical biosensors in chemotherapy

Chemotherapy is an important weapon for the treatment of cancer. A large number of compounds have been developed as potential candidates for anticancer drugs, but only handful of them have become effective in clinical protocols. As such, the need to develop drugs which can effectively treat various forms of cancer is widely recognized. The development of new antineoplastic drugs (anticancer drugs) requires a clear cut understanding of the mechanism of action of the drug at the cellular and molecular levels. Cancer (neoplasias) are the diseases in which the growth of the cells, exceeds that of healthy tissue, suppressing the organic reserves surrounding the normal tissue. The potential targets for antineoplastic drugs are essentially the four nucleic acids, specific enzymes, microtubules and hormone/growth factor receptors. When the target of the drug are nucleic acids, the DNA damage causes cell death (cytotoxic and genotoxic drugs).

The antineoplastic drugs can bind DNA through several mechanisms. One of the mechanism suggests alkylation of nucleophilic sites with in the double helix. The clinically effective alkylating agents have two moieties capable of producing transient carbocations, which combine covalently to the electron rich sites of DNA like N7 position of guanine. The bifunctional alkylating agents produce cross linking of two strands of DNA which prevents the use of DNA as a template for further DNA and RNA synthesis, causing inhibition of replication and transcription leading to cell death. A large number of alkylating agents are known which have shown antitumor activity. They include nitrogen mustards (mechlorethamine, cyclophosphamide etc), aziridines and epoxides (thiotepa, mitomycin C etc), alkyl sulphonates (busulfan and its analogues), triazenes, hydrazines and related compound etc.

Another mechanism of drug-DNA binding is intercalation i.e. the insertion of a planar (generally aromatics) ring molecule between two adjacent nucleotides of DNA. Many antitumor antibiotics work through this mechanism. The antibiotic molecule (doxorubicin, daunorubicin etc) is noncovalently but firmly bound to DNA, distorting the shape of the DNA double helix. Thus, inhibiting DNA replication and RNA transcription.

Bleomycins also cause DNA damage through intercalation. These glycopeptides intercalate between guanine, cytosine, DNA base pairs and the end of the peptide binds Fe (II), which is capable to catalyze molecular oxygen reduction to superoxide or hydroxyl radicals, which causes DNA strand scission due to oxidative stress.

Since, the antitumor effect of a drug depends upon its efficiency to interact with DNA. Therefore, the molecular recognition of nucleic acids by low molecular weight compounds is an area of fundamental interest. This very fact has encouraged scientists working in the field of pharmaceutical and biomedical analysis to design experiments using a proper physiochemical technique for the study of interaction of small molecules with DNA.

1.5 Electrochemical methods for biomedical analysis

Among the physiochemical techniques, some modern electrochemical methods have attracted interest of scientists working in the field of biomedical and pharmaceutical analysis. Due to the simplicity and reliability of electrochemical methods, they offer advantages over biological and chemical assays. Since a large number of organic molecules have a tendency to exhibit redox activity, the microelctroanalytical methods have a potential to provide a useful compliment to the previously listed methods of investigation in the field. The use of electrochemical techniques are mainly based on the differences in the redox behavior of organic molecules i.e. nucleic acid binding molecules in the absence and presence of the DNA. The change in the redox behavior of the molecule under study results in the change of formal potential of the redox couple and the decrease of the peak current, which results due to the dramatic change in the diffusion coefficient after the combination of the molecule with DNA. On the other hand, since, DNA is also electrochemically active (Palacek, 1983) the drug-DNA interaction can also be described by means of variation of redox behavior of (DNA) nucleobases, such as guanine and adenine in the presence of interacting molecule.

For fabricating an electrochemical biosensor a successful marriage between the transducer, generally a microelectrode (glassy carbon fiber electrode, carbon paste electrode, carbon nanotube electrode etc) and the biological element/chemical (drug) is the primary requirement. The interactions of target analyte with the receptors on transducer (electrode) surface produce characteristic (current/potential) signals. The sensitivity, selectivity, response time and stability of the electrochemical biosensor are the important parameters, which decide the practical utility of the developed biosensor for biomedical analysis and also in the study of in-vivo mechanism of action of the drug. It is a challenging task before the scientists working in the field to design comprehensive analytical procedures setting experiments that are parallel to the expected *in-vivo* interaction conditions.

Quite a good number of compounds have a tendency to interact with DNA, causing changes in its structure and base sequence, which results in disturbing the DNA cross linking reaction. As such, in the field of medicinal science, the drug-DNA interaction can be highly useful for evaluating the damage caused to DNA by carcinogens and oxidizing substances (Perry,1996, Blackburn,1996). In recent years, the use of modified microfaradaic biosensors has proved to be highly significant for the study of interaction mechanism between substances of medicinal relevance (Brett,1999). They also work as electrochemical biosensors (Niu,2006) as a simple and inexpensive technology for the diagnosis of genetic diseases and the detection of pathogenic biological species (Erdem,2005, Rauf,2005). We know that some DNA intercalators (Ozkan,2004, Karadeniz,2003, Pang,2000, Ju,2003, Girousi,2004) which generally work as anticancer drugs are helpful in detection of the sequence specific hybridization of nucleic acids.

1.6 The anticancer drug-epirubicin

Epirubicin, an antibiotic drug of anthracyclines family, possesses a wide spectrum chemotherapeutic applications and antineoplasic action. Antitumor properties of Epirubicin are known for more than two decades but, the pharmacokinetic and biochemical studies to establish its in-vivo mechanism of action and to improve its administration and anticancer activity are still important goals to achieve. A survey of literature records that Epirubicin and other analogous anthracyclines behave as DNA intercalators and their activity accumulates in nuclear genome (Ozkan ,2003, Martinez, 2005).

Since the mid 1980's epirubicin has been extensively used for both early stage and metastatic breast cancer. Epirubicin is the 4'-epimer of the popular anthracyclin antitumor antibiotic, doxorubicin. A number of mechanisms have been suggested to explain the antineoplastic effect of epirubicin; First, it intercalates between DNA nucleotide base pairs, which results in the inhibition of DNA, RNA and protein synthesis. Second, the intercalation leads to topoisomerase II cleavage of DNA, resulting in cytocidal activity and the third mechanism suggests that epirubicin inhibits DNA helicase activity which finally interacts with DNA, RNA replication and transcription.

Due to reorientation of the hydroxyl group in the 4'-position of daunosamine (Figure 4) ring equatorial for epirubicin and axial for doxorubicin, epirubicin possesses several different pharmacological properties as compared to doxorubicin. Its pKa value is lower than that of doxorubicin. Consequently, it is more lipophilic and better able to penetrate cells. Besides, the glucuronidation of epirubicin and epirubicinol to inactivate metabolites results in a shorter terminal half life for epirubicin as compared to doxorubicin.

The below structural difference between epirubicin and doxorubicin is responsible for different safety profiles for the two antineoplastic drugs. Larger doses of epirubicin are required to produce the same degree of toxicity as doxorubicin. The doze ratios for similar toxicities for doxorubicin: epirubicin are 1:1.8 for cardiac, 1:1.5 for nonhematologic and 1:1.2 for hematologic. As such, the superior safety profile of epirubicin compared with that of doxorubicin allows for greater doze escalation that can be achieved safely which clearly means that epirubicin has a greater therapeutic window.

Chemically modified electrodes (CME) as voltammetric biosensors (Shrivastava,2004) accumulate analytes selectively and protect them from interference from other ions/electrochemical species, have played a leading role in the analysis of biosynthetic polynucleotides containing adenine/ guanine residues, using species sensitive DPV method. (Palacek,1983). As such, looking at the importance of the use of epirubicin, as a anticancer and the usefulness of electrochemical biosensors we have fabricated DNA modified and epirubicin adsorbed GCFE biosensors and studied the interaction of epirubicin in situ with ds-DNA at its surface. Since, the literature also reports that the in-vivo interaction of the anticancer drug epirubicin with DNA takes place at charged phospholipid membranes and proteins, the studied interaction would be parallel to the in-vivo DNA- epirubicin complex situation, where DNA is in close contact with charged phospholipid membranes and proteins. A suitable mechanism to the above reaction has been proposed.

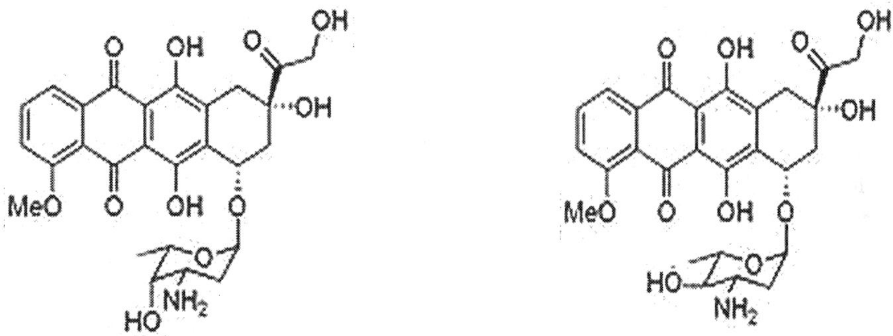

Doxorubicin Epirubicin

Fig. 4. Chemical structures of doxorubicin and doxorubicin

2. Experimental

2.1 Chemicals and instrumental

Deionised water was used to prepare the solutions of Calf thymus DNA (Himedia ltd. Mumbai) and epirubicin hydrochloride (gift sample supplied by M/S. Dabur Pharma. Ltd. Baddi distt. Solan H.P.).

An Elico (Hyderabad, India) µp-polarographic analyser model CL-362 was used for all voltammetric studies. Glassy carbon fibers (NF-12, Sigity Elititigoitit, U.K.) were used for the fabrication of glassy carbon fiber electrode (GCFE) as working electrode, a saturated calomel electrode and a coiled platinum wire electrode was used as reference and counter electrode, respectively. The pH-measurements were made on a systronic (India) µ-pH system-361. All experiments were performed at room temperature and dissolved oxygen was removed by passing pure nitrogen through the solutions.

For all the DPV (differential pulse voltammetry) experiments the instrumental parameters were used as follows: scan rate 12mV/s, sensitivity 10µA, and pulse amplitude 50mV.

2.2 Fabrication of modified electrodes

2.2.1 Epirubicin adsorbed GCFE

Epirubicin adsorbed GCFE was fabricated by dipping the electrode in a voltammetric cell containing solution of the drug (80µg/ml) for ten min., at a deposition potential of +0.40V. The electrode was taken out of solution, thoroughly rinsed with distilled water and then used for voltammetric measurements. To study the drug-DNA interaction the modified electrode was dipped in a voltammetric cell containing 80µg/ml DNA and 0.1M acetate buffer at pH 4.5±0.1, and the DP Voltammogram was recorded.

2.2.2 Thin layer ds-DNA modified GCFE

For the fabrication of thin layer ds-DNA modified GCFE, the electrode was immersed in 80μg/ml ds-DNA solution at +0.40V applied potential for ten min. This ds-DNA modified GCFE was washed with distilled water and then dipped in epirubicin solution for three min. It was then rinsed with water and transferred to a voltammetric cell containing acetate buffer solution at pH 4.5±0.1 and the differential pulse voltammogram was recorded.

2.2.3 Thick layer ds-DNA modified GCFE

For the fabrication of thick layer ds-DNA modified GCFE, the electrode was dipped in 25mg/ml solution of ds-DNA for ten min. It was taken out of solution and allowed to dry. The electrode was then dipped in (20μg/ml) solution of epirubicin for varying time intervals. Each time the electrode was taken out of the solution, washed with distilled water and dried. The dried electrode was dipped in a solution of acetate buffer (0.1M) at pH 4.5±0.1 and the voltammogram was recorded.

3. Results and discussion

3.1 DPV analysis of epirubicin at bare GCFE

Epirubicin produces two reduction peaks (Table 1) at Ep value -0.46V and -0.62V (Figure 5) due to the reduction of its 5,12-diquinone groups to produce a highly reactive semiquinone radical were observed. However, if the solution is electrolyzed performing positive potential scanning of the working electrode, the resulting differential pulse voltammogram produced a well defined peak at +0.54V (Figure 6), due to the oxidation of 6,11-dihydroquinone of epirubicin. On recording the DP Voltammogram (oxidation peak) for varying concentration of epirubicin (from 5μg/mL to 120μg/mL) under above experiment conditions, a linear relationship between the peak height of the voltammogram and epirubicin concentration was observed. Thus, enabling the quantitative determination of epirubicin. The minimum detection limit was found to be 5μg/mL of the analyte, with good accuracy and precision of determination.

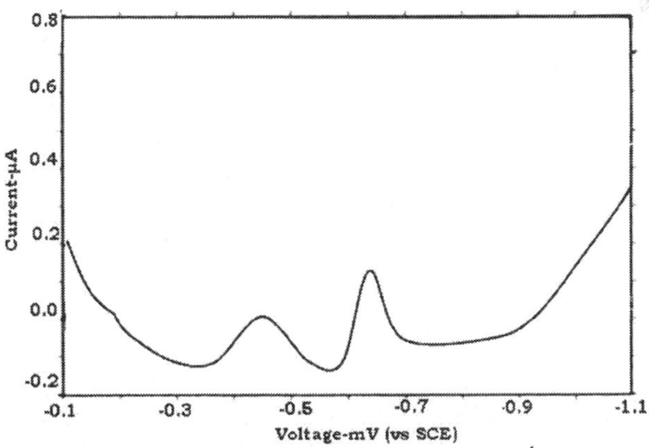

Fig. 5. Differential Pulse Voltammogram for 80μg/ml epirubicin (reduction) in 0.1M acetate buffer at pH 4.5±0.1 at bare GCFE.

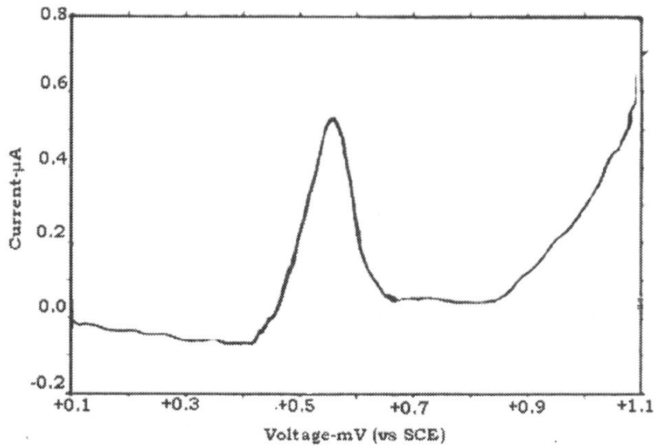

Fig. 6. Differential Pulse Voltammogram for 80μg/ml epirubicin (oxidation) in 0.1M acetate buffer at pH 4.5±0.1 at bare GCFE.

S. No	Drug/DNA Solutions	Working Electrode	Voltammetric Experimental Sequence	Ep V vs SCE I II III
1	80μg/ml Epirubicin	Bare GCFE	Cathodic potential scanning (reduction)	-0.46 -0.62 --
2	80μg/ml Epirubicin	Bare GCFE	Anodic potential scanning (oxidation)	+0.54 -- --
3	80μg/ml ds-DNA	Epirubicin modified GCFE	Applying a potential -0.60V for 60 s, followed by anodic potential scanning	+0.45
4	20μg/ml Epirubicin	Thin layer ds-DNA modified GCFE	Electrode immersed in 20μg/ml Epirubicin for 180 s followed by anodic scanning	+0.54
5	20μg/ml Epirubicin	Thin layer ds-DNA modified GCFE	Applying a potential of -0.60V for 60 s, followed by anodic scanning	+0.40 +0.54 +0.90
6	20μg/ml Epirubicin	Thick layer ds-DNA modified GCFE	Scanning the potential of the working electrode from -0.70V to -0.00V	-0.45 -0.60
7	20μg/ml Epirubicin	Thick layer ds-DNA modified GCFE	Electrode immersed in Epirubicin solution for 300 s, then applied a potential of -0.60V for 60 s, followed by anodic scanning	+0.54 +0.80 +1.1

Table 1. Summary of Voltammetric Experimental Conditions and Observed Data (in 0.1 acetate buffer at pH 4.5, Scan rate 12mV/S, Pulse amplitude- 50mV)

3.2 DPV analysis of epirubicin-DNA interaction at bare GCFE

The first set i.e. without DNA, produced a DPV oxidation peak for epirubicin at +0.54V, which shifted to more electro-positive potential with increasing DNA concentration and the peak current shortened. The shift in Ep value and shortening of peak current may be explained on the basis of change of species that is oxidized at the GCFE surface, i.e. due to the formation of drug-DNA complex.

Although, the above experimental results confirm the formation of Epirubicin-DNA complex, but, to have a clear-cut understanding on the mechanism of the drug-DNA interaction at charged surfaces, the GCFE has been modified in three different ways:

3.3 Epirubicin-DNA interaction at epirubicin adsorbed GCFE

It showed a big peak at +0.54V due to oxidation of adsorbed epirubicin and the other peaks may be due to oxidation of purine bases of DNA. This explanation of the observed voltammogram is based on the presumption that DNA diffuses from bulk of the solution to electrode surface and the chemisorbed epirubicin is intercalated into its double helix. As such, the distortion of double strand takes place, which allows the oxidation of purine bases. However, after the first scan if a potential of -0.60V was applied for 60 s, and then the voltammogram was recorded, it produced a peak at +0.45V (Figure 7). The appearance of this peak is due to the interaction of epirubicin with ds-DNA through guanine rich region.

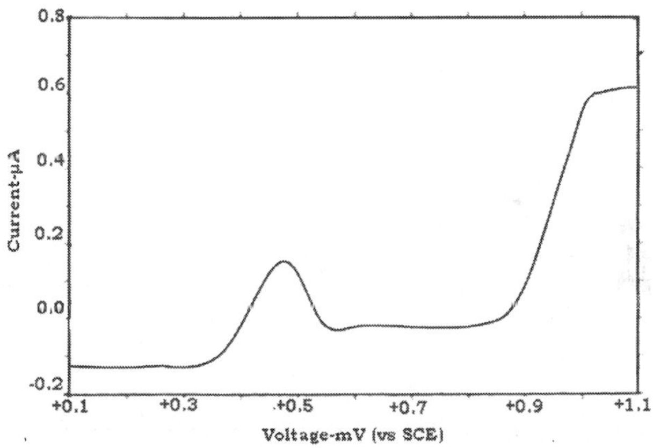

Fig. 7. Differential Pulse Voltammogram for 80µg/ml ds-DNA solution in 0.1M acetate buffer at pH 4.5±0.1, after applying a potential of -0.60V during 60 s, at epirubicin modified GCFE.

3.4 Epirubicin-DNA interaction at thin layer ds-DNA modified GCFE

The DPV for the oxidation of epirubicin, showed a well defined peak with peak potential +0.54V. The peak may be attributed to the oxidation of 6,11-dihydroquinone group of epirubicin molecule.

However, after recording the oxidation peak, a negative potential of -0.60V was applied on the modified electrode for 60 s, followed by recording of DP Voltammogram with positive potential scanning of the working electrode. The resulting voltammogarm showed two new peaks in addition to the epirubicin oxidation peak. The peak at +0.90V (Figure 8) may be attributed as due to 8-oxo-Guanine (8-oxo-G) oxidation and that at +0.40V may be due to the oxidation of purine bases of DNA. A clear separation of the peak due to 8-oxo-G and epirubicin can be explained on the basis of non-uniform coverage of the GCFE surface by DNA and adsorption of epirubicin at these uncovered surfaces. [The results are in good agreement with those observed using thick layer DNA modified GCFE]. This shift of 8-oxo-G peak to less positive potential informs about the DNA-epirubicin interaction (damage to DNA).

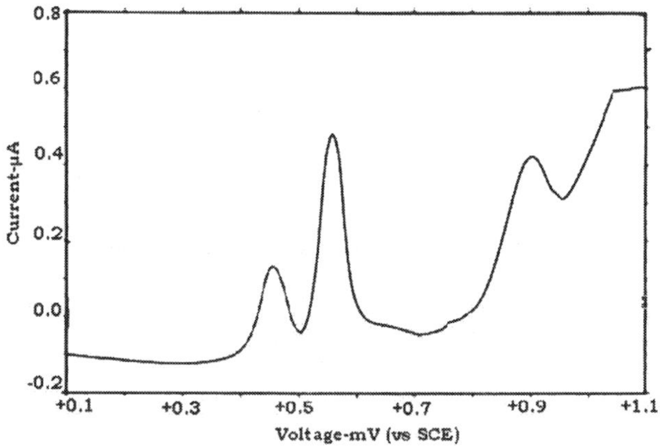

Fig. 8. Differential Pulse Voltammogram in 0.1M acetate buffer at pH 4.5±0.1, obtained with a thin layer ds-DNA modified GCFE after being immersed in 20µg/ml epirubicin solution during 180 s, after applying a potential -0.60V during 60 s.

3.5 Epirubicin-DNA interaction at thick layer ds-DNA modified GCFE

Epirubicin produced a well-defined voltammetric oxidation peak with Ep value +0.54V. The height of the epirubicin oxidation peak with respect to the time of immersion of the thick layer ds-DNA modified GCFE in epirubicin solution was investigated. The results showed a linear relationship between the peak height and time of immersion of the electrode in epirubicin solution i.e.0.00 to 60 min, and then it attained a constant value. Thus, indicating the preconcentration of epirubicin at the thick layer ds-DNA modified electrode surface.

It is important to note that reproducible peak currents were observed for the similar time of immersion of the thick layer ds-DNA modified GCFE in epirubicin solution for the first scan only. However, if the differential pulse voltammogram is recorded using the same modified electrode, an abrupt decrease in the peak current was observed. This suggests a fast consumption of the neoplasic drug at the modified electrode surface.

However, on performing the above voltammetric experiments separately using bare GCFE and thick layer ds-DNA modified GCFE as working electrode and scanning the potential from -0.70V to -0.00V, the resulting DPV curve with bare GCFE produced only one peak at -0.56V. Whereas, using thick layer ds-DNA modified GCFE two peaks were observed at -0.60V and -0.45V, respectively. The observed new peak at -0.45V speaks of a different interaction mechanism of epirubicin-DNA, at the modified GCFE surface.

Since, epirubicin is irreversibly adsorbed at the bare GCFE surface, it becomes necessary to clean the electrode each time before use. Whereas, the thick layer ds-DNA modified GCFE

did not require cleaning. This clearly reveals that the epirubicin is intercalated inside ds-DNA film and could not reach the electrode surface. On the basis of above observations it could be concluded that the voltammetric peaks are observed due to epirubicin which is intercalated into thick layer of ds-DNA. Since, the voltammograms were recorded in acetate buffer supporting electrolyte solution only, the possibility of any contribution to the voltammetric peaks from epirubicin present in solution is ruled out. As such, the observed new peak at -0.45V may be attributed to the epirubicin-guanine site (in DNA) interaction leading to a charge transfer reaction to from epirubicin semiquinone and guanine radical cation. However, the peak at -0.60V may be attributed to the reduction of the epirubicin. As mentioned earlier, epirubicin at bare GCFE produces a peak at -0.56V, the shift in the peak potential for epirubicin reduction at the two different electrode surfaces may be explained due to the change in the electrode surfaces.
However, if the ds-DNA modified GCFE after being dipped in epirubicin for 300s, rinsed and immersed in a buffer solution at pH 4.5±0.1, was subjected to a potential of -0.60V for about 60s and then the voltammogram was recorded by positive potential scanning of the modified electrode, the resulting voltammogram produced two new peaks, one at +0.80V and other at +1.1V (Figure 9). The former peak may be attributed to guanine oxidation and the later due to adenine oxidation.

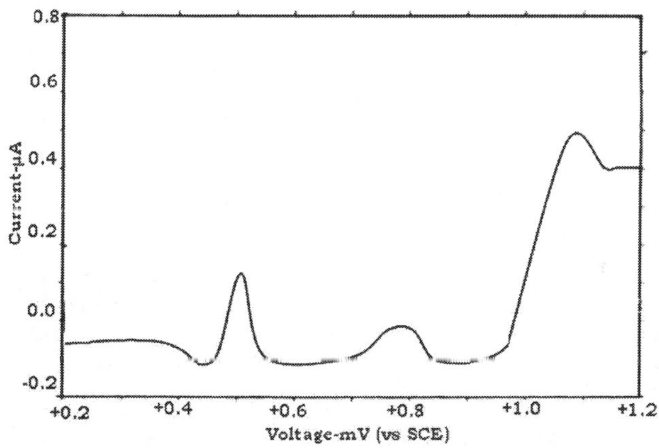

Fig. 9. Differential Pulse Voltammogram in 0.1M acetate buffer at pH4.5±0.1 obtained with a thick later ds-DNA modified GCFE after being immersed in 20µg/ml epirubicin solution for 60 s at potential -0.60V.

4. Mechanism

Epirubicin transfers an electron to its quinone portion (Perry, 1996) to generate a free radical. The highly reactive free radical formed at -0.60V may oxidize the guanine site of ds-DNA in which it is intercalated within the double helix, forming drug-DNA complex. Besides, the study on drug-DNA interaction at bare GCFE showed that the peak at +0.54V as observed in case of pure epirubicin oxidation, at bare GCFE shifts to less positive side i.e.+0.45V, on its complexation with ds-DNA, which may be explained as due to interaction between epirubicin and 8-oxo-G which is formed as a result of interaction of epirubicin with guanine rich region of ds-DNA. As such, one electron transfer from guanine moiety to quinone leading to guanine cation formation appears to be the probable reaction. However, due to the tendency of guanine cation to undergo hydrolysis, finally the semiquinone is further reduced to form epirubicin and 8-oxo-G.

Mechanism model

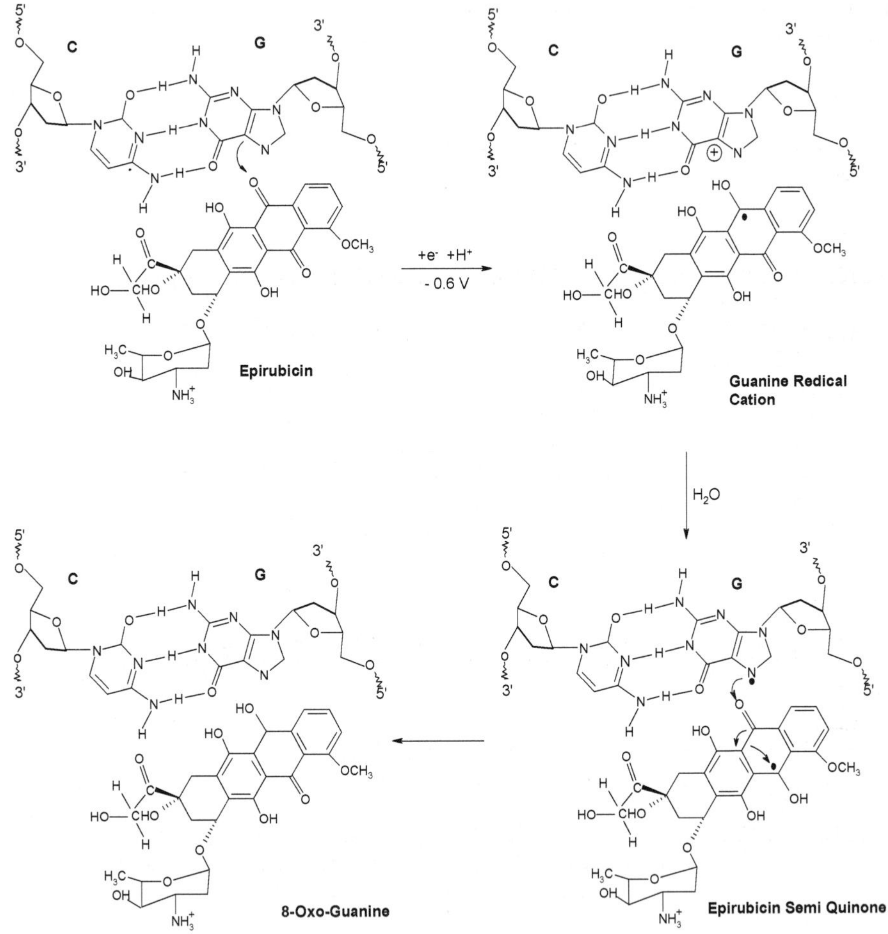

Mechanism model : Mechanism of electrochemical epirubicin oxidative damage to DNA

5. Conclusion

Voltammetric in-situ sensing of DNA oxidative damage caused by reduced epirubicin intercalated into DNA is possible using ds-DNA modified GCFE microfaradaic biosensor. The results show that epirubicin intercalated in double helix of DNA can undergo oxidation or reduction and react specifically with the guanine moiety and thus forms mutagenic 8-oxo-G residue. A mechanism model for the reaction may be proposed. The fabricated microfaradaic biosensors are of utmost relevance because the mechanism of interaction of DNA-epirubicin at charged interfaces is parallel to in-vivo DNA-drug complex reaction, where DNA is in close contact with charged phospholipid membranes and proteins rather then when intercalation is in solution. It also promises the use of voltammetric techniques for in situ generation of reaction intermediates. As such, is a complementary tool for the study of biomolecular interaction mechanism of medicinal relevance.

6. Acknowledgment

University Grants Commission, New Delhi, India, for financial support under its special assistance program (SAP) level-1.

7. References

Blackburn, GM. & Gair, MJ. (1996). Nucleic acids in chemistry and biology, Oxford University Press, UK.

Brett. OM.; Serrano, SP., & Piedade, JP. (1999). Comprehensive chemical kinetics compton, R.G. Hancock (Eds), Elsevier, Amsterdam.

Bousse, L. (1996). Whole cell biosensors. Sensors Actuators, Vol. B34, pp. 270–275.

Clark, LC. & Lyons, C. (1962). Electrode systems for continuous monitoring of cardiovascular surgery. Ann. NY. Acad. Sci., Vol. 102, pp. 29–35.

Erdem, A.; Kosmider, B.; Osiecka, R.; Zyner, E.; Ochocki, J., & Ozsoz, M. (2005). Electrochemical genosensing of the interaction between the potential chemotherapeutic agent, cis-bis (3-aminoflavone) dichloroplatinum (II) and DNA in comparison with cis-DDP. J. Pharm. Biomed. Anal., Vol. 38, pp. 645-652.

Gil, ES. & Melo GR. (2010). Electrochemical biosensors in pharmaceutical analysis. Brazilian J. Pharma. Scien., Vol. 46, pp. 375-391.

Girousi, ST.; Gherghi, IC., & Karava, MK. (2004). DNA-modified carbon paste electrode applied to the study of interaction between rifampicin (RIF) and DNA in solution and at the electrode surface. J. Pharm. Biomed. Anal., Vol. 36, pp. 851-858.

Ju, HX.; Ye, YK.; Zhao, JH., & Zhu, YL. (2003). Hybridization biosensor using di (2,2'-bipyridine) osmium (III) as electrochemical indicator for detection of polymerase chain reaction product of hepatitis B virus DNA. Anal. Biochem., Vol. 313, pp. 255-261.

Karadeniz, H.; Gulmez, B.; Sahinci, F.; Erdem, A.; Kaya, GI.; Unver, N.; Kivcak, B., & Ozsoz, M. (2003). Disposable electrochemical biosensor for the detection of the interaction between DNA and lycorine based on guanine and adenine signals. J. Pharm. Biomed. Anal., Vol. 33, pp. 295-302.

Lojou, E. & Bianco, P. (2006). Application of the electrochemical concepts and techniques to amperometric biosensor devices. J. Electroceram., Vol. 16, pp. 79-91.

Martínez, R. & Chacón-García, L. (2005). The search of DNA-intercalators as antitumoral drugs: What it worked and what did not work. Curr. Med. Chem., Vol. 12, pp. 127-151.

Meadows, D. (1996). Recent developments with biosensing technology and applications in the pharmaceutical industry. Adv. Drug Deliv. Rev., Vol. 21, pp. 179–189.

Nakamura, H. & Karube, I. (2003). Current research activity in biosensors. Anal. Bioanal. Chem., Vol. 377, pp. 446-468.

Niu, S.; Li, F.; Zhang, S.; Wang, L.; Li, X., & Wang, S. (2006). Studies on the interaction mechanism of 1,10-phenanthroline cobalt (II) complex with DNA and preparation of electrochemical DNA biosensor. Sensor, Vol. 6, pp. 1234-1244.

Ozkan, A. & Fiskin, K. (2003). Cytotoxicity of low dose epirubicin-HCI combined with lymphokine activated killer cells against hepatocellular carcinoma cell line hepatoma G2. Turk. J. Med. Sci., Vol. 34, pp. 11-19.

Ozkan, D.; Karadeniz, H.; Erdem, A.; Mascini, M., & Ozsoz, M. (2004). Electrochemical genosensor for Mitomycin C–DNA interaction based on guanine signal. J. Pharm. Biomed. Anal., Vol. 35, pp. 905-912.

Paddle, BM. (1996). Biosensors for chemical and biological agents of defence interest. Biosens. Bioelectron., Vol. 11, pp. 1079–1113.

Palacek, E. (1983). Modern polarographic (voltammetric) techniques part (ii) in biochemistry and molecular biology, In: Topics in Bioelectrochemistry and Bioenergetics, G. Milazzo (Eds), John Wiley & Sons, New York.

Pang, DW. & Abruna, HD. (2000). Interactions of benzyl viologen with surface-bound single and double-stranded DNA. Anal. Chem., Vol. 72, pp. 4700-4706.

Perry, MC. (1996). The Chemotherapy Source Book, Williams and Wilkins, Baltimore, USA.

Rauf, S.; Gooding, JJ.; Akhtar, K.; Ghauri, MA.; Rahman, M.; Anwar, MA., & Khalid, AM. (2005). Electrochemical approach of anticancer drugs–DNA interaction. J. Pharm. Biomed. Anal., Vol. 37, pp. 205-217.

Ravishankara, MN.; Pillai, AD., & Handral, RD. (2001) Biosensor and its application. East. Pharm., Vol. 44, pp. 21-25.

Shrivastava, AK. (2004). Electrochemical sensors based on macrocyclic compounds in International Conference on electroanalytical chemistry and allied topics, January 18-23, 2004 Dona Paula, Goa (India), Indian Soc. Electroanal. Chem., Mumbai (India).

Silley, P. & Forsythe, S. (1996). Impedance microbiology: a rapid change for microbiologists. J. Appl. Bacteriol., Vol. 80, pp. 233–243.

Yuqing, M.; Jianquo, G., & Jianrong C. (2003). Ion sensitive field effect transducer-based biosensors. Biotechnol. Adv., Vol. 21, pp. 527–534.

Yuqing, M.; Jianrong, C., & Keming, F. (2005). New technology for the detection of pH. J. Biochem. Biophys. Methods, Vol. 63, pp. 1–9.

Ziegler, C. & Göpel, W. (1998). Biosensor development. Curr. Opin. Chem. Biol., Vol. 2, pp. 585–591.

16

Light Addressable Potentiometric Sensor as Cell-Based Biosensors for Biomedical Application

Hui Yu, Qingjun Liu and Ping Wang*
Biosensor National Special Lab, Key Lab of Biomedical Engineering of Ministry of Education, Department of Biomedical Engineering, Zhejiang University China

1. Introduction

One of most enduring topics in the field of biosensors and bioelectronics is cell-based biosensors, which are able to convert cellular biological effects to electrical signals, via living cells. As the archetypal interface between a biological and an electronic system, the research and development of cell-based biosensors are essentially dependent on the combined knowledge of engineers, physicists, chemists and biologists. In recent years, the miniaturization and expanding applications of cell-based biosensors in biology, environment and medicine fields, have drawn extensive attention.

Light addressable potentiometric sensor (LAPS) is a semiconductor device proposed by Hafeman in 1988, and it is now as commonly used as ISFET (Hafeman et al., 1988). LAPS indicates a heterostructure of silicon/silicon oxide/silicon nitride, excited by a modulated light source to obtain a photocurrent. The amplitude of this light induced photocurrent is sensitive to the surface potential and thus LAPS is able to detect the potential variation caused by an electrochemical even. Therefore, in principle, any event that results in the change of surface potential can be detected by LAPS, including the change of ion concentration (Parce et al., 1989), redox effect (Piras et al., 1996), etc. LAPS shows some advantages comparing to ISFET while constructing cell-based biosensor. The easier fabrication process of LAPS is fully compatible with the standard microelectronics facilities. The encapsulation of LAPS is much less critical since no metal contact is formed on the surface. Besides, the extremely flat surface makes it compatible to incorporate into very small volume chamber, which is important for small dose measurement. Therefore, LAPS seems promising for biomedical application.

Due to the spatial resolving power, LAPS also has an advantage for array sensing application (Shimizu et al., 1994). Usually, no additional sensor structure is needed to realize the LAPS array sensing. In fact, LAPS is an integrated sensor itself, whose integration level is defined by the spatial resolution and the illuminating system. Thus, miniaturization with high integration level can be achieved. Many efforts have been drawn on the integration of LAPS (Men et al., 2005; Wang et al., 2005). Among these attempts, most are focused on the

*Corresponding address: cnpwang@zju.edu.cn

multi-sensing of different ions. Our lab proposed an electronic nose with MLAPS for environmental detection, which can detect H^+, Fe^{3+} and Cr^{6+} simultaneously (Men et al., 2005). Schooning et al. proposed a 16-channel handheld pen-shaped LAPS which can detect pH of 16 spots on the surface (Schooning et al., 2005). For biomedical sensing, our lab reported a novel microphysiometer to detect several different ions in cell metabolism (Wu et al., 2001a). Besides integrating LAPS to detect different ions, other possible attempts are also performed to integrate both abilities of ion concentration detection and extracellular potential signal detection, although it is still a long term from realistic application (Yu et al., 2009).

While constructing cell-based biosensors, one of the biggest obstacles is that the target cells are required to be deposited on predetermined electrodes. Due to the light addressing ability, the light addressable potentiometric sensor (LAPS) can overcome this geometrical restrict, which makes LAPS an outstand candidate among various cell-based biosensors. LAPS show great potential for constructing miniaturized and integrated biosensors. One promising solution is the LAPS array for integrated cell-based biosensors. By combining the IC techniques, mechanisms, and signal sampling methods, the LAPS array system has been greatly improved and miniaturized for biomedical applications.

LAPS as cell-based biosensors are able to perform longtime monitoring of several different cell physiology parameters, including extracellular acidification rate, various metabolites in extracellular microenvironment and action potential. These distinguish functions provide LAPS some promising applications in biomedical fields, such as cell biology, pharmacology, toxicology, etc (Parce et al., 1989; Mcconnell et al., 1992; Wada et al., 1992; Hafner, 2000; Wille et al., 2003). Furthermore, the multi functions of LAPS array as integrated cell-based biosensors makes the LAPS array system a good platform for drug analysis.

This chapter covers design and fabrication rules, systems and applications of LAPS. LAPS as cell-based biosensors are described in details, including principle, developments, and applications. Promising aspects and developments in miniaturization of LAPS array systems are introduced for cell-based biosensors. Applications of LAPS as cell-based biosensors are provided in biomedical fields, including the interaction of ligands and receptors, drug analysis, etc. Some future developments of LAPS as cell-based biosensors are proposed in the last part of this chapter.

2. Principle

LAPS is a semiconductor based potential sensitive device that usually consists of the metal-insulator-semiconductor (MIS) or electrolyte-insulator-semiconductor (EIS) structure. As for constructing cell-based biosensor, electrolyte is needed for cells living, thus LAPS with EIS structure is always adopted. LAPS with EIS structure is schematically shown in Figure 1A. The LAPS consists of the heterostructure of $Si/SiO_2/Si_3N_4$. An external DC bias voltage is applied to scan the EIS structure to form accumulation, depletion and inversion layer at the interface of the insulator (SiO_2) and semiconductor (Si), sequentially. When a modulated light pointer illuminates the bulk silicon, light induced charge carriers are separated by the internal electric field and thus photocurrent can be detected by the peripheral circuit. The amplitude of the photocurrent depends on the local surface potential. By detecting the photocurrent of LAPS, localized surface potential can be obtained (Hafeman et al., 1988).

The basic function of LAPS is for pH detection. Usually, a layer of Si_3N_4 is fabricated on the surface of LAPS as the H^+-sensitive layer. According to the site-binding theory, a potential difference which is related to the concentration of H^+ in the electrolyte forms at the interface of insulator (Si_3N_4/SiO_2) and solution (Siu et al., 1979; Bousse et al., 1982). This potential is coupled to the bias voltage applied to the sensor. Larger concentration of H^+ provides a larger value of this potential difference, causing the I-V curve to shift along the axis of bias voltage (Figure 1B). When the bias voltage keeps constant in the middle region, change of the photocurrent indicates the pH change of the electrolyte. With the microchamber specified for biological assay, the extracellular acidification rate of cells can be monitored in the microenvironment by the commercialized Cytosensor™ Microphysiomter system.

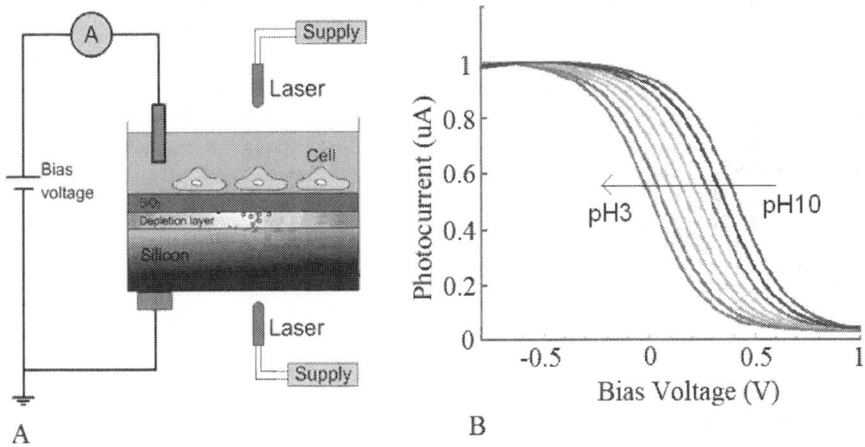

Fig. 1. (A) Working principle of the LAPS. (B) Characteristic I-V curves of n-type LAPS

Beside the pH detection, attempt has been made for the extracellular detection of electrical signals. LAPS is a surface potential detector with spatial resolution. Light pointer used for LAPS detection can be focused by microscope and optical lens, which suggests the LAPS possible for cell analysis on any non-predetermined testing site. After cells are cultured on the LAPS, a focused laser, 10 μm in diameter, is used to illuminate the front side of the chip to address the cells to be monitored. Excitable cells such as cardiac myocytes or neuron cells can generate extracellular action potential. This potential is coupled to the bias voltage applied to the LAPS, which correspondingly changes the amplitude of the photocurrent. Thus, by monitoring the photocurrent at a constant bias voltage, extracellular potential signals can be detected (Xu et al., 2005).

Illuminating different sensing areas with modulated lights of different frequencies generates a photocurrent signal, from which corresponding information of each testing site can be obtained by FFT (Fast Fourier Transform) methods (Cai et al., 2007). Comparing with conventional surface potential detectors such as FET or MEA, integration of LAPS array has many advantages. The most important feature of LAPS array is the great reduction of the required leads. For MEA, the number of required leads is the same as the number of electrodes, while for LAPS array, only one lead is necessary, regardless of the number of testing sites, which is important for high level integration (George et al., 2000). Besides, LAPS can detect extracellular potential as well as ion concentrations (Wu et al., 2001b), which makes it suitable for multi-functional integration. Sensing surface of LAPS is extremely flat and free of metal contact. Thus it's easy for encapsulation of LAPS array and fabrication of micro testing chamber.

3. Device and system

The LAPS device is a typical EIS structure. Fabrication procedure is easy and fully compatible with standard microelectronics facilities. We have introduced in our publications the most commonly used LAPS device and system (Xu et al., 2005). In this section, we mainly introduce the devices and fabrication process of LAPS array sensors.

3.1 Devices

As mentioned before, the LAPS can be treated as an array sensor with no extra structures due to the spatial resolution. However, since only a little part of the LAPS surface is illuminated with the modulated light pointer, unilluminated parts, where no photocurrent flows, act as stray capacitance and cause noises. Therefore, the smaller the total capacitance of the device is, the better the potential sensitivity will be. Small effective areas as well as a thick insulating layer reduce the total capacitance, and thus improve the potential sensitivity. Nevertheless, by reducing the effective LAPS surface to small areas, the advantage of the LAPS against surface potential detectors with discrete active sites is lost (George et al., 2000). According to our experience in cell experiments, we found 200μm×200μm a compromised size between cell culture and the noise level (Xu et al., 2006).

One typical structure of the integrated LAPS array sensor reported for multifunctional detection of extracellular pH detection and extracellular potential signals is schematically shown in Fig.2 (a). (Yu et al., 2009) The chip has a total area of about 1cm×2cm. Testing areas of two different sizes are fabricated on the same silicon chip by heavily doping the silicon between the testing areas. For extracellular potential signal detection, about 400 small square wells were fabricated in size of 200μm×200μm and the plateau between two adjacent testing areas was 100μm in width. Cells were cultured on the areas with small wells for potential detection. The depth of the well shaped structure was about several hundred nanometers, and we found that cells are more likely to grow on the testing areas of the arrays, which had lower altitude. Four larger wells for detection of cell acidification were 3mm×3mm in size and 1mm away from each other.

The fabrication process of such LAPS array structures was shown in Fig.2(b). A p-type silicon wafer (thickness of 450μm) with <100> crystal orientation was used. First, a thick layer of silicon oxide was thermally grown on the surface. Then, after the pattern was transferred to the surface using photolithography, all silicon oxide, except that grown on testing areas (acting as a protector of substrate at testing areas from being doped in the following step), was removed by etching. Thermal diffusion doping was then carried out. As the silicon wafer is p-type, boron was selected as the impurity. There were two steps in doping process. First, a glass layer containing boron was pre-deposited on the sensing surface. Then pre-diffusion doped the surface of silicon to a small depth. After pre-diffusion, the glass layer was removed, followed by the redistribution step. During the redistribution step, a thick layer of silicon oxide about several hundred nanometers formed on the surface of doped areas, which participated in forming a well shaped structure. The doped part of the semiconductor was several micrometers in depth to cut off the depletion layer of adjacent detection sites. After the doping procedure, silicon oxide layer on testing areas was removed. Instead, a thin layer of silicon oxide, 30nm in thickness, was thermally grown on testing sites and then a 60nm silicon nitride layer as the sensitive layer to H+ was deposited on the sensor chip by PECVD. At last, a thin layer of aluminum (thickness of 200nm) was evaporated on the backside of the silicon chip to form an ohm contact.

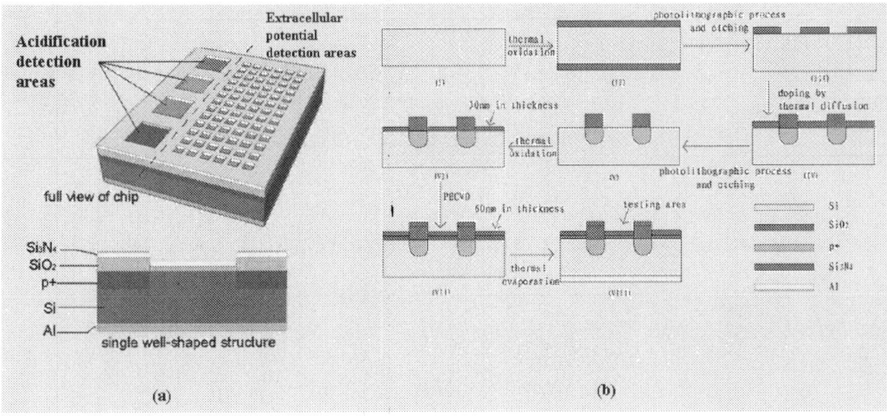

Fig. 2. (a) Schematic diagram of LAPS array sensor structure: the upper one is the full view of chip; the lower one is the well-shaped structure of single testing area. (b) Fabrication process of the LAPS array.

3.2 System

The LAPS system usually requires LED driver, chemical working station, lock-in amplifier, sampling card, flow control system, etc. In our work, a potentiostat (EG&G Princeton Applied Research, M273A) is employed to control the bias voltage across the silicon bulk to form the depletion layer inside. In running process, the bias voltage of LAPS is applied to the platinum counter electrode versus the silicon working electrode and the photocurrent flows through the working electrode to be detected by peripheral equipment. Preamplification is also performed in the potentiostat, which transforms the current signal into potential signal.

In LAPS system, the surface potential signal is amplitude modulated by the high frequency light signal, resulting in the high frequency photocurrent signal. Thus, to obtain the original surface potential signal, demodulation is required after preamplification. Lock-in amplifier is always used for small signal detection, as it can greatly increase the signal to noise ratio (SNR), usually an improvement of the SNR for over 10^6 times. In Our system, the lock-in amplifier (Stanford Research System, SR830) is employed. The lock-in amplifier only detects the signals in narrow band near the object frequency, determined by the reference frequency. Thus, in order to get corresponding surface potential signal from the photocurrent signal, it is important to keep the internal reference frequency exactly the same as the carrier frequency of the photocurrent signal, which is the light frequency. The laser generator supply is controlled by external reference signal generated by lock-in amplifier, which has the same frequency as the internal reference signal used for demodulation. Therefore, the result of the lock-in amplifier includes the amplitude and phase information of the photocurrent signal, which reflects the change of the surface potential signal of the

LAPS chip. After signal demodulation by lock-in amplifier, data is then sampled by a 16-bit acquisition card to the computer for data screening and further processing by the software. Programming can be performed with different programming languages, among which, labVIEW is recommended.

For LAPS array detection, different LAPS array system were established. The simple way is to scan the light pointer along the LAPS devices. Each sample contained information at corresponding detecting area. However, this solution suffered from low resolution and long scanning time, which prevented it from wide application (Nakao et al., 1996). An alternative way to perform the LAPS array detection is using multi light sources as the illumination. Several light sources were modulated at different frequencies and illuminating different area of the LAPS devices. In this situation, each sample contained information of several detecting areas. To extract each signal from the overall mixed signal, Fast Fourier Transform (FFT) technique is a preferred way. Our lab has reported a novel design that could significantly increase the measurement rate of LAPS (Zhang et al., 2001). By illuminating the LAPS simultaneously at several different positions, each of which is illuminated with a light pointer modulated with different frequencies, the surface potential at all illuminated regions can be measured simultaneously by analyzing the resulting photocurrent. Using this method, the rate to obtain a complete image of the surface potential distribution across a LAPS wafer can be drastically increased compared to the conventional system. However, the multi-light LAPS needs to equip a signal generator for each light source. To obtain an 8×8 image, the system needs to provide 64 signal generators. With LEDs as the light sources, this system has a lower resolution and precision. So this method is unsuitable for accurate imaging. Moreover, the problem lies in the big volume of the illuminating system, which was a main obstacle for highly integrated system, and the longer time for digital demodulation, which is not suitable for fast detection such as the detection of extracellular action potential.

Researchers have paid attentions in solving the problems in constructing LAPS array system. Our lab also has presented a novel imaging system, shown in Figure 3. With microlens array, a single laser is separated into a focused laser line array. Every focused laser is modulated separately to a different settled frequency. With a line-scanning control, an 8×8 image can be obtained that only needs 8 scanning. Moreover, with different sensing materials, this device can be used to detect several components of sample in parallel. (Cai et al., 2007)

To illustrate the constructing of LAPS array system for cell-based biosensors, our system for multi detection of cellular parameters were shown in Fig.4 (Yu et al., 2009). A laser light with the wavelength at 690nm (red) was used for illumination of extracellular potential detection. The laser was modulated at 10kHz by the lock-in amplifier (SR830, Stanford Research System), and the power is about 0.2mW. The laser was focused to about 10μm in diameter through an optimized microscope so that it can be used to address a cluster of cells on the sensor chip. Four LEDs with the wavelength at 625nm (red) were respectively driven at four different frequencies of crime numbers to avoid harmonic interference with a power of 50mW. These LEDs illuminated the relative four testing areas for acidification detection. These five lights illuminated the sensor chip at the same time. A photocurrent signal including signals at all these five different frequencies was generated, respectively representing information of the five different testing sites. The detecting system was designed to sample the overall signal and extract signals at the five different frequencies.

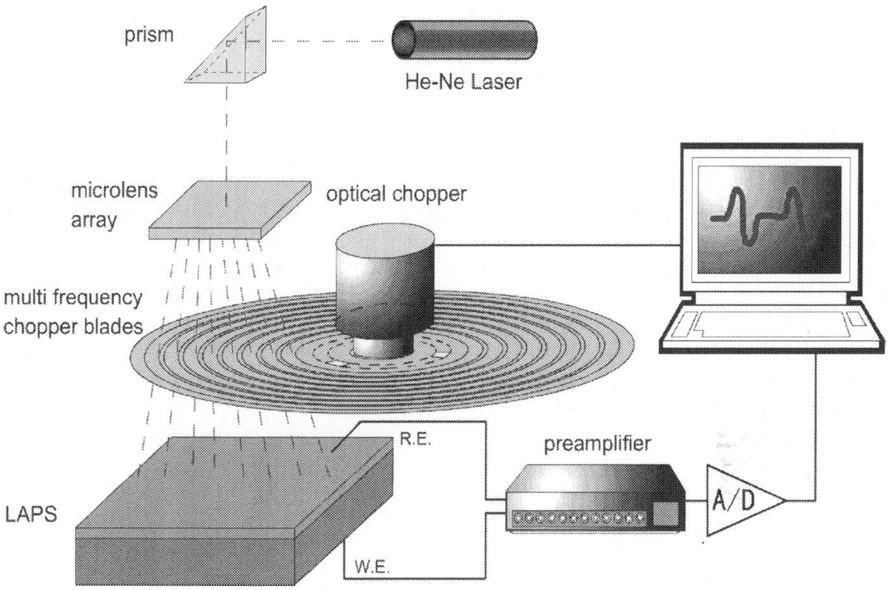

Fig. 3. Schematic diagram of the line-scanning light sources based on microlens array.

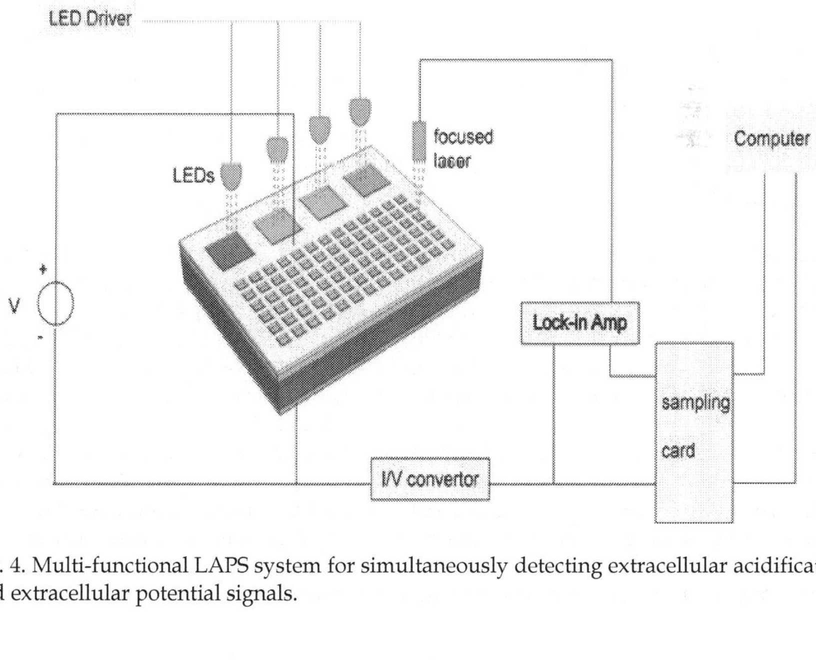

Fig. 4. Multi-functional LAPS system for simultaneously detecting extracellular acidification and extracellular potential signals.

Basically, single spike of action potential recorded lasts only several hundred milliseconds or even less (Sprössler et al., 1999; Fromherz.P et al., 2002; Sprössler et al.,1998). Thus, the sampling frequency should be high enough not to miss any action potential signals. Besides, for real-time monitoring of extracellular potential signals, time delay between sensing and display was preferred to be as small as possible. It's a different situation for acidification detection. Usually, the extracellular pH change is a long time effect. Accumulation of H+ in extracellular environment will not cause significant signals until several minutes (Hafner, 2000). Thus, for acidification detection, time delay between sampling and display was less critical.

Usually, there were several seconds interval between two times of sampling. A potentiostat (Model 273A, EG&G) was used to apply the bias voltage to the sensor chip and perform the I/V-converting. Due to the different requirements in the time delay, two different methods were combined for signal recording. For extracellular potential detection, after the overall photocurrent signal was I-V converted, the lock-in amplifier was used. As the laser was modulated at 10kHz by the internal reference signals of the lock-in amplifier, the output of the lock-in amplifier was also the component at 10kHz. Thus, only the signal generated at the testing site illuminated by the focused laser was preserved and demodulated, which indicated the extracellular potential signal. High sampling frequency up to 100kHz was set to monitor the action potential. The lock-in amplifier can perform a fast demodulation of signals, and thus little delay was introduced for real-time monitoring.

For acidification detection, after the overall photocurrent signal of five different frequencies was converted to a potential signal, it was directly sampled to the computer for analysis. Signals generated at the four different sensing areas were gained separately by digitally demodulating the signal by software with FFT methods (Cai et al., 2007) at respective illuminating frequencies of the four LEDs, which were four different crime numbers. The overall signal was also sampled at 100kHz. Data of one second was sampled every five seconds. Thus, there was four seconds for the software to perform digital demodulation of the signals at these four different frequencies and then display each part.

4. Application

LAPS has many advantages for constructing cell-based biosensors. Since the first publishing of the Cytosensor™ Microphysiometer, it has been widely used by researchers. Besides, the newly proposed cell-semiconductor LAPS device for extracellular potential detection is considered as a useful tool for cell electric biology study. Applications of LAPS for cell-based biosensor are introduced in cell biology, pharmacology, toxicology, environment measurement, etc. Several reviews have been published to introduce the applications of the microphysiometer (Parce et al., 1989; Mcconnell et al., 1992; Wada et al., 1992; Hafner, 2000; Wille et al., 2003). In this section, the application of LAPS sensors, especially the LAPS array biosensors for drug analysis, was introduced.

4.1 Multi-parameter monitoring of cell physiology by LAPS array for drug analysis

The primary functions of LAPS as cell-based biosensors are monitoring the extracellular acidification. Researchers have been working with the Cytosensor Microphysiometer on various aspects including the ligand/receptor binding, pharmacology, toxicology, etc. However, the microphysiometer suffered a major problem that only H^+ can be monitored. In recent work, the microphysiometer was usually used together with other instruments for biological detection. To solve this problem, getting more information about the multi-functional cellular processing of input- and output-signals in different cellular plants is essential for basic research as well as for various fields of biomedical applications. Therefore, research work with LAPS for extracellular potential detection and multi-parameter detection of cell physiology was preferred.

Liu et al. have constructed a cell-semiconductor hybrid device for some applications in drug analysis (Liu et al., 2007a). As an agent of β-adrenoceptor agonist that contributes to cardio-activity, isoproterenol (ISO) enhances the L-type calcium channel activity, which caused an increase in Ca^{2+} signal. As shown in Figure 5, it is obvious that after administration of ISO, the beating frequency, amplitude and duration of cardiomyocytes were all increased in a dose-depended manner (0.1, 1, 10 μM). The cellular contractibility all recovered after washing drugs out at above concentrations. Whereas, as a negative one, carbamylcholine (CARB) had opposite effect to ISO, increasing K^+ conductance in cardiacmyocytes, and signals indicated a decreasing trend. Figure 5A showed the changes of curves to ISO and CARB at concentration of 1 μM. We could see that the parameters display the two drugs distinct. Furthermore, if we differentiated parameters to each stroke shown in Figure 5BCD, more approving results could be got. According to those changes, we know that ISO and CARB have direct effects on the duration and amplitude of the strokes 2 and 3, which accord with the pharmacological increase of the Ca^{2+} or K^+ ion current, respectively. Thus, cooperated with Na^+, K^+ and Ca^{2+}, targets of a concrete drug can be evaluated synchronously by the biosensor system.

The concentrations of the extracellular ions, such as Na^+, K^+, Ca^{2+}, may change along with the alteration of cell physiology. In order to analyze simultaneously the relations of the extracellular environmental H^+, Na^+, K^+, Ca^{2+} under the effects of drugs, our lab has developed a novel microphysiometer based on multi-LAPS (Wu et al., 2001a; Wu et al., 2001b). The surface of the LAPS is deposited with different sensitive membranes by silicon microfabrication technique and the poly- (PVC) membrane technique. Three different sensitive membranes are illuminated in parallel with light sources at different frequencies, and measured on-line by parallel processing algorithm, Figure 6A. Different sensitive (H^+, K^+, Ca^{2+}) membrane is illuminated on the sensor, simultaneously with three light sources at different frequencies (3kHz for K^+, 3.5kHz for Ca^{2+}, 4kHz for H^+). The photocurrent comprises these three frequency components, and the amplitude of each frequency component might be measured on-line by software FFT analysis, as shown in Figure 6B. Dilantin, i.e. phenytoin sodium, a sort of anti-epilepsy drugs, has significant effects of transqulizing and hypnotic and anti-seizure. Moreover, dilantin is also one of the anti-arrhythmia drugs. It is proved that dilantin has membrane stabilizing action on neural cells because it can reduce pericellular membrane ions (Na^+, Ca^{2+}) permeability, inhibit Na^+ and Ca^{2+} influx, stave K^+ efflux, thus, prolong refractory period, stabilize pericellular membrane, decrease excitability (Figure 6C).

Besides combining detection of different metabolites, integration of different functional biosensors is also attractive. In our work, we have proposed a LAPS array system for simultaneously detection of both the acidification rate and the extracellular signals []. Although this system is some distance from realistic application for drug screening, this integrated cell-based biosensor can be used for simultaneously detection of both the acidification rate and the extracellular signals under certain drug effect. Comparing to conventional microphysiometer, this system combined both the electrical signal and the metabolism signals of cells, which could be of great help in analyzing the cellular response to drugs.

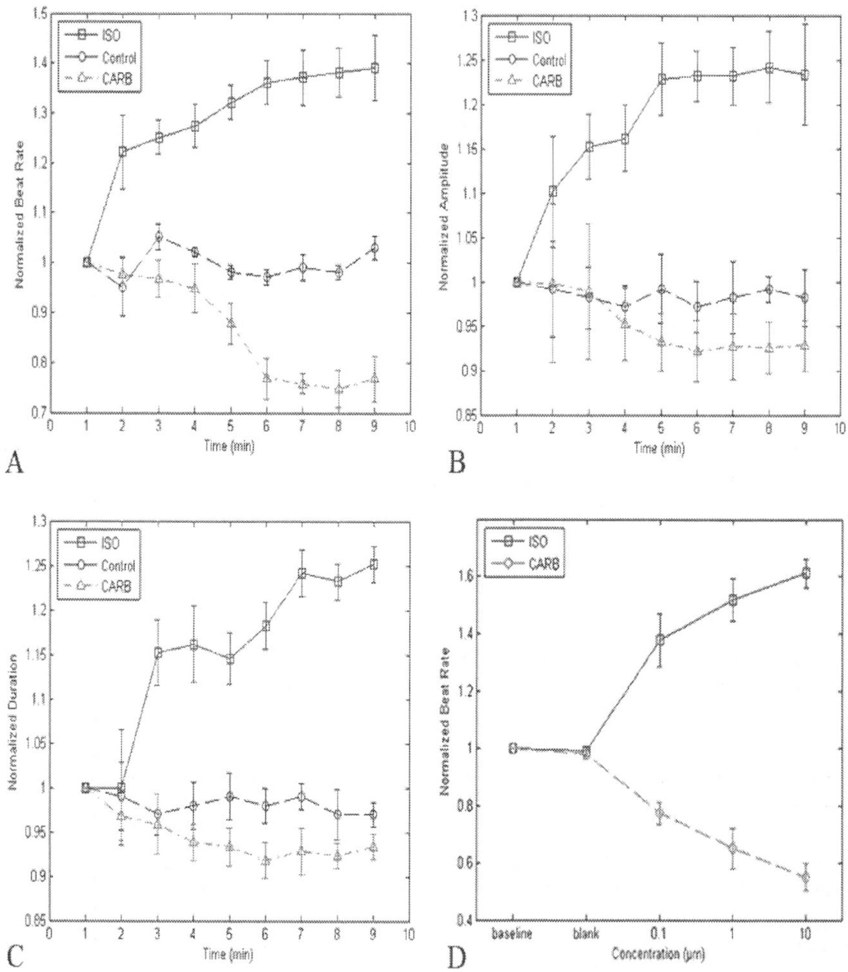

Fig. 5. Plots comparing the response of cardiomyocytes to the carbamylcholine (CARB), isoproterenol (ISO) and physiological solution as control. The concentration of drugs are all 1 μM. Drugs effect on the beat rate (A), amplitude (B) and duration (C) of each extracellular potential. Effect of different drug concentration to beat rate (D). Each data point represents an average over 50 s. The experimental data is the average value of six times of repetition.

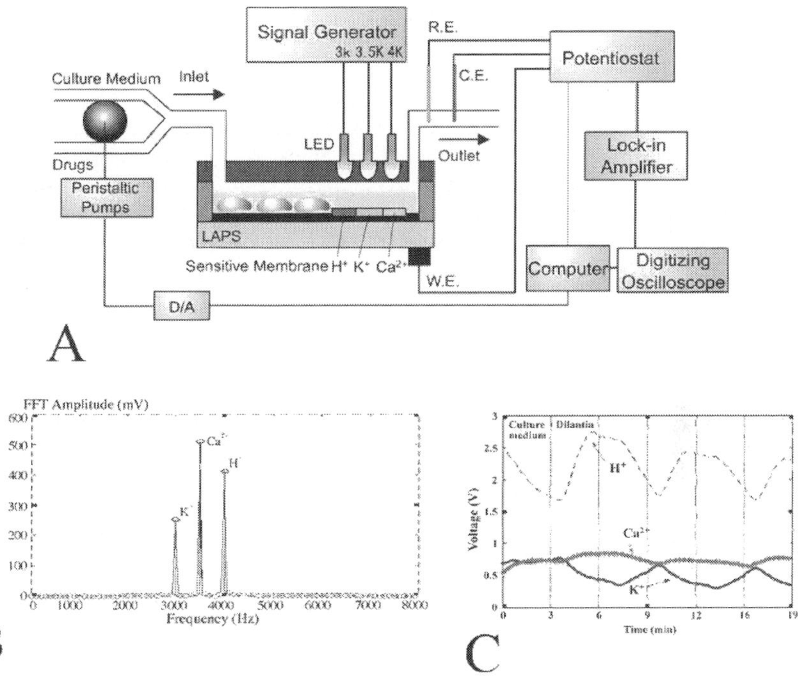

Fig. 6. Microphysiometer studies based on multi-LAPS. (A) The schematic drawing of the system of the multi-LAPS to different extracellular ions (H^+, K^+, and Ca^{2+}). (B) Illuminate simultaneously at the three sensitive membranes with three light sources at different modulated frequencies. (C) H^+, K^+, Ca^{2+} analyzed simultaneously by multi-LAPS.

4.2 LAPS for environment monitoring

Environment monitoring is a very important aspect in LAPS application. In our work, we mainly treated situation with heavy metal ion. We have reported the electronic tongue system with LAPS for heavy metal ions monitoring in sea water [][]. However, this system requires the ion sensitive membranes of corresponding heavy metal ions which increases the cost and was indirect to study the effect of the target sea water to the biological object.

The LAPS biosensor system has been reported to detect heavy metal ions according to changes in parameters describing spontaneous beating of cardiomyocytes under the different toxic effects (Liu et al., 2007b). The effects of heavy metal ions on cell function were evaluated by comparing the changes of the sensor signals before and after the cells were exposed to the toxins. Figure 7 shows the change of frequency, duration and amplitude of the signals after the addition of 10 μM heavy metals for each type (Fe^{3+}, Hg^{2+}, Pb^{2+}, Cd^{2+}, Cu^{2+} and Zn^{2+}). Exposure of beating cardiomyocytes to 10 μM Fe^{3+} decreases the frequency, amplitude and duration to about 50% of the basal signal. Similar curves were found for Pb^{2+} and Cd^{2+} solutions with a smaller decrease of amplitude and duration, however a slight progressive increase of frequency was observed. On the contrary, the three parameters all increased in Hg^{2+} solution. There were no apparent trends with regard to Cu^{2+} and Zn^{2+} toxic effects on measured parameters (only duration on Zn^{2+} showed a slight increase). Comparing with biosensors using pure enzymes, cell-based biosensors, which use whole cells as the bio-recognition elements, LAPS for biosensors can detect agents functionally (Bousse, 1996; Stenger et al., 2001). Metal ions are found to have effects on the cellular organelles and components, such as cell membrane, mitochondrial, lysosome, endoplasmic reticulum, nuclei, and some enzymes involved in metabolism, detoxification, and damage repair (Squibb and Fowler, 1981). All these systems are considered to influence metal induced cellular responses simutaneously. Therefore, incorporated with whole cells, cell based biosensors would offer potential physiological monitoring advantages over devices based on isolated enzymes or proteins. And with the help of living cells, especially mammalian cells, we could not only detect but also evaluate toxicities of heavy metals with cellular physiological changes.

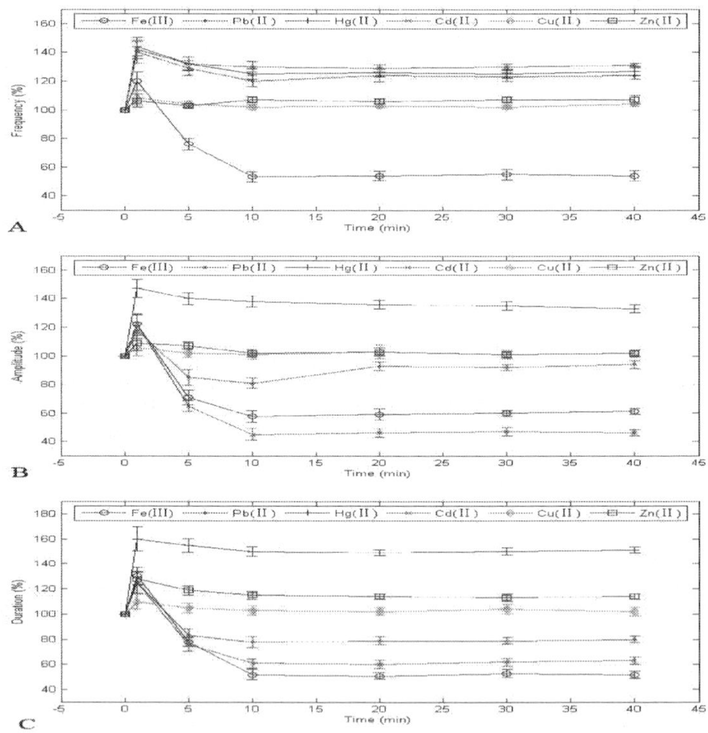

Fig. 7. Plots comparing the response of cardiomyocytes to the carbamylcholine (CARB), isoproterenol (ISO) and physiological solution as control. The concentration of drugs are all 1 μM. Drugs effect on the beat rate (A), amplitude (B) and duration (C) of each extracellular potential. Effect of different drug concentration to beat rate (D). Each data point represents an average over 50 s. The experimental data is the average value of six times of repetition.

4.3 LAPS as bioelectronic nose and bioelectronic tongue

Göpel and his colleague first proposed utilizing olfactory neurons as sensitive materials to develop a bioelectronic nose (Gopel et al., 1998; Ziegler et al., 1998; Gopel et al., 2000). They suggested the biomolecular function units can be used to develop highly sensitive sensors (like the dog's nose to sense drugs or explosives) as one of independent trends for electronic nose or tongue chip.

When olfactory receptors were expressed on the membrane of a heterologous cell system, the binding of olfactory receptors with specific odorant molecules can be detected by QCM or SPR. However, these cells were not excitable, so the action potentials produced by the interaction of receptors and glands can not be detected. Here will present the olfactory and taste cell-based biosensors in our laboratory. The implementation of olfactory and taste cell sensors system based on LAPS with artificial olfactory and artificial taste sensor system for odor and ion sensor array are described (Liu et al., 2006; Wang et al., 2007; Zhang et al., 2008).

Besides the cell-based biosensors, tissue-based biosensors with LAPS were reported as the bioelectronic nose, shown in Figure 8 (Liu et al.,2010a; Liu et al., 2010b). The study engaged in designing an olfactory epithelium tissue and semiconductor hybrid neuron chip to investigate the firing modes of the olfactory receptor neurons under different odor stimulations, shown in Figure 9. The theory model of olfactory epithelium coupled to LAPS surface after odor stimulation was established and simulated. Extracellular potentials obtained before and during odor stimulation could be analyzed on basis of local field potentials and differentiated by PCA. All the results reported suggest that the olfactory receptor cells respond to odors in a tissue and semiconductor hybrid neuronchip will be a novel bioelectronics nose with great potential development.

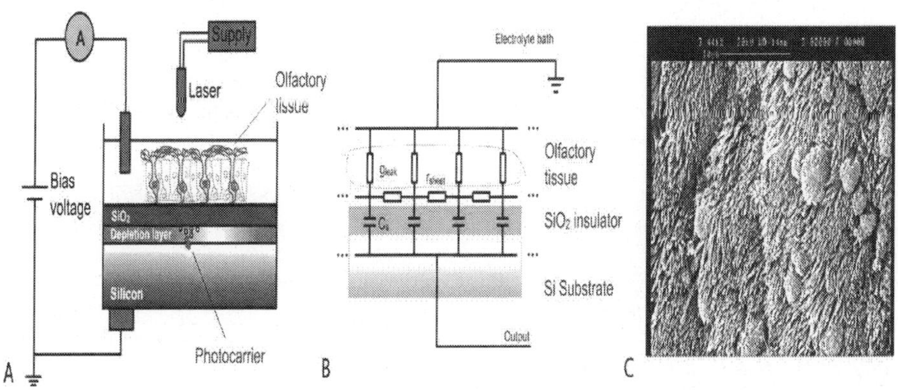

Fig. 8. Olfactory epithelium tissue hybrid with LAPS. (A) LAPS system with the olfactory epithelium on the sensor surface. (B) Sheet conductor model on extracellular potentials recording of the tissue layer between electron conductor and electrolyte bath on LAPS. (C) Olfactory epithelium tissue fixed on the surface of LAPS observed by the scanning electron microscope.

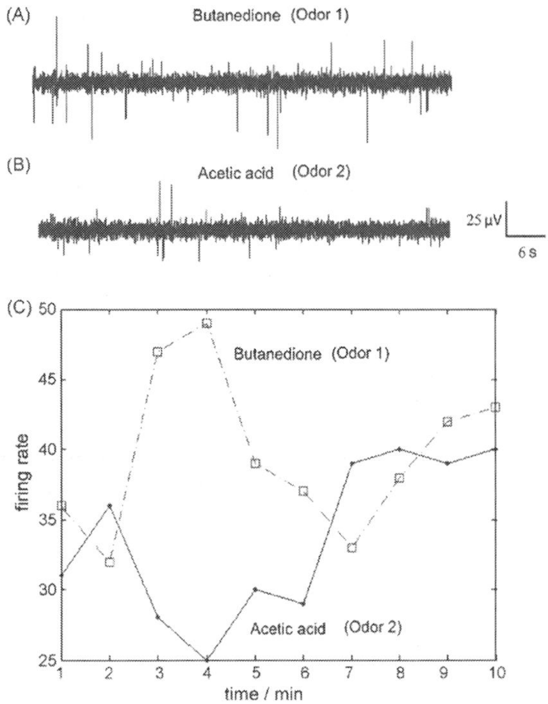

Fig. 9. Responses of the extracellular potential changes of olfactory mucosa tissue to odors of butanedione (A) and acetic acid (B), with different discharge models (C).

5. Conclusion

In this chapter, we engaged the light addressable potentiometric sensor (LAPS) as the cell-based biosensors for biomedical application. The main purpose was to introduce the principle, devices, fabrications, detection systems and applications of the LAPS sensor, especially the recent concept of constructing LAPS array for biomedical application. LAPS has its own advantages while constructing cell-based biosensors and showed promising prospect for application in various areas such as biomedical, environmental, food safety, etc. LAPS array can be used for highly integrated sensors system, which is essential in high throughput drug screening. By improving the sensitivity, spatial resolution, sampling rate, LAPS array could be a super candidate for constructing sensor systems, especially cell-besed biosensors.

6. References

Bousse, L., 1996. Whole cell biosensors. Sensor. Actuat. B-Chem. 34: 270-275.
Fromherz, P., 2002. Electrical interfacing of nerve cells and semiconductor chips. Chem. Phys. Chem. 3: 276-284.

George, M., Parak, W.J., Gaub, H.E., 2000. Highly integrated surface potential sensors. Sensor. Actuat. B-Chem. 9, 266-275.

Hafeman, D.G., Parce, J.W., McConnell, H.M., 1988. Light-addressable potentiometric sensor for biochemical systems. Science 240: 1182-1185.

Hafner, F., 2000. Cytosensor® Microphysiometer: technology and recent applications. Biosens. Bioelectron. 15: 149-158.

Liu, Q.J., Cai, H., Xu, Y., Xiao, L.D., Yang, M., Wang, P., 2007b. Detection of heavy metal toxicity using cardiac cell-based biosensor. Biosens. Bioelectron. 22: 3224-3229.

Liu, Q.J., Huang, H.R., Cai, H., Xu, Y., Li, Y., Li, R., Wang, P., 2007a. Embryonic stem cells as a novel cell source of cell-based biosensor. Biosens. Bioelectron. 22: 810-815.

Liu, Q.J., Cai, H., Xiao, L.D., Li, R., Yang, M., Wang, P., 2007c. Embryonic stem cells biosensor and its application in drug analysis and toxin detection. IEEE Sens. J. 7: 1625-1631.

Liu, Q.J., Ye, W.W., Hu, N., Cai, H., Yu, H., Wang, P., 2010a. Olfactory receptor cells respond to odors in a tissue and semiconductor hybrid neuron chip. Biosen. Bioelectron., 26: 1672-1678. Liu, Q.J., Ye, W.W., Yu, H., Hu, N., Du, L., Wang, P., Yang, M., 2010b. Olfactory mucosa tissue-based biosensor: A bioelectronic nose with receptor cells in intact olfactory epithelium. Sensor. Actuat. B-Chem. 146: 527-533.

McConnell, H.M., Owicki, J.C., Parce, J.W., Miller, D.L., Baxter, G.T., Wada, H.G., Pitchford, S., 1992. The Cytosensor microphysiometer: biological application of silicon technology. Science 257: 1906-1912.

Men, H., Zou, S.F., Li, Y., Wang, Y.P., Ye, X.S., Wang, P., 2005. A novel electronic tongue combined MLAPS with stripping voltammetry for environmental detection. Sensor. Actuat. B-Chem. 110: 350-357.

Nakao, M., Inoue S., Yoshinobu, T., Iwasaki, H., 1996. pH imaging sensor for microscopic observation of microorganisms. Actuat. B-Chem. 34: 234-239.

Parce, J.W., Owicki, J.C., Kercso, K.M., Sigal, G.B., Wada, H.G., Muir, V.C., Bousse, L.J., Ross, K.L., Sikic, B.I., McConnell, H.M., 1989. Detection of cell-affecting agents with a silicon biosensor. Science 246: 243-247.

Shimizu, M., Kanai Y., Uchida H., Katsube, T., 1994. Integrated biosensor employing a surface photovoltage technique. Sensor. Actuat. B-Chem. 20: 187-192

Piras, L., Adami, M., Fenua, S., Dovisb, M., Nicolini, C., 1996. Immunoenzymatic application of a redox potential biosensor. Anal. Chim. Acta. 335: 127-135.

Schooning, M.J., Wagner, T., Wang C., Otto, R., Yoshinobu, T., 2005. Development of a handheld 16 channel pen-type LAPS for electrochemical sensing. Sensor. Actuat. B-Chem. 108: 808-814.

Siu, W.M., Cobbold, R.S.C., 1979. Basic properties of the electrolyte-SiO2-Si system: physical and theoretical aspects. IEEE. Trans. Electron. Dev. 26: 1805-1815.

Sprossler, C., Denyer, M., Britland, S., Knoll, W., Offenhausser, A., 1999. Electrical recordings from rat cardiac muscle cells using field-effect transistors. Phys. Rev. E 60: 2171-2176.

Sprössler, C., Denyer, M., Offenhäusser, A., 1998. Biosensors & Bioelectronics 13, 613-618.

Stenger, D.A., Gross, G.W., Keefer, E.W., Shaffer, K.M., Andreadis, J.D., Ma, W., Pancrazio, J.J., 2001. Detection of physiologically active compounds using cell-based biosensors. Trends Biothchnol. 19: 304-309.

Squibb, K.S., Fowler, B.A., 1981. Relationship between metal toxicity to subcellular systems and the carcinogenic response. Environ. Health. Persp. 40: 181-188.

Wada, H.G., Owicki, J.C., Bruner, L.H., Miller, K.R., Raley-Susman, K.M., Panfili, P.R., Humphries, G., Parce, J.W., 1992. Measurement of cellular responses to toxic agents using a silicon microphysiometer. AATEX. 1: 154-164.

Wang, P., Liu, Q.J., Xu, Y., Cai, H., Li, Y., 2007. Olfactory and taste cell sensors and its applications in biomedicine. Sens. Actuators A: Phys. 139: 131-138.

Wille, K., Paige, L.A., Higgins, A.J., 2003. Application of the Cytosensor Microphysiometer to drug discovery. Receptor. Channel., 9(2): 125-131.

Wang, P., Xu, G.X., Qin, L.F., Xu, Y., Li, Y., Li, R., 2005. Cell-based biosensors and its application in biomedicine. Sensor. Actuat. B-Chem. 108: 576-584.

Wu, Y.C., Wang, P., Ye, X.S., Zhang, G.Y., He, H.Q., Yan, W.M., Zheng, X.X., Han, J.H., Cui, D.F., 2001a. Drug evaluations using a novel microphysiometer based on cell-based biosensors. Sensor. Actuat. B-Chem. 80: 215-221.

Wu, Y.C., Wang, P., Ye, X.S. Zhang, Q.T., Li, R., Yan, W.M., Zheng, X.X., 2001b. A novel microphysiometer based on MLAPS for drug screening, Biosens. Bioelectron. 16: 277-286.

Yu, H., Cai H., Zhang, W., Xiao, L., Liu, Q., Wang, P., 2009. A novel design of multifunctional integrated cell-based biosensors for simultaneously detecting cell acidification and extracellular potential. Biosens. Bioelectron. 24(5): 1462-1468.

Xu, G.X., Ye, X.S., Qin, L.F., Xu, Y., Li, Y., Li, R., Wang, P., 2005. Cell-based biosensors based on light-addressable potentiometric sensors for single cell monitoring. Biosens. Bioelectron. 20: 1757-1763.

Zhang, Q.T., Wang, P., Wolfgang, J.P., George, M., Zhang, G.Y., 2001. A novel design of multi-light LAPS based on digital compensation of frequency domain. Sensor. Actuat. B-Chem. 73: 152-156.

Zhang, W., Li, Y.., Liu, Q.J. Xu, Y., Cai, H., Wang, P., 2008. A Novel experimental research based on taste cell chips for taste transduction mechanism. Sensor. Actuat. B-Chem. 131(1): 24-28.

Ziegler, C., Gopel, W., Hammerle, H., Hatt, H., Jung, G., Laxhuber, L., Schmidt, H.L., Schutz, S., Vogtle, F., Zell, A., 1998. Bioelectronic noses: a status report. Part II, Biosen. Bioelectron. 13: 539-571.

17

Sol-Gel Technology in Enzymatic Electrochemical Biosensors for Clinical Analysis

Gabriela Preda, Otilia Spiridon Bizerea and Beatrice Vlad-Oros
West University of Timişoara, Faculty of Chemistry-Biology-Geography, Department of Chemistry, Timişoara, Romania

1. Introduction

Enzymes are without question the most powerful, versatile and efficient, wide-spread biocatalysts in the biological world, being responsible for remarkable reaction rate enhancements. Enzymes are also very specific, able to discriminate between substrates with quite similar structures. They exhibit different types of selectivity (chemo-, enantio-, regio- and diastereoselectivity) and can catalyse a broad range of reactions. Moreover they are environmentally friendly, acting under mild conditions. They are used in many biotechnological domains, as isolated enzymes or whole cells, in free or immobilized form. The dual character of an enzyme, as both protein and catalyst, brings face to face the special properties of proteins like activity, selectivity, inhibition phenomena, unfolding in a harsh environment with the need for stability, reproducibility, long term reusability of the catalyst. The catalytic activity of enzymes depends on the integrity of their native protein conformation. If an enzyme is denatured or dissociated into its subunits, catalytic activity is usually lost. Thus the primary, secondary, tertiary, and quaternary structures of protein enzymes are essential to their catalytic activity. Therefore, enzymes cannot be used at high temperature, extreme pH or high ionic strength, operation parameters that could lead to enzyme deactivation. Another issue that limits the efficiency of the enzymatic reactions is the substrate or product inhibition - the enzyme stops working at higher substrate and/or product concentration (Chibata, 1978; Smith, 2004).
So, reliable techniques for protein stabilization are of great practical importance (Rothenberg, 2008). Enzymes in biosensors are used in an "immobilized" form. Even though at the beginning of the 21th century immobilization of biomolecules may be at a first glance a solved problem, reality shows that work has yet to be done in order to obtain stable, long-living robust and active biocatalysts, even if they are isolated biomolecules (enzymes, proteins, nucleic acids), whole cells or other biological species.
A lot of immobilization methods are available. Among them, sol-gel technology application in biosensing has been of great interest in the last two decades. Sol-gel technology (Brinker & Scherer, 1990) opens a simple route to produce materials like glasses, monoliths, powders, thin films in mild conditions. Inorganic and hybrid organic-inorganic micro and nano-structered matrices based mainly on silica gels will be briefly described. Enzymes

entrapment in silica gels by sol-gel route is now history (Avnir et al., 1994; Gill & Ballesteros, 2000; Livage et al., 2001; Retz et al., 2000). Application of sol-gel technique in biosensing has been a logical consequence (Kunzelmann & Bottcher., 1997; de Marcos et al., 1999; Wang, 1999). In recent years, the research has been focused on new sol-gel-derived materials to make the network more compatible with the biomolecules (Gupta & Chaudhury, 2007; Smith et al., 2007). The most important applications are in biocatalysis and biosensing, in clinical, environmental, food or process analysis. Till 1992, about 3000 enzymes have been recognized by The International Union of Biochemistry, but only a small percent of them is commercially available, so the potential of these powerful biocatalysts is not fully exploited remaining that future research to increase their use (Faber, 2000).

This chapter will focus on enzyme biosensors with application in clinical analysis, mainly on glucose sensing based on glucose oxidase. Why glucose sensing? Why glucose oxidase? More than 60% of research in biosensors is focused on this analyte and this enzyme (Newman & Turner, 2005; Yoo & Lee, 2010). Glucose/glucose oxidase system could be, no doubt, a case study. The enzyme is very "suited" for sensing, accessible, with very high specificity, versatile and, most of all, the subject is of tremendous public importance.

2. Biosensors – short overview

2.1 Concepts and definitions

In a modern, suggestive and concise context, a biosensor is a sensor that incorporates a biological sensitive element, i.e. an analytic device that converts a biological response in an analytical signal (Velusamy et al., 2010). In a larger acceptation, a biosensor can be defined as a compact, self-contained, reversible, integrated bioanalytical device, having a biological sensitive component or a biological derivative directly connected to a compatible physicochemical transducer. Together, they transpose the concentration of a certain analyte or a group of similar analytes, in a measurable response, and are connected to a processor of the provided electronic signal (Matrubutham & Sayler, 1998; Rogers & Mascini, 2009; Sing & Choi, 2009; Thévenot et al., 1999; Turner et al., 1987; Urban, 2009).

According to the standard definition given by the International Union of Pure and Applied Chemistry (IUPAC), a biosensor is an integrated self-contained receptor-transducer device, able to provide selectively quantitative or semi-quantitative analytical information using a biologic recognition element, which is in direct spatial contact with a transducer element (Justino et al., 2010; Thévenot et al., 1999), or a device based on specific biochemical reaction catalyzed by isolated enzymes, immunosystems, tissues, organelles, or whole cells to detect chemical compounds, usually by electric, thermal or optical signals, respectively (Nayak et al., 2009).

A biosensor can be schematically presented as in Figure 1 considering that integrates a biological recognition element (*bioreceptor*) with a physicochemical *transducer* generating a measurable electronic signal, proportional with the concentration of the determined analyte, which is then *amplified*, *processed* and *displayed* (Belkin, 2003; Lei et al., 2006; Su et al., 2010; Wilson & Gifford, 2005).

2.2 Components

It is already known, that biosensors are composed of two main components connected in series: a molecular recognition system (*biorecognition element* or *biocatalyst* generically called *bioreceptor*) that detects the analyte of interest intimately connected or integrated to a

physicochemical transducer (detector), converting the spot target in a measurable electric signal (Bergveld, 1996; Justino et al., 2010; Singh & Choi, 2009; Tothill, 2009; Velusamy et al., 2010).
The *biological recognition element* of a biosensor is a molecular species that uses a specific biochemical mechanism, mediated by enzymes, nucleic acids, antibodies, cellular systems, microorganisms etc., to detect the target analyte from biological samples. The *biorecognition elements* can be classified in two broad categories: *bioligands* (antibodies, nucleic acids, lectins etc.) and *biocatalysts* (enzymes, hormones, vitamins, microorganisms, tissues etc.). The *bioligands* are responsible for binding the considered analyte to the biosensor, for detection and measurement of the target compounds from the sample, usually by transforming them in an electric, thermal or optical signal. *Biocatalysts* are substances with activating role in biological reactions, in the transformation of substrates to products. After the interaction with target species, the physicochemical properties of the sensitive layer (weight, optical properties, resistance) are changed. The modified parameter is taken over by the *transducer* and converted in an equivalent, measurable electrical signal which is then *amplified*. The amplified signal, proportional with the concentration of the substance or set of analyzed substances, is *processed* by a signal processor that provides a digital electronic signal which can be *saved, displayed* and *analyzed* with a proper hardware and software (Castillo et al., 2004; Justino et al., 2010; Singh & Choi, 2009; Velusamy et al., 2010).
Many biological recognition elements, which provide the specificity and sensitivity required to sense low levels of the sample analyte, are used as *bioreceptors* to detect bioanalytes such as: *enzymes, hormones, vitamins, proteins, nucleic acids, antibodies/antigens, whole cells from superior organisms, tissues, organelles, liposomes, bacteria, viruses, other microorganisms, cofactors, biomimethics etc.* (Singh & Choi, 2009; Su et al., 2010; Tothill, 2009; Velusamy et al., 2010;).
The transducer can be *electrochemical* (i.e. ion-selective electrodes), *heat sensitive* (i.e. calorimetric), *piezoelectric* (i.e. acoustic sounds), *optical* (i.e. optical fibers), *magnetic* and *micromechanical* or any other *combination of these* (Velusamy et al., 2010).
The bioreceptor is responsible for the selectivity and specificity of biosensor towards a certain analyte. The detector is not selective but has a great influence on the sensitivity of the biosensor.
Very often, optimal functioning of biosensors requires the presence of an intermediate compound, called *mediator*, which shuttles redox equivalents between bioreceptor and transducer. Depending on the type of contact and integration level of biological recognition element and transducer, biosensors have mainly known *three generations* of development. *First generation* of biosensors have the biorecognition element physically bound or entrapped into a membrane fixed on the transducer surface. Electrochemical biosensors of this generation include only the biorecognition element and the transducer. *Second generation* of biosensors have the biologically active component directly adsorbed or covalently bound on the transducer surface without a semipermeable membrane. In this case, the diffusion of mediators, which are not immobilized on the transducer surface, may take place freely. In case of *third generation* of biosensors, the bioreceptor is directly bound on an electronic device which transforms and amplifies the signal. The biosensors based on conducting polymers belong to this category.
Even if, apparently, the difference between *second* and *third generation* of biosensors does not seem significant, setting up the whole sensing chemistry on the transducer surface is a complex task. Generally, the methods utilized to immobilize biomolecules on the electrode surface are used also for redox mediators (e.g. adsorption, covalent binding to conducting or non-conducting polymer backbones, mixing with the electrode material (e.g. carbon paste)

or entrapment into a polymeric matrix by ion exchange) to ensure a suitable electron transfer pathway (Castillo et al., 2004; Singh & Choi, 2009).

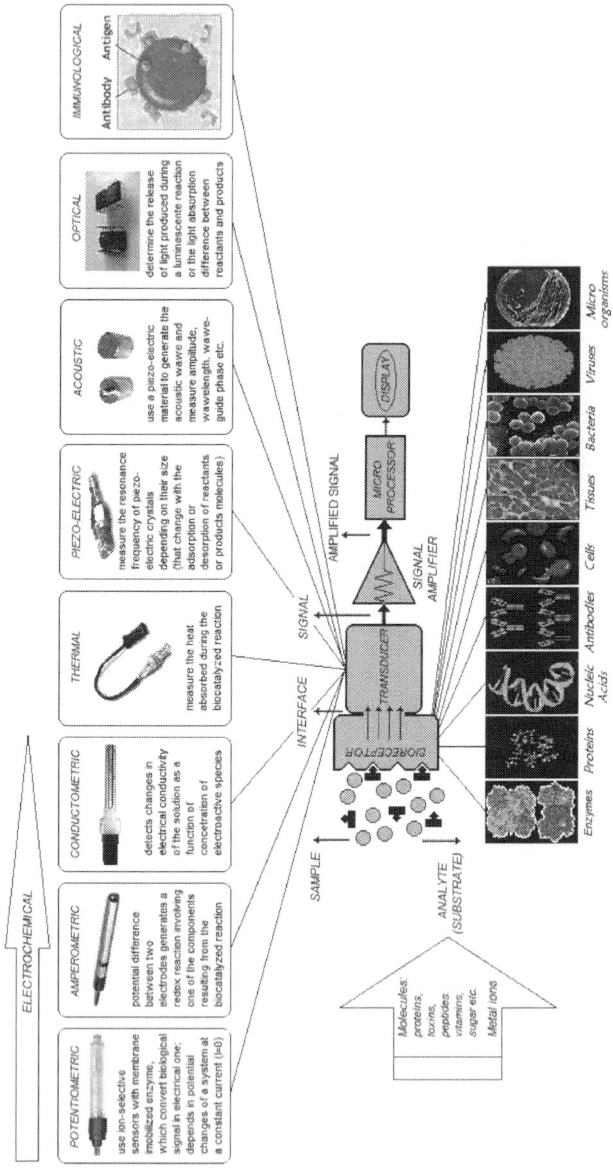

Fig. 1. Biosensor device

The analyte molecules may comprise proteins, toxins, peptides, vitamins, sugars, metal ions etc. The most common signalling principles/elements can be electrons, ions (voltammetry, potentiometry, conductivity), protons - pH changes, optical (SPR, ELM, IR), electromechanical (QCM), magnetic, heat, pressure, light, mass variation, fluorescence. Response variables can be: the potential, current, frequency, mass, temperature and pressure, respectively. Typical sensing techniques for biosensors are fluorescence, DNA microarray, Surface Plasmon Resonance (SPR), impedance spectroscopy, Scanning Probe Microscopy (SPM, AFM, STM), Quartz Crystal Microbalance (QCM), Surface Enhanced Raman Spectroscopy (SERS), electrochemical.

2.3 Classification

Biosensors can be classified according to many criteria, out of which we mention the followings:

- the bioactive/bioreceptor material
- the transducer
- the immobilization technique.

In general, the bioreceptors or the recognition biological materials can be classified in five major classes, as it is shown in Figure 2. The enzymes, antibodies and nucleic acids are the main bioreceptor classes that are mostly used in biosensors applications. In general, they are immobilized on a support which can be the detector surface, its vicinity or a transporter (Ivnitski et al., 2000; Lazcka et al., 2007; Oh et al., 2005; Radke & Alocilja, 2005; Velusamy et al., 2010).

The biosensors classification according to the nature of the variable parameter converted by the transducer in electric signal can be seen in Figure 1, but a more complete classification is given in Figure 3.

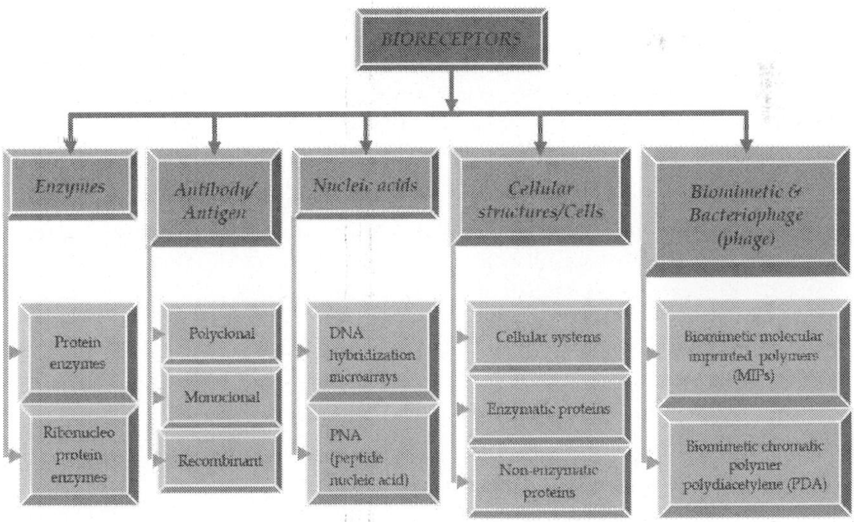

Fig. 2. Biosensors classification according to the bioreceptor type

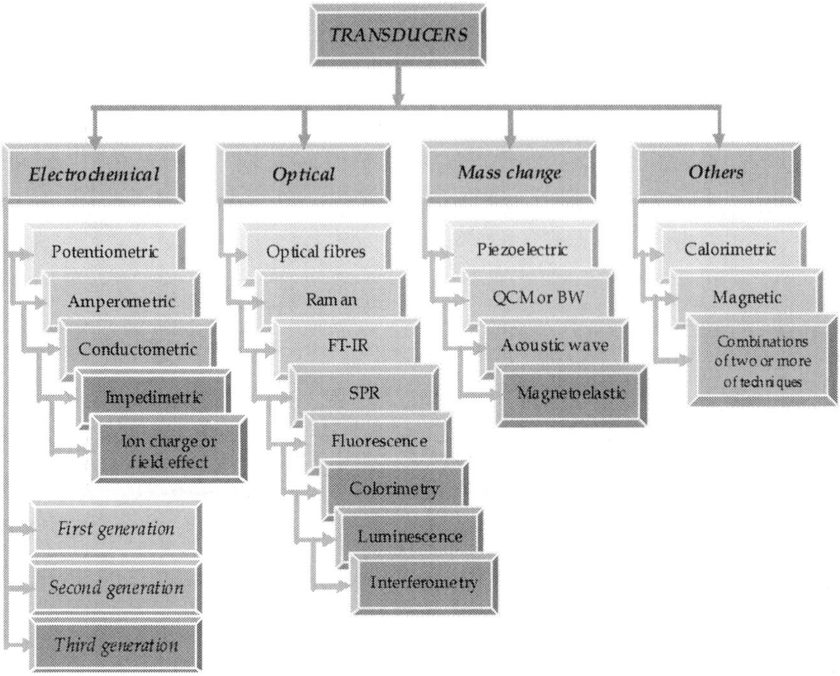

Fig. 3. Biosensors classification according to the transducer type

During the biochemical transformation, the modified parameters that can be detected with the *electrochemical transducer* are: electric current, potential, impedance and conductance.
Optical transducers are based on the optical properties of the substances, as: absorption, reflection, refraction, light scattering, fluorescence, chemiluminescence, phosphorescence etc. Due to their sensitivity, the most used optical detection techniques are Raman and Fourier Transform Infrared Spectroscopy (FT-IR), Surface Plasmon Resonance (SPR) and Fluorescence. The most used types of biosensors are amperometrical, potentiometrical and optical ones. The foremost methods based on *mass exchanges detected with biosensors transducer,* depend on the use of piezoelectric crystals. The two major types of sensors based on mass variation are Bulk Wave (BW), also called Quartz Crystal Microbalance (QCM), and Surface Acoustic Wave (SAW), respectively (Velusamy et al., 2010).

2.4 Biosensors mechanisms

According to the interaction mechanism, three types of biosensors can be identified: 1. *biocatalytic (enzymatic/metabolic) biosensors* (the recognition element is represented by *enzymes*); 2. *biosensors that act based on bioaffinity or biocomplexation* (based on recognition mechanisms with *antibodies, nucleic acids, lectins* etc.). 3. *biosystems based on microorganisms.* (Rogers & Mascini, 2009; Thévenot et al., 1999).
In case of biocatalysis, biorecognition reaction is catalyzed by macromolecules that can be present in a biologic environment or have been previously isolated. The substrate interacts

with the immobilized biocatalyst on the sensor (surface), then a biocatalyst-substrate complex is formed and after the reaction takes place, the product is released and the catalyst is regenerated. The substrate consumption or the product release is continuously measured and the biological response is converted into an electrically quantifiable signal monitored by the integrated detector of the biosensor. These types of biosensors (biocatalytic sensors) usually use *enzymes, whole cells* (cellular microorganisms as bacteria, fungi etc.), *cellular organelles* (mithocondria, cell walls) or *tissues* (vegetal or animal). Generally, biocatalysts based biosensors depend on the use of enzymes. These biological catalysts can be comprised in one of the six classes: oxidoreductases (dehydrogenases, oxidases, peroxidases, oxygenases), transferases, hydrolases, lyases, isomerases and ligases. Biocatalysis underlying mechanisms involve either the catalytic conversion of an analyte from an undetectable form in a detectable one or the detection of an analyte that inhibits or mediates the enzymatic activity (Rogers & Mascini, 2009; Thévenot et al., 1999).

In case of bioaffinity, operation of biosensors relies on selective interactions between the analyte of interest and biomolecules or organized molecular assemblies, either (present) in their biological environment or previously isolated. After the biocomplexing reaction, equilibrium is achieved and the analyte is no longer consumed. The equilibrium responses are monitored by the integrated detector. The antibodies capacity to specifically recognize different molecular structures confers high selectivity to biosensors based on bioaffinity (Rogers & Mascini, 2009; Thévenot et al., 1999; Velusamy et al., 2010).

The class of *biosensors based on microorganisms* is used for analytes that form a respiratory substrate. These can detect either biodegradable organic compounds measured as biological oxygen demand or respiration inhibition caused by the analyte of interest. The biosensors based on Genetically Modified Microorganisms (GMMs) recognize and report the presence of a specific analyte (Rogers & Mascini, 2009).

2.5 Functional characteristics

The main *functional characteristics* of a biosensor are shown in Figure 4.

The assessment of the functionality of any biosensor must begin with its calibration. This is generally performed using standard solutions of the analyte followed by the plot of the steady-state response against the analyte concentration or its logarithm. Exceptions are the biosensors causing a continuous change in the concentration of the analyte standard solutions because they trigger a reaction that takes place throughout the measurement till the depletion of the substrate. An example is the glucose potentiometric biosensor based on glucose oxidase. In this case the biosensor monitors the ongoing reaction following the variation of a parameter which is continuously changing and, at time considered optimal, calibration curve is plotted. The value of the followed parameter at optimal time depends on the concentration of standard solution in which monitoring is made (Thévenot et al., 1999; Bizerea-Spiridon et al., 2010a; Bizerea-Spiridon et al., 2010b; Vlad-Oros et al., 2009;).

2.6 Applications

Biosensors represent a rocketed developing field, with an enormous potential in terms of detection and control of a large number of analytes with important applications in health, agriculture, food industry, environmental monitoring etc. With an annual growth rate estimated at 60% (Chaplin & Bucke, 1990), biosensors and analytical techniques in which they are involved will play an increasingly important role in the future technology. Some of the

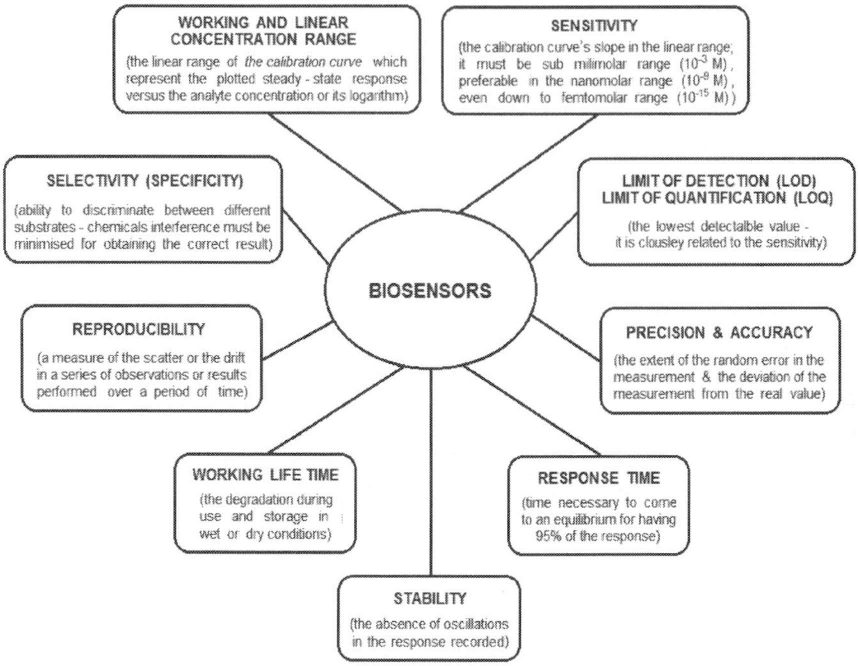

Fig. 4. The main functional features of a biosensor

most important applications of biosensors are presented in Table 1 (Castillo et al., 2004; Justino et al., 2010; Lazcka et al., 2007; Mello & Kubota, 2002; Nayak et al., 2009; Rodriguez-Mozaz et al., 2005; Rodriguez-Mozaz et al., 2006; Rogers, 2006; Tothill, 2009; Verma & Singh, 2005).

The recent progress in micro- and nanoscale technologies shows high promises in enabling a number of new applications in biosensing. Based on enzyme immobilization techniques, in the shape of capsules, beads, columns or membranes, many types of biosensors have been developed on a laboratory or even on a commercial scale (Rothenberg, 2008).

3. Enzyme immobilization by sol-gel technique for biosensing applications

3.1 Fundamentals of enzyme immobilization for biosensing

In vivo, nature produces enzymes when they are needed in the biochemical pathways. *In vitro*, in biocatalytic transformations, they have to be recovered and efficiently reused. This may be done by immobilization (Lalonde & Margolin, 2002). Immobilized enzymes are defined as "*enzymes physically confined or localized in a certain defined region of space with retention of their catalytic activities, and which can be used repeatedly and continuously*" (Chibata, 1978).

In the last six decades, several methods of immobilization have been developed, starting with binding onto natural or synthetic carriers (Chibata, 1978), inclusion in organic or inorganic polymeric networks, or cross-linking, sometimes in the presence of inert molecules (Murty et al., 2002; Kennedy & Cabral, 1987; Khan & Alzohairy, 2010; Sheldon, 2007; Ullmann, 1987).

Realm	*Applications*	*Analyte*	*Transducer*	*Limitations*
Healthcare Medical diagnosis	***Diagnostic tests for personalized needs (clinical and laboratory analyses)*** ***Glucose detection in vivo*** ***Bacterial urinary tract infections*** ***Human immuno-deficiency virus (HIV) detection*** ***Cancer clinical testing*** ***Drug delivery and monitoring***	pH, Sodium; Potassium; Calcium; Urea, Penicillin; Glucose, Lactate, Cholesterol, Creatinine, Uric acid, L-Glutamate, Ethanol, Oxalat; Catecholamines: DA, EPI, NEPI; C-Reactive Protein, Insulin; Hepatitis B; Toxic substances, Pathogenic bacteria *Candida albicans*; Pathogens (*Mycobacterium tuberculosis, Vibriocholerae, Treponema palladium*); Biomarkers for cancer type disease	Glass ion-selective electrodes; Ion-exchange-selective electrodes; Liquid membrane ion-selective electrodes; Potentiometric enzymatic biosensors; Amperometric enzymatic biosensors; Optical fiber enzymatic biosensors; Immunosensors; Chemiluminescentimmunosensors; Antigen-antibody immunosensors; Piezoelectric immunosensors; Amperometric immunosensors using screen printed electrodes, Electrochemical DNA biosensors; Electrochemical, Optical, Mass sensitive immunosensors	Measurements are often invasive Sterile environment is required Biocompatibility is necessary Toxicity is not well known Miniaturization is difficult Stability is often reduced Lifetime is limited Electrochemical interferences are frequent

Table 1. Important domains for biosensors usage

Realm	*Applications*	*Analyte*	*Transducer*	*Limitations*
Environmental monitoring	***Detection of environmental pollutants*** *Air pollution* *Water pollution* *Soil pollution*	Anions & Cations;	Solid and liquid membrane ion-selective electrodes;	Miniaturization is difficult Lifetime is limited Electrochemical interferences are frequent Sterile environment is required
		Inorganic phosphate;	Amperometric trienzymatic biosensors;	
		Ammonia , Nitrit, Nitrate;	Amperometric enzymatic, Optical fluorescent biosensors;	
		Heavy metals (Cu^{2+}, Hg^{2+}, Pb^{2+}, Cd^{2+}, Zn^{2+}, Co^{2+}, $Cr^{3+,6+}$, $As^{3+,5+}$);	Amperometric enzymatic, Optical bioluminescent, Calorimetric, Conductometric, Mass signal biosensors;	
		Heavy metals (Cu^{2+}, Hg^{2+}, Pb^{2+}, Cd^{2+}, Zn^{2+});	Non-enzyme proteins biosensors;	
		Heavy metals (Cu^{2+}, Pb^{2+}, Cd^{2+}, Ni^{2+}, Co^{2+});	Genetically engineered microorganisms biosensors;	
		Formaldehyde, Phenols, Organophosphorous compounds;	Amperometric enzymatic, Optical biosensors, Quartz Crystal Microbalance;	
		Benzene and its derivatives, Naphthalene, Phenanthrene, Aromatic amines;	Optical fluorescent and bioluminescent biosensors;	
		Pesticides, Herbicides;	Amperometric enzymatic, Optical fluorescent biosensors, Quartz Crystal Microbalance;	
		Pathogens (*Escherichia coli, Lysteria monocytogenes, Chlamydia trachomatis, Salmonella typhymurium, Salmonella enteriditis*)	Electrochemical potentiometric & chronopotentiometric, Optical, Acoustic biosensors	

Table 1. Important domains for biosensors usage cont'

Realm	*Applications*	*Analyte*	*Transducer*	*Limitations*
Food and beverage quality monitoring	***Food analyses*** *Fish, Sea food, Chicken and egg, Meat, Fruit and vegetables Spinach samples Olive oil, Sauces*	Inorganic ions; Nitrate, Phosphate, Sulfite, Oxalate; Glucose, Fructose, Galactose, Lactose, Sucrose, Aspartame, Cholesterol, Glycerides, Cadaverine, Histamine, Ethanol, Methanol, Ascorbic acid, Citric acid, Acetic acid, Acetate, Amino acids, Acethaldehyde;	Ion-selective electrodes (ISE); Amperometric enzymatic biosensors; Potentiometric and Amperometric enzymatic biosensors;	Toxicity is not well known Sterile environment is required Sensitivity is low Lifetime is limited Miniaturization is difficult
	Beverage analyses *Milk, Fruit juices, Soft drinks, Wine, Beer, Alcoholic beverages, Monitoring fermentation*	Carbohydrates, Alcohols, Pesticide; Carbohydrates, Sucrose, Alcohols, Lipids, Amines; Carbohydrates, Vitamins, Contaminants (Antibiotics, Fungicides, Pesticides);	Optical fluorescent biosensors; Thermal biosensors; Piezoelectric biosensors;	
	Synthetic samples ***Drinking water***	Pathogenic microorganisms (*Escherichia coli, Lysteria monocytogenes, Salmonella typhimurium, Legionella pneumophila, Enterobacter*)	Amperometric enzymatic, Optical chemiluminescent biosensors, Quartz Crystal Microbalance	

Table 1. Important domains for biosensors usage cont'

For a successful immobilization procedure, three elements have to be considered: a) the enzyme, b) the support and c) the nature of enzyme binding to the support (Kennedy & Cabral, 1987). The immobilization methods can be divided considering the interaction between enzyme and support in: a) *physical binding* or b) *covalent binding* to a solid carrier, c) *entrapment* in gel networks or d) *cross-linking* using (bi)functional agents (Smith, 2004).

These methods are widely used for enzymes immobilization. Physically, enzymes are adsorbed onto insoluble supports, entrapped within gel networks or encapsulated within microcapsules or in/behind semi-permeable membranes. Chemically, enzymes are either covalently bound to organic or inorganic carriers or cross-linked with functional agents.

In the *physical binding* the interaction between enzyme molecules and solid supports consists of stronger, ionic and hydrogen forces or weaker, van der Waals or hydrophobic forces, respectively. The physical methods are simple, inexpensive and usually they do not affect the catalytic activity of enzymes. The main disadvantage is the reversible binding of enzyme to the support (leading to enzyme leaching)(Lalonde &Margolin, 2002; Smith, 2004).

The *entrapment in a gel network* is obtained by polymerization or precipitation/coagulation reactions in the presence of enzyme. The process is usually very simple, the enzymes structure is not affected, but sometimes activity loss may occur. The enzymes are captured in the pores network, while smaller or larger substrate or product molecules can diffuse throughout the gel towards/from the catalyst. If environmental changes disturb the porous network, enzyme leakage could happen. The diffusional limitations due to the polymeric matrix are usually problematic. A very important characteristic of entrapment is that it may be applied for cell fragments or even whole cells immobilization (Chibata, 1978; Lalonde & Margolin, 2002; Smith, 2004).

In order to perform the coupling the enzymes by *covalent binding* to inorganic or organic, natural or synthetic carriers, a huge number of chemical reactions have been used (Kennedy & Cabral, 1987; Sheldon, 2007). The most important advantage is that chemical binding, stronger than the methods previously described, leads to more stable biocatalysts. The covalent binding is non-specific and activity loss is observed if residues from the active site are involved.

Even though there is an enormous experience in the realm, it is obvious that no general rule is available to obtain active, stable, efficient, advanced immobilized biocatalysts with high yield and low costs. Stability vs. activity is a perpetual target in all applications.

An immobilized enzyme has to fulfil a sort of requirements for a good overall activity, such as reasonable immobilization yields, high activity and catalytic efficiency, high operational stability, limited mass transfer effect, easy handling and reusability (Bickerstaff, 1997; Khan & Alzohairy, 2010; Krajewska, 2004; Sheldon, 2007).

Enzyme immobilization may change the kinetics and other properties essential for catalysis (optimum pH or temperature), usually with a decrease of the specific activity. An enhancement of enzymes stability (pH, thermal, storage and operational stability) upon immobilization is commonly observed - key advantage in enzyme immobilization (Mateo et al., 2007; Murty et al., 2002; Petkar et al., 2006).

The special characteristics of the immobilized enzymes have made them suitable for many applications in bioconversion processes or as biomaterials for health and biosensors (Coradin et al., 2006; Gupta & Chaudhury, 2007; Khan & Alzohairy, 2010; Kim et al., 2006; Li & Takahashi, 2000). The main techniques for enzymes immobilization applied to biosensors are shown in Figure 5.

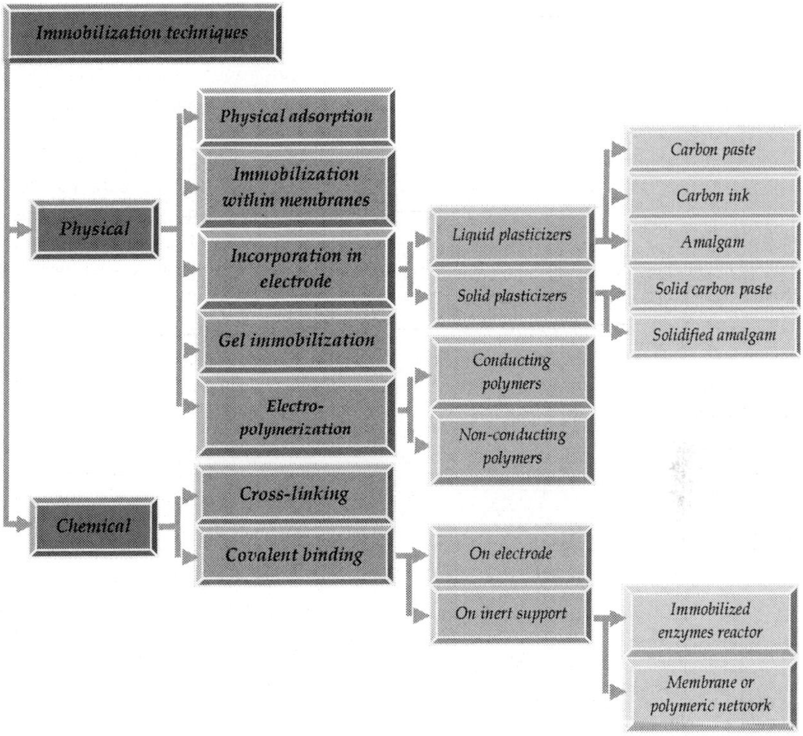

Fig. 5. Enzyme immobilization applied to enzymatic biosensors

In biosensing, immobilization is a key step in coupling of enzyme to electrode. The biosensor efficiency relies on solving problems such as: enzyme loss caused by the binding procedure, diminished availability of enzyme molecule within the carrier, slow diffusion of substrate molecules and active species within the pore network, good transfer of the chemical signal to the electrode. Furthermore, in biosensors, reproducibility, rapid answer, operational stability, enzyme molecule availability, kinetic parameters are essential for a good response (Coradin et al., 2006; Gupta & Chaudhury, 2007; Khan & Alzohairy, 2010; Kim et al., 2006).

3.2 Sol-gel entrapment – a versatile tool for enzyme immobilization

Although practice shows that a universal carrier is not known, some characteristics are desirable to any material considered for immobilizing enzymes: large surface area, hydrophilicity, permeability, insolubility, chemical, thermal and mechanical stability, resistance to microbial attack, etc. (Kennedy & Cabral, 1987; Ullmann, 1987).

Gel entrapment of biomolecules is a well-established method for many years. Gels as agar, agarose, gelatin, alginate, chitin, chitosan, carrageenan or polyvinyl alcohol are highly biocompatible, accessible, easy to handle and largely used in very different applications. The most important disadvantages reside in their organic nature: some of them are mechanically fragile, cannot stand for biological attack or are highly toxic (Smith, 2004).

Due to their physical properties, inorganic carriers have some important advantages over their organic counterparts: high mechanical strength, good thermal stability, high resistance to organic solvents and microbial attack, easy handling and regeneration. Inorganic supports are stable and do not alter their structure at environmental changes (pH or temperature) (Coradin et al., 2006; Kennedy & Cabral, 1987; Ullmann, 1987).

This chapter will deal with immobilization of enzymes using inorganic carriers. In order to make them compatible with organic and bio-molecules, mild synthesis methods are needed. Sol-gel synthesis of inorganic gels in conditions as harmless as possible is such an option. Silica sol-gel materials have been developed starting with the 1990's as a versatile and viable alternative to classical immobilization methods (Avnir et al., 1994; Reetz et al., 2000, Reetz et al., 2003). The sol-gel synthesis of silica gels is a chemical synthesis of amorphous inorganic solids starting from metal-organic precursors ($Si(OCH_3)_4$ or $Si(OC_2H_5)_4$ being the most commonly used) which undergo numerous catalytic hydrolysis and condensation reactions that can be written schematically as follow (Brinker & Scherer, 1990; Park & Clark, 2002):

- hydrolysis/esterification

$$\equiv Si{-}OR + H_2O \rightleftharpoons \equiv Si{-}OH + ROH \tag{1}$$

- water condensation/hydrolysis

$$\equiv Si{-}OH + HO{-}Si\equiv \rightleftharpoons \equiv Si{-}O{-}Si\equiv + H_2O \tag{2}$$

- alcohol condensation/alcoholysis

$$\equiv Si{-}OH + RO{-}Si\equiv \rightleftharpoons \equiv Si{-}O{-}Si\equiv + ROH \tag{3}$$

Sol-gel technique implies the silica matrix synthesis, at room temperature and mild conditions, around biomolecules or even larger biological species, without altering the biological activity (Bhatia et al., 2000; Gupta & Chaudhury, 2007). Biomolecules like proteins, enzymes, hormones, antibodies, cell components or even viable whole cells remain active in the porous network. Smaller species from the environment may diffuse within the matrix and interact with the entrapped biomolecules (Yoo & Lee, 2010).

This method avoids problems such as covalent modification (strong binding which can affect residues involved in the catalytic site) or desorbtion (van der Waals, hydrogen or ionic binding). Due to its inorganic nature, silica is a chemically, thermally, mechanically and biologically inert material. The high hydrophilicity and porosity make it compatible with biological species. More than that, synthesis of sol-gel materials is simple, fast and flexible (Avnir et al., 1994; Jin & Breman, 2002; Livage et al., 2001).

The result of hydrolysis and polycondensation reactions is a colloidal sol that contains siloxane bonds (Si-O-Si network) and that, in presence of the target biomolecules or biological species, undergoes further condensation reactions till the gelation point is reached, in a time lasting from seconds to days. At the gelation point, the silica matrix forms a continuous solid throughout the whole volume, with an interstitial liquid phase, containing the biomolecules or biological species. The most important property of this material is its dynamic structure. The hydrolysis and condensation reactions continue as far as unreacted hydroxy or alkoxy groups are still present in the system, in the aging phase. A nano- or a mesostructured material is formed. The water and the alcohol introduced or produced can be removed stepwise, in a drying process that leads to a solid in which the pores collapse as solvent is removed. The shrinkage of the wet matrix may alter the protein. Fortunately, most applications imply function in aqueous environment so complete drying can be avoided.

The three-dimensional Si-O-Si bonds are formed around the biomolecule which, even though is trapped in the cage, remains active in the porous network. The sol-gel matrices preserve the native stability and reactivity of biological macromolecules for sensing. More than that, they can be obtained as powders, fibers, monoliths or thin films. This versatility makes them suitable for biosensing. The formation of thin films is a rather complex process. Sol viscosity, gelation time, solvent evaporation, film collapse may influence the microstructure of the thin film. This microstructure is essential for the access of small molecules and analytes. Dip-coating or spin-coating may be used to obtain thin films with reproducible properties.

Metal alkoxides are the typical precursors for sol-gel technology. The development of silica based sol-gels in the materials sciences is mainly based on tetraalkoxysilanes $Si(OR)_4$ or organoalkoxysilanes $R'_{(4-x)}Si(OR)_x$, where x = 1-4 and R is an organic residue (R: CH_3-, C_2H_5-, C_6H_5-, R′: CH_3-, C_2H_5-, C_6H_5-, etc.) (Brinker & Scherer, 1990; Gupta & Chaudhury, 2007). Hydrolysis and condensation reactions of organoalkoxysilanes occur in a similar manner:

- hydrolysis/esterification

$$R'Si(OR)_3 + H_2O \rightleftharpoons (RO)_2R'Si{-}OH + ROH \qquad (4)$$

- water condensation/hydrolysis

$$(RO)_2R'Si{-}OH + HO{-}SiR'(OR)_2 \rightleftharpoons (RO)_2R'Si{-}O{-}SiR'(OR)_2 + H_2O \qquad (5)$$

- alcohol condensation/alcoholysis

$$(RO)_2R'Si{-}OH + RO{-}SiR'(OR)_2 \rightleftharpoons (RO)_2R'Si{-}O{-}SiR'(OR)_2 + ROH \qquad (6)$$

Precursors containing R′ hydrophobic residues modify the polymeric network. Other precursors, containing functions such as vinyl, methacryl or epoxy, may act as network forming precursors, due to their reactive monomers (Table 2).

Organically modified alkoxides act in the hydrolysis and polycondensation reactions identically with un-substituted alkoxides. Their reactivity increases in the order: TEOS < VTES < MTES. By far the most largely used precursors for the sol-gel matrixes are TMOS and TEOS. Due to their low water solubility, an alcohol is needed to avoid phase separation. Also, during the hydrolysis and polycondensation processes, an alcohol is released, which may cause enzyme inactivation. Tetrakis (2-hydroxiethyl) orthosilicate (THEOS) is a completely water soluble precursor which can avoid thermal effects or enzyme unfolding, due to biocompatibility of the ethylene glycol released in reaction (Shchipunov et al., 2004).

Network modifying precursors	Network forming precursors
Methyltriethoxysilane (MTES) 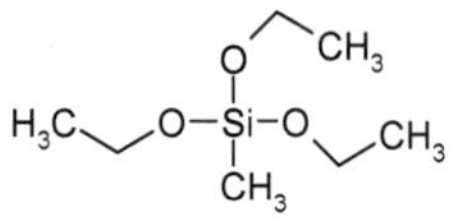	Metallic alkoxides $M(OEt)_4$, M = Si, Ti, Zr
Propyltriethoxysilane (PTES) 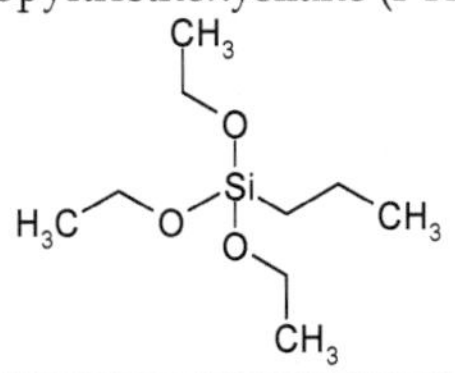	Vinyltriethoxysilane (VTES) 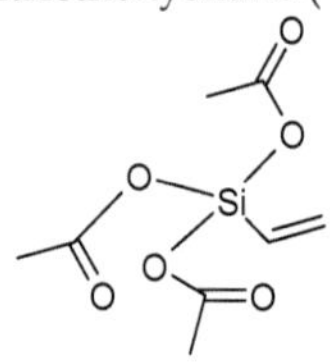
Phenyltriethoxysilane (PTES) 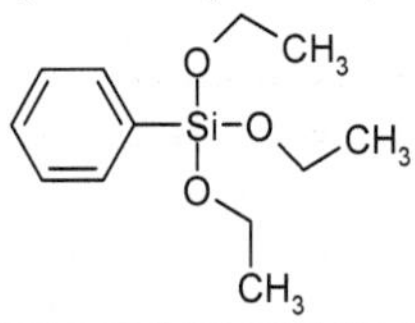	Methacryloxypropyltriethoxysilane 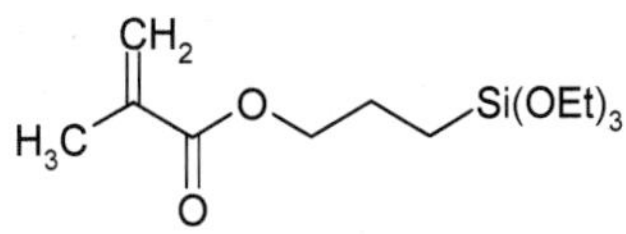
3-aminopropyltriethoxysilane (APTES) 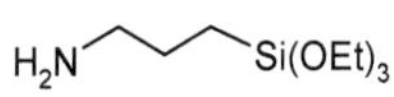	3-(Glycidoxypropyl)triethoxysilane (GPTES) 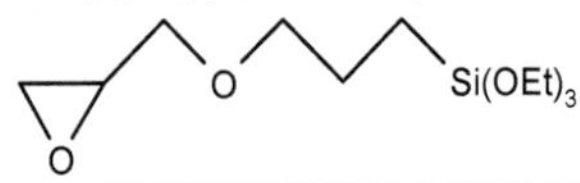
Mercaptopropyltriethoxysilane 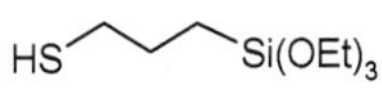	3-(trimethoxysilyl)propyl acrylate 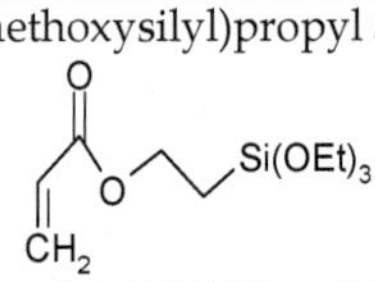

Table 2. Examples of network forming and modifying precursors

To make the sol-gel synthesis compatible with the biomolecules, less invasive reaction conditions are needed. Usually to avoid thermal effects, the sol is produced before the enzyme is added. TMOS derived gels shrink very much, the enzyme being physically restricted in a limited space, which leads to activity loss. Hybrid organic-inorganic matrices shrink less. The properties of sol-gel matrices (porosity, surface aria, polarity, rigidity) depend on the hydrolysis and polycondensation reactions. They are influenced by the precursors, water - precursor molar ratio, solvent, concentrations of the reaction mixture components, pressure, temperature, maturation and drying conditions and different additives, as pore forming or imprinting agents (Coradin et al., 2006).

Polymers like alginate, xanthan, gelatin, chitin, chitosan, carrageenan, hydroxyethyl cellulose, polyvinyl alcohol, polyethylene glycol, polyacrylamide, 2-hydroxyethyl methacrylate or polyethylene oxide may be added in the sol-gel matrix. In this hybrid sol-gel materials covalent, hydrogen, van der Waals bindings or electrostatic interactions may occur between the inorganic and organic components. The macromolecular additives may act as pore forming agents. The porosity can be tailored by using detergents, ionic liquids, crown-ethers, cyclodextrines, etc. D-glucose was used as imprinting agent, being easy to eliminate. Additionally PEG and PVA may avoid pores collapse (Avnir et al., 1994; Coradin et al., 2006).

3.3 Glucose biosensors based on sol-gel immobilized glucose oxidase

Enzymes applications in health care are of remarkable impact (Table 3). Among them, glucose sensing with enzymes is of tremendous importance. Blood glucose level is one of the most important parameters in clinical practice, with continuous monitoring in diabetes, as one of the most important diseases in humans. Sedentary lifestyle and bad eating habits which lead to obesity are important causes of vascular diseases. Glucose level monitoring is important also in insulin therapy, dietary regimes or hypoglycemia (Yoo & Lee, 2010).

Glucose can be measured using three enzymes: hexokinase, glucose oxidase (GOx) and glucose-dehydrogenase (GDH). Glucose oxidase (β-D-glucose:oxygen-1-oxidoreductase, E.C.1.1.3.4.), discovered by Muller in 1928, is the most used oxidoreductase for glucose assay. This enzyme can be isolated from algae, citrus fruits, insects, bacteria or fungi. Most studies were carried out with microbial enzymes obtained by fermentation of *Aspergillus niger* and *Penicillum notatum* strains (Turdean et al., 2005; Wilson & Turner, 1992). Glucose oxidase has high substrate specificity for glucose, high activity, high accessibility (mainly from *Aspergillus niger*).

The glucose biosensor is based on the ability of glucose oxidase to catalyse the oxidation of glucose by molecular oxygen to gluconic acid and hydrogen peroxide:

$$\beta\text{-D-glucose} + O_2 + H_2O \xrightarrow{\text{Glucose oxidase}} \text{D-gluconic acid} + H_2O_2 \quad (7)$$

$$H_2O_2 \longrightarrow O_2 + 2H^+ + 2e^- \quad (8)$$

Glucose oxidase, a flavoprotein, as a redox reaction catalyst, requires a cofactor, FAD, which is regenerated by reaction with molecular oxygen, so no cofactor regeneration is needed.

The molecular oxygen consumption or the hydrogen peroxide production during the reaction is proportional with the glucose concentration. Hydrogen peroxide is oxidized at the electrode and the electron exchange between the enzyme and the electrode (the current generated) can be detected amperometrically. On the other hand, D-gluconic acid is released in the reaction, the pH decay being proportional with the glucose consumption. The pH can be monitored by potentiometric measurements, with a pH-sensitive glass electrode. In both cases, the enzyme has to be attached to the sensitive surface of the electrode. So, the electrode has a double function: to support the enzyme and to detect a change of a parameter (molecular oxygen consumption, pH change) related to the change of the analyte concentration. Alternatively, the enzyme can be incorporated in the electrode (carbon paste).

Three generations of glucose biosensors are described in literature. While H_2O_2 and D-gluconic acid production can be monitored potentiometrically, the oxygen consumption can be measured amperometrically, for example with a Pt electrode, similarly with the oxygen electrode invented by Clark in 1962 (first-generation biosensors). Also, a redox mediator can be used to facilitate electrons transfer from GOx to electrode surface. A variety of mediators were used to enhance biosensor performances: ferrocenes, ferricyanides, quinines and their derivatives, dyes, conducting redox hydrogels, nanomaterials (second-generation biosensors).

Enzyme	E.C. number	Application
		Markers for disease
Acetyl cholinesterase (AChE)	E.C.3.1.1.7	important in controlling certain nerve impulses
Creatine kinase (CK)	E.C.2.7.3.2	indicates a stroke or a brain tumour (heart attack)
Lactate dehydrogenase (LDH)	E.C.1.1.1.27	indicates a tissue damage (heart attack)
		Clinical diagnoses of diseases
Alanine aminotransferase (ALT)	E.C.2.6.1.2	sensitive liver-specific indicator of damage
Alkaline phosphatase (ALP)	E.C.3.1.3.1	involved in bone and hepatobiliary diseases
Aspartate aminotransferase (AST)	E.C.2.6.1.1	myocardial, hepatic parenchymal and muscle diseases in humans and animals
Butylcholinesterase (ButChE)	E.C.3.1.1.8	acute infection, muscular dystrophy, chronic renal disease and pregnancy, insecticide intoxication
Creatine kinase (CK)	E.C.2.7.3.2	myocardial infarction and muscle diseases
Lactate dehydrogenases (LDH)	E.C.1.1.1.27	myocardial infarction, haemolysis and liver disease
Serum pancreatic lipases (triacylglycerol lipase)	E.C.3.1.1.3	pancreatitis and hepatobiliary disease
Sorbitol dehydrogenase (SDH)	E.C.1.1.1.14	hepatic injury
Trypsin	E.C.3.4.21.4	pancreatitis, biliary tract and fibrocystic diseases
α-Amylase (AMY)	E.C.3.2.1.1	diagnostic aid for pancreatitis
γ-Glutamyltransferase (GGT)	E.C.2.3.2.2	hepatobiliary disease and alcoholism
Acid phosphatase (ACP)	E.C.3.1.3.2	prostate carcinoma
		Therapeutic agents
Asparaginase	E.C. 3.5.1.1	leukaemia
		Clinical chemistry
Glucose oxidase	E.C.1.1.3.4	D-glucose content; diagnosis of diabetes mellitus
Lactate dehydrogenase	E.C.1.1.1.27	blood lactate and pyruvate
Urease	E.C.3.5.1.5	blood urea
Cholesterol oxidase	E.C.1.1.3.6	blood cholesterol
Luciferase	EC.1.13.12.7	adenosine triphosphate (ATP) (e.g. from blood platelets); Mg^{2+} concentration
		Immunoassays
Horseradish peroxidise	E.C.1.11.1.7	enzyme-linked immunosorbent assay (ELISA)
Alkaline phosphatise	E.C.3.1.3.1	

Table 3. Enzymes applications in health care (Soetan et al., 2010)

Conducting organic polymers, conducting organic salts, polypyrrole based electrodes were used in the third generation of glucose biosensors, which allowed a direct transfer of electrons between enzyme and electrode (Yoo & Lee, 2010). Sol-gel technology may be present in all three biosensors generations. Some characteristic examples on how sol-gel immobilization is involved in several enzyme biosensors construction are shown in Table 4.

Both largely used amperometric biosensors or less extended potentiometric biosensors have yet to pass efficient, long term functioning exams in time. The main problems that have to be overcome:

a. Amperometric biosensors

The high polarizing voltage needed may cause interferences. Substances such as ascorbic acid, uric acid or other drugs, often present in biological fluids, are oxidized at high potential. To avoid this, either redox mediators or modified electrodes are used.

b. Potentiometric biosensors

The enzymatic reaction is based on oxidation of β-D-glucose to D-glucono-β-lactone catalyzed by glucose oxidase. Three inherent problems may occur. First, molecular oxygen is the electron acceptor which produces hydrogen peroxide as product. But, in biological fluids, the dissolved oxygen concentration controls the glucose detection limit. Second, potentiometric biosensors detect the hydrogen ions produced by the dissociation of D-gluconic acid. Its low dissociation constant is responsible for the low sensitivity of the method. Third, product inhibition by hydrogen peroxide on enzyme activity may occur. Though simple and economical, potentiometric biosensors have to find solutions for all this problems (better pH sensors and immobilization method, solutions to overcome oxygen deficiency and enzyme inhibition) (Liao et al., 2007).

4. New trends in sol-gel immobilized glucose oxidase biosensors

Recent studies are focused now on nano- and bio-nanomaterials. Enzyme immobilization using methods based on sol-gel combined with smart materials (carbon nanotubes, conducting polymers, metal or metal oxide nanoparticles, self assembled systems) could be an interesting alternative (Table 4).

a. Conducting polymers

New generation of mediator-free (reagentless) biosensors based on direct electron transfer uses immobilized enzymes on conducting substrates. Many methods and materials have been used to promote the electron transfer from oxidoreductases directly to the electrode surface. Among them, conducting biopolymers, nanostructures combined with sol-gel matrices are included. Due to their conductivity and electroactivity, they may act as electrons mediators between enzyme active site and electrode surface, leading to short response time and high operational and storage stability (Teles & Fonseca, 2008).

Silica conducting polymer hybrids may be synthesized by co-condensation of organosilanes, post-coupling of functional molecules on silica surface or non-covalent binding of different species. A strategy for silica conducting polymer hybrids synthesis is to modify silica with organic functional moieties and then, these functionalized precursors may react to form polymer chains in the pores or channels of the silica.

Polyaniline (PA) is one of the most important conducting polymers. A glucose biosensor (PA-GOx/Pt) modified using a sol-gel precursor containing sulphur ((3-mercaptopropyl) trimethoxysilane, MPTMS) has good analytical characteristics and does not respond to interferences (Yang et al., 2008).

Sol-gel immobilization method	Enzyme(s)	Analyte	Ref.
TEOS derived sol–gel matrixes	Glucose oxidase	Glucose	Chang et al., 2010
Single TEOS sol–gel matrix coupled to *N*-Acetyl-3,7-dihydroxy-phenoxazine	Horseradish peroxidase Superoxide dismutase Xanthine oxidase	Xanthyne	Salinas-Castillo et al., 2008
Thin sol–gel film derived from TEOS sol–gel system	Acetylcholinesterase	Organophos-phorous pesticides	Anitha et al., 2004
MTOS sol-gel chitosan/silica and MWCNT organic–inorganic hybrid composite film	Chlolesterol oxidase	Cholesterol	Tan et al., 2005
TMOS sol-gel/chitosan inorganic-organic hybrid film	Horseradish peroxidase	H_2O_2	Miao et al., 2001
One-pot covalent immobilization in a biocompatible hybrid matrix based on GPTMS and chitosan	Horseradish peroxidase	H_2O_2	Li et al., 2009
Sol-gel organic-inorganic hybrid material based on chitosan and THEOS	Horseradish peroxidase	H_2O_2	Wang et al., 2006
Chitosan/silica sol-gel hybrid membranes obtained by cross-linking of APTES with chitosan	Horseradish peroxidase	H_2O_2	Li et al., 2008
Immobilization in multi-walled carbon nanotubes (MWCNTs) embedded in silica matrix (TEOS)	Urease	Urea	Ahuja et al., 2011
Immobilization in MTOS sol-gel chitosan/silica hybrid composite film	Glucose oxidase	Glucose	Tan et al., 2005
Encapsulation within sol-gel matrix based on (3-aminopropyl) triethoxy silane, 2-(3,4-epoxycyclohexyl)-ethyltrimetoxy silane	Glucose oxidase	Glucose	Couto et al., 2002
Immobilization in sol-gel films obtained from (3-aminopropyl) trimethoxysilane, 2-(3,4-epoxy-cyclohexyl) ethyl-trimethoxysilane	Lactate oxidase	Lactate	Gomes et al., 2007
Covalent immobilization onto TEOS sol–gel films	Cholesterol esterase, cholesterol oxidase	Cholesterol	Singh et al., 2007
Immobilization of the enzyme in a TMOS derived silica sol-gel matrix	Yeast hexokinase	Glucose	Hussain et al., 2005

Table 4. Sol-gel technique adapted to different enzyme biosensors

A mediatorless bi-enzymatic amperometric glucose biosensor with two enzymes (GOx and horseradish peroxidase (HRP)) co-immobilized into porous silica-polyaniline hybrid composite was obtained by electrochemical polymerization of N[3-(trimethoxysilyl) propyl]aniline (TMSPA). The method revealed the advantages of using both conducting polymers and silica matrices synergistically in one-pot polymerization and immobilization (Manesh, 2010). The co-immobilization of both GOx and HRP, which acts in cascade, allows both a glucose measurement that avoids interferences and a signal amplification that increases biosensor efficiency.

b. Carbon nanotubes

In the last 20 years, carbon nanotubes have been a subject of intense studies. Carbon nanotubes (CNT) are carbon cylinders obtained by folding of graphite sheets in single (single-walled carbon nanotubes (SWCNT)) or several coaxial shells (multi-walled carbon nanotubes (MWCNT)). SWCNT and MWCNT have found important applications in biosensing due to some valuable properties, which make them compatible with sensing and biomolecules: ordered nanostructure, capacity to be functionalized with reactive groups and to link biomolecules and, very important in sensing, enhancement of electron transfer from enzyme to electrode. MWCNT were used in hybrid organic-inorganic matrices combined with sol-gel and other materials, in sandwich-type structures (Ahuja et al., 2011; Kang et al., 2008; Mugumura, 2010).

c. Metal nanoparticles and self-assembled systems

Since 1970s, we are witnesses of a rapid growth in nanocience interest for metal nanoparticles, such as Au, Pt, Ag, Cu, due to their enormous potential applications in catalysis, chemical sensors and biosensors. The biocompatibility of metal nanoparticles is based on their property to bind different ligands which, at their turn, can bind different biomolecules including enzymes. These nanoparticles have special electronic and photonic properties which make them extremely suitable in sensing.

Self-assembled systems are used in simple and versatile procedures to immobilize enzymes on metal or metal oxide surfaces. Organoalkoxysilanes or organochlorosilanes are able to undergo processes of self-assembly on glass, silicon or alumina surfaces. Sulphur containing molecules have a special well-known affinity to noble metal surfaces. Sulphur containing alkoxysilanes can be used as sol-gel precursors to facilitate the binding of not only enzymes but also nanoparticles and redox active species to surfaces of Pt, Au, Cu or glassy carbon.

Biosensors can be fabricated by means of self-assembled double-layer networks obtained from (3-mercaptopropyl)-trimethoxysilane (MPS) polymerized on gold electrode. Then, gold nanoparticles are attached by chemosorbtion on the double-layer polymer-gold electrode and, finally, GOx is bound to gold nanoparticles. Due to very low background current, such biosensors exhibit high sensitivity and short response time. The biosensors show a linear dependence at very low glucose concentrations and have a very low detection limit ($1x10^{-10}$ M). No interferences are observed. The performances of such biosensors may be explained considering that the nanoparticle – MPS network produces an increased surface area, thus increasing the enzyme loading (Barbadillo et al., 2009; Zhong et al., 2005).

5. Conclusions

Research for advanced technologies, including highly efficient enzymes and immobilization strategies, based on new materials and improved electrodes continue to be performed.

Future trends in the design of robust biological sensors should include new goals such as:

1. Research for new strains to produce more versatile enzymes with improved compatibility, operational activity and stability.
2. A deeper understanding of matrix–enzyme interaction, protein folding/unfolding and mobility phenomena to prevent inactivation. Other goals are: a tight and more specific bond of enzyme to matrix, a more tunable pore size distribution, new matrices, with improved properties, reduced diffusional barriers and minimal enzyme leaching to obtain an efficient and fast response from an operationally stable system.
3. New electrodes with enhanced analytical characteristics (high operational stability and sensibility, long life-time and low detection limit), active in hostile environment. High rate response and quick electron transfer from the enzyme to the transducer are problems that still wait for better solutions.
4. Improved immobilization methods for enzymes, a more efficient attachment of the enzyme - matrix assembly to the physical transducer, considering that the matrix is the key link between enzyme and transducer. A new view of geometry at nano and micro scale, to facilitate a better link among biocatalyst, matrix and transducer, based on biocompatibility.
5. Better non-invasive, portable settings for continuous *in vivo* monitoring. Miniaturization, biocompatibility, long term stability, specificity, and, first of all, higher accuracy are needed.

Due to their excellent biocompatibility, silica matrices may contribute to the development of new applications for more specific biosensing devices.

6. References

Ahuja,T.; Kumar, D.; Singh, N.; Biradar, A. M. & Rajesh (2011). Potentiometric urea biosensor based on multi-walled carbon nanotubes (MWCNTs)/silica composite material, *Mater. Sci. Eng. C* 31 (2) 90-94.

Anitha, K.; Mohan, S.V. & Reddy, S.J. (2004). Development of acetylcholinesterase silica sol-gel immobilized biosensor-an application towards oxydemeton methyl detection, *Biosens. Bioelectron.*, 20 (4) 848-856.

Avnir, D.; Braun, S.; Lev, O. & Ottolenghi M. (1994). Enzymes and other proteins entrapped in sol-gel materials, *Chem. Mater.* 6, 1605-1614.

Barbadillo, M.; Casero, E.; Petit-Dominguez, M. D.; Vazquez, L., Pariente, F. & Lorenzo, E. (2009). Gold nanoparticles-induced enhancement of the analytical response of an electrochemical biosensor based on an organic-inorganic hybrid composite material, *Talanta* 80 (2), 797 - 802.

Belkin, S. (2003). Microbial whole-cell sensing systems of environmental pollutants, *Curr. Opin. Microbiol.* 6 (3), 206-212.

Bergveld, P. (1996). The future of biosensors, *Sensors and Actuators A: Physical*, 56 (1-2) 65-73.

Bhatia, R.B.; Brinker, C.J.; Gupta, A.K. & Singh, A.K. (2000). Aqueous sol-gel process for protein encapsulation, *Chem. Mater.*, 12 (8), 2434-2441.

Bickerstaff, G. F. (1997), *Immobilization of Enzymes and Cells*, 2nd Ed., Humana Press, New Jersey, ISBN 0-89603-386-4.

Bizerea-Spiridon, O.; Vlad-Oros, B.; Preda, G. & Vintilă, M. (2010a). Studies regarding the membranous support of a glucose biosensor based on GOx, *Animal Sciences and Biotechnologies*, 43 (1), 354-357.

Bizerea-Spiridon, O.; Vlad-Oros, B.; Preda, G. & Vintilă, M. (2010b). The optimal composition of PVA membranar support of a glucose biosensor based on GOx, *Annals of West University of Timişoara, Series of Chemistry*, 19 (1), 97-104.

Brinker, C. J. & Scherer, G. W. (1990). *Sol Gel Science. The Physics and Chemistry of Sol–Gel Processing*, Academic Press, Boston.

Castillo, J.; Gáspár, S.; Leth, S.; Niculescu, M.; Mortari, A.; Bontidean, I.; Soukharev, V.; Dorneanu, S. A.; Ryabov, A. D. & Csöregi, E. (2004). Biosensors for life quality. Design, development and applications, *Sensor Actuat B-Chem.*, 102 (2), 179-194.

Chang, G.; Tatsu, Y.; Goto, T.; Imaishi, H.& Morigaki, K. (2010). Glucose concentration determination based on silica sol-gel encapsulated glucose oxidase optical biosensor arrays, *Talanta* 83 (1) 61-65.

Chaplin, M.& Bucke, C. (1990). *Enzyme Technology*, Cambridge University Press, Cambridge, ISBN 0521344298.

Chibata, I. (1978) in *Immobilized Enzymes*, Ed. I. Chibata, John Wiley, New York, 1-73.

Coradin, T.; Allouche, J.; Boissière, M. & Livage, J. (2006). Sol-gel biopolymer/silica nanocomposites in biotechnology, *Curr. Nanosci.*, 2, 219–230.

Couto, C.M.C.M.; Araujo, A. N.; Montenegro, M. C. B. S. M.; Rohwedder, J.; Raimundo, I. & Pasquini, C. (2002). Application of amperometric sol-gel biosensor to flow injection determination of glucose, *Talanta* 56 (6) 997-1003.

de Marcos, S.; Galindo, J.; Sierra, J. F.; Galban, J. & Castillo, J. R. (1999). An optical glucose biosensor based on derived glucose oxidase immobilised onto a sol-gel matrix, *Sensor Actuat B-Chem.*, 57 (1-3), 227 - 232.

Faber, K., (2000). *Biotransformation in Organic Chemistry*, 4th Ed., Springer, Berlin, 21.

Gill, I. & Ballesteros, A. (2000). Bioencapsulation within synthetic polymers (Part 1): sol-gel encapsulated biologicals, *Trends Biotechnol.* 18, 282-296.

Gomes, S.P.; Odlozilikova, M.; Almeida, M. G.; Araujo,A. N.; Couto, C.M.C.M. & Montenegro, M. C. B. S. M. (2007). Application of lactate amperometric sol-gel biosensor to sequential injection determination of l-lactate, *J. Pharmaceut. Biomed.* 43(4) 1376-1381.

Gupta, R. & Chaudhury, N.K. (2007). Entrapment of biomolecules in sol–gel matrix for applications in biosensors: Problems and future prospects, *Biosens. Bioelectron.* 22, 2387–2399.

Hussain, F.; Birch, D. J. S. & Pickup, J. C. (2005). Glucose sensing based on the intrinsic fluorescence of sol-gel immobilized yeast hexokinase, *Anal.Biochem.* 339 (1) 137-143.

Ivnitski, D.; Abdel-Hamid, I.; Atanasov, P.; Wilkins, E. & Stricker, S. (2000). Application of electrochemical biosensors for detection of food pathogenic bacteria, *Electroanalysis*, 12 (5), 317-325.

Jin, W. & Breman, J. D. (2002). Properties and applications of proteins encapsulated within sol - gel derived materials, *Anal. Chim. Acta*, 461, 1-36.

Justino, C .I. L.; Rocha-Santos, T. A. & Duarte, A. C (2010). Review of analytical figures of merit of sensors and biosensors, *TRAC - Trend. Anal. Chem.*, 29 (10), 1172-1183.

Kang, X.; Mai, Z.; Zou, X.; Cai, P. & Mo, J. (2008). Glucose biosensors based on platinum nanoparticles-deposited carbon nanotubes in sol-gel chitosan/silica hybrid, *Talanta* 74 (4), 879 - 886.

Kennedy, J. F. & Cabral, J. M. S. (1987) in *Biotechnology*, vol. 7a, *Enzyme Technology*, Ed. J. F. Kennedy, VCH, Weinheim, 349-400.

Khan, A. A. & Alzohairy, M. A. (2010). Recent Advances and applicationa of immobilized enzyme technologies, *Res. J. Biol. Sci.*, 5(8), 565-575.

Kim J.; Grate J. W. & Wang P. (2006). Nanostructures for Enzyme Stabilization, *Chem. Eng. Sci.* 61, 1017-1026.

Krajewska, B. (2004) Application of chitin- and chitosan-based materials for enzyme immobilizations: a review, *Enzyme Microb. Technol.*, 35, 126–139.

Kunzelmann, U. & Bottcher, H. (1997). Biosensor properties of glucose oxidase immobilized within SiO_2 gels, *Sensor Actuat. B-Chem.*, 39(1-3), 222 - 228.

Lalonde J. & Margolin A. (2002) in *Enzyme Catalysis in Organic Synthesis*, Ed. Drauz K. & Waldmann H., 2nd Ed., Wiley-VCH, Weinheim, 163-185.

Lazcka, O.; Del Campo, F. J. & Munoz, F. X. (2007). Pathogen detection: a perspective of traditional methods and biosensors, *Biosens. Bioelectron.*, 22, 1205-1217.

Lei, Y.; Chen, W. & Mulchandani, A. (2006). Microbial biosensors, *Anal. Chim. Acta*, 568 (1-2), 200-210.

Liao, C.-W.; Chou, J.-C.; Sun, T.-P.; Hsiung, S.-K.; Hsieh, J.-H. (2007). Preliminary investigations on glucose biosensor based on the potentiometric principle, *Sensor Actuat B-Chem* 123, 720-726.

Li, B. & Takahashi, H. (2000). New immobilization method for enzyme stabilization involving a mesoporous material and an organic/inorganic hybrid gel, *Biotechnol. Lett.*, 22, 1953–1958

Li, F.; Chen,W.; Tang,C. & Zhang, S. (2009). Development of hydrogen peroxide biosensor based on in situ covalent immobilization of horseradish peroxidase by one-pot polysaccharide-incorporated sol-gel process, *Talanta* 77(4), 1304-1308.

Li, W.; Yuan, R.; Chai,Y.; Zhou, L.; Chen, S. & Li,N. (2008). Immobilization of horseradish peroxidase on chitosan/silica sol-gel hybrid membranes for the preparation of hydrogen peroxide biosensor, *J. Biochem. Biophys. Methods* 70 (6), 830-837.

Livage, J.; Coradin, T. & Roux, C. (2001). Encapsulation of biomolecules in silica gels, *J. Phys.: Condens. Matter.* 13, 673-691.

Manesh, K. M.; Santhosh, P.; Uthayakumar, S.; Gopalan, A. I. & Lee, K. P. (2010). One-pot construction of mediatorless bi-enzymatic glucose biosensor based on organic-inorganic hybrid, *Biosens. Bioelectron.* 25(7), 1579 - 1586.

Mateo, C.; Palomo, J. M.; Fernandez-Lorente, G.; Guisan , J. M. & Fernandez-Lafuente, R. (2007). Improvement of enzyme activity, stability and selectivity via immobilization techniques, *Enzyme Microb. Technol.*, 40, 1451–1463.

Matrubutham, U.& Sayler, G.S. (1998). Microbial biosensors based on optical detection, in *Enzyme and Microbial Biosensors: Techniques and Protocols,* Methods in Biotechnology, Vol. 6, Mulchandani, A., Rogers K. R., Eds., Humana Press, Totowa, 249-256.

Mello, L. D. & Kubota, L. T. (2002). Analytical, nutritional and clinical methods - review of the use of biosensors as analytical tools in the food and drink industries, *Food Chem.* 77(2), 237–256.

Miao,Y. & Tan, S.N. (2001). Amperometric hydrogen peroxide biosensor with silica sol-gel/chitosan film as immobilization matrix, *Anal. Chim. Acta*, 437 (1) 87-93.

Mugumura, H. (2010). Amperometric Biosensor Based on Carbon nanotube and Plasma Polymer, in *Biosensors,* Ed. Serra, P.A., INTECH, 47-72, ISBN 978-953-7619-99-2.

Murty, V. R.; Bhat, J. & Muniswaran, P. K. A. (2002). Hydrolysis of oils by using immobilized lipase enzyme: a review, *Biotechnol. Bioprocess Eng.*, 7, 57-66.

Nayak, M.; Kotian, A.; Marathe, S. & Chakravortty, D. (2009). Detection of microorganisms using biosensors - A smarter way towards detection techniques, *Biosens. Bioelectron.*, 25 (4) 661-667.

Newman, J.D.; Turner, A.P. (2005). Home blood glucose biosensors: a commercial perspective, *Biosens. Bioelectron.*, 20, 2435-2453.

Oh, B. K.; Lee, W.; Chun, B. S.; Bae,Y.M.; Lee, W. H. & Choi, J. W. (2005). The fabrication of protein chip based on surface plasmon resonance for detection of pathogens, *Biosens. Bioelectron.*, 20 (9) 1847-1850.

Park, C. B. & Clark, D. S. (2002). Sol-gel encapsulated enzyme arrays for high-throughput screening of biocatalytic activity, *Biotechnol. Bioeng.*, 78 (2), 229-235.

Petkar, M.; Lali, A.; Caimi, P. & Daminati, M. (2006). Immobilization of lipases for non-aqueous synthesis, *J. Mol. Catal., B Enzym.*, 39, 83–90.

Radke, S. M. & Alocilja, E. C. (2005). A high density microelectrode array biosensor for detection of *E. coli* O157:H7, *Biosens. Bioelectron.*, 20 (8) 1662-1667.

Reetz, M. T.; Wenkel, R. & Avnir, D. (2000). Entrapment of lipases in hydrophobic sol-gel materials: Efficient heterogenous biocatalysts in aqueous medium, *Synthesis* 6, 781-783.

Reetz, M. T.; Tielmann, P.; Wiesenhöfer, W.; Könen, W. & Zonta, A. (2003). Second Generation Sol - Gel Encapsulated Lipases: Robust Heterogeneus Biocatalysts, *Adv. Synt. Catal.*, 345, 717-728.

Rodriguez-Mozaz, S.; López de Alda, M. J.; Marco, M. P. & Barceló, D. (2005). Biosensors for environmental monitoring. A global perspective, *Talanta*, 65 (2) 291–297.

Rodriguez-Mozaz, S.; López de Alda, M. J.; Marco, M. P. & Barceló, D. (2006). Biosensors as useful tools for environmental analysis and monitoring, *Anal. Bioanal. Chem.* 386 (4) 1025–1041.

Rogers, K. R. (2006). Recent advances in biosensor techniques for environmental monitoring, *Anal. Chim. Acta*, 568, (1-2) 222–231.

Rogers, K. R. & Mascini, M. (2009). Biosensors for Analytical Monitoring - General Introduction and Review, in *US Environmental Protection Agency*, 05.01.2011, http://www.epa.gov/heasd/edrb/biochem/intro.html

Rothenberg G. (2008). *Catalysis, Concepts and Green Applications*, Wiley-VCH, Weinheim, ISBN 978-3-527-31824-7

Salinas-Castillo, A.; Pastor, I.; Mallavia, R. & Mateo, C. R. (2008). Immobilization of a trienzymatic system in a sol-gel matrix: A new fluorescent biosensor for xanthine, *Biosens. Bioelectron.*, 24 (4), 1053-1056.

Shchipunov, Y. A.; Karpenko, T. Y.; Bakunina, I. Y.; Burtseva, Y. V. & Zvyagintseva T. N. (2004). A new precursor for the immobilization of enzymes inside sol-gel derived hybrid silica nanocomposites containing polysaccharides, *J. Biochem. Biophys. Meth.* 58 (1), 25-38.

Sheldon, R. (2007). Enzyme Immobilization: The quest for optimum performance, *Adv. Synth. Catal.*, 349, 1289–1307.

Singh, R. P. & Choi, J.W. (2009). Biosensors development based on potential target of conducting polymers, *Sensors & Transducers Journal*, 104 (5) 1-18.

Singh, S.; Singhal, R. & Malhotra, B. D. (2007). Immobilization of cholesterol esterase and cholesterol oxidase onto sol-gel films for application to cholesterol biosensor, *Anal. Chim. Acta*, 582 (2), 335-343.

Smith, J.E. (2004). *Biotechnology*, Cambridge University Press, Cambridge, ISBN 0521833329.

Smith, S.; Mukundan, P.; Krishna Pillai, P. & Warrier, K. G. K. (2007). Silica-gelatin bio-hybrid and transparent nano-coatings through sol-gel technique, *Mater. Chem. Phys.* 103 (2-3), 318 – 322.

Soetan, K. O.; Aiyelaagbe, O. O. & Olaiya, C. O, (2010). A review of the biochemical, biotechnological and other applications of enzymes, *Afr. J. Biotechnol.*, 9 (4), 382-393.

Su, L.; Jia, W.; Hou, C. & Lei, Y. (2010). Microbial biosensors: A review, *Biosens. Bioelectron.*, 26(5), 1788-1799.

Tan, X.; Li, M.; Cai, P.; Luo, L. & Zou, X. (2005). An amperometric cholesterol biosensor based on multiwalled carbon nanotubes and organically modified sol-gel/chitosan hybrid composite film, *Anal. Biochem.* 337 (1) 111-120.

Teles, F. R. R. & Fonseca, L. P. (2008). Applications of polymers for biomolecule immobilization in electrochemical biosensors, *Mater. Sci. Eng.* C 28 (8), 1530-1543.

Thévenot, D. R.; Toth, K.; Durst, R. A. & Wilson, G. S.. (1999). Electrochemical biosensors: Recommended definitions and classification (Technical Report), *Pure Appl. Chem.* 71 (12), 2333-2348.

Tothill, I. E. (2009). Biosensors for cancer markers diagnosis, *Seminars in Cell & Developmental Biology*, 20 (1), 55-62.

Turdean, G. L.; Stanca, S. E. & Popescu, I. C. (2005). *Biosenzori Amperometrici. Teorie si Aplicatii*, Presa Universitara Clujeana, Cluj-Napoca, 5 – 242, ISBN 973-610-359-5

Turner A. P. F.; Karube I. & Wilson G. S. (1987). *Biosensors: Fundamentals and Applications*, Oxford University Press, Oxford, ISBN 0198547242

Ullmann's Enciclopedia of Industrial Chemistry, (1987). Ed. V, vol. A14, Ed. Kandy, L.; Rounsaville J. F.; Schutz, G., VCH, Weinheim, 1-48.

Urban, G. A. (2009). Micro- and nanobiosensors - state of the art and trends, *Meas. Sci.Technol.* 20 (1) 1-18.

Velusamy, V.; Arshak, K.; Korostynska, O.; Oliwa, K. & Adley, C. (2010). An overview of foodborne pathogen detection: In the perspective of biosensors, *Biotechnol. Adv.* 28 (2), 232-254.

Verma, N. & Singh, M. (2005). Biosensors for heavy metals, *BioMetals*, 18 (2), 121–129.

Vlad-Oros, B.; Bizerea-Spiridon, O.; Preda, G. & Chiriac, A. (2009). Studies regarding the influence of the enzyme immobilization methods on the electrodic surface upon the performances of the glucose biosensor, *Rev. Chim.-Bucharest*, 60 (7), 693-698.

Wang, G. H. & Zhang, L. M. (2006) Using novel polysaccharide-silica hybrid material to construct an amperometric biosensor for hydrogen peroxide, *J. Physical Chem. B* 110 (49), 24864-24868.

Wang, J. (1999). Sol-gel materials for electrochemical biosensors, *Anal. Chim. Acta*, 399 (1-2), 21-27.

Wilson, G. S. & Gifford, R. (2005). Biosensors for real-time in vivo measurements, *Biosens. Bioelectron.*, 20 (12), 2388-2403.

Wilson, R. & Turner, A. P. F. (1992). Glucose oxidase: an ideal enzyme, *Biosens. Bioelectron.*, 7 (3), 165-185.

Yang, Y.L.; Tseng, T.F.; Yeh, J. M.; Chen, C. A. & Lou, S. L. (2008). Performance characteristic studies of glucose biosensors modified by (3-mercaptopropyl)trimethoxysilane sol-gel and non-conducting polyaniline, *Sensor Actuat B-Chem.* 131 (2), 533 - 540.

Yoo, E.-H. & Lee, S.-Y. (2010). Glucose biosensors: An overview of use in clinical practice, *Sensors*, 10, 4558-4576.

Zhong, X.; Yuan, R.; Chai, Y.; Liu, Y.; Dai, J. & Tang, D. (2005), Glucose biosensor based on self-assembled gold nanoparticles and double-layer 2d-network (3-mercapto-propyl)-trimethoxysilane polymer onto gold substrate, *Sen. Actuators B-Chem.*, 104 (2), 191 - 198.

18

Giant Extracellular Hemoglobin of *Glossoscolex paulistus*: Excellent Prototype of Biosensor and Blood Substitute

Leonardo M. Moreira et al.*
Departamento de Engenharia de Biossistemas (DEPEB),
Universidade Federal de São João Del Rei (UFSJ)
Brazil

1. Introduction

Porphyrins and their metal complexes have been investigated for many years because the richness of the properties of these compounds is of interest to a wide range of scientific disciplines, from medicine to materials science (Figure 1). Metalloporphyrins in living systems play many functions that are essential for life, and the elucidation of both the geometric and electronic structures of these compounds is of extreme relevance to a detailed understanding of their roles in biological systems. Moreover, the possibility of mimicking the complex chemistry exhibited by metalloporphyrins in living organisms with synthetic models propitiates the possibility of exploiting then in a wide range of different applications, from medical diagnostics and treatments to catalysts and sensors (Walker, 2006).

The heme groups (iron porphyrins) sites are involved in a range of biological functions. These roles are developed through various biochemical processes, such as electron transfer (e.g., cytochromes *a*, *b*, *c*, and *f*), in which the heme cycle between low-spin Fe(II) and low-spin Fe(III) small-molecule binding and transport, catalysis, and O_2 activation (e.g. peroxidases and cytochromes P450), where high-valent iron centers are involved in several chemical reactions, such as hydrogen atom abstraction, hydroxylation, and epoxide formation (Figure 1). Heme sites are significantly different from non-heme iron sites in which the porphyrin ligand allows the delocalization of the iron d-electrons into the porphyrin π system. This distribution of electronic density changes the properties of the iron with respect to the flexibility of the central coordination site, the energetics of reactivity, and, consequently, to its biological function (Hocking et al., 2007).

Alessandra L. Poli[2], Juliana P. Lyon[3], Pedro C. G. de Moraes[1], José Paulo R. F. de Mendonça[1], Fábio V. Santos[4], Valmar C. Barbosa[5] and Hidetake Imasato[2]
[1]*Departamento de Engenharia de Biossistemas (DEPEB), Universidade Federal de São João Del Rei (UFSJ), Brazil*
[2]*Instituto de Química de São Carlos (IQSC), Universidade de São Paulo (USP), Brazil*
[3]*Departamento de Ciências Naturais (DCNAT), Universidade Federal de São João Del Rei (UFSJ),Brazil*
[4]*Campus Centro Oeste Dona Lindu, Universidade Federal de São João Del Rei (UFSJ), Brazil*
[5]*Instituto de Fìsica (IF), Universidade Federal do Rio de Janeiro (UFRJ), Brazil*

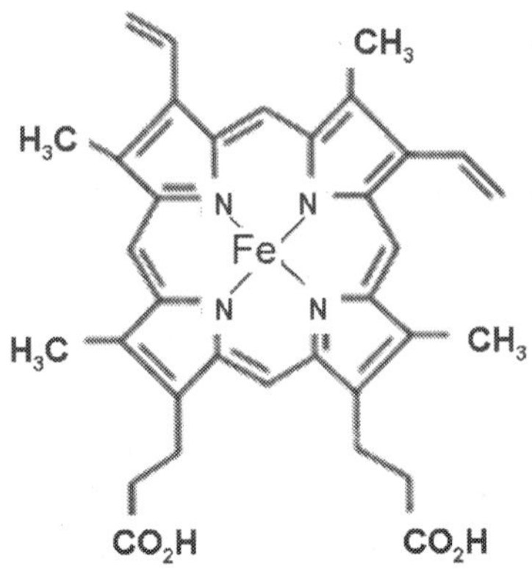

Fig. 1. Protoporphyrin IX (PpIX) demonstrating the ferrous íon as coordination Center and the nitrogens of the four pyrrolic rings acting as coordinating sites (Lewis basis).

The heme groups (iron porphyrins) sites are involved in a range of biological functions. These roles are developed through various biochemical processes, such as electron transfer (e.g., cytochromes *a, b, c,* and *f*), in which the heme cycle between low-spin Fe(II) and low-spin Fe(III) small-molecule binding and transport, catalysis, and O_2 activation (e.g. peroxidases and cytochromes P450), where high-valent iron centers are involved in several chemical reactions, such as hydrogen atom abstraction, hydroxylation, and epoxide formation (Figure 1). Heme sites are significantly different from non-heme iron sites in which the porphyrin ligand allows the delocalization of the iron d-electrons into the porphyrin π system. This distribution of electronic density changes the properties of the iron with respect to the flexibility of the central coordination site, the energetics of reactivity, and, consequently, to its biological function (Hocking et al., 2007).

The structure-activity relationship of iron-porphyrins as well as the activity-function relation of globins is still a great challenge to several researchers. Understanding the function of macromolecular complexes is related to a precise knowledge of their structure. These large complexes are often fragile high molecular mass noncovalent multimeric proteins (Bruneaux et al., 2008). This extraordinary hemoprotein system is widely distributed in nature, presenting slight differences between the several types of heme proteins. In spite of the various similar physico-chemical properties, the apparently small significant differences are responsible for a diversity of characteristics that becomes quite distinct the biochemical behavior of these proteins. In this way, the association of instrumental tools is essential to elucidate intricate aspects involving the structure-function relationship of these protein systems. By combining native mass and subunit composition data, structural models can be proposed for large edifices such as annelid extracellular hexagonal bilayer hemoglobins (HBL-Hb) and crustacean hemocyanins (Hc) (Bruneaux et al., 2008). Association/dissociation mechanisms, protein-protein interactions, structural diversity among species and environmental adaptations can also be addressed with these methods (Bruneaux et al., 2008). An example of these light structural differences that provoke significantly distinct functions is the case of the nitrophorins that are NO-carrying hemoproteins, being significantly different of the O_2-carrying hemoproteins, such as hemoglobin (Figure 2). Nitrophorins constitute an example of this complex reality, since that these proteins are a group of NO-carrying hemoprotein encountered in the saliva of, at least, two species of blood-sucking insects, *Rhodnius prolixus* and *Cimex lectularius*, which present very elaborated physico-chemical properties deeply associated to its complex biochemical role (Berry & Walker, 2007; Knipp et al., 2007). These hemoproteins sequester nitric oxide (NO) that is produced by a nitric oxide synthase (NOS) present in the cells of the salivary glands, which is a protein similar to vertebrate constitutive NOS. NO is kept stable for long periods by ligation as sixth ligand of the ferriheme center. Upon injection into the tissues of the victim, NO dissociates, diffuses through the tissues to the nearby capillaries to cause vasodilatation, and thereby allows more blood to be transported to the respective site of the wound. At the same time, histamine, which causes swelling, itching, and initiates the immune response, is released by mast cells and platelets of the victim. In the case of the *Rhodnius* proteins, this histamine binds to the heme iron sites of the nitrophorins, hence preventing the victim`s detection of the insect for a period of time, which allows it to obtain a sufficient blood meal (Berry & Walker, 2007; Knipp et al., 2007). It is important to notice that great and crescent number of studies that employees porphyrin-like compounds in different chemical contexts denotes the extraordinary interdisciplinary and multidisciplinary characters of these macrociclic compounds. The applications of porphyrin-like compounds, metallated or not, in PDT (Moreira et al., 2008), catalysis, electrochemical studies, biomimetic studies, and others are a definitive fingerprint of the great biochemical and physico-chemical relevance of this chemical system.

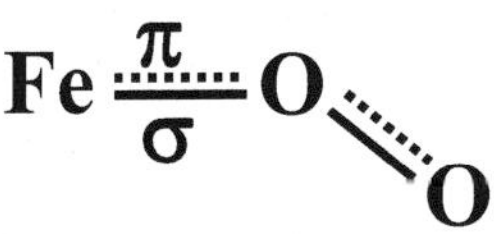

(1.3)

Fig. 2. Iron-Oxygen bound, with the Oxygen molecule (oxygen-oxygen bound axix) presenting significant inclination in relation to the iron-oxygen bound axis.

2. Electronic properties of heme groups

The delocalization of the Fe d-electrons into the porphyrin ring and its effect on the redox chemistry and reactivity of these systems has been difficult to study by optical spectroscopies due to the dominant porphyrin п-п* transitions, which obscure the metal center (Hocking et al., 2007). In any case, the information obtained from Ligand-to-Metal Charge Transfer (LMCT) transitions can be accessed in several cases, mainly when this electronic band occurs above 600 nanometers. In this situation, it is possible to infer a higher number of relevant physico-chemical data from electronic spectra. Recently, Hocking and co-workers (Hocking et al., 2007) developed a methodology that allows the interpretation of the multiplet structure of Fe L-edges in terms of differential orbital covalency (i.e., differences in mixing of the d-orbitals with ligand orbitals) using a valence bond configuration interaction (VBCI) model. This method can be considered an interesting alternative to obtain significant information about the heme properties, principally when these data are not accessible through UV-VIS spectroscopy. In fact, when this methodology is applied to low-spin heme systems, this method allows experimental determination of the delocalization of the Fe d-electrons (Figure 3) into the porphyrin (P) ring in terms of both

PfFe ó and ð-donation and FefP ð back-bonding. We find that ð-donation to Fe(III) is much larger than ð back-bonding from Fe(II), indicating that a hole superexchange pathway dominates electron transfer (Hocking et al., 2007).

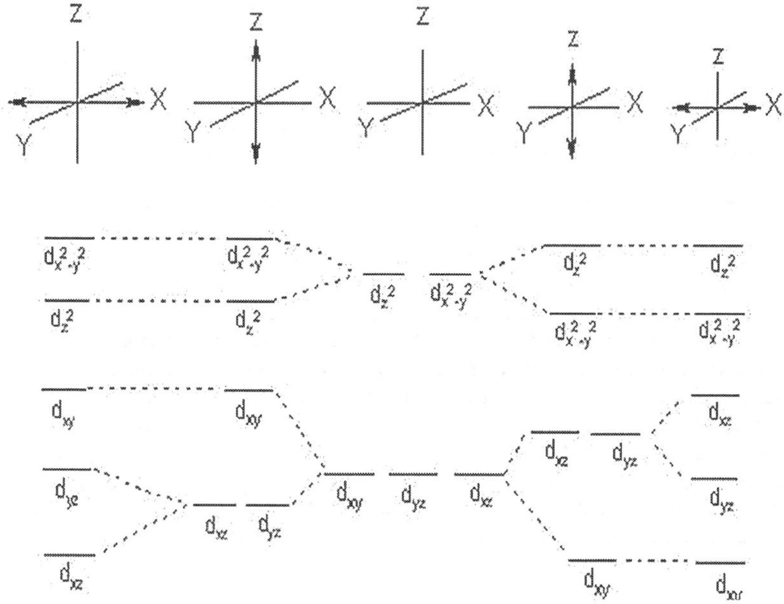

Fig. 3. 3*d* orbitals splitting related to octaedric complexes that present tetragonal and rhomboedric distortions complexos octaédricos devido às distorções. Right side: Assymetric distribution of d_{xz} e d_{yz} orbitals intensifies the Jahn-Teller distortions provoking the rhombic symmetry. The tetragonal symmetry is favored in the absence of steric precluding.

3. Hydrophobic isolation of the heme pocket in hemoproteins and the aqueous solvent role in the structure-activity relationship

Binding of water to hemoglobin is the determinant step in the mechanism of allosteric regulation (Pereira et al., 2005). An analytical method known as osmotic stress has been developed based on this inclusion/exclusion process for situations of low macromolecular concentrations. This methodology is being extensively applied to analyze the hydration water involved in the interaction of macromolecules (Pereira et al., 2005). Furthermore, the water action upon the hemoglobin structure is deeply associated to the native hydrophobic isolation inherent to the heme pockets of hemoproteins. This hydrophobic isolation limits significantly the access of aqueous solvent to the metallic center, which implicates in a more stable redox state as well as lower number of ligand changes of the first coordination sphere of the metallic center. Consequently, when the natural hydrophobicity of the native heme pocket is maintained, it is limited the occurrence of hemoglobin autoxidation (Figure 4), which would be accentuated by the presence of anionic ions in the heme pocket (Figure 5)

$$Fe^{2+}\text{—}O_2 \longrightarrow Fe^{2+} + O_2$$
$$Fe^{2+}\text{—}O_2 \longrightarrow Fe^{3+} + O_2^{-\cdot}$$

Fig. 4. Oxygen ligand exit from the first coordination sphere of the ferrous ion, which can occur as superoxide anion (autoxidation) or neutral oxygen molecule

4. pH influence on the oligomeric structure of hemoproteins

The effect of pH on biological systems has been widely investigated using various models to gain insights into the role of protons in modulating biochemical processes. Analysis of the stability of high protein aggregates using hydrostatic pressure (>250 MPa) to promote protein dissociation has shown that protein aggregation is strongly pH-dependent (Bispo et al., 2005). The ability of protons to cause protein conformational changes, including allosteric phenomena, means that the study of pH is important for understanding normal protein folding and function. In hemoglobins (Hbs), the role of protons in oxygen affinity (Bohr effect) has been extensively studied in the physiologic pH range and at extreme conditions. The cooperativity in ligand binding is also pH-dependent, with a decrease in cooperativity as pH increases. This behavior is responsible for the sigmoidal nature of the plot of Hb saturation versus oxygen pressure, with a tendency to assume a hyperbolic shape at alkaline pH (Bispo et al., 2005). These properties demonstrated the high sensitivity of the oligomeric structure of hemoglobins to the environmental changes.

$$\mathbf{MbFe(II)(O_2) + X^- \longrightarrow \left[MbFe \begin{matrix} X^- \\ O_2 \end{matrix} \right] \longrightarrow MbFe(III)(X^-) + O_2^{-\cdot}} \quad (1.8)$$

Fig. 5. Autoxidation mechanism favored by the presence of anionic ligand

5. The interface between redox and oligomeric properties of hemoproteins

Studies focused on the evaluation of redox potential of human hemoglobins have demonstrated a negative value of redox to the couple of *quasi*-reversible redox peaks, such as -0.38 V (*versus* SCE) in 0.1 M pH 7.0 PBS obtained through a Hb/gelatin/GCE system (Yao et al., 2006). Zhao and co-workers performed their direct electrochemistry with the formal potential of -0.032V for hemoglobin and system of ZrO_2 nanoparticles with heme proteins on functional glassy carbon electrode (Zhao et al., 2005). In fact, the determination of redox potential in hemoproteins is frequently associated to complex methodologies, since the polypeptide chains and the hydrophobic isolation of the heme pocket preclude the direct contact between the electrode and the main redox site of hemoproteins, which is the metallic center of heme (ferrous or ferric ion). These redox potentials strongly suggest that the heme group of several heme proteins, especially hemoglobins, would be easily oxidized in a short time interval, mainly if the accessibility of oxidant agents into heme pocket would not deeply precluded.Considering these redox potentials, it is plausible to infer that only the

hydrophobic isolation would not be able to avoid the oxidation of the ferrous ion. The limitation propitiated by the lateral chains of the aminoacid residues of the heme pocket neighborhood is not sufficient to maintain, at least, 95% of heme species in its ferrous form. In fact, in mammalian organisms, only 1% of ferric species is considered a normal physiological condition, being that the minimum of 99% is reached by the action of reductase enzymes, which limits significantly the concentration of ferric form in the organism. In any case, the redox potential of most hemoproteins would suggest a more representative percentage of oxidized heme species in the respective organisms. However, this fact does not occur as function, mainly, of the great compaction that constitutes the native state (wild configuration) of the hemoproteins, especially in hemoproteins with great supramolecular mass, which is the case of the giant extracellular hemoglobins. This high level of compaction of the globin chains limits pronouncedly the accessibility of ions into heme pocket. In fact, it is well established that the more intense accessibility of potential ligands to the metallic center is a decisive factor to improve the autoxidation rate (Figure 5).
Liu and co-workers (Liu et al., 1996) claims that the major difference between the Im-cyt and cyt *c* lies in their respective redox potential (-178 mV for Im-cyt *c* versus 260 mV for cyt *c*). In this context, the functional relevance of the axial Met80 ligand can be emphasized. In summary, the variation in the redox potentials of cytochrome *c* can be accounted for by differences in two effects: (a) the nature of the axial ligation to the iron; (b) the effects of the surrounding protein environment. The substitution of axial methionine by imidazole has been indicated to decrease the redox potential of cytochrome *c* by 160 mV. Since the imidazole ligated cyt *c* has a potential of 438 mV lower than the native cyt *c*, it appears that environmental factors may be most important. In fact, axial ligands provided by the side chains of His-18 and Met-80 as well as the covalently attached heme not only are essential for the structure and function of cytochrome *c* (cyt *c*), but they also play an important role in the folding process. It has been demonstrated by optical and NMR spectroscopy that one of the axial ligands in native oxidized cyt *c*, Met-80, dissociates more readily, and can be displaced by the intrinsic or extrinsic ligands, for instance, in the zinc cyt *c* used in the electron transfer studies or in the alkaline form of the protein (Shao et al., 1996). The high reduction potential of cyt *c* is also caused by exclusion of water from the heme environment by the surrounding hydrophobic and bulky amino acids. In Im-cyt *c*, apparent changes have happened to the heme hydrophobic pocket including heme-contact residues within 60 s helix, the region around Met80 and the lower left side of the molecule which is near be accounted for by changes in the secondary structures for example, the absence of 3_{10} helix from Tyr67 to Asn70, the type II turn form from Ile75 to Thr78 and distorted 50s helix from 51 to 54 (Liu et al., 1996).
Previous data focused on giant extracellular hemoglobins demonstrated that the initial protein unfolding provoked by interaction with low concentration of ionic surfactants promotes a surprising increase in the size of the supramolecular protein arrangement, probably caused by the discompaction of the chains. Interestingly, only after this slight polypeptide chains separation, it is possible to differentiate the physico-chemical and spectroscopic behaviors of each chain. Therefore, besides the protection against oxidation, the compaction would be the main cause of a very peculiar phenomenon, which is the equalization of heme groups, due to the intense compactness of the quaternary structure. This proposal is supported by several studies found on autoxidation kinetics that demonstrated that an initial loss of intra- and inter-chains contacts is a fundamental pre-requisite to the initial oxidation of the heme groups. The oxidation phenomenon has

demonstrated to be very dependent of the occurrence of some medium perturbation. For example, we can mention the pH changes, which, affecting the relation of ionic charges that involves the intra- and inter-chains contacts, decrease the compaction level of the quaternary arrangement of the protein. In fact, all factors that can perturb the global spatial configuration of the polypeptide chains can be considered as potential inductors of oxidation, since that the oligomeric alteration of the native form tends to originate a less compacted configuration. In this way, pH changes, surfactant addition and oxidant agents presence between others, constitute decisive influences that gradually decrease the native characteristics of the hemoglobin quaternary and tertiary configurations. Thus, an initial discompaction must to occur with concomitant increase of the protein size previously to a more representative unfolding process. This gradual process of loss of compaction would be the predominant phenomenon if the protein perturbation is small, which can occur when, for example, the surfactant concentration or the pH change is low (small distance of the neutrality). In more drastic processes, including drastic pH transitions and addition of high surfactant concentration, the discompaction is already accompanied by a very pronounced protein unfolding and until, in some cases, of an initial chains separation. Probably, in these drastic processes, the interaction of surfactants with the protein is a micelle-like phenomenon, being characterized by a significant concentration of the ionic surfactants molecules on each ionic site of opposite charge situated on the protein surface. On the other hand, low concentration of surfactants propitiates a more specific and individual interaction between the surfactant molecules and the sites of opposite ionic charge that are encountered on the protein surface.

6. The redox-dependent structure change in hemoproteins: Comparative analysis between ferrous and ferric forms

Many studies focused on understanding the structure-function problem in several hemoproteins, such as cytochrome *c*, have revealed that *ferricytochrome c* is different from *ferrocytochrome c* in several physical and chemical properties, including global stability, compressibility, molecular extent evaluated by low-angle X-ray scattering, hydrogen-exchange behavior and the chemical reactivity of specific groups (Feng et al., 1990). Therefore, the redox state change generates a sequence of relevant events that can alter drastically the protein activity. The cytochrome *c* protein favors the reduced form of its bound heme, which means that the heme binds more strongly to the protein in the reduced form and therefore makes reduced cytochrome *c* the more stable form. The higher structural free energy level of the oxidized proteins reveals itself when structural stability is measured, e.g., in equilibrium denaturation experiments which measure overall stability and, at higher resolution, in the hydrogen-exchange rates of individual hydrogens, which depend upon local unfolding reactions (Feng et al., 1990).

7. The iron ligands and the structural implications regarding the configuration of the first coordination sphere

The ligand affinities for O_2 and CO in monomeric hemoglobin (Hb) and myoglobin (Mb) are exquisitely modulated over wide ranges by relatively few residues within a largely conserved globular fold consisting of 7-8 helices with the heme wedged between helices E and F and ligated by His(F8) (Kolczak et al., 1997) (Figure 6). Various direct influences have been proposed to modulate the stability of the "ligated protein" in comparison with unligated protein, including hydrogen-bond stabilization by the ubiquitous His(E7) of the bound O_2 (observed in neutron diffraction of MbO_2) (Figure 6), steric destabilization by Val (E11) for bound CO (observed by tilt or bend of Fe-CO in X-ray diffraction of MbCO or HbCO), and pocket polarity as determined by residues such as B10. A more indirect mechanism proposed to modulated ligand affinity in general is the control of the spacing between the F-helix and the heme, which must be significantly reduced in ligated form when compared with the unligated state (Kolczak et al., 1997).

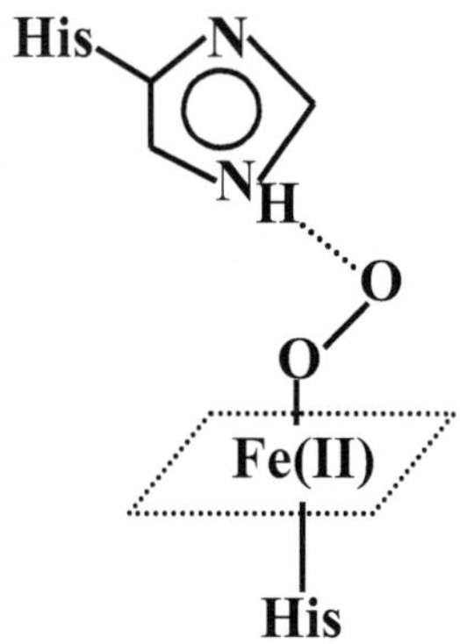

Fig. 6. Distal histidine E7 generating stability to the iron-oxygen bound through the formation of a hydrogen bound between the NH group of imidazole and the molecular oxygen.

8. Hemoglobins

Among the four types of existing respiratory proteins: (a) hemocyanins; (b) hemerytrins; (c) chlorocruorins; and (d) hemoglobins, the latter is widely distributed in the vertebrate and invertebrate animals (Arndt & Santoro, 1998). In the mollusks, the main oxygen carrier is the copper containing hemocyanin and extracellular hemoglobins (erythrocruorins) are restricted to two families of clams, Astartidae and Carditidae and one family of freshwater snails, the Planorbidae (Arndt & Santoro, 1998). The snail extracellular hemoglobins are multi-subunit proteins with reported molecular weights varying between 1.65 and 2.25_103 kDa. They contain 10 to 12 polypeptide chains of 175–200 kDa linked in pairs by disulfide bridges forming five to six subunits of 350– 400 kDa. Each of these chains comprises 10 to 12 heme binding domains based in its minimum molecular weight of 17.0–22.5 kDa (Arndt & Santoro 1998). This pattern is also observed in the branchiopod crustacean *Artemia sp* which contains 9 domains per polypeptide chain and corresponds to the multi-domain, multi-subunit structure reviewed by Vinogradov (Arndt & Santoro, 1998). This kind of structure denotes the relevance of the polypeptide contacts, which are decisive to determine the intensity of compaction of the hemoprotein, generating the tertiary and quaternary structure that are peculiar to each protein. Hemoglobin (Hb) occurs in all the kingdoms of living organisms. Its distribution is episodic among the nonvertebrate groups in contrast to vertebrates. Nonvertebrate Hbs range from single-chain globins found in bacteria, algae, protozoa, and plants to large, multisubunit, multidomain Hbs found in nematodes, molluscs and crustaceans, and the giant annelid and vestimentiferan Hbs comprised of globin and nonglobin subunits. Chimeric hemoglobins have been found recently in bacteria and fungi. Hb occurs intracellularly in specific tissues and in circulating red blood cells (RBCs) and freely dissolved in various body fluids (Weber & Vinogradov, 2001).

9. Mammalian hemoglobins

Mammalian adult hemoglobin (HbA) is a tetramer of two Hb and two Hb subunits (Figure 7), which is produced in extremely high concentrations (340 mg mL^{-1}) in red blood cells (Gell et al., 2009). Numerous mechanisms exist to balance and coordinate HbA synthesis in normal erythropoiesis, and problems with the production of either HbA subunit give rise to thalassemia, a common cause of anemia worldwide (Gell et al., 2009). In this context, it is interesting to notice that Hematrocrit (Ht) levels higher or lower than the normal range can influence the physiological function and increase the risk of cardiovascular disease. The Ht level is indicative of the proportion of blood occupied by red blood cells, and is normally 40.7-50.3% for males and 36.1-44.31% for females (Sakudo et al., 2009).

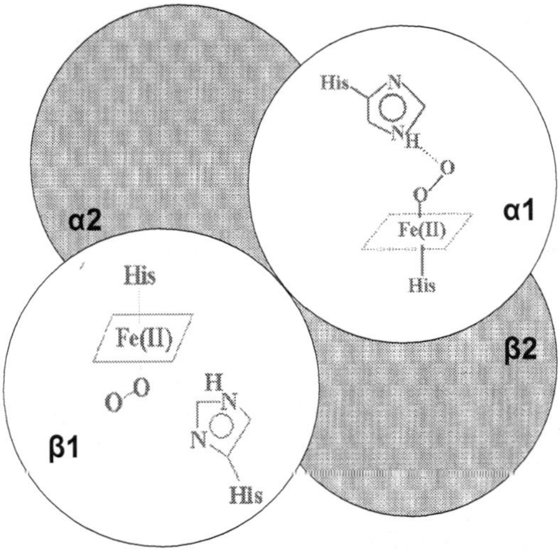

Fig. 7. Scheme of the contact $\alpha_1\beta_1$, which favors the inclination of the distal histidine of β chain of the human hemoglobin.

10. Extracellular hemoglobins

The hemoglobin from Biomphalaria glabrata is an extracellular respiratory protein of high molecular mass composed by subunits of 360 kDa, each one containing two 180 kDa chains linked by disulfide bridges, being that data regarding the structural and biochemical properties indicate that the multisubunit structure of this hemoglobin is compatible with a tetrameric arrangement (Arndt et al., 2003). However, there is a great number of extracellular hemoglobins that presents a much more complex quaternary structure, preseting a higher number of oligomeric subunits, which are called giant extracellular hemoglobins (HBLs).

11. Giant extracellular hemoglobins (HBLs)

Assembly of protein subunits into large complexes is an important mechanism employed to attain greater efficiency and regulatory control of biological processes. Annelid erythrocruorins pose key problems in the design of such large macromolecular assemblages. The extracellular nature and giant size of these molecules have made them ideal systems for a number of seminal investigations into protein structure (Royer et al., 2000). Natural acellular polymeric hemoglobins (Hb) provide oxygen transport and delivery within many terrestrial and marine invertebrate organisms. These natural acellular Hbs may serve as models of therapeutic hemoglobin-based oxygen carriers (HBOC) (Harrington et al., 2007). For instance, acellular Hb from the terrestrial invertebrate Lumbricus terrestris (Lt) possesses a unique hierarchical structure and a peculiar ability to function extracellularly without oxidative damage. Lumbricus Hb as well as Arenicola Hb is resistant to autoxidation, chemical oxidation by potassium ferricyanide, and have low capability to transfer electrons to Fe(III)complexes at 37°C. An understanding of how these invertebrate acellular oxygen carriers maintain their structural integrity and redox stability in vivo is vital for the design of a safe and effective red cell substitute. In fact, this hemoglobin presents positive redox potential (Harrington et al., 2007). Homotropic and heterotropic allosteric interactions are important mechanisms that regulate protein function. These mechanisms depend on the ability of oligomeric protein complexes to adopt different conformations and to transmit conformation-linked signals from one subunit of the complex to the neighboring ones (Hellmann et al., 2008). An important step in understanding the regulation of protein function is to identify and characterize the conformations available to the protein complex. This task becomes increasingly challenging with increasing numbers of interacting binding sites. However, a large number of interacting binding sites allows for high homotropic interactions (cooperativity) and thus represents the most interesting case (Hellmann et al., 2008). Giant extracellular hemoglobins are examples of very large and cooperative protein complexes. This class of hemoglobins is found in annelid worms that contain 144 oxygen-binding sites, such as the giant extracellular hemoglobins of *Lumbricus terrestris* and *Glossoscolex paulistus*. These proteins show strict hierarchy in structure, being that the interaction of various ligands, such as O_2, CO and NO, and the principle binding behavior of these protein complexes has been considered the main topics to the understanding of the respective structure-function relationship (Hellmann et al., 2008).

12. Giant extracellular hemoglobin of *glossoscolex paulistus*

The hemoglobin (Hb) of the annelid *Glossoscolex paulistus* is a giant extracellular Hb (erythrocruorin) that dissociates into low affinity subunits after incubation under pressure (with stabilization of the dissociated products), alkalization (mainly around pH 9.0) of acidification of medium or surfactant addition (Bispo et al., 2007).

13. The influence of ions on the structure-activity relationship: A comparative evaluation between vertebrate and invertebrate hemoproteins

Elucidation of the detailed thermodynamics of heme site ligation and its linkages to heterotropic effectors has required circumvention of the following obstacles: (i) lability of the heme iron-oxygen bond precludes the isolation and study of most intermediates; (ii) high binding cooperativity greatly reduces the populations of intermediates in equilibrium with the end-state species; and (iii) dissociation of tetramers into dimmers leads to their reassembly into tetramers with rearranged configurations of occupied sites (Huang et al., 1997). The oxygen binding properties of extracellular giant hemoglobins (Hbs) in some annelids exhibit features significantly different from those of vertebrate tetrameric Hbs. Annelid giant Hbs show cooperative oxygen binding properties in the presence of inorganic cations, while the cooperativities of vertebrate Hbs are enhanced by small organic anions or chloride ions (Numoto et al., 2008). This interesting difference must be associated to several aspects of the distinct structure-function relationship found in vertebrate and invertebrate hemoglobins, respectively. Giant extracellular hemoglobins are known by their acid isoelectric points (pI), which is deeply related to several oligomeric and physico-chemical properties that are peculiar to this hemoprotein systems, when compared with mammalian hemoproteins. In contrast to mammalian or vertebrate tetrameric Hb, invertebrate Hbs show remarkable varieties in terms of quaternary structure and oxygen binding properties. Two types of extracellular giant Hbs occur in some annelids. Earthworm *Lumbricus terrestris* has a 3600 kDa Hb designated as hexagonal bilayer (HBL) Hb, which also occurs in many other annelids. *Lumbricus* Hb shows moderate oxygen affinity and highly cooperative oxygen binding properties coupled with inorganic cations and protons (Numoto et al., 2008). The heterotropic interactions involving inorganic cations are commonly observed features among annelid HBL Hbs. Cations and protons preferably bind to the R state and increase the ligand affinity of HBL Hbs; the heterotropic effectors in the annelid HBL Hbs differ markedly from those of vertebrate Hbs. Another giant Hb from an annelid is a 400 kDa Hb that occurs in some siboglinid polychaetes. *Oligobrachia mashikoi*, a frenulate beard worm, has a 400 kDa Hb composed of four globin subunits (A1, A2, B1, and B2) that form a 24-mer hollow-spherical structure. The oxygen binding properties of *Oligobrachia* Hb are qualitatively similar to those of annelid HBL Hbs. It is important to notice that both the oxygen affinity and cooperativity of *Oligobrachia* Hb are enhanced by the addition of Ca2+ and/or Mg2+, or by an increase in pH (Numoto et al.,, 2008). Oxygenation properties of hemoglobin (Hb) from Oligobrachia mashikoi were extensively investigated. Compared to human Hb, Oligobrachia Hb showed a high oxygen affinity (P50 = 1.4 mmHg), low cooperativity (n = 1.4), and a small Bohr effect (dH+ =_0.28) at pH 7.4 in the presence of minimum salts (Aki, et al., 2007). Addition of NaCl caused no change in the oxygenation properties of Oligobrachia Hb, indicating that Na^+ and Cl^- had no effect. Mg^{2+} and Ca^{2+} remarkably increased the oxygen affinity and cooperativity. Thus, unlike the vertebrate Hbs, but like the annelid extracellular Hbs, the oxygen binding properties of Oligobrachia Hb are regulated by divalent cations which preferentially bind to the oxy form (Aki, et al., 2007).

14. Why the intensity of polypeptide compaction is decisive to the physico-chemical properties of HbGp?

The oligomeric compaction, which is dependent of the level of polypeptide compressibility, is a fundamental aspect of the structure-activity relationship of HbGp. Probably this fact occurs as consequence of two factors: The extraordinarily high hydrophobicity of the compacted arrangement, i.e., the native configuration, and the high restriction to the accessibility of ions, which can induce the occurrence of autoxidation mechanisms.The dielectric constant of the heme pocket neighborhood affects pronouncedly the hydrogen bonds developed by the aminoacid residues around the heme, including the distal and proximal histidines. These two histidines are extraordinarily important in several processes that control the structure-function of hemoglobins, such as the ligand exchange on the first coordination sphere of the metallic center. The physico-chemical properties of these important residues can be intensely altered when the polarity of medium is modified, which can affect the influence of these residues upon the heme reactivity.

15. The peculiarities of the unfolding mechanism in alkaline and acid media

Venkatesh and co-workers (Venkatesh, 1999), studying hemoglobins reconstituted with Cu-porphyrin and Ni-porphyrin as function of pH, provide significant insight about the mechanism of conservation of the native configuration in hemoproteins. In any case, the work of these authors supports that the alkaline medium propitiates a higher complexity in the equilibria of species when compared with the acid medium (Venkatesh, et al., 1999). The higher complexity of species in alkaline medium when compared with the acid conditions would be associated to some factors. Firstly, the several specific disprotonation processes, which can occur with the different aminoacid residues in alkaline medium, offers a great number of potential ligands to the metallic center, together with the aqueous solvent molecules, which can to coordinate the metallic center as well as its disprotonated form, i.e., the hydroxyl ion.

In acid medium, the potential ligands can be protonated, depending of their respective isoelectric points (pI). This fact limits the number and the efficacy as ligands of the aminoacid residues.An interesting example of the influence of the protonation state on the properties as ligands can be encountered in the evaluation of the histidine as ligand. Actually, histidine is very important ligand to heme proteins, mainly hemoglobins, where can to form the bis-histidine complexes, which are commonly called "hemichromes". In alkaline conditions, some configuration can be considered effective ligands to the metallic center, while in acidic medium, the number of active states as ligands is pronouncedly lower. In this context, it is relevant to notice that the extraordinary level of compaction of the polypeptide chains probably is related to an intense and well organized interaction between opposite charges. The slight and gradual loss of intra- and inter-chains contacts lightly initiates a process of discompaction that is very difficult to be reversed, mainly in giant extracellular hemoglobins as function of the extraordinarily large supramolecular mass of this class of hemoproteins (approximately 3.6 MDa to *Lumbricus terrestris* and *Glossoscolex paulistus* hemoglobins). In our previous article, which is focused on drastic pH transitions of heme species, it is possible to infer that HbGp presents high level of irreversibility in more drastic pH changes.

16. What are the predominant ferric heme configurations in HbGp?

Bis-imidazole and bis-pyridine complexes of Fe(III) porphyrins,1-3 including the octaalkyltetraphenylporphyrins provide excellent models for bis-histidine coordinated heme centers involved in a number of cytochrome-containing systems, examples of which include cytochromes *b* of mitochondrial Complexes II5 and III6-20 and of chloroplast cytochrome *b6f* (Yatsunyk et al., 2006). In fact, these model complexes, which allow a study focused on the first coordirnation sphere as well as the hemoproteins, such as HbGp, that present more global information, demonstrates that aquomet, hemichrome and pentacoordinate (mono-histidine) species are the predominant forms in heme systems. The tendency of hemichrome hexacoordinated species formation immediately after light medium perturbation in the neighborhood of the protein suggests a deeply high sensitivity of the F helix, permitting a significant approach of the distal histidine in relation to the metallic center. Nevertheless, after this slight spatial modification, the predominant part of the polypeptide chains tends to lose great number of intra- and inter-chains subunits contacts, favoring a labilization process of the two helices bounded axially to the metallic center through the distance increase between the helices that constitute the secondary protein structure. This mechanical influence compromises the stability of these axial ligations of the metallic center, favoring the respective breakage of one of them, with consequent appearance of a significant presence of pentacoordinated ferric species. Obviously, in a very large supramolecular system, including 180 biological macromolecules, which are the polypeptide chains, depending of the unfolding mechanism, the tension on the axial helices would be significantly different to each subunit, which can justify the coexistence of several heme species. In other words, we can propose that, in spite of some general properties, the polypeptide chains are not submitted strictly to the same unfolding process. This fact can explain the coexistence of distinct ferric heme species in each pH value, mainly when the medium conditions are very distant of the neutrality (pH=7.0).

17. The interaction between HbGp and surfactants as resource of physico-chemical informations

Surfactants are surface-active agent and belong to the category of amphiphilic molecules. They are capable of forming aggregates known as micelles and the concentration at which they form is known as the critical micellar concentration (cmc). Surfactants are widely employed in biochemistry and biotechnology for the purpose of protein solubilization, purification, characterization, and protein structure determination (Miksovska, et al., 2006). Surfactant-protein interactions are very common in the fields of medicine, chemistry, biology and so on (Liu et al., 2007; van der Veen et al., 2004; Orioni et al., 2006; Vasilescu et al., 1999; Stenstam et al., 2003). Many approaches have been focused such as the kind of protein-surfactant interaction, the influence of the aggregation state of the surfactant (monomer, pre-micellar aggregate and micelle) on the protein structure, the properties of the surfactant-protein system, the characterization of the interaction sites on the protein surface, the identification of the intermediate protein conformations, etc (Liu et al., 2007; Liu et al., 2005; Ajloo et al., 2002). Research involving interaction of cationic and anionic surfactants with macromolecules, especially proteins, have been developed (Maulik et al., 1998; Tofani et al., 2004), being the interaction of charged headgroups the main focus of these works. Furthermore, depending of the concentration, surfactants can act as unfolding and denaturant agents, which can be used to evaluate the structural properties of the different proteins and their active sites. Studies of the interaction of globular proteins with surfactants, in particular with sodium dodecyl sulphate (SDS), have been carried on with the aim to understand details of the structure and function of proteins (Yang et al., 2003; Tanford et al., 1973; Gebicka& Gebick, 1999; Chattopadhyay & Mazumbar, 2003). Three ranges of surfactant concentrations associated to different effects on the protein should be mentioned. The first one, at stoichiometric surfactant concentration, is related to the finding that occurs to specific sites on the protein, due to, mainly, electrostatic interactions (Dayer et al., 2002; Moosavi-Movahedi, 2003 et al., Decker et al., 2001). At higher surfactant concentrations, near to the surfactant critical micellar concentration (cmc), where pre-micellar aggregates are formed and a massive increase in protein binding due to cooperative

ligand interactions takes place (Turro, 1995 et al., Jones, 1995). Above the cmc, at milimolar surfactant concentrations, the protein-surfactant interaction is an extremely complicated phenomenon.
Generally, surfactants induce a decrease of the α-helix content, and this effect is smaller for cationic than for anionic ones (Tofani et al., 2004). However, in the case of the giant extracellular hemoglobins, which are also called erytrocruorins, such as *Glossoscolex paulistus* hemoglobin, this is not true (Santiago et al., 2007). Probably, this is associated to the decisive influence of the value of isoelectric point (pI) in the control of the interaction with ionic surfactants, since the erytrocruorins are proteins with very acid pI, differently of the most of the hemoproteins. Otzen and Oliveberg (Otzen et al., 2002), studying a small protein S6 in the presence of SDS, argue that monomeric SDS binds to the native state, but global unfolding would occur only above the critical micelle concentration (cmc). Indeed, this verification is corroborated for various works about interaction between surfactants and hemoproteins (Oellerich et al., 2003; Tofani et al., 2004; Das et al., 1999). Oellerich and co-workers (Oellerich et al., 2003), analyzing the interaction between SDS and cytochrome *c*, explain that the differences observed below and above the cmc are due to the different modes of binding of SDS monomers and micelles. These authors argue that alterations of the heme structure are common to both modes of interaction, implying that the sites of electrostatic and hydrophobic contacts should be located in the vicinity of the cytochrome c heme pocket. In agreement with this discussion, Tofani and co-workers (Tofani et al., 2004) observed for Horse myoglobin (MbH), that only in a SDS/MbH ratio higher than 400, would occur a more significant protein unfolding and, for consequence, a more exposed and accessible heme pocket. Studies focused on the SDS-cytochrome *c* interaction at neutral pH have demonstrated that the unfolded state is stabilized when occur the bis-histidine (hemichrome) species formation, being that subsequent modifications of the secondary structure are rate-limited by the histidine dissociation rate (Das et al., 1999). Therefore, the hemichrome formation anchors the E helix into the ferric center, and, with the E and F helices maintained connected to the metallic center, the new polypeptide chains arrangement is stabilized, at least partially. This observation illustrates the correlation between the oligomeric assembly changes with the modifications that occur in the first coordination sphere of the metal in hemoproteins.
The dependence of the kind of protein-surfactant interaction with the surfactant concentration is also found to other types of protein. Bovine Serum Albumin (BSA), for example, presents initial high affinity binding sites for surfactants, which correspond to an intense electrostatic binding, characteristic for anionic compounds and BSA, at higher surfactant concentrations become some sort of nucleation sites for binding of "micelle-like" aggregates (Gelamo et al., 2004). In spite of the great predominance of the electrostatic contribution in the interaction of SDS with hemoproteins, the hydrophobic contacts present a significant importance to the total interaction. Gebicka and co-workers (Gebicka & Gebicki, 1999) argue that the hydrocarbon part geometry from the surfactant in the SDS-cytochrome *c* interaction is responsible for great influence on the spatial configuration of the heme pocket. Polar lipids of biological membranes are predominantly zwitterionic phophatidylcholine and phophatidyllethanolamine. Therefore, micelles of the zwitterionic surfactant N-hexadecyl-N,N-dimethyl-3-ammonio-1-propanesulfonate (HPS) may be considered as a convenient model of lipid aggregates (Yushmanov et al., 1994). In spite of this significant biological relevance, the number of works in the literature focusing on the interaction of zwitterionic surfactants, such as HPS, with hemeproteins is significantly lower

as compared to the studies regarding the interactions of hemeproteins and cationic and anionic surfactants.

18. Technological applications of hemoproteins

The understanding of interactions between proteins and surfaces is critically important in many fields of biochemical science, from biosensors to biocompatible materials. The development of biosensors, for instance, presents a critical step that is the immobilization of proteins with intact functions onto the surface of a transducer. Although many proteins spontaneously adsorb onto solid surfaces, the adsorbed proteins often denature or adapt undesirable orientation on the surfaces. In order to avoid these problems, various methods have been developed, each with its own advantages and disadvantages (Boussaad & Tao, 1999).

In recent years, a novel technique of layer-by-layer self-assembly has aroused more interests among researchers and has been developed into a general approach for fabricating ultrathin films on solid surfaces. This molecular architecture method is fundamentally based on the alternate adsorption of oppositely charged species from their solutions with precise thickness control on the nanometer scale. The layer-by-layer assembly has been extended to building up protein or other biomacromolecules films and has been successfully employed for the design and construction of biodevices (Shen & Hu, 2005). It is important to notice, for example, the development of a novel method for fabricating hydrogen peroxide (H_2O_2) sensor, which has been presented based on the self-assembly of ZrO_2 nanoparticles with heme proteins on functional glassy carbon electrode (Zhao et al., 2005). The immobilized proteins performed their direct electrochemistry with the formal potential of -0.032 V for hemoglobin and -0.026 V for myoglobin in pH 6.0, respectively. In fact, the resultant heme-protein electrode exhibited fast amperometric response (within 10 seconds) to H_2O_2, excellent stability, long-term life (more than one month) and good reproducibility (Zhao et al., 2005). Another interesting study was elaborated by Yao and co-workers (Yao et al., 2006), which made a electrochemical and electrocatalytic system of hemoglobin immobilized on glass carbon electrode containing gelatine films that displayed a fast amperometric response to the reduction of H_2O_2 and nitrite (Yao et al., 2006).

19. Hemoproteins as oxygen carrier substitutes and biossensors: Future perspectives

The infusion of Hb-based O_2 carriers (HBOCs) generally causes vasoconstriction and hypertension due to their ability to efficiently scavenge endothelial-derived nitric oxide (NO) and attenuates the vasodilatory NO signal to the vascular smooth muscle (Olson et al., 2004; Cole et al., 2009). However, great efforts are being developed in order to avoid or, at least, attenuate this limitation, altering some variables associated to the application of the hemoproteins as artificial blood. Indeed, the increasing perspectives of this area are motivating several research groups to test the giant extracellular hemoglobins due to its autoxidation resistance and immunological suitability. The applications as biosensor are also interesting employments of this class of hemoglobin due to great affinity to several ligands with great biological relevance, such as NO, CO, O_2, CN-, and several aminoacids and peptides. This kind of iron ligands constitutes a very important group to the physiological medium of several various species. Moreover, these ligands are relevant chemical species to several types of environmental conditions, implying that the giant extracellular hemoglobins, such as HbGp, could be applied as biosensor in physiological and environmental media.

20. Technological applications of surfactant-hemoprotein systems

Several applications have been developed employing the interactions between proteins and surfactants (Shan et al., 2008; Hu et al., 2007). An interesting work was developed by Shan and co-workers (Shan et al., 2008), which elaborated a self-assembled electroactive layer-by-layer film of heme proteins with anionic surfactant dihexadecyl phosphate. This film grown on pyrolytic graphite (PG) electrodes, showing a pair of well-defined and nearly reversible cyclic voltammetry peaks at around -0.35 V vs SCE at pH 7.0, which is characteristic of the heme protein Fe(III)/Fe(II) redox couples. Hu and co-workers (Hu, 2007) developed similar film using the cationic surfactant didodecyldimethylammonium bromide (DDAB) on PG electrodes and demonstrated two pairs of nearly reversible redox peaks at approximately -0.22 and -1.14 V vs SCE at pH 7.0, which are typical of the hemoglobin Fe(III)/Fe(II) and Fe(II)/Fe(I) redox couples, respectively. Based on the direct electrochemistry of heme proteins, the films could also be applied to electrochemically catalyze reduction of oxygen, hydrogen peroxide and nitrite with significant lowering of reduction overpotentials.

21. Conclusions

The hemoglobin-surfactant interactions also produces oxidation of the metallic center, originally in the ferrous form, into the ferric state. The complex oligomeric assembly of HbGp subunits may influence the autoxidation rate and the exponential decay behavior. In fact, a synergic process in the sequence dissociation-oxidation-dissociation takes place, which means that an initial dissociation favors the occurrence of a more intense oxidation that, in its time, favors a secondary dissociation process. Subsequently, this synergic cycle continues uninterruptedly until a substantial dissociation of the protein fractions, characterizing a kind of oxidation-dissociation cooperative effect. This point is very interesting, since the hemes present a very similar behavior in terms of ligand affinity and spectroscopic profile to the native form of HbGp, in spite of their significant structural differences. This distinction can be observed in the recent studies employing MALDI-TOF-MS, which denote the great number of coexistent isoforms in each subunit (Oliveira et al., 2007; Oliveira et al., 2008). In fact, the oligomeric compaction of the native form works as a kind of equalization of the different hemes. When the dielectric constant of the medium increases as function of the higher freedom of the polypeptide chains, which provokes higher aqueous solvent accessibility into heme pocket, the kinetic behavior of the chains becomes significantly altered. In this way, it is possible to infer that the global environment around the hemes is useful to preclude the iron oxidation as well as to equalize the heme properties. Indeed, an extraordinarily complex arrangement with 180 polypeptide chains represents effective shielding to all hemes of the integral HbGp. This analysis would explain the extraordinarily simple and "pure" RPE spectrum obtained at pH 7.0 with HbGp in a native state, in spite of the evident difference between the heme groups, which is demonstrated when the aqueous solvent accessibility into heme pocket is intensified. These data are in agreement with Moreira and co-workers (Moreira et al., 2006), which demonstrate representative presence of aquomet species until pH 4.0. This ferric species is very sensitive to perturbations in the heme pocket neighborhood, being very unstable in alkaline medium (Moreira et al., 2008), which reinforces the higher oligomeric stability of HbGp in acid medium when compared with the basic environment. It is important to register that the mono-aquo ferric pentacoordinate species can be encountered into the heme pocket or free in the aqueous solvent, being very difficult to differentiate both pentacoordinate species as function of their similarities with respect to their spectroscopic data. In fact, the ferric porphyrins, which is free in water solvent maintains its pentacoordinated configurations, i.e., the number of coordination continues being five (5). This occurs due to the electronic configuration of metallic centers d^5, which usually are more stable when compared with tetracoordinated configurations (number of coordination four (4). Therefore, it is plausible to infer that the compaction level of the whole HbGp is much more conserved in acid medium, when compared with alkaline one. Furthermore, the level of assembly of the globin chains must be responsible to the difficult of heme distinction, when the native state of this protein is well conserved. The present article demonstrates that the high level of oligomeric compaction is a determinant factor to the "equalization" of the 180 hemes of HbGp. In fact, in spite of their different properties when dissociated, the hemes present very similarity in the native state of HbGp at pH 7.0. However, the interaction with small concentration of ionic surfactants (CTAC and SDS) generates a significant increase in the size of the supramolecular system, denoting a representative loss of oligomeric compaction. Indeed, this original fact is comprehensible in a protein with an extraordinary molecular mass around 3.6 MDa, such as HbGp. This point is decisive to the structure-function relationship to HbGp, and probably to others giant extracellular hemoglobins, since is associated to several relevant phenomenons, such as ligand exchange, oligomeric dissociation and autoxidation. In addition, our present results demonstrate the importance of the isoelectric point in the modulation of protein-surfactant interactions, especially the electrostatic contribution at low surfactant concentrations, suggesting that this parameter is decisive to determine the oligomeric arrangement, as well as the structure-activity relationships.

22. References

Aki, Y., Nakagawa, T., Nagai, M., Sasayama, Y., Fukumori, Y. & Imai, K. (2007). Oxigenation properties of extracellular giant hemoglobin from *Oligobrachia mashikoi*. *Biochemical and Biophysical Research Communications*, Vol. 360, pp. 673-678.

Arndt, M.H.L. & Santoro, M.M. (1998). Structure of the extracellular hemoglobin of *Biomphalaria glabrata*. *Comparative Biochemistry and Physiology B*, Vol. 119, pp. 667-675.

Arndt, M.H.L., de Oliveira, C.L.P. &, Regis, W.C.B. (2003). Torriani IL, Santoro MM, Small angle X-ray scattering of the hemoglobin from *Biomphalaria glabrata*. *Biopolymers*, Vol. 69, PP. 470-479.

Berry, E.A. & Walker, F.A. (2008). Bis-histidine-coordinated hemes in four-helix bundles:how the geometry of the bundle controls the axial imidazole plane orientations in transmembrane cytochromes of mitochondrial Complexes II and III and related proteins. *Journal of Biological Inorganic Chemistry*, Vol.13, pp.481-498.

Bispo, J.A.C., Landini, G.F., Santos, J.L.R., Norberto, D.R. & Bonafe, C.F.S. (2005). Tendency for oxidation of annelid hemoglobin at alkaline pH and dissociated states probed by redox titration. *Comparative Biochemistry and Physiology B*, Vol. 141, pp. 498-504.

Bispo, J.A.C., Santos, J.L.R., Landini, G.F., Gonçalves & J.M., Bonafe, C.F.S. (2007). pH dependence of the dissociation of multimeric hemoglobin probed by high hydrostatic pressure. *Biophysical Chemistry*, Vol. 125, pp. 341-349.

Boussaad, S. & Tao, N.J. (1999). Electron Transfer and Adsorption of Myoglobin on Self-Assembled Surfactant Films: An Electrochemical Tapping-Mode AFM study. *Journal of the American Chemical Society*, Vol. 121, pp. 4510-4515.

Bruneaux, M., Rousselot, M., Leize, E., Lallier, F.H. & Zal, F. (2008). The structural analysis of large noncovalent oxygen binding proteins by MALLS and ESI-MS: A review on annelid hexagonal bilayer hemoglobin and crustacean hemocyanin. *Current Protein & Peptide Science*, Vol. 9, pp. 150-180.

Chattopadhyay, K. & Mazumbar, S. (2003). Stabilization of partially folded states of cytochrome C in aqueous surfactant: effects of ionic and hydrophobic interactions. *Biochemistry*, Vol. 42, pp. 14606-14613.

Cole, R.H., Malavalli, A. & Vandegriff, K.D. (2009). Erythrocytic ATP release in the presence of modified cell-free hemoglobin. *Biophysical Chemistry*, Vol. 144, pp.119-122.

Das, T. P., Boffi, A., Chiancone, E. & Rousseau, D. L. (1999). Hydroxide Rather Than Histidine Is Coordinated to the Heme in Five-coordinate Ferric *Scapharca inaequivalvis*Hemoglobin *J. Biol. Chem.* 1999, 274, 2916.

Dayer, M.R. ,Moosavi-Movahedi, A.A., Norouzi, P., Ghourchian, H.O. & Safarian, S. (2002). Inhibition of human hemoglobin autoxidation by sodium n-dodecyl sulphate. *Journal of Biochemical and Molecular Biology*, Vol. 35, pp.364-370.

Decker, H., Ryan, M., Jaenicke, E. & Terwilliger, N. (2001). SDS-induced phenoloxidase activity of hemocyanins from *Limulus polyphemus, Eurypelma californicum,* and *Cancer magister*. *The Journal of Biological Chemistry*, Vol. 276, pp. 17796-17799.

Feng, Y., Roder, H. & Englander, S.W. (1990) Redox-Dependent Structure Change and Hyperfine Nuclear Magnetic Resonance Shifts in Cytochrome *c*. *Biochemistry* , Vol. 29, pp. 3494-3504.

Gebicka, L. & Gebicki, J.L. (1999). Kinetic studies on the interaction of ferricytochrome C with anionic surfactants. *Journal of Protein Chemistry*, Vol. 18, pp.165-172.

Gelamo, E. L., Itri, R. & Tabak, M. (2004). Small Angle X-Ray Scattering (SAXS) Study of the Extracellular Hemoglobin of Glossoscolex paulistus: Effect of pH, Iron Oxidation State and Interaction With Anionic SDS Surfactant. *The Journal of Biological Chemistry*, Vol. 279, pp. 33298-33305.

Gell, D.A., Feng, L., Zhou, S., Jeffrey, P.D., Bendak, K., Gow, A., Weiss, M.J., Shi, Y. & Mackay, J.P. (2009). A *cis*-Proline in Hemoglobin Stabilizing Protein Directs the Structural Reorganization of Hemoglobin. *The Journal of Biological Chemistry*,Vol. 284, pp. 29462-29469.

Harrington, J.P., Kobayashi, S., Dorman, S.C., Zito, S.L., & Hirsch, R.E. (2007). Acellular invertebrate hemoglobins as model therapeutic oxygen carriers: Unique redox potentials. *Artificial Cells Blood Substitutes and Biotechnology* , Vol. 35, pp. 53-67.

Hellmann, N., Weber, R.E. & Decker, H. (2008). Linker analysis of large cooperative, allosteric systems: The case of the giant HBL hemoglobins, Globins and other nitric oxide-reactive proteins. *Methods in Enzymology*, Vol. 436, pp. 436-485.

Hocking, R.K., Wasinger, E.C., Yan, Y., deGroot, F.M.F., Walker, F.A. Hodgson, K.O., Hedman, B. & Solomon, E.I. (2007). Fe L-Edge X-ray Absorption Spectroscopy of Low-Spin Heme Relative to Non-heme Fe Complexes: Delocalization of Fe d-Electrons into the Porphyrin Ligand, *Journal of the American Chemical Society*, Vol.129, pp.113-125.

Hocking, R.K., Wasinger, E.C., Yan, Y.L., deGroot, F.M.F., Walker, F.A., Hodgson, K.O. & Hedman, B. (2007). Solomon EI, Fe L-edge x-ray absorption spectroscopy of low-spin heme relative to non-heme Fe complexes: Delocalization of Fe d-electrons into the porphyrin ligand. *Journal of the American Chemical Society*, Vol. 129, pp.113-125.

Hu, Y., Sun, H. & Hu, N. (2007). Assembly of layer-by-layer films of electroactive hemoglobin and surfactant didodecyldimethylammonium bromide. *Journal of Colloid and Interface Science*, Vol. 314, pp. 131-140.

Huang, Y.W., Koestner, M.L. & Ackers, G.K. (1997). Tertiary and quaternary chloride effects of the partially ligated (CN-met) hemoglobin intermediates. *Biophysical Chemistry*, Vol. 64, pp. 157-173.

Jones, M.N. (1992). Surfactant interactions with biomembranes and proteins. *Chemical Society Reviews*, Vol. 21, pp. 127-136.

Knipp, K., Yang, F., Berry, R.E., Zhang, H., Shokhirev, M.N. & Walker, F.A. (2007). Spectroscopic and Functional Characterization of Nitrophorin 7 from the Blood-Feeding Insect *Rhodnius prolixus* Reveals an Important Role of Its Isoform-Specific N-Terminus for Proper Protein Function. *Biochemistry*, Vol. 46, pp. 13254-13268.

Kolczak, U., Han, C. Sylvia, L.A. & La Mar, G.N. (1997). Approaches to the Solution NMR Characterization of Active Sites for 65 kDa Tetrameric Hemoglobins in the Paramagnetic Cyanomet State. *Journal of the American Chemical Society*, Vol. 119, pp. 12643-12654.

Liu, G., Shao, W., Huang, X., Wu, H. & Tang, W. (1996). Structural studies of imidazole-cytochrome *c*: resonance assignments and structural comparison with cytochrome *c*, *Biochimica et Biophysica Acta*, Vol. 1277, pp. 61-82.

Liu, W., Guo, X. & Guo, R. (2007). The Interaction of Hemoglobin with two Surfactants of Different Charges, *International Journal of Biological Macromolecules*, Vol. 41, pp. 548-557.

Maulik, S., Dutta, P., Chattoraj, D.K. & Moulik, S.P. (1998). Biopolymer-surfactant interactions: 5 Equilibrium studies on the binding of cethyltrimethyl ammonium bromide and sodium dodecyl sulfate with bovine serum albumin, β-lactoglobulin, hemoglobin, gelatin, lysozyme and deoxyribonucleic acid. *Colloids and Surfaces B*, Vol.11, pp. 1-8.

Miksovska, J., Yom, J., Diamond, B. & Larsen, R.W. (2006). Spectroscopic and Phototermal Study of Myoglobin Conformational Changes in the Presence of Sodium Dodecyl Sulfate. *Biomacromolecules*, Vol. 7, pp.476-482.

Moosavi-Movahedi, A.A., Dayer, M.R., Norouzi, P., Shamsipur, M., Yeganeh-faal, A., Chaichi, M.J. & Ghourchian, H.O. (2003). Aquamethemoglobin reduction by sodium n-dodecyl sulfate via coordinated water oxidation. *Colloids and Surfaces B*, Vol. 30, pp. 139-146.

Moreira, L. M., Lima Poli, A., Costa Filho, A. & Imasato, H. (2006). Pentacoordinate and hexacoordinate ferric hemes in acid medium: EPR, UV Vis and CD studies of the giant extracellular hemoglobin of Glossoscolex paulistus. *Biophysical Chemistry*, Vol. 124, pp. 62-72.

Moreira, L., Poli, A., Costa Filho, A. & Imasato, H. (2008). Ferric species equilibrium of the giant extracellular hemoglobin of Glossoscolex paulistus in alkaline medium: HALS hemichrome as a precursor of pentacoordinate species. *International Journal of Biological Macromolecules*, Vol. 42, pp. 103-110.

Numoto, N., Nakagawa, T., Kita, A., Sasayama, Y., Fukumori, Y. & Miki, K. (2008). Structural Basis for Heterotropic and Homotropic Interactions of Invertebrate Giant Hemoglobin. *Biochemistry*, Vol. 47, pp.11231-11238.

Oliveira, M., Moreira, L. & Tabak, M. (2007). Partial characterization of giant extracellular hemoglobin of Glossoscolex paulistus: A MALDI-TOF-MS study. *International Journal of Biological Macromolecules*, Vol. 40, pp. 429-436.

Oliveira, M., Moreira, L., Tabak, M. (2008). Interaction of giant extracellular Glossoscolex paulistus hemoglobin (HbGp) with ionic surfactants: A MALDI-TOF-MS study. *International Journal of Biological Macromolecules*, Vol. 42, pp. 111-119, 2008

Olson, J.S., Foley, E.W., Rogge, C., Tsai, A.L., Doyle, M.P. & Lemon, D.D. (2004). NO scavenging and the hypertensive effect of hemoglobin-based blood substitutes. *Free Radical in1 Biological Medicine*, Vol. 36, pp. 685–697.

Orioni, B., Roversi, M., La Mesa, C., Asaro, C., Asaro, F., Pellicer, G. & D´Errico, G. (2006). Polymorphic behavior in protein-surfactant mixtures: the water-bovine serum albumin-sodium taurodeoxycholate system. *Journal of Physical Chemistry B*, Vol 110, pp.12129-12140.

Pereira, M.T., Silva-Alves, J.M., Martins-José, A., Lopes, J.C.D. & Santoro, M.M. (2005). Thermodynamic evaluation and modeling of proton and water exchange associated with benzamidine and berenil binding to ß-trypsin. *Brazilian Journal of Medical and Biological Research*, Vol. 38, pp. 1593-1601.

Royer, W.E., Strand, K. M. & Hendrickson, W.A. (2000). Structural hierarchy in erythrocruorin, the giant respiratory assemblage of annelids, *PNAS*, Vol. 97, pp. 7101-7111.

Sakudo, A., Kato, Y.H., Kuratsune, H. & Ikuta, K. (2009). Non-invasive prediction of hematocrit levels by portable visible and near-infrared spectrophotometer. *Clinica Chimica Acta*, Vol. 408, pp. 123-127.

Santiago, P.S., Moreira, L. M., de Almeida, E.V. & Tabak, M. (2007). Giant extracellular *Glossoscolex paulistus* Hemoglobin (HbGp) upon interaction with cethyltrimethylammonium chloride (CTAC) and sodium dodecyl sulphate (SDS) surfactants: Dissociation of oligomeric structure and autoxidation. *Biochimica et Biophysica Acta. G, General Subjects* (Print), vol. 1770, pp. 506-517.

Shan, W., Liu, H., Shi, J., Yang, L. & Hu, N. (2008). Self-assembly of electroactive layer-by-layer films of heme proteins with anionic surfactant dihexadecyl phosphate. *Biophysical Chemistry*, Vol. 134, pp. 101-109.

Shao, W. , Liu, G., Huang, X. , Wu, H. & Tang, W. (1996) 2D-NMR studies of the effects of axial substitution on two helices in horse cytochrome *c*, *Biochimica et Biophysica Acta*,Vol. 1295, pp. 44-50.

Shen, L. & Hu, L.N. (2005). Electrostatic Adsorption of Heme proteins Alternated with Polyamidoamine Dendrimers for Layer-by-Layer Assembly of Electroactive Films. *Biomacromolecules*, Vol. 6, pp.1475-1483.

Stenstam, A., Montalvo, G., Grillo, I. & Gradzielski, M. (2003). A sans study of lysozyme-sds aggregates, *Journal of Physical Chemistry B*, Vol. 107, pp.12331-12338.

Tanford, C. The Hydrophobic Effect: Formation of Micelles and Biological Membranes, Wiley, New York, 1973.

Tofani, L., Feis, A., Snoke, R.E., Berti, D., Baglioni, P. & Smulevich, G. (2004). Spectroscopic and interfacial properties of myoglobin/surfactant. *Biophysical Journal*, Vol. 87, pp. 1186-1195.

Turro, N.J., Lei, X.G., Ananthapadmanabhan, K.P. & Aronson, M. (1995). Spectroscopic probe analysis of protein-surfactant interactions - The BSA/SDS System. *Langmuir*, Vol. 11, pp. 2525-2533.

van der Veen, M., Norde, W. & Stuart, M.C. (2004). Electrostatic interactions in protein adsorption probed by comparing lysozyme and succinylated lysozyme. *Colloids and Surfaces B*, Vol. 35, pp. 33-40.

Vasilescu, M., Angelescu, D., Alegren, M. & Valstar, A. (1999). Interactions of globular proteins with surfactants studied with fluorescence probe methods . *Langmuir*, Vol.15, pp.2635-2643.

Venkatesh, B., Ramasamy, S., Mylrajan, M., Asokan, R., Manoharan, P.T. & Rifkind, J.M. (1999). Fourier transform Raman approach to structural correlation in hemoglobin derivatives. *Spectrochimica Acta A*, Vol. 55, pp. 1691-1697.

Walker, F.A. (2006). The heme environment of mouse neuroglobin: histidine imidazole plane orientations obtained from solution NMR and EPR spectroscopy as compared with X-ray crystallography. *Journal of Biological Inorganic Chemistry*, Vol. 11, pp. 391-397.

Weber,R.E.& Vinogradov, S.N. (2001). Nonvertebrate Hemoglobins: Functions and Molecular Adaptations, Vol. 81, pp. 569-628.

Yang, X., Guo, X. & Li, H. (2003). Fluorimetric determination of hemoglobin using spiro form rhodamine B hydrozide in a micellar medium. *Talanta*, Vol.61, pp.439-445.

Yao, H., Li, N., Xu, J. & Zhu, J. (2007). Direct electrochemistry and electrocatalysis of hemoglobin in gelatine film modified glassy carbon electrode. *Talanta*, Vol. 71, pp. 550-554.

Yatsunyk, L.A., Dawson, A., Carducci, M.D., Nichol, G.S. & Walker, F.A. (2006). Models of the Cytochromes: Crystal Structures and EPR Spectral Characterization of Low-Spin Bis-Imidazole Complexes of (OETPP)FeIII Having Intermediate Ligand Plane Dihedral Angles. *Inorganic Chemistry*, Vol. 45, pp. 5417-5428.

Yushmanov, V. E., Perussi, J. R., Imasato, H., Ruggiero, A. C. & Tabak, M. (1994). Ionization and binding equilibria of papaverine in ionic micelles studied by 1H-NMR and optical absorption spectroscopy. *Biophysical Chemistry*, Vol. 52, pp. 157-163. Estados Unidos, v. 52, p. 157-163, 1994.

Zhao, G., Feng, J., Xu, J. & Chen, H. (2005). Direct electrochemistry and electrocatalysis of heme proteins immobilized on self-assembled ZrO_2 film. *Electrochemistry Communications*, Vol. 7, pp. 724-729.

Mitochondria as a Biosensor for Drug-Induced Toxicity – Is It Really Relevant?

Ana C. Moreira[1,2], Nuno G. Machado[2], Telma C. Bernardo[2], Vilma A. Sardão[2] and Paulo J. Oliveira[2]
[1]*Doctoral Programme in Experimental Biology and Biomedicine, University of Coimbra*
[2]*Center for Neuroscience and Cell Biology, Department of Life Sciences, University of Coimbra*
Portugal

1. Introduction

Mitochondria, from the Greek *mito* (thread) and *chondros* (grains) are small organelles that exist as a network in the cytoplasm of eukaryotic cells, performing a variety of important functions including energy production, calcium homeostasis, fatty acid metabolism or heme and pyrimidine biosynthesis (Pereira, Moreira et al., 2009). Moreover, mitochondria play a critical role in programmed cell death (apoptosis) (Jeong & Seol, 2008; Wang & Youle, 2009). Mitochondrial structure comprises two different membranes, the outer (OMM) and the inner membrane (IMM) that functionally separate two distinct compartments, the inter-membrane space (IMS) and the matrix (Jezek & Plecita-Hlavata, 2009) (Fig. 1). The outer membrane encloses mitochondria and it is somewhat identical to other cell membranes, including cholesterol in its composition, and is permeable to a large variety of ions and metabolites. The inner membrane lacks cholesterol, is rich in the tetra fatty acid-containing phospholipid cardiolipin, and basically controls the entry of metabolites and ions into mitochondria, through the action of specific transport proteins (Scatena, Bottoni et al., 2007). Inner membrane invaginations and membrane enclosed structures which can exist connected to the IMM or freely in the mitochondrial matrix are called *cristae*. It is in these latter structures that most of the membrane-bound metabolic proteins and energy-producing respiratory complexes (complexes I–V) exist (Fig. 1) (Zick, Rabl et al., 2009).

1.1 Organization and genomics

Also considered as a *reticulum*, the mitochondrial network continuously moves, fuses and divides in a process tightly regulated by cellular stimuli and disturbances inside this organelle (Detmer & Chan, 2007). The shape greatly varies depending on the tissue, developmental and physiological state. Within a cell, the distribution of mitochondria is unequal depending on the cellular energetic or metabolic demands (Grandemange, Herzig et al., 2009). The overall shape of mitochondrial network results from an equilibrium between fusion and fission events (Wallace & Fan, 2010). These events allow the exchange of organelle contents such as membrane lipids, proteins, solutes, metabolites and even mitochondrial DNA (Detmer & Chan, 2007), as well as to provide a balance of the electrochemical gradient (Twig, Graf et al., 2006). Balanced mitochondrial fusion and fission is crucial to preserve mitochondrial integrity and functionality (Wallace & Fan, 2010). Three distinct proteins seem to be involved in mitochondrial fusion: Mitofusins 1 and 2 (Mfn1 and Mfn2) and Optic Atrophy-1 (OPA-1). Mfn 1 and 2 are GTPases proteins that are localized in the OMM and form homo- and hetero-oligomeric complexes between themselves and with counterparts in adjacent mitochondria, which mediate their tethering (Arnoult, 2007). OPA-1 is a dynamin-related protein that can be found in a soluble form in the IMS or tightly associated with the IMM, being a key protein for the fusion of this mitochondrial membrane (Arnoult, Grodet et al., 2005). Evidence also suggests that OPA-1 controls *cristae* morphology and is implicated in the complete release of cytochrome c during apoptosis (Jourdain & Martinou, 2009; Perkins, Bossy-Wetzel et al., 2009). Fusion of both membranes is a two-step process that occurs in a coordinate fashion, although the precise mechanism remains unclear (Malka, Guillery et al., 2005). Mitochondrial fission requires the recruitment of dynamin-related protein 1 (Drp1) from the cytosol to the OMM where it forms multimeric rings and spiral-like structures that surround and constrict the organelle in a GTP-dependent manner (Sheridan & Martin, 2010). The mechanism that triggers this recruitment is still unknown, however, Fis1, a small mitochondrial transmembrane protein, seems to be responsible for this mobilization (Sheridan & Martin, 2010).

Mitochondria are the only organelles outside of the nucleus that contain their own genome and replicate itself in an independent manner from the nuclear genome. A single DNA polymerase (polymerase-gamma), with base excision repair activity, ensures the replication of the mitochondrial DNA (mtDNA). Moreover, mtDNA has a particular feature since it is exclusively maternally inherited. Each mitochondrion contains approximately 10-15 copies of a small circular chromosome that are organized into one or more structures called nucleoids. Mitochondrial DNA encodes for 13 proteins that are essential for the electron transport and ATP generation by oxidative phosphorylation (OXPHOS) and 2 rRNA and 22 tRNA (Van Houten, Woshner et al., 2006). The remaining proteins required for mitochondrial activity are encoded by the nucleus, synthesized in the cytosol and translocated to mitochondria (Wallace, 2008). Mitochondrial DNA undergoes a mutation rate that seems to be between 5- to 20- fold higher than what occurs in nuclear DNA mutations, although this is not consensual (Malka, Lombes et al., 2006; Scatena, Bottoni et al., 2007). The high rate of mutations, if indeed real, can be explained for both the lack of mtDNA protective proteins and its proximity to the electron transport chain, where the majority of, free-radical production occurs (Fruehauf & Meyskens, 2007). Furthermore, the repair mechanism of mitochondrial DNA is less efficient than of nuclear DNA (Berneburg, Kamenisch et al., 2006).

1.2 Oxidative phosphorylation and energy production

Production of energy within a living cell is performed by the conversion of dietary fats and carbohydrates into reducing equivalents. Mitochondria are considered the powerhouses of the cell, due to a variety of important energy-producing metabolic pathways in their interior. Pyruvate is formed in the cytosol as an end-product of glucose metabolism (glycolysis) and can undergo lactic acid or alcoholic fermentation in the absence of oxygen (anaerobic conditions). Under aerobic conditions, pyruvate is converted into acetyl coenzyme A (acetyl-CoA) by pyruvate dehydrogenase (PDH) in the mitochondrial matrix (Pereira, Moreira et al., 2009).

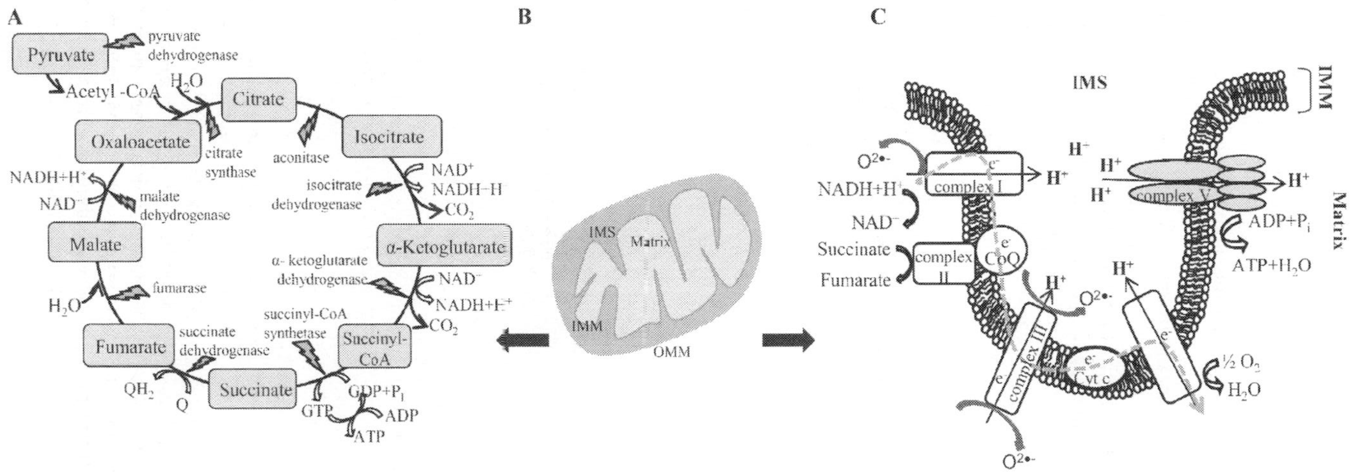

Fig. 1. Mitochondria play a critical role in ATP production, biosynthesis, calcium homeostasis and cell death. The figure represents some of the functions referred to in the text: (**A**) The Krebs cycle occurs in the matrix and supplies reducing equivalents for oxidative phosphorylation, besides participating as intermediate in several biosynthetic pathways. (**B**) Overall view of mitochondria morphology: The outer mitochondrial membrane (OMM) encloses the organelle within the cell; the inner mitochondrial membrane (IMM) separates functionally the matrix from the mitochondrial inter-membrane space (IMS). (**C**) Oxidative phosphorylation (OXPHOS): electrons from the Krebs cycle are transferred along the respiratory chain. The energy derived from electron transfer is used to pump out protons across the inner membrane at complexes I, III and IV, creating a proton electrochemical gradient between both sides of inner membrane. This electrochemical gradient forms a proton-motive force, which is use to drive the re-entry of protons to the matrix through complex V (ATP synthase). A small amount of electrons can leak towards the matrix through complex I and complex III due to an one electron transfer reduction of molecular oxygen forming superoxide anion ($O_2^{\bullet-}$). Figure adapted from (Pereira, Moreira et al., 2009), with permission.

Acetyl-CoA enters the Krebs cycle, being oxidized to generate several intermediates including NADH and succinate (Fig. 1). Other intermediates of the Krebs cycle are also important in several metabolic pathways, including biosynthesis of heme and amino acids (Shadel, 2005). Mitochondria can be involved in the β-oxidation of fatty acids (Vockley & Whiteman, 2002). The end product of this pathway is, once again, Acetyl-CoA, which is used in the Krebs cycle. NADH and succinate, among other intermediates that are produced by different pathways are oxidized by the electron transport chain, ultimately leading to the production of adenosine triphosphate (ATP) in a process known as OXPHOS (Zick, Rabl et al., 2009; Hebert, Lanza et al., 2010) (Fig. 1). Electrons derived from reduced substrates are transferred through several multi-protein complexes (mitochondrial complexes I to IV), down their redox potentials and the energy derived from electron transfer is used to pump out protons across the IMM at complexes I, III and IV which creates an electrochemical gradient between both sides of the IMM. This electrochemical gradient is a proton-motive force driving the re-entry of protons towards the matrix through complex V (ATP synthase), which is coupled to ATP synthesis (Hebert, Lanza et al., 2010). ATP that is produced is exported from the mitochondria by the mitochondrial ADP/ATP translocator (ANT). Molecular oxygen is the final electron acceptor in the mitochondrial respiratory chain, which is reduced via a sequential four-electron transfer into water by complex IV (cytochrome c oxidase, COX). However, some of the electrons that are transferred across the mitochondrial electron transport chain can escape and perform a single electron reduction of molecular oxygen. This phenomenon occurs continuously even in normal conditions leading to formation of superoxide anion ($O_2^{\bullet-}$) and it will be discussed in the next section of this chapter.

1.3 Generation of free radicals

Among the reactive species that are produced within a living cell, reactive oxygen species (ROS) are the most significant. Mitochondrial complexes I and III account for a significant proportion of intracellular ROS formation, although complex I is considered the major contributor (Adam-Vizi & Chinopoulos, 2006; Soubannier & McBride, 2009). The mitochondrial electron transport chain contains several redox centers, which can react with molecular oxygen. As a result, a small amount of electrons leaks from complex I (NADH dehydrogenase) and complex III (CoQ cycle), performing a one-electron reduction of molecular oxygen that gives rise to superoxide anion ($O_2^{\bullet-}$). Approximately 1-2% of the oxygen consumed during OXPHOS under physiological conditions is converted into this product (Solaini, Baracca et al., 2010). Superoxide anion produced by respiratory complex I is released in the mitochondrial matrix and transformed into hydrogen peroxide (H_2O_2) spontaneously or via manganese superoxide dismutase (MnSOD). In turn, $O_2^{\bullet-}$ generated by complex III can be released in both sides of the IMM but in the IMS, the dismutation into H_2O_2 is achieved via Cu/Zn-dependent SOD (Cu/ZnSOD). Hydrogen peroxide can be converted into water in the mitochondrial matrix by catalase or glutathione peroxidase (GSH). Mitochondrial thioredoxin, glutaredoxin and even cytochrome c are other relevant ROS scavengers (for a review see (Fruehauf & Meyskens, 2007)). The H_2O_2 produced can also diffuse to the cytosol and trigger the activation of some transcription factors and various enzymatic cascades (Cadenas, 2004). General oxidative stress arises when an imbalance in the redox steady-state occurs and ROS production exceeds the capacity of the cell for detoxification. If H_2O_2 encounters a reduced transition metal (Fe^{2+} or Cu^{2+}) or $O_2^{\bullet-}$ it can be further reduced in a highly reactive and toxic hydroxyl radical (•OH) by a Fenton or Haber-Weiss reaction, respectively (Brandon, Baldi et al., 2006), which is the most potent ROS. Although very short-lived, •OH can damage cellular macromolecules including proteins, lipids and nucleic acids. The oxidation of proteins can inactivate and target them for degradation; oxidative damage to DNA causes single and double strand-breaks, cross-link to other molecules and base modifications, while lipid oxidation can generate membrane disturbances. As described above, mtDNA represents a critical target of oxidative damage since it does not contain histones and it is located in proximity to the production site of ROS (Hebert, Lanza et al., 2010). Once damaged, mtDNA can indirectly amplify oxidative stress since transcription of critical mitochondrial proteins is defective, leading to a vicious cycle of ROS production and eventually triggering cell death. Oxidative stress is largely related with aging (Balaban, Nemoto et al., 2005) and is often associated with some disorders such as cancer and diabetes (Van Houten, Woshner et al., 2006). Reactive nitrogen species (RNS), including nitric oxide and peroxynitrite, can also contribute for a regulation of mitochondrial function (especially the former (Brown & Borutaite, 2007)), as well for increased mitochondrial damage during pathological conditions (Poderoso, 2009).

1.4 Cell death

Unlike what was thought during several years, cell death is not a process only observed when cell tissues are injured by external factors. Actually, cell death is an evolutionary conserved and genetically regulated process that is crucial for development, morphogenesis and homeostasis in tissues (Martin & Baehrecke, 2004). Programmed cell death (PCD) was the first designation attributed to this regulated process. Later, Kerr *et al.* introduced the term apoptosis (Kerr, Wyllie et al., 1972) to designate programmed cell death and these designations remain synonymous until now. Cell death was classified into two types: apoptosis (programmed cell death) and necrosis (accidental cell death). Nowadays, other types of cell death have been identified, including autophagy. Although it has become clear that autophagy can work as an adaptive response to nutrient starvation, cell death can occur due to autophagy over-stimulation (Rami, 2009). Autophagy is a spatially restricted phenomenon characterized by the absence of chromatin condensation and in which parts of the cytoplasm are engulfed by specialized double membrane vesicles, so-called autophagosomes, and digested by lysosomal hydrolases (Ulivieri, 2010). Mitophagy is a specific autophagic elimination of mitochondria, identified in yeast and mammals and regulated by PINK-1, among others (Youle & Narendra, 2011). However, if for some reason the clearing of old/damaged mitochondria is insufficient, a malignant transformation may occur (Morselli, Galluzzi et al., 2009). Necrotic cell death is characterized by a moderate or null chromatin condensation and by an increase in cell volume that culminates in loss of plasma membrane integrity and swelling of cytoplasmic organelles (Galluzzi, Maiuri et al., 2007). The disruption of cell membranes leads to the release of cell contents usually resulting in local inflammatory reactions and damage to contiguous cells. Several studies have already demonstrated that mitochondria can be involved in this type of cell death due to a phenomenon called mitochondrial permeability transition (MPT), which results from the opening of unspecific protein pores in the IMM. The MPT results in dissipation of mitochondrial membrane potential ($\Delta\Psi$) and leads to an uncoupling of OXPHOS and decreased ATP, leading cells to necrosis (Sharaf El Dein, Gallerne et al., 2009; Zorov, Juhaszova et al., 2009). Apoptosis is the best-studied modality of cell death and plays an essential role in the maintenance of homeostasis by eliminating damaged, infected or superfluous cells in a regulated form that minimizes inflammatory reactions and damage to neighboring cells (Jeong & Seol, 2008; Schug & Gottlieb, 2009; Sheridan & Martin, 2010). Apoptotic imbalance may contribute to the development of neurodegenerative disorders, autoimmune disorders, cancer or even viral infections (Arnoult, 2007; Jourdain & Martinou, 2009). Apoptotic cells exhibit specific changes, including chromatin condensation, nuclear fragmentation, and plasma membrane blebbing. The late stages of apoptosis are characterized by fragmentation of the cell-membrane into vesicles called apoptotic bodies which contain intact cytoplasmatic organelles or nuclear fragments. These vesicles are recognized by the immune system macrophages, preventing inflammatory responses (Martin & Baehrecke, 2004; Jeong & Seol, 2008; Tait & Green, 2010). There are two main pathways by which a cell can engage apoptosis: the extrinsic (or cell death receptor-mediated) apoptotic pathway and intrinsic (or mitochondrial-mediated) apoptotic pathway (Tait & Green, 2010) (Fig. 2). In both pathways, the apoptotic process is driven by a family of cysteine proteases that are expressed as pro-enzymes and are activated by proteolysis.

These proteases, known as caspases, specifically cleave their substrates at aspartic residues and are categorized into initiators (such as caspases -8 and -9) and effectors or executioners (such as caspases -3 and -7) (Arnoult, 2007; Jeong & Seol, 2008). Mitochondria are central players in the intrinsic apoptotic pathway; in fact, mitochondria retain a pool of pro-apoptotic factors in the IMS. During the development of the intrinsic pathway, pores are formed in the OMM in a process called outer mitochondrial membrane permeabilization (OMMP, different from the mitochondrial permeability transition). The OMMP results in the release of pro-apoptotic factors, such as cytochrome *c* and the apoptotic-inducing factor, AIF, to the cytosol (Saelens, Festjens et al., 2004; Sheridan & Martin, 2010). Although the effects of pro-apoptotic factors that are released in the cytosol are well characterized, the mechanisms underlying the OMMP remains controversial (Martinou & Green, 2001) and there are currently several mechanisms that have been proposed. One of these mechanisms involves members of Bcl-2 proteins family, which comprises three subgroups; the anti-apoptotic family members such as Bcl-2 and Bcl-xL, the pro-apoptotic Bax/Bak sub-family and the pro-apoptotic BH3-only proteins such as Bim, Bad, Bid, Puma and Noxa. BH3-only proteins links cell death signals to mitochondria, where the interplay between various members of the Bcl-2 family determines the fate of the cell (Martinou & Green, 2001; Wong & Puthalakath, 2008). A mild change in the dynamic balance of these proteins may result either in inhibition or exacerbation of cell death. The intrinsic and extrinsic pathways can interact with each other at the mitochondrial level where signal amplification occurs (Fig. 2) (Saelens, Festjens et al., 2004).

2. Mitochondria and disease

As it was discussed in the previous sections, mitochondria are organelles with crucial importance in cell bioenergetics, signaling and survival, among others. Mitochondrial dysfunction is associated with several diseases, as it will be discussed in the present section.

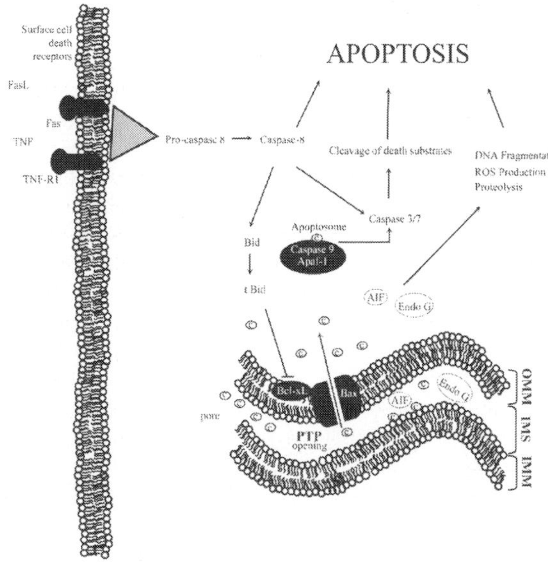

Fig. 2. An overview of the extrinsic and intrinsic pathways of apoptosis. The intrinsic and extrinsic pathways can crossroad in mitochondria, which leads to signal amplification. IMM, inner mitochondrial membrane; IMS, intermembrane space; OMM, outer mitochondrial membrane. Figure adapted from (Pereira, Moreira et al., 2009), with permission.

2.1 Cancer

As described above, the impact of mitochondria on cellular physiology is not limited to ATP production. Due to the importance of mitochondria for cellular functions and cell fate, the role of these small organelles in cancer cell biology is becoming increasingly recognized. The first suggestion about the role of mitochondria in tumor metabolism appeared in 1920's, when Otto Warburg observed increased glycolysis in tumor cells, even in the presence of abundant oxygen. Following this observation, Warburg hypothesized that tumor cells tend to obtain most of their energy through aerobic glycolysis (Warburg, 1930). This phenomenon, known as the Warburg effect, is considered one of the major metabolic alterations observed during cancer development (Warburg, 1956). Since then, several hypotheses have been suggested in order to explain the aerobic glycolysis observed in some (but not all) cancer cells. An irreversible respiratory impairment was first proposed by Warburg (Warburg, 1956). In fact, the author suggested that the origin of cancer cells was in an irreversible damage to the respiration apparatus (Warburg, 1956). However, Warburg results were questioned when Boyland observed an increase in respiration after addition of succinate or fumarate to tumor slices (Boyland & Boyland, 1936). Also, it was described that neoplasias can have a normal oxidative phosphorylation capacity when supplemented with NAD^+ (Wenner & Weinhouse, 1953). More recently, it was demonstrated that oxidative phosphorylation can be improved in cancer cells by changing substrate availability (Rossignol, Gilkerson et al., 2004). Despite all the arguments against the hypotheses raised by Warburg, the truth is the Warburg effect was an important discovery that allowed for an important progress in cancer research and prognosis (Ak, Stokkel et al., 2000). Being mitochondria the organelle where several cellular metabolic reactions occur and where the majority of cellular energy is produced, the role of mitochondria in cancer development is indubitable. For example, mutations in mitochondrial and nuclear genes encoding proteins involved in oxidative phosphorylation have been observed in several cancers, suggesting a role for defective mitochondrial oxidative phosphorylation in tumorigenesis (for a review see (Chandra & Singh, 2010)). Mutations can be acquired during or after oncogenesis and result in an inhibition of oxidative phosphorylation, increased ROS production, tumor cells proliferation and adaptation to tumor microenvironments (Hung, Wu et al., 2010; Lee, Chang et al., 2010). Also, decreased mtDNA copy number has been associated with resistance to apoptosis and increased invasiveness (Chandra & Singh, 2010). The loss of function of mitochondrial-specific enzymes, such as succinate dehydrogenase and fumarate dehydrogenase, results in the accumulation of specific metabolites in the cytosol, that can favor the activation of transcription factors (eg. hypoxia-inducible factor, HIF), directing the metabolism to aerobic glycolysis (Yeung, Pan et al., 2008; Bellance, Lestienne et al., 2009; Marin-Hernandez, Gallardo-Perez et al., 2009) establishing a possible correlation between mitochondrial alterations and the Warburg effect observed in cancer cells.

2.2 Mitochondrial DNA diseases

Besides the nucleus, mitochondria have their own functional genome (Reich & Luck, 1966). Mutations in mtDNA are associated with the development of different pathologies. Although the mtDNA of an individual is usually identical in all cell types (homoplasmy), variations may occur, causing dissimilarities between wild type and mutant mtDNA (heteroplasmy). Progressive accumulation of mutant mtDNA in affected tissue will increase the severity of the phenotype associated with those mutations. Besides the rate of heteroplasmy, the age, gender and environment clearly contribute for the high diversity of phenotypes (McFarland, Taylor et al., 2002). The so-called mitochondrial diseases are caused by mutations in mtDNA or in nuclear genes that codify for proteins involved in the mitochondrial respiratory chain or in overall mitochondrial biology. For the sake of simplicity, we will focus now in diseases that are the result from mtDNA mutations. The degree of severity of mtDNA alterations and the impact on organ phenotype is determined by the threshold effect, or in other words, the dependency of the organ on the mutated protein, or on the mitochondrial function itself (Dimauro & Davidzon, 2005). Simplifying, this means that organs that are more dependent on energy will be first affected by alterations of mitochondrial function caused by mtDNA mutations (Rossignol, Faustin et al., 2003). Mitochondrial DNA diseases can be divided in two main categories based on the genomic origin of the disorder: 1) syndromes due to mtDNA rearrangements or 2) syndromes based on mtDNA point mutations. Kearns-Sayre (KSS) and Person Marrow-Pancreas Syndromes are classical examples of disorders associated with mtDNA rearrangements. KSS is characterized by external progressive opthalmoplegia and pigmentary retinopathy and is associated with heteroplasmatic mtDNA deletions. Pearson Marrow-Pancreas Syndrome is commonly diagnosed during infancy or postmortem and is caused by deletions or duplications in mtDNA. It is rarely diagnosed during pregnancy, but should be suspected in the presence of severe anemia or lactic acidosis (Morel, Joris et al., 2009). Mitochondrial myopathy, encephalopathy, lactic acidosis and stroke-like episodes (MELAS) is a multisystem mitochondrial maternally inherited disease. It is caused by a point mutation characterized by a A to G transition at the position 3260 of the mitochondrial genome. It is normally associated with frequent episodes of migraine and intraventricular conduction disturbances and syncopal episodes based on paroxysmal atrioventricular block have been found already (Connolly, Feigenbaum et al., 2010). Leigh Syndrome is a maternal-inherited point mutation in polypeptide-encoding genes based disorder. Although still largely unknown, it is suggested that the Leigh Syndrome is caused by defects in genes coding for the pyruvate dehydrogenase complex, cytochrome *c* oxidase, ATP synthase subunit 6 or complex I subunits (Quintana, Kruse et al.; Naess, Freyer et al., 2009; Quintana, Mayr et al., 2009).

2.3 Diabetes

Diabetes mellitus (DM) is a metabolic disease characterized by hyperglycemia and alterations in carbohydrate, lipid and protein metabolism due to disturbances in insulin secretion, having as a long-term consequence, the failure in several organs. As in previous cases, mitochondrial multi-tasking suggests an important role of this organelle not only in the pathogenesis of this condition, but also in the development of long-term complications. Several mitochondrial alterations have been described during the progress of diabetes mellitus, including respiratory alterations and altered induction of the MPT (reviewed in (Oliveira, 2005)). Besides the heart (Oliveira, Rolo et al., 2001; Oliveira, Seica et al., 2003; Santos, Palmeira et al., 2003; Bugger & Abel, 2011), alterations of mitochondrial function have been recorded in liver (Ferreira, Seica et al., 2003), kidney (Oliveira, Esteves et al., 2004), brain (Moreira, Santos et al., 2004) and testis mitochondria (Palmeira, Santos et al., 2001; Amaral, Oliveira et al., 2008; Amaral, Mota et al., 2009), which show a multi-organ scope of hyperglycaemia-induced mitochondrial alterations. Oliveira *et al.* demonstrated that streptozotocin (STZ)-induced diabetes results in inhibition of cardiac mitochondrial respiration and increased susceptibility to calcium-induced MPT (Oliveira, Seica et al., 2003). In theory, this means that heart mitochondria from diabetic animals are less able to withstand a metabolic stress, mimicked in this work by the addition of ADP and calcium. Interestingly, heart mitochondria from Goto-Kakizaki (GK) rats have decreased susceptibility to the MPT (Oliveira, Rolo et al., 2001). GK rats are an animal model for non-obese type 2 diabetes, developing hyperglycaemia earlier in life, suggesting that the severity/duration of the hyperglycaemic period is important for cardiac mitochondrial alterations. Interestingly, different alterations in terms of hepatic mitochondrial respiratory activity were found in both STZ-treated and GK rats, such alterations being modulated by the age of the animals (Ferreira, Palmeira et al., 2003; Ferreira, Seica et al., 2003). Alterations in MPT induction are also widespread to other tissues. Lumini-Oliveira *et al.* reported that 18 weeks of STZ treatment lead to a decrease in gastrocnemius mitochondrial respiratory control ratio and to decreased calcium-dependent MPT, which may counteract the negative effects of hyperglycaemia. It is still unclear what may cause mitochondrial alterations during the course of diabetes and why such alterations appear to be organ and age-specific. Increased oxidative stress due to increased mitochondrial generation of ROS and/or depression of mitochondrial antioxidant defenses may be an attractive mechanism

(Kucharska, Braunova et al., 2000; Turko, Li et al., 2003; Kowluru, Atasi et al., 2006; Ren, Li et al., 2008; Munusamy & MacMillan-Crow, 2009). A growing body of evidence also suggests that mitochondrial dysfunction in pancreatic beta-cells may be also one of the initiation factors responsible for depressed insulin release (Mulder & Ling, 2009). In fact, mitochondria in beta-cells have a critical role in the release of insulin. Beta cell mitochondria play a key role in this process, not only by providing ATP to support insulin secretion when required, but also by synthesizing metabolites that can couple glucose sensing to insulin exocytosis. ATP alone or possibly modulated by several coupling factors, triggers closure of the ATP-sensitive potassium channel, resulting in membrane depolarization that increases intracellular calcium and insulin secretion (Liu, Okada et al., 2009; Jitrapakdee, Wutthisathapornchai et al., 2011). In several models for diabetes, mitochondrial defects in beta-cells have been found (reviewed in (Maechler, Li et al., 2011)), including altered expression of the voltage-dependent anion-channel (Ahmed, Muhammed et al., 2011) and altered respiratory activity and oxidative stress (Lu, Koshkin et al., 2011). In beta-cell mitochondria, increased oxidative stress may be critically important in the pathogenesis of the disease (Nishikawa & Araki, 2007), although what exactly leads to that is still a matter of debate. What is interesting is that some forms of diabetes are originated by defects on mitochondrial DNA, present in pancreatic beta-cells (de Andrade, Rubi et al., 2006; Mezghani, Mkaouar-Rebai et al., 2011). Other mitochondrial-relevant alterations in beta-cells include enhanced apoptosis in some forms of auto-immune type I and type II diabetes (Johnson & Luciani, 2011).

3. Drug-induced mitochondrial toxicity

Toxic compounds can interfere and modify physiological mechanisms, leading to cell alterations and ultimately damage. In many cases of drug-induced toxicity, mitochondria are the preferential target for toxic compounds and one important initiator of cell damage. In this section, we will focus on the present knowledge regarding the mechanism of action of some selected drugs, whose mechanism of toxicity has a clear mitochondrial component.

3.1 Anti-cancer drugs

For five decades, anthracycline antibiotics have played an important role in the treatment of a variety of cancer types, due to their efficacy and broad spectrum of activity (Sawyer, Peng et al., 2010). The anti-tumor activity of anthracyclines is based on their ability to intercalate DNA and to inhibit enzymes involved in DNA replication and transcription such as topoisomerase II and RNA polymerases, respectively (Sawyer, Peng et al., 2010). Disturbance of DNA function is thought to be the main responsible for tumor cell death, a typical behavior shared by other anti-cancer drugs (Singal, Iliskovic et al., 1997). However, anthracycline therapy is associated with significant side effects, including cardiotoxicity (Chen, Peng et al., 2007; Sawyer, Peng et al., 2010). A particular leading drug of this group, Doxorubicin (DOX), has been intensively studied and rapidly stood out from other analog molecules due to its efficacy. Unfortunately, its cardiotoxicity also stood out, although the molecular mechanisms are still far of being completely understood (Arola, Saraste et al., 2000; Horenstein, Vander Heide et al., 2000). The onset of DOX-induced cardiomyopathy is characterized by several forms of tachycardia (Bristow, Minobe et al., 1981), altered left ventricular function (Hrdina, Gersl et al., 2000), and severe histological changes such as vacuolization of the cytoplasm, loss of myofibrils, altered sarcoplasmic reticulum, deposition of lipid droplets, and mitochondrial swelling (Lefrak, Pitha et al., 1973; Olson & Capen, 1978; Iwasaki & Suzuki, 1991; Sardao, Oliveira et al., 2009). More evidence suggests that mitochondria are a critical target in the development of DOX-induced cardiomyopathy (Yoon, Kajiyama et al., 1983; Praet & Ruysschaert, 1993; Jung & Reszka, 2001; Wallace, 2003; Berthiaume & Wallace, 2007). Numerous mechanisms for the toxicity of DOX on cardiac mitochondrial function have been proposed, such as generation of free radicals (Muraoka & Miura, 2003), interaction with mitochondrial DNA (L'Ecuyer, Sanjeev et al., 2006), disruption of cardiac gene expression (Berthiaume & Wallace, 2007), alteration of calcium homeostasis (Lebrecht, Kirschner et al.), lipid peroxidation mediating disturbance of mitochondrial membranes (Mimnaugh, Trush et al., 1985), and inhibition of mitochondrial respiration chain, decreasing both intracellular ATP and phosphocreatine (PCr) (Tokarska-Schlattner, Zaugg et al., 2006). DOX can also interfere with mitochondrial function in other targets, including by inhibiting phosphorylation steps (Marcillat, Zhang et al., 1989) or by exerting partial uncoupling (Bugger, Guzman et al.). Although several hypotheses have been proposed to explain cardiac DOX toxicity, oxidative stress is the most widely accepted; in fact, data from the literature indicate that the cardiac tissue is particularly susceptible to free radicals due to reduced levels of enzymatic antioxidants defenses when compared with other tissues (Hrdina, Gersl et al., 2000). DOX is able to increase ROS through both an enzymatic mechanism involving a redox cycle and cellular oxidoreductases such as NADH dehydrogenase of complex I or cytochrome P-450 reductase, and through a non-enzymatic pathway involving complexes with iron (Fe^{3+}) (Davies & Doroshow, 1986; Doroshow & Davies, 1986; Jung & Reszka, 2001; Minotti, Recalcati et al., 2004). DOX-induced oxidative stress can also be related with induction of the MPT (Ascensao, Lumini-Oliveira et al.; Zhou, Starkov et al., 2001; Oliveira, Santos et al., 2006; Oliveira & Wallace, 2006), which is observed in both *in vivo* and *in vitro* studies (Pereira & Oliveira, 2010). *In vitro*, DOX-induced MPT pore opening results in mitochondrial depolarization, respiratory inhibition, matrix swelling, pyridine nucleotides depletion and release of intermembrane proteins, including cytochrome c (Oliveira, Bjork et al., 2004; Berthiaume, Oliveira et al., 2005; Oliveira, Santos et al., 2006).

3.2 Nucleoside-analog reverse transcriptase inhibitors

Nucleoside reverse transcriptase inhibitors (NRTIs), a class of anti-retroviral drugs, are specifically prescribed as a therapy to Acquired Immune Deficiency Syndrome (AIDS). Several studies indicate that these drugs induce mitochondrial toxicity by interfering with mitochondrial DNA (mtDNA) synthesis (Lund & Wallace, 2004; Lewis, Kohler et al., 2006). The targets of NRTIs are reverse transcriptase enzymes but due to the similarities with substrates for the mitochondrial enzyme DNA polymerase-gamma, NRTIs also inhibit this mitochondrial enzyme, affecting mtDNA copy number (Lewis, Simpson et al., 1994). As described above, mitochondrial DNA depletion may be clinically manifested in one or several main targets tissues, depending on the energy requirements of that same tissue (Rossignol, Faustin et al., 2003). Liver mitochondrial complications as hepatomegaly and increased lipid deposits have been primarily observed with dideoxynucleosidesdidanosine, stavudine, and zalcitabin. mtDNA depletion has been demonstrated in the liver of HIV patients, with each of dideoxynucleosides inducing a time- and concentration-dependent mtDNA depletion (Walker, Bauerle et al., 2004). Several NRTIs were shown to directly interfere with cardiac mitochondrial respiratory chain decreasing membrane potential and decreasing mitochondrial calcium buffer capacity (Lund & Wallace, 2004). Zidovudine (AZT) is the most well-known antiviral and its side effects have been subject of several studies focused on studying mitochondrial interactions (Lewis, Simpson et al., 1994). Competitive inhibition of thymidine phosphorylation (Lynx, Bentley et al., 2006; Lynx & McKee, 2006), induction of superoxide anion formation (Szabados, Fischer et al., 1999; de la Asuncion, Del Olmo et al., 2004), inhibition of adenylate kinase activity (Barile, Valenti et al., 1994), and inhibition of the ANT both in heart (Valenti, Barile et al., 2000) and liver (Barile, Valenti et al., 1997) are some of the effects observed in isolated mitochondria incubated with AZT and other NRTIs. Inhibition of phosphate transport in rat heart mitochondria by AZT was found to be related with increased superoxide anion production, as shown by the protective effects of several ROS scavengers (Valenti, Atlante et al., 2002). Oxidative stress probably plays the most important role in AZT-induced mitochondrial dysfunction. Indeed, a 2-week treatment of rats with AZT leads to increased ROS and peroxynitrite production and induced single-strand DNA breaks (Szabados, Fischer et al., 1999). Lipid peroxidation and oxidation of cell proteins, determined from protein carbonyl content, increased as a consequence of AZT treatment (Szabados, Fischer et al., 1999). Depletion of mitochondrial glutathione was also found in mitochondria isolated from the hearts of AZT-treated rats (de la Asuncion, Del Olmo et al., 2004). Furthermore, NRTIs are able to indirectly inhibit the regulation of mitochondrial complex I by cyclic adenosine monophosphate (cAMP). This type of inhibition may explain disturbances observed in many patients regarding ROS production, $NADH/NAD^+$ ratio, and high lactate levels (Lund & Wallace, 2008).

3.3 Anti-diabetic agents

Treatment of hyperglycemia during diabetes involves the use of hypoglycemic drugs. Initially, biguanide agents such as metformin, phenformin and buformin were used for the management of hyperglycemia in type 2 diabetes mellitus (T2D). However, these anti-diabetic drugs rapidly resulted into a number of serious adverse effects, which made the pharmacological management of hyperglycemia still a challenge to the clinic.

Both buformin and phenformin were withdrawn from the market in the 1970´s due to high incidence of lactic-acidosis-associated mortality and gastrointestinal symptoms, although phenformin is still available in some countries. Metformin is now believed to be the most widely prescribed anti-diabetic drug in the world (Correia, Carvalho et al., 2008). The anti-diabetic effect of metformin and phenformin and increased lactic acidosis observed during treatment are suggested to result from a single mechanism, the inhibition of mitochondrial complex I (El-Mir, Nogueira et al., 2000; Correia, Carvalho et al., 2008). Other investigators described that inhibition of hepatocyte complex I not only caused not only a reduction of blood glucose levels in human subjects but also a complete inhibition of hepatic gluconeogenesis, a metabolic process that is significantly increased in T2D contributing to the observed fasting hyperglycemia (Hundal, Krssak et al., 2000). In intact cells, metformin increases AMP-activated protein kinase (AMPK) activity, resulting in increased fatty acid oxidation, down-regulation of lipogenic genes, decreased hepatic glucose production and stimulation of glucose uptake (Zhou, Myers et al., 2001). Beyond biguanides, thiazolidinediones (TZD) is a class of oral antihyperglycemic drugs also known as glitazones that have been used as an auxiliary therapy for diabetes mellitus (Petersen, Krssak et al., 2000; Mudaliar & Henry, 2001). Glitazones includes troglitazone, rosiglitazone, and pioglitazone, which are used to ameliorate hyperglycemia by increasing insulin-stimulated glucose removal by skeletal muscle (Petersen, Krssak et al., 2000; Mudaliar & Henry, 2001). Indeed, TZDs can also be considered insulin sensitizers because they are able to lower glucose levels in models of insulin resistance without increasing pancreatic insulin production (Kliewer, Xu et al., 2001). The ability of TZD to lower serum glucose levels and promote an increase in glucose utilization by accelerating glycolytic flux, can lead to excessive lactic acid production. Although lowering glucose efficiently is considered a desired effect of TZD, lactic acidosis seems to be a compensatory mechanism to a decrease in mitochondrial generated ATP, something that is often observed in diabetic individuals. These drugs are known to bind and activate the nuclear peroxisome proliferation receptor γ (PPARγ), and interestingly to also inhibit mitochondrial complex I. The efficacy of TZD to inhibit complex I or to cause lactate release in skeletal muscle or rat liver homogenates follows the sequence troglitazone, rosiglitazone, and metformin, being the latter less efficient (Brunmair, Staniek et al., 2004). Several studies reveal that TZDs may increase the risk of heart failure (Delea, Edelsberg et al., 2003; Karter, Ahmed et al., 2004), which limits their clinical application. The risk for heart failure may lie on mitochondrial impairment as consequence of TZD toxicity. In this case, disruption of NADH oxidation by mitochondrial complex I tends to occur, although the toxicity effect may also be the mechanism for the pharmacological benefits observed (Scatena, Martorana et al., 2004). This means the border line between a desired pharmacological effect and a toxic consequence is very blurred, and in fact, long-term and/or large-scale inhibition of complex I activity can lead to ATP depletion, oxidative burst and ultimately cell death (Li, Ragheb et al., 2003). An example of TZD which had high impact in the clinic is troglitazone (TRO), introduced in 1997 but soon withdrawn from the market because of reports of serious hepatotoxicity, receiving a black box warning from the U.S. Food and Drug Administration (FDA). In fact, TRO, when incubated with HepG2 cells, decreased cellular ATP and $\Delta\Psi$ (Tirmenstein, Hu et al., 2002; Bova, Tam et al., 2005). Lim *et al.* also demonstrated that TRO increases intramitochondrial oxidative stress that activates the Trx2/Ask1 pathway, leading to mitochondrial permeabilization (Lim, Liu et al., 2008). More recently, data indicate that significant mtDNA damage caused by TRO is a prime initiator of the hepatoxicity caused by this drug (Rachek, Yuzefovych et al., 2009). Overall, the data suggest that the reported mitochondrial effects of anti-diabetic drugs, especially complex I inhibition are worth of further attention, not only to explain some of its pharmacological effects but also to predict safety during drug development.

3.4 Anti-depressant agents

Tricyclic antidepressants (TCAs) are heterocyclic chemicals discovered in the early 1950s and which have been primarily used to relieve depressive symptoms. Fluoxetine (Prozac), an antidepressant of the selective serotonin reuptake inhibitor (SSRI) class, presents some cardiovascular side effects and drug-drug interactions. Interestingly, some studies show that fluoxetine indirectly affects electron transport and F_1F_o-ATPase activity inhibiting OXPHOS in isolated rat brain and liver mitochondria (Souza, Polizello et al., 1994; Curti, Mingatto et al., 1999). The results obtained by Curti *et al.*, suggested that these effects are mediated by the drug interference with the physical state of lipid bilayer of the IMM (Curti, Mingatto et al., 1999). In turn, nefazodone is a TCA with a more favorable side effect profile when compared to fluoxetine and even with other drugs commonly used to mitigate depressive conditions. Nefazodone was initially considered very advantageous among several other TCAs (Davis, Whittington et al., 1997). Initially, the incidence of specific organ toxicity was considered very low, and related fatalities by severe toxicity were non-existent on several hundred of patients during long periods of treatment (Lader, 1996; Robinson, Roberts et al., 1996; Davis, Whittington et al., 1997). Among other physiological advantages, nefazodone had the ability to treat some patients who did not respond to other TCAs (Ellingrod & Perry, 1995; Robinson, Roberts et al., 1996). However, some cardiovascular complications such as asymptomatic reduced systolic blood pressure and asymptomatic sinus bradycardia, started to be detected and considered as markers for cardiotoxicity (Robinson, Roberts et al., 1996). Despite the possible therapeutic advantages, the drug was withdrawn from the U.S. market in 2004, based on cardiotoxicity and later on some severe cases of adverse hepatoxicity as well. Indeed, more recent data show that when compared to buspirone, nefazodone is more toxic to hepatic mitochondrial function (Dykens, Jamieson et al., 2008). Dykens *et al.* demonstrated that nefazodone promoted inhibition of mitochondrial respiration and increased glycolysis in isolated rat liver mitochondria and in intact HepG2 cells, respectively (Dykens, Jamieson et al., 2008). Two other anti-depressant drugs, amineptine and tianeptine, can also lead to hepatitis associated with microvesicular steatosis, in fact, their heptanoic acid side chain may be responsible for reversibly inhibiting mitochondrial fatty acid oxidation by a competitive mechanism (Fromenty, Freneaux et al., 1989).

3.5 Statins and fibrates

Statins (or HMG-CoA reductase inhibitors) are a class of drugs used to decrease cholesterol levels by inhibiting the enzyme HMG-CoA reductase, which plays a central role in the production of cholesterol in the liver. Statins are generally safe and well tolerated, but the major side effect, which occurs in about 1% of patients, is skeletal myopathy (Davidson, 2001). Interestingly, many congenital myopathies are associated with defects in mitochondrial enzymes (Cornelio & Di Donato, 1985; Wallace, 2000) and bio-accumulation of statins by fast twitch skeletal muscle cells can increase the risk of mitochondrially-induced rhabdomyolysis (Westwood, Bigley et al., 2005). Several reports describe acute effects of statins on skeletal muscle mitochondria. Lovastatin and simvastatin were reported to induce the MPT *in vitro* and decrease the content of total membrane thiol groups in mitochondria isolated from mouse hind limb (Velho, Okanobo et al., 2006). Mitochondrial degeneration was observed on rat skeletal muscle fibers treated with cerivastatin (Seachrist, Loi et al., 2005). A variety of other statins are known to induce the MPT leading to irreversible collapse of the transmembrane potential and release of pro-apoptotic factors (Cafforio, Dammacco et al., 2005; Kaufmann, Torok et al., 2006), in a Bcl-xL-preventable manner (Blanco-Colio, Justo et al., 2003). Kaufman and colleagues also reported inhibition of β-oxidation and swelling of isolated skeletal muscle mitochondria by statins (Kaufmann, Torok et al., 2006). Ubiquinone coenzyme Q10 (CoQ_{10}) depletion is another hypothetic contributor to statin-induced myopathy (Folkers, Langsjoen et al., 1990). Thus, CoQ_{10} depletion can contribute to mitochondrial dysfunction leading to statin-induced myopathy since CoQ_{10} acts as an electron carrier in the mitochondrial respiratory chain (Schaars & Stalenhoef, 2008). Besides the effects on skeletal muscle, lovastatin and simvastatin inhibit mitochondrial respiration of isolated liver mitochondria by a direct effect on complexes II, III, IV and V (Nadanaciva, Dykens et al., 2007). Fibrates, in turn, are used as accessory therapy in many forms of hypercholesterolemia, usually in combination with statins

(Steiner, 2007). Fibrates are structurally related to the thiazolidinediones, and pharmacologically act on PPARγ, impairing mitochondrial function (Barter & Rye, 2006). In an *ex vivo* experiment with isolated mitochondria, fenofibrate inhibits complex I activity and disturbs rat mitochondrial function (Brunmair, Lest et al., 2004). The fibrates ciglitizone, bezafibrate, gemfibrozil, and clofibric acid were reported to increase lactate and acetate levels due to increase anaerobic glycolysis and fatty acid beta-oxidation, to inhibit NADH-cytochrome *c* reductase activity, and show a correlation between mitochondrial toxicity and inhibition of HL-60 cell growth (Scatena, Martorana et al., 2004). In opposition, Scatena *et al.* argued that fibrates induce toxicity by disrupting mitochondrial function through a mechanism partly independent on PPARs (Scatena, Bottoni et al., 2004).

4. Environmental pollutants

Humans are daily exposed to a variety of molecules, which can be present in food, beverages and even in the atmosphere. Although most are harmless, either due to their intrinsic safety or to the decreased exposure levels, the truth is that some of those molecules disturb several biological systems, including mitochondria, leading to short or long-term organ toxicity (Wallenborn, Schladweiler et al., 2009).

Heavy metal toxicity is widespread in the world due to the very large amount of industrial activities that release these compounds in nature. Heavy metal toxicity can have different aspects and result into different pathologies, including carcinogenesis and vascular diseases (Nash, 2005). As expected, the toxicity of heavy metals also impacts mitochondria. Cadmium, for example, which has been associated with learning impairments and neurological disorders, has been described to cause mitochondrial-dependent apoptosis in oligodendrocytes (Hossain, Liu et al., 2009) and in a skin cell line (Son, Lee et al., 2011). Cadmium accumulation in the kidney involves alteration of mitochondrial function, which results into increased generation of mitochondrial free radicals (Gobe & Crane, 2011), similarly to what occurs in other target organs (Cannino, Ferruggia et al., 2009). As expected, cadmium, similarly to as mercury and copper, induces the MPT, resulting in mitochondrial swelling and activation of basal respiration, as well as in membrane depolarization (Belyaeva, Glazunov et al., 2004). Mercury also caused apoptosis in several biological models by interfering with mitochondrial function (Shenker, Guo et al., 1998). In fact, low concentrations of methylmercury cause inhibition of mitochondrial function, which progresses to apoptotic cell death (Carranza-Rosales, Said-Fernandez et al., 2005). Mitochondrial respiration in hepatoma AS-30D cells is initially uncoupled for lower concentrations and progressively inhibited for higher concentrations, resulting also in increased generation of ROS (Belyaeva, Dymkowska et al., 2008). Although in this same model, copper (Cu^{2+}) was not as toxic (Belyaeva, Dymkowska et al., 2008), other works have shown that copper causes toxicity in astrocytes, due to increased MPT induction and oxidative stress (Reddy, Rao et al., 2008). Also, copper decreased $\Delta\Psi$, followed by apoptosis in MES23.5 dopaminergic cells (Shi, Jiang et al., 2008). Interestingly, at least a significant part of copper toxicity in non-human species can also be explained by inhibition of mitochondrial function, including activation of the MPT, as observed in trout hepatocytes (Krumschnabel, Manzl et al., 2005). Iron has been considered a significant pro-oxidant metal due to its role in the formation of hydroxyl radical via Fenton reactions (Stohs & Bagchi, 1995). Although iron is essential for life, it can pose serious health risks with the liver being the most relevant target. Heavy iron overload, as described during primary (hereditary) or secondary forms of hemochromatosis, may cause cirrhosis, liver failure, and hepatocellular carcinoma (Bonkovsky & Lambrecht, 2000). In addition, iron can contribute to the development or progression of alcoholic liver disease, nonalcoholic liver steatohepatitis, chronic viral hepatitis and prophyria cutanea tarda, among other diseases (Bonkovsky & Lambrecht, 2000). In thalassemia major, one of the clinical end-points is an iron overload resulting from diverse factors. The excess of iron results in ROS formation, damaging several intracellular organelles, including mitochondria (Hershko, 2011). The observed effects are very close to what has been observed in rats subjected to a single injection of a massive dose of iron-dextran. In this case, mitochondria from treated rats showed decreased respiratory control ratio (Pardo Andreu, Inada et al., 2009). In another different model, rats diet-supplemented with iron lactate showed decreased ATP content in the liver and spleen, which was suggested to occur due to mitochondrial alterations (Fujimori, Ozaki et al., 2004). An interesting hypothesis is drawn from the work of Liang *et al.* The authors suggest that mitochondrial aconitase may be an important early source of mitochondrial iron accumulation in a model for experimental Parkinson's disease, with an oxidative inactivation of that enzyme occurring due to iron-mediated oxidative stress (Liang & Patel, 2004). The role of iron in exacerbating the toxic effects of clinically used drugs is demonstrated, among other examples, by the fact that the iron chelator dexrazoxane protects cardiac myocytes against the toxicity of DOX (see above), via a mitochondrial mechanism (Hasinoff, Schnabl et al., 2003).

Dioxins are environmental pollutants with a large impact on human health, being by-products of incineration processes and of production of several chloro-organic chemicals (Sweeney & Mocarelli, 2000; Parzefall, 2002). 2,3,7,8-Tetrachlorodibenzo-p-dioxin (TCDD) is the best studied and the most toxic dioxin and data are vast describing clear direct effects of this compound on mitochondria. Several works identified the inhibition of the mitochondrial electron chain and increased generation of ROS as one mechanism by which TCDD exerts its toxicity in the heart (Nohl, de Silva et al., 1989) and liver (Stohs, Alsharif et al., 1991; Latchoumycandane, Chitra et al., 2002; Senft, Dalton et al., 2002). Senft *et al.* demonstrated that mitochondria are the source of TCDD-induced ROS, although the exact mechanism was still not clearly identified (Senft, Dalton et al., 2002). TCDD treatment resulted in an increased hydrogen peroxide release by the respiratory chain, although no alterations in mitochondrial superoxide dismutase or glutathione peroxidase were observed (Senft, Dalton et al., 2002). Interestingly, one week after treating mice with TCDD, coenzyme Q levels in the liver decreased, while activities of some of the mitochondrial complexes were increased (Shertzer, Genter et al., 2006). These and other results, led to the proposal that TCDD causes a defect on the ATP synthase in the liver, resulting in decreased ATP levels in the liver (Shertzer, Genter et al., 2006). Results in isolated rat hepatocytes confirmed the mitochondrial role on oxidative stress caused by TCDD (Aly & Domenech, 2009). It was also demonstrated by using a knock-out model that mitochondrial reactive oxygen production is dependent on the aromatic hydrocarbon receptor (Senft, Dalton et al., 2002) and causes direct damage to mtDNA (Shen, Dalton et al., 2005). Interestingly, TCDD induces apoptosis of human lymphoblastic T-cells, which do not express the aromatic hydrocarbon receptor; the mechanism being the triggering of mitochondrial-mediated intrinsic apoptotic pathway, mediated by calcium/calmodulin (Kobayashi, Ahmed et al., 2009). Another interesting possibility regarding the linkage between mitochondria and TCDD toxicity is the perturbation of reproductive function by that dioxin (Wu, Li et al., 2001). Reported data indicate that low doses of TCDD cause increased oxidative stress, including depletion of antioxidant enzymes, in mitochondria and microsomal fractions from rat testis, which can alter the mitochondrial ability to supply energy to male germ cells (Latchoumycandane, Chitra et al., 2002). Mitochondrial interactions of TCDD and the possible carcinogenesis associated with dioxin exposure (Knerr & Schrenk, 2006; Jenkins, Rowell et al., 2007) (although others disagree, (Cole, Trichopoulos et al., 2003)) were also demonstrated to be related since TCDD causes mitochondrial depolarization, stress signaling and tumor invasion, besides altering calcium homeostasis (Biswas, Srinivasan et al., 2008). Besides, TCDD directly targets mitochondrial transcription and causes a mitochondrial phenotype which is similar to what is observed in rho0 cells (Biswas, Srinivasan et al., 2008).

5. Mitochondrial liability in drug development and safety assessment

Mitochondria are indeed, the crossroad for many cellular pathways, which explains the growing number of publications dealing with the mitochondrial role in cell life and death (Pereira, Moreira et al., 2009). As a result of the increased efforts focused on the role of mitochondria on a variety of human disorders as cancer, neurodegenerative, cardiovascular diseases, obesity, and diabetes, "mitochondrial medicine" emerged as a whole new field of biomedical research. Based on the recent developments in this field, a large effort is underway to understand how different molecules regulate or damage mitochondrial function, with the ultimate goal to improve human health. Two distinct and important mechanisms/endpoints by which drugs may inhibit mitochondrial function, can be considered (Fig. 3): a) direct interference with mitochondrial respiration/ATP synthesis (inhibition of respiratory complex activity, damage by ROS production, uncoupling activity, MPT induction) and b) inhibition of mtDNA synthesis. Regardless of the initial trigger, inhibition of ATP synthesis and bioenergetic failure of the tissue are severe manifestations of mitochondrial impairment. Several drugs or other xenobiotics can drive mitochondrial to an irreversible collapse via formation of the MPT pore leading to release of pro-apoptotic factors such as cytochrome *c*. Drugs that alter the normal equilibrium between pro-apoptotic and anti-apoptotic proteins, such as Bak/Bax and Bcl-2, can also induce mitochondrial failure and eventually cell death. Additional information for drug development and safety, as well for toxicity assessments may be achieved by the use of targeted approaches, affinity for overexpressed/subexpressed mitochondrial proteins during different diseases types, or selective mitochondrial accumulation of delocalized lipophilic molecules with positive charge and with different redox actions. Nevertheless, further investigation in these endpoints or guidelines of the molecular mechanisms of mitochondria-drug interaction will be needed for a better understanding of the mechanism of action involved in mitochondrial toxicity, allowing an improvement in the design of safer drugs or hazard assessment of xenobiotics with relevant human exposure. Notwithstanding these concerns, until now, several high-throughput techniques have been used to test and screen drug safety on mitochondrial function and could easily be studied to improve basic knowledge in drug development and associated toxicity.

6. High throughput methods – the faster the better?

High throughput methods have been developed with the ultimate objective of allowing company and research laboratories to perform large-scale screening or biochemical analyses for a certain research or commercial objective. During many decades, low throughput methods were used in most research laboratories, including the Clark-type electrode or the tetraphenylphosphonium electrode to measure mitochondrial membrane potential or $\Delta\Psi$, respectively (Pereira, Moreira et al., 2009; Pereira, Pereira et al., 2009). Other low-throughput methods to investigate mitochondrial toxicity of several agents involved the measurement of activities of components of the mitochondrial respiratory chain by using polarographic, spectrophotometric or blue-native gel techniques (Barrientos, Fontanesi et al., 2009; Diaz, Barrientos et al., 2009). Although such methods are still in use in many laboratories worldwide (and in our own as well), profit-thirsty pharmaceutical companies require faster and cheaper methods to screen thousands of compounds per month in an attempt to uncover mitochondrial liabilities. For example, in the context of mitochondrial toxicity screening in drug development and safety, a fluorescence-based oxygen consumption assay was developed to analyze the ability of certain compounds to cause mitochondrial dysfunction. This approach provides detailed and specific information about the possible mechanisms of toxicity based on measurements of respiratory states 3 and 4 by means of oxygen-sensitive probes. The advantages of this particular fluorescence method are the simplicity and large-scale of measurement, since it can be adapted to a plate reader system. The results can be visualized in real time and quantified in plate reader software (Hynes, Marroquin et al., 2006). A later development included a combination of five high-throughput assays adding important information by identifying enzymes which can be target of the test compounds (Nadanaciva, Bernal et al., 2007). A set of immunocapture-based assays to identify compounds that directly inhibit oxidative phosphorylation can be used in the early evaluation of compound for clinical trials (Nadanaciva, Bernal et al., 2007). The same research group improved a method based on fluorescent probes for the study of oxygen consumption. The advantage is the possibility of screening several compounds simultaneously, being further up-scaled, automated and adapted for other enzyme- and cell-based screening applications (Will, Hynes et al., 2006). To test compounds that interfere with the synthesis of mitochondrial DNA or mtDNA-encoded proteins, a 96-well plate format method, that measures complex IV subunit 1, a protein encoded by mtDNA and complex V subunit 1, an nuclear DNA- encoded protein was developed (Nadanaciva, Dillman et al., 2010).

The literature is getting richer in terms of new methods for high-throughput methods to evaluate mitochondrial function in different applications. When comparing fibroblasts from patients with mtDNA diseases with control subjects, a decrease in ATP production rate in muscle with normal OXPHOS enzyme activities was observed (Jonckheere, Huigsloot et al., 2010). This and other types of assays allow finding primary and secondary mitochondrial dysfunction, which can facilitate the search for genetic defects that can lead to mitochondrial diseases (Jonckheere, Huigsloot et al., 2010). Although in a smaller scale, the Seahorse Bioscience analyzer can be used for a multi-end point of cell and mitochondrial metabolism. In one particular study, the authors measured the mitochondrial function of renal proximal tubular cells observing that several nephrotoxicants alter mitochondria function before altering the basal respiration (Beeson, Beeson et al., 2010). The future will no doubt yield new fast and cost-effective high-throughput methods to quickly investigate mitochondrial toxicity of xenobiotics in order not only to produce safer drugs but also to perform safety screenings on many compounds that humans are daily exposed to.

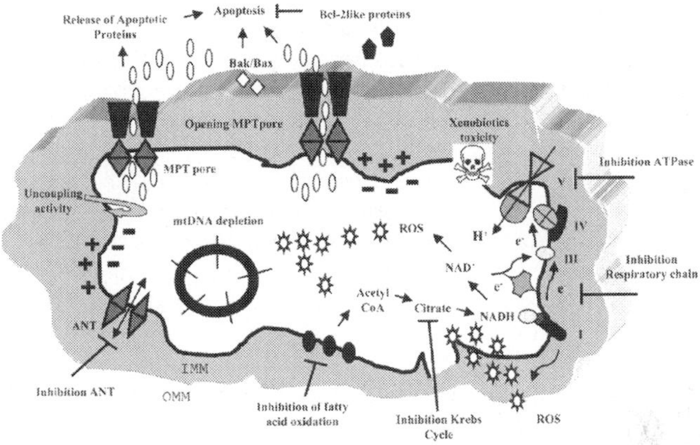

Fig. 3. Drugs or environmental xenobiotics can impair mitochondrial function through affecting different targets, including mitochondrial oxidative phosphorylation and ATP production. Oxidative stress and calcium overload increase the probability of irreversible mitochondrial failure via MPT pore, leading to release of pro-apoptotic factors such as cytochrome *c*. In addition, drugs that alter the ratio pro-apoptotic and anti-apoptotic proteins, such as Bak/Bax and Bcl-2, can also induce mitochondrial failure. OMM, Outer mitochondrial membrane; IMM, Inner mitochondrial membrane; NADH, Nicotinamide adenine dinucleotide reduced form; NAD^+, Nicotinamide adenine dinucleotide oxidized form.

7. Concluding remarks

The question in the title suggests that doubts would still exist regarding the use of mitochondria as a biosensor for drug-induced toxicity. Hopefully, the present chapter provides enough evidence that mitochondria are a critical target in the toxicity of a wide variety of agents, ranging from clinically-relevant drugs, to environmental poisons. Moreover, it has been here demonstrated that failure of mitochondrial function originates several pathologies, which by its turn, contribute to amplify mitochondrial damage. Idiosyncratic drug reactions have also been proposed to involve mitochondria as well (Lucena, Garcia-Martin et al.). In fact, an individual who has a lower mitochondrial power may succumb first to the toxicity of mitochondrial-directed toxicants, even if the original mild mitochondrial alterations are asymptomatic. This is extremely critical for patients with diagnosed mitochondrial DNA diseases, who are in a high risk of suffering mitochondrial failure upon a second hit with a toxicant, either a clinically used drug or an environmental pollutant.

The large number of mitochondrial targets, some of which were not even explored in this chapter, and the growing list of compounds presenting mitochondrial liabilities, clearly answers our initial question. The field of mitochondrial pharmacotoxicology (Scatena, Bottoni et al., 2007) is now critical for many pharmaceutical companies and for a large number of research laboratories which work on basic toxicology (Chan, Truong et al., 2005; Dykens, Marroquin et al., 2007; Wallace, 2008; Nadanaciva & Will, 2009; Pereira, Moreira et al., 2009; Pereira, Pereira et al., 2009). Some for the sake of profit, others for the good of science itself, but all focusing on that little organelle that is in the spotlight right now.

8. Acknowledgements

Mitochondrial research at the authors' laboratory is funded by the Foundation for Science and Technology (FCT), Portugal (research grants PTDC/SAU-OSM/104731/2008, PTDC/QUI-BIQ/101052/2008, PTDC/QUI-QUI/101409/2008, PTDC/AGR-ALI/108326/2008 and PTDC/SAU-FCF/101835/2008). Ana C. Moreira and Nuno G. Machado are funded by FCT (Ph.D. fellowships SFRH/BD/33892/2009 and SFRH/BD/66178/2009, respectively). Vilma A. Sardão is recipient of a Pos-Doc fellowship from the FCT (SFRH/BPD/31549/2006).

9. References

Adam-Vizi, V., & Chinopoulos, C. (2006). Bioenergetics and the formation of mitochondrial reactive oxygen species. *Trends Pharmacol Sci* 27. 12: 639-45.

Ahmed, M., Muhammed, S. J., Kessler, B., & Salehi, A. (2011). Mitochondrial proteome analysis reveals altered expression of voltage dependent anion channels in pancreatic beta-cells exposed to high glucose. *Islets* 2. 5: 283-92.

Ak, I., Stokkel, M. P., & Pauwels, E. K. (2000). Positron emission tomography with 2-[18F]fluoro-2-deoxy-D-glucose in oncology. Part II. The clinical value in detecting and staging primary tumours. *J Cancer Res Clin Oncol* 126. 10: 560-74.

Aly, H. A., & Domenech, O. (2009). Cytotoxicity and mitochondrial dysfunction of 2,3,7,8-tetrachlorodibenzo-p-dioxin (TCDD) in isolated rat hepatocytes. *Toxicol Lett* 191. 1: 79-87.

Amaral, S., Mota, P. C., Lacerda, B., Alves, M., Pereira Mde, L., Oliveira, P. J., & Ramalho-Santos, J. (2009). Testicular mitochondrial alterations in untreated streptozotocin-induced diabetic rats. *Mitochondrion* 9. 1: 41-50.

Amaral, S., Oliveira, P. J., & Ramalho-Santos, J. (2008). Diabetes and the impairment of reproductive function: possible role of mitochondria and reactive oxygen species. *Curr Diabetes Rev* 4. 1: 46-54.

Arnoult, D. (2007). Mitochondrial fragmentation in apoptosis. *Trends Cell Biol* 17. 1: 6-12.

Arnoult, D., Grodet, A., Lee, Y. J., Estaquier, J., & Blackstone, C. (2005). Release of OPA1 during apoptosis participates in the rapid and complete release of cytochrome c and subsequent mitochondrial fragmentation. *J Biol Chem* 280. 42: 35742-50.

Arola, O. J., Saraste, A., Pulkki, K., Kallajoki, M., Parvinen, M., & Voipio-Pulkki, L. M. (2000). Acute doxorubicin cardiotoxicity involves cardiomyocyte apoptosis. *Cancer Res* 60. 7: 1789-92.

Ascensao, A., Lumini-Oliveira, J., Machado, N. G., Ferreira, R. M., Goncalves, I. O., Moreira, A. C., Marques, F., Sardao, V. A., Oliveira, P. J., & Magalhaes, J. Acute exercise protects against calcium-induced cardiac mitochondrial permeability transition pore opening in doxorubicin-treated rats. *Clin Sci (Lond)* 120. 1: 37-49.

Balaban, R. S., Nemoto, S., & Finkel, T. (2005). Mitochondria, oxidants, and aging. *Cell* 120. 4: 483-95.

Barile, M., Valenti, D., Hobbs, G. A., Abruzzese, M. F., Keilbaugh, S. A., Passarella, S., Quagliariello, E., & Simpson, M. V. (1994). Mechanisms of toxicity of 3'-azido-3'-deoxythymidine. Its interaction with adenylate kinase. *Biochem Pharmacol* 48. 7: 1405-12.

Barile, M., Valenti, D., Passarella, S., & Quagliariello, E. (1997). 3'-Azido-3'-deoxythmidine uptake into isolated rat liver mitochondria and impairment of ADP/ATP translocator. *Biochem Pharmacol* 53. 7: 913-20.

Barrientos, A., Fontanesi, F., & Diaz, F. (2009). Evaluation of the mitochondrial respiratory chain and oxidative phosphorylation system using polarography and spectrophotometric enzyme assays. *Curr Protoc Hum Genet* Chapter 19. Unit19 3.

Barter, P. J., & Rye, K. A. (2006). Cardioprotective properties of fibrates: which fibrate, which patients, what mechanism? *Circulation* 113. 12: 1553-5.

Beeson, C. C., Beeson, G. C., & Schnellmann, R. G. (2010). A high-throughput respirometric assay for mitochondrial biogenesis and toxicity. *Anal Biochem* 404. 1: 75-81.

Bellance, N., Lestienne, P., & Rossignol, R. (2009). Mitochondria: from bioenergetics to the metabolic regulation of carcinogenesis. *Front Biosci* 14. 4015-34.

Belyaeva, E. A., Dymkowska, D., Wieckowski, M. R., & Wojtczak, L. (2008). Mitochondria as an important target in heavy metal toxicity in rat hepatoma AS-30D cells. *Toxicol Appl Pharmacol* 231. 1: 34-42.

Belyaeva, E. A., Glazunov, V. V., & Korotkov, S. M. (2004). Cd2+ -promoted mitochondrial permeability transition: a comparison with other heavy metals. *Acta Biochim Pol* 51. 2: 545-51.

Berneburg, M., Kamenisch, Y., Krutmann, J., & Rocken, M. (2006). 'To repair or not to repair - no longer a question': repair of mitochondrial DNA shielding against age and cancer. *Exp Dermatol* 15. 12: 1005-15.

Berthiaume, J. M., Oliveira, P. J., Fariss, M. W., & Wallace, K. B. (2005). Dietary vitamin E decreases doxorubicin-induced oxidative stress without preventing mitochondrial dysfunction. *Cardiovasc Toxicol* 5. 3: 257-67.

Berthiaume, J. M., & Wallace, K. B. (2007). Adriamycin-induced oxidative mitochondrial cardiotoxicity. *Cell Biol Toxicol* 23. 1: 15-25.

Berthiaume, J. M., & Wallace, K. B. (2007). Persistent alterations to the gene expression profile of the heart subsequent to chronic Doxorubicin treatment. *Cardiovasc Toxicol* 7. 3: 178-91.

Biswas, G., Srinivasan, S., Anandatheerthavarada, H. K., & Avadhani, N. G. (2008). Dioxin-mediated tumor progression through activation of mitochondria-to-nucleus stress signaling. *Proc Natl Acad Sci U S A* 105. 1: 186-91.

Blanco-Colio, L. M., Justo, P., Daehn, I., Lorz, C., Ortiz, A., & Egido, J. (2003). Bcl-xL overexpression protects from apoptosis induced by HMG-CoA reductase inhibitors in murine tubular cells. *Kidney Int* 64. 1: 181-91.

Bonkovsky, H. L., & Lambrecht, R. W. (2000). Iron-induced liver injury. *Clin Liver Dis* 4. 2: 409-29, vi-vii.

Bova, M. P., Tam, D., McMahon, G., & Mattson, M. N. (2005). Troglitazone induces a rapid drop of mitochondrial membrane potential in liver HepG2 cells. *Toxicol Lett* 155. 1: 41-50.

Boyland, E., & Boyland, M. E. (1936). Studies in tissue metabolism: The effect of fumarate and succinate on tumour respiration. *Biochem J* 30. 2: 224-6.

Brandon, M., Baldi, P., & Wallace, D. C. (2006). Mitochondrial mutations in cancer. *Oncogene* 25. 34: 4647-62.

Bristow, M. R., Minobe, W. A., Billingham, M. E., Marmor, J. B., Johnson, G. A., Ishimoto, B. M., Sageman, W. S., & Daniels, J. R. (1981). Anthracycline-associated cardiac and renal damage in rabbits. Evidence for mediation by vasoactive substances. *Lab Invest* 45. 2: 157-68.

Brown, G. C., & Borutaite, V. (2007). Nitric oxide and mitochondrial respiration in the heart. *Cardiovasc Res* 75. 2: 283-90.

Brunmair, B., Lest, A., Staniek, K., Gras, F., Scharf, N., Roden, M., Nohl, H., Waldhausl, W., & Furnsinn, C. (2004). Fenofibrate impairs rat mitochondrial function by inhibition of respiratory complex I. *J Pharmacol Exp Ther* 311. 1: 109-14.

Brunmair, B., Staniek, K., Gras, F., Scharf, N., Althaym, A., Clara, R., Roden, M., Gnaiger, E., Nohl, H., Waldhausl, W., & Furnsinn, C. (2004). Thiazolidinediones, like metformin, inhibit respiratory complex I: a common mechanism contributing to their antidiabetic actions? *Diabetes* 53. 4: 1052-9.

Bugger, H., & Abel, E. D. (2011). Mitochondria in the diabetic heart. *Cardiovasc Res* 88. 2: 229-40.

Bugger, H., Guzman, C., Zechner, C., Palmeri, M., Russell, K. S., & Russell, R. R., 3rd. Uncoupling protein downregulation in doxorubicin-induced heart failure improves mitochondrial coupling but increases reactive oxygen species generation. *Cancer Chemother Pharmacol.*

Cadenas, E. (2004). Mitochondrial free radical production and cell signaling. *Mol Aspects Med* 25. 1-2: 17-26.

Cafforio, P., Dammacco, F., Gernone, A., & Silvestris, F. (2005). Statins activate the mitochondrial pathway of apoptosis in human lymphoblasts and myeloma cells. *Carcinogenesis* 26. 5: 883-91.

Cannino, G., Ferruggia, E., Luparello, C., & Rinaldi, A. M. (2009). Cadmium and mitochondria. *Mitochondrion* 9. 6: 377-84.

Carranza-Rosales, P., Said-Fernandez, S., Sepulveda-Saavedra, J., Cruz-Vega, D. E., & Gandolfi, A. J. (2005). Morphologic and functional alterations induced by low doses of mercuric chloride in the kidney OK cell line: ultrastructural evidence for an apoptotic mechanism of damage. *Toxicology* 210. 2-3: 111-21.

Chan, K., Truong, D., Shangari, N., & O'Brien, P. J. (2005). Drug-induced mitochondrial toxicity. *Expert Opin Drug Metab Toxicol* 1. 4: 655-69.

Chandra, D., & Singh, K. K. (2010). Genetic insights into OXPHOS defect and its role in cancer. *Biochim Biophys Acta.*

Chen, B., Peng, X., Pentassuglia, L., Lim, C. C., & Sawyer, D. B. (2007). Molecular and cellular mechanisms of anthracycline cardiotoxicity. *Cardiovasc Toxicol* 7. 2: 114-21.

Cole, P., Trichopoulos, D., Pastides, H., Starr, T., & Mandel, J. S. (2003). Dioxin and cancer: a critical review. *Regul Toxicol Pharmacol* 38. 3: 378-88.

Connolly, B. S., Feigenbaum, A. S., Robinson, B. H., Dipchand, A. I., Simon, D. K., & Tarnopolsky, M. A. (2010). MELAS syndrome, cardiomyopathy, rhabdomyolysis, and autism associated with the A3260G mitochondrial DNA mutation. *Biochem Biophys Res Commun* 402. 2: 443-7.

Cornelio, F., & Di Donato, S. (1985). Myopathies due to enzyme deficiencies. *J Neurol* 232. 6: 329-40.

Correia, S., Carvalho, C., Santos, M. S., Seica, R., Oliveira, C. R., & Moreira, P. I. (2008). Mechanisms of action of metformin in type 2 diabetes and associated complications: an overview. *Mini Rev Med Chem* 8. 13: 1343-54.

Curti, C., Mingatto, F. E., Polizello, A. C., Galastri, L. O., Uyemura, S. A., & Santos, A. C. (1999). Fluoxetine interacts with the lipid bilayer of the inner membrane in isolated rat brain mitochondria, inhibiting electron transport and F1F0-ATPase activity. *Mol Cell Biochem* 199. 1-2: 103-9.

Davidson, M. H. (2001). Safety profiles for the HMG-CoA reductase inhibitors: treatment and trust. *Drugs* 61. 2: 197-206.

Davies, K. J., & Doroshow, J. H. (1986). Redox cycling of anthracyclines by cardiac mitochondria. I. Anthracycline radical formation by NADH dehydrogenase. *J Biol Chem* 261. 7: 3060-7.

Davis, R., Whittington, R., & Bryson, H. M. (1997). Nefazodone. A review of its pharmacology and clinical efficacy in the management of major depression. *Drugs* 53. 4: 608-36.

de Andrade, P. B., Rubi, B., Frigerio, F., van den Ouweland, J. M., Maassen, J. A., & Maechler, P. (2006). Diabetes-associated mitochondrial DNA mutation A3243G impairs cellular metabolic pathways necessary for beta cell function. *Diabetologia* 49. 8: 1816-26.

de la Asuncion, J. G., Del Olmo, M. L., Gomez-Cambronero, L. G., Sastre, J., Pallardo, F. V., & Vina, J. (2004). AZT induces oxidative damage to cardiac mitochondria: protective effect of vitamins C and E. *Life Sci* 76. 1: 47-56.

Delea, T. E., Edelsberg, J. S., Hagiwara, M., Oster, G., & Phillips, L. S. (2003). Use of thiazolidinediones and risk of heart failure in people with type 2 diabetes: a retrospective cohort study. *Diabetes Care* 26. 11: 2983-9.

Detmer, S. A., & Chan, D. C. (2007). Functions and dysfunctions of mitochondrial dynamics. *Nat Rev Mol Cell Biol* 8. 11: 870-9.

Diaz, F., Barrientos, A., & Fontanesi, F. (2009). Evaluation of the mitochondrial respiratory chain and oxidative phosphorylation system using blue native gel electrophoresis. *Curr Protoc Hum Genet* Chapter 19. Unit19 4.

Dimauro, S., & Davidzon, G. (2005). Mitochondrial DNA and disease. *Ann Med* 37. 3: 222-32.

Doroshow, J. H., & Davies, K. J. (1986). Redox cycling of anthracyclines by cardiac mitochondria. II. Formation of superoxide anion, hydrogen peroxide, and hydroxyl radical. *J Biol Chem* 261. 7: 3068-74.

Dykens, J. A., Jamieson, J. D., Marroquin, L. D., Nadanaciva, S., Xu, J. J., Dunn, M. C., Smith, A. R., & Will, Y. (2008). In vitro assessment of mitochondrial dysfunction and cytotoxicity of nefazodone, trazodone, and buspirone. *Toxicol Sci* 103. 2: 335-45.

Dykens, J. A., Marroquin, L. D., & Will, Y. (2007). Strategies to reduce late-stage drug attrition due to mitochondrial toxicity. *Expert Rev Mol Diagn* 7. 2: 161-75.

El-Mir, M. Y., Nogueira, V., Fontaine, E., Averet, N., Rigoulet, M., & Leverve, X. (2000). Dimethylbiguanide inhibits cell respiration via an indirect effect targeted on the respiratory chain complex I. *J Biol Chem* 275. 1: 223-8.

Ellingrod, V. L., & Perry, P. J. (1995). Nefazodone: a new antidepressant. *Am J Health Syst Pharm* 52. 24: 2799-812.

Ferreira, F. M., Palmeira, C. M., Seica, R., Moreno, A. J., & Santos, M. S. (2003). Diabetes and mitochondrial bioenergetics: alterations with age. *J Biochem Mol Toxicol* 17. 4: 214-22.

Ferreira, F. M., Seica, R., Oliveira, P. J., Coxito, P. M., Moreno, A. J., Palmeira, C. M., & Santos, M. S. (2003). Diabetes induces metabolic adaptations in rat liver mitochondria: role of coenzyme Q and cardiolipin contents. *Biochim Biophys Acta* 1639. 2: 113-20.

Folkers, K., Langsjoen, P., Willis, R., Richardson, P., Xia, L. J., Ye, C. Q., & Tamagawa, H. (1990). Lovastatin decreases coenzyme Q levels in humans. *Proc Natl Acad Sci U S A* 87. 22: 8931-4.

Fromenty, B., Freneaux, E., Labbe, G., Deschamps, D., Larrey, D., Letteron, P., & Pessayre, D. (1989). Tianeptine, a new tricyclic antidepressant metabolized by beta-oxidation of its heptanoic side chain, inhibits the mitochondrial oxidation of medium and short chain fatty acids in mice. *Biochem Pharmacol* 38. 21: 3743-51.

Fruehauf, J. P., & Meyskens, F. L., Jr. (2007). Reactive oxygen species: a breath of life or death? *Clin Cancer Res* 13. 3: 789-94.

Fujimori, H., Ozaki, K., Matsuura, T., Matsushima, S., Narama, I., & Pan-Hou, H. (2004). Effect of iron lactate overloading on adenine nucleotide levels and adenosine 3'-monophosphate forming enzyme in rat liver and spleen. *Biol Pharm Bull* 27. 9: 1371-5.

Galluzzi, L., Maiuri, M. C., Vitale, I., Zischka, H., Castedo, M., Zitvogel, L., & Kroemer, G. (2007). Cell death modalities: classification and pathophysiological implications. *Cell Death Differ* 14. 7: 1237-43.

Gobe, G., & Crane, D. (2011). Mitochondria, reactive oxygen species and cadmium toxicity in the kidney. *Toxicol Lett* 198. 1: 49-55.

Grandemange, S., Herzig, S., & Martinou, J. C. (2009). Mitochondrial dynamics and cancer. *Semin Cancer Biol* 19. 1: 50-6.

Hasinoff, B. B., Schnabl, K. L., Marusak, R. A., Patel, D., & Huebner, E. (2003). Dexrazoxane (ICRF-187) protects cardiac myocytes against doxorubicin by preventing damage to mitochondria. *Cardiovasc Toxicol* 3. 2: 89-99.

Hebert, S. L., Lanza, I. R., & Nair, K. S. (2010). Mitochondrial DNA alterations and reduced mitochondrial function in aging. *Mech Ageing Dev* 131. 7-8: 451-62.

Hershko, C. (2011). Pathogenesis and management of iron toxicity in thalassemia. *Ann N Y Acad Sci* 1202. 1-9.

Horenstein, M. S., Vander Heide, R. S., & L'Ecuyer, T. J. (2000). Molecular basis of anthracycline-induced cardiotoxicity and its prevention. *Mol Genet Metab* 71. 1-2: 436-44.

Hossain, S., Liu, H. N., Nguyen, M., Shore, G., & Almazan, G. (2009). Cadmium exposure induces mitochondria-dependent apoptosis in oligodendrocytes. *Neurotoxicology* 30. 4: 544-54.

Hrdina, R., Gersl, V., Klimtova, I., Simunek, T., Machackova, J., & Adamcova, M. (2000). Anthracycline-induced cardiotoxicity. *Acta Medica (Hradec Kralove)* 43. 3: 75-82.

Hundal, R. S., Krssak, M., Dufour, S., Laurent, D., Lebon, V., Chandramouli, V., Inzucchi, S. E., Schumann, W. C., Petersen, K. F., Landau, B. R., & Shulman, G. I. (2000). Mechanism by which metformin reduces glucose production in type 2 diabetes. *Diabetes* 49. 12: 2063-9.

Hung, W. Y., Wu, C. W., Yin, P. H., Chang, C. J., Li, A. F., Chi, C. W., Wei, Y. H., & Lee, H. C. (2010). Somatic mutations in mitochondrial genome and their potential roles in the progression of human gastric cancer. *Biochim Biophys Acta* 1800. 3: 264-70.

Hynes, J., Marroquin, L. D., Ogurtsov, V. I., Christiansen, K. N., Stevens, G. J., Papkovsky, D. B., & Will, Y. (2006). Investigation of drug-induced mitochondrial toxicity using fluorescence-based oxygen-sensitive probes. *Toxicol Sci* 92. 1: 186-200.

Iwasaki, T., & Suzuki, T. (1991). Ultrastructural alterations of the myocardium induced by doxorubicin. A scanning electron microscopic study. *Virchows Arch B Cell Pathol Incl Mol Pathol* 60. 1: 35-9.

Jenkins, S., Rowell, C., Wang, J., & Lamartiniere, C. A. (2007). Prenatal TCDD exposure predisposes for mammary cancer in rats. *Reprod Toxicol* 23. 3: 391-6.

Jeong, S. Y., & Seol, D. W. (2008). The role of mitochondria in apoptosis. *BMB Rep* 41. 1: 11-22.

Jezek, P., & Plecita-Hlavata, L. (2009). Mitochondrial reticulum network dynamics in relation to oxidative stress, redox regulation, and hypoxia. *Int J Biochem Cell Biol* 41. 10: 1790-804.

Jitrapakdee, S., Wutthisathapornchai, A., Wallace, J. C., & MacDonald, M. J. (2011). Regulation of insulin secretion: role of mitochondrial signalling. *Diabetologia* 53. 6: 1019-32.

Johnson, J. D., & Luciani, D. S. (2011). Mechanisms of pancreatic beta-cell apoptosis in diabetes and its therapies. *Adv Exp Med Biol* 654. 447-62.

Jonckheere, A. I., Huigsloot, M., Janssen, A. J., Kappen, A. J., Smeitink, J. A., & Rodenburg, R. J. (2010). High-throughput assay to measure oxygen consumption in digitonin-permeabilized cells of patients with mitochondrial disorders. *Clin Chem* 56. 3: 424-31.

Jourdain, A., & Martinou, J. C. (2009). Mitochondrial outer-membrane permeabilization and remodelling in apoptosis. *Int J Biochem Cell Biol* 41. 10: 1884-9.

Jung, K., & Reszka, R. (2001). Mitochondria as subcellular targets for clinically useful anthracyclines. *Adv Drug Deliv Rev* 49. 1-2: 87-105.

Karter, A. J., Ahmed, A. T., Liu, J., Moffet, H. H., Parker, M. M., Ferrara, A., & Selby, J. V. (2004). Use of thiazolidinediones and risk of heart failure in people with type 2 diabetes: a retrospective cohort study: response to Delea et al. *Diabetes Care* 27. 3: 850-1; author reply 852-3.

Kaufmann, P., Torok, M., Zahno, A., Waldhauser, K. M., Brecht, K., & Krahenbuhl, S. (2006). Toxicity of statins on rat skeletal muscle mitochondria. *Cell Mol Life Sci* 63. 19-20: 2415-25.

Kerr, J. F., Wyllie, A. H., & Currie, A. R. (1972). Apoptosis: a basic biological phenomenon with wide-ranging implications in tissue kinetics. *Br J Cancer* 26. 4: 239-57.

Kliewer, S. A., Xu, H. E., Lambert, M. H., & Willson, T. M. (2001). Peroxisome proliferator-activated receptors: from genes to physiology. *Recent Prog Horm Res* 56. 239-63.

Knerr, S., & Schrenk, D. (2006). Carcinogenicity of 2,3,7,8-tetrachlorodibenzo-p-dioxin in experimental models. *Mol Nutr Food Res* 50. 10: 897-907.

Kobayashi, D., Ahmed, S., Ishida, M., Kasai, S., & Kikuchi, H. (2009). Calcium/calmodulin signaling elicits release of cytochrome c during 2,3,7,8-tetrachlorodibenzo-p-dioxin-induced apoptosis in the human lymphoblastic T-cell line, L-MAT. *Toxicology* 258. 1: 25-32.

Kowluru, R. A., Atasi, L., & Ho, Y. S. (2006). Role of mitochondrial superoxide dismutase in the development of diabetic retinopathy. *Invest Ophthalmol Vis Sci* 47. 4: 1594-9.

Krumschnabel, G., Manzl, C., Berger, C., & Hofer, B. (2005). Oxidative stress, mitochondrial permeability transition, and cell death in Cu-exposed trout hepatocytes. *Toxicol Appl Pharmacol* 209. 1: 62-73.

Kucharska, J., Braunova, Z., Ulicna, O., Zlatos, L., & Gvozdjakova, A. (2000). Deficit of coenzyme Q in heart and liver mitochondria of rats with streptozotocin-induced diabetes. *Physiol Res* 49. 4: 411-8.

L'Ecuyer, T., Sanjeev, S., Thomas, R., Novak, R., Das, L., Campbell, W., & Heide, R. V. (2006). DNA damage is an early event in doxorubicin-induced cardiac myocyte death. *Am J Physiol Heart Circ Physiol* 291. 3: H1273-80.

Lader, M. H. (1996). Tolerability and safety: essentials in antidepressant pharmacotherapy. *J Clin Psychiatry* 57 Suppl 2. 39-44.

Latchoumycandane, C., Chitra, K. C., & Mathur, P. P. (2002). The effect of 2,3,7,8-tetrachlorodibenzo-p-dioxin on the antioxidant system in mitochondrial and microsomal fractions of rat testis. *Toxicology* 171. 2-3: 127-35.

Lebrecht, D., Kirschner, J., Geist, A., Haberstroh, J., & Walker, U. A. Respiratory chain deficiency precedes the disrupted calcium homeostasis in chronic doxorubicin cardiomyopathy. *Cardiovasc Pathol* 19. 5: e167-74.

Lee, H. C., Chang, C. M., & Chi, C. W. (2010). Somatic mutations of mitochondrial DNA in aging and cancer progression. *Ageing Res Rev* 9 Suppl 1. S47-58.

Lefrak, E. A., Pitha, J., Rosenheim, S., & Gottlieb, J. A. (1973). A clinicopathologic analysis of adriamycin cardiotoxicity. *Cancer* 32. 2: 302-14.

Lewis, W., Kohler, J. J., Hosseini, S. H., Haase, C. P., Copeland, W. C., Bienstock, R. J., Ludaway, T., McNaught, J., Russ, R., Stuart, T., & Santoianni, R. (2006). Antiretroviral nucleosides, deoxynucleotide carrier and mitochondrial DNA: evidence supporting the DNA pol gamma hypothesis. *AIDS* 20. 5: 675-84.

Lewis, W., Simpson, J. F., & Meyer, R. R. (1994). Cardiac mitochondrial DNA polymerase-gamma is inhibited competitively and noncompetitively by phosphorylated zidovudine. *Circ Res* 74. 2: 344-8.

Li, N., Ragheb, K., Lawler, G., Sturgis, J., Rajwa, B., Melendez, J. A., & Robinson, J. P. (2003). Mitochondrial complex I inhibitor rotenone induces apoptosis through enhancing mitochondrial reactive oxygen species production. *J Biol Chem* 278. 10: 8516-25.

Liang, L. P., & Patel, M. (2004). Iron-sulfur enzyme mediated mitochondrial superoxide toxicity in experimental Parkinson's disease. *J Neurochem* 90. 5: 1076-84.

Lim, P. L., Liu, J., Go, M. L., & Boelsterli, U. A. (2008). The mitochondrial superoxide/thioredoxin-2/Ask1 signaling pathway is critically involved in troglitazone-induced cell injury to human hepatocytes. *Toxicol Sci* 101. 2: 341-9.

Liu, S., Okada, T., Assmann, A., Soto, J., Liew, C. W., Bugger, H., Shirihai, O. S., Abel, E. D., & Kulkarni, R. N. (2009). Insulin signaling regulates mitochondrial function in pancreatic beta-cells. *PLoS One* 4. 11: e7983.

Lu, H., Koshkin, V., Allister, E. M., Gyulkhandanyan, A. V., & Wheeler, M. B. (2011). Molecular and metabolic evidence for mitochondrial defects associated with beta-cell dysfunction in a mouse model of type 2 diabetes. *Diabetes* 59. 2: 448-59.

Lucena, M. I., Garcia-Martin, E., Andrade, R. J., Martinez, C., Stephens, C., Ruiz, J. D., Ulzurrun, E., Fernandez, M. C., Romero-Gomez, M., Castiella, A., Planas, R.,

Duran, J. A., De Dios, A. M., Guarner, C., Soriano, G., Borraz, Y., & Agundez, J. A. Mitochondrial superoxide dismutase and glutathione peroxidase in idiosyncratic drug-induced liver injury. *Hepatology* 52. 1: 303-12.

Lund, K. C., & Wallace, K. B. (2004). Direct, DNA pol-gamma-independent effects of nucleoside reverse transcriptase inhibitors on mitochondrial bioenergetics. *Cardiovasc Toxicol* 4. 3: 217-28.

Lund, K. C., & Wallace, K. B. (2008). Adenosine 3',5'-cyclic monophosphate (cAMP)-dependent phosphoregulation of mitochondrial complex I is inhibited by nucleoside reverse transcriptase inhibitors. *Toxicol Appl Pharmacol* 226. 1: 94-106.

Lynx, M. D., Bentley, A. T., & McKee, E. E. (2006). 3'-Azido-3'-deoxythymidine (AZT) inhibits thymidine phosphorylation in isolated rat liver mitochondria: a possible mechanism of AZT hepatotoxicity. *Biochem Pharmacol* 71. 9: 1342-8.

Lynx, M. D., & McKee, E. E. (2006). 3'-Azido-3'-deoxythymidine (AZT) is a competitive inhibitor of thymidine phosphorylation in isolated rat heart and liver mitochondria. *Biochem Pharmacol* 72. 2: 239-43.

Maechler, P., Li, N., Casimir, M., Vetterli, L., Frigerio, F., & Brun, T. (2011). Role of mitochondria in beta-cell function and dysfunction. *Adv Exp Med Biol* 654. 193-216.

Malka, F., Guillery, O., Cifuentes-Diaz, C., Guillou, E., Belenguer, P., Lombes, A., & Rojo, M. (2005). Separate fusion of outer and inner mitochondrial membranes. *EMBO Rep* 6. 9: 853-9.

Malka, F., Lombes, A., & Rojo, M. (2006). Organization, dynamics and transmission of mitochondrial DNA: focus on vertebrate nucleoids. *Biochim Biophys Acta* 1763. 5-6: 463-72.

Marcillat, O., Zhang, Y., & Davies, K. J. (1989). Oxidative and non-oxidative mechanisms in the inactivation of cardiac mitochondrial electron transport chain components by doxorubicin. *Biochem J* 259. 1: 181-9.

Marin-Hernandez, A., Gallardo-Perez, J. C., Ralph, S. J., Rodriguez-Enriquez, S., & Moreno-Sanchez, R. (2009). HIF-1alpha modulates energy metabolism in cancer cells by inducing over-expression of specific glycolytic isoforms. *Mini Rev Med Chem* 9. 9: 1084-101.

Martin, D. N., & Baehrecke, E. H. (2004). Caspases function in autophagic programmed cell death in Drosophila. *Development* 131. 2: 275-84.

Martinou, J. C., & Green, D. R. (2001). Breaking the mitochondrial barrier. *Nat Rev Mol Cell Biol* 2. 1: 63-7.

McFarland, R., Taylor, R. W., & Turnbull, D. M. (2002). The neurology of mitochondrial DNA disease. *Lancet Neurol* 1. 6: 343-51.

Mezghani, N., Mkaouar-Rebai, E., Mnif, M., Charfi, N., Rekik, N., Youssef, S., Abid, M., & Fakhfakh, F. (2011). The heteroplasmic m.14709T>C mutation in the tRNA(Glu) gene in two Tunisian families with mitochondrial diabetes. *J Diabetes Complications* 24. 4: 270-7.

Mimnaugh, E. G., Trush, M. A., Bhatnagar, M., & Gram, T. E. (1985). Enhancement of reactive oxygen-dependent mitochondrial membrane lipid peroxidation by the anticancer drug adriamycin. *Biochem Pharmacol* 34. 6: 847-56.

Minotti, G., Recalcati, S., Menna, P., Salvatorelli, E., Corna, G., & Cairo, G. (2004). Doxorubicin cardiotoxicity and the control of iron metabolism: quinone-dependent and independent mechanisms. *Methods Enzymol* 378. 340-61.

Moreira, P. I., Santos, M. S., Moreno, A. M., Proenca, T., Seica, R., & Oliveira, C. R. (2004). Effect of streptozotocin-induced diabetes on rat brain mitochondria. *J Neuroendocrinol* 16. 1: 32-8.

Morel, A. S., Joris, N., Meuli, R., Jacquemont, S., Ballhausen, D., Bonafe, L., Fattet, S., & Tolsa, J. F. (2009). Early neurological impairment and severe anemia in a newborn with Pearson syndrome. *Eur J Pediatr* 168. 3: 311-5.

Morselli, E., Galluzzi, L., Kepp, O., Vicencio, J. M., Criollo, A., Maiuri, M. C., & Kroemer, G. (2009). Anti- and pro-tumor functions of autophagy. *Biochim Biophys Acta* 1793. 9: 1524-32.

Mudaliar, S., & Henry, R. R. (2001). New oral therapies for type 2 diabetes mellitus: The glitazones or insulin sensitizers. *Annu Rev Med* 52. 239-57.

Mulder, H., & Ling, C. (2009). Mitochondrial dysfunction in pancreatic beta-cells in Type 2 diabetes. *Mol Cell Endocrinol* 297. 1-2: 34-40.

Munusamy, S., & MacMillan-Crow, L. A. (2009). Mitochondrial superoxide plays a crucial role in the development of mitochondrial dysfunction during high glucose exposure in rat renal proximal tubular cells. *Free Radic Biol Med* 46. 8: 1149-57.

Muraoka, S., & Miura, T. (2003). [Free radicals mediate cardiac toxicity induced by adriamycin]. *Yakugaku Zasshi* 123. 10: 855-66.

Nadanaciva, S., Bernal, A., Aggeler, R., Capaldi, R., & Will, Y. (2007). Target identification of drug induced mitochondrial toxicity using immunocapture based OXPHOS activity assays. *Toxicol In Vitro* 21. 5: 902-11.

Nadanaciva, S., Dillman, K., Gebhard, D. F., Shrikhande, A., & Will, Y. (2010). High-content screening for compounds that affect mtDNA-encoded protein levels in eukaryotic cells. *J Biomol Screen* 15. 8: 937-48.

Nadanaciva, S., Dykens, J. A., Bernal, A., Capaldi, R. A., & Will, Y. (2007). Mitochondrial impairment by PPAR agonists and statins identified via immunocaptured OXPHOS complex activities and respiration. *Toxicol Appl Pharmacol* 223. 3: 277-87.

Nadanaciva, S., & Will, Y. (2009). The role of mitochondrial dysfunction and drug safety. *IDrugs* 12. 11: 706-10.

Naess, K., Freyer, C., Bruhn, H., Wibom, R., Malm, G., Nennesmo, I., von Dobeln, U., & Larsson, N. G. (2009). MtDNA mutations are a common cause of severe disease phenotypes in children with Leigh syndrome. *Biochim Biophys Acta* 1787. 5: 484-90.

Nash, R. A. (2005). Metals in medicine. *Altern Ther Health Med* 11. 4: 18-25.

Nishikawa, T., & Araki, E. (2007). Impact of mitochondrial ROS production in the pathogenesis of diabetes mellitus and its complications. *Antioxid Redox Signal* 9. 3: 343-53.

Nohl, H., de Silva, D., & Summer, K. H. (1989). 2,3,7,8, tetrachlorodibenzo-p-dioxin induces oxygen activation associated with cell respiration. *Free Radic Biol Med* 6. 4: 369-74.

Oliveira, P. J. (2005). Cardiac mitochondrial alterations observed in hyperglycaemic rats--what can we learn from cell biology? *Curr Diabetes Rev* 1. 1: 11-21.

Oliveira, P. J., Bjork, J. A., Santos, M. S., Leino, R. L., Froberg, M. K., Moreno, A. J., & Wallace, K. B. (2004). Carvedilol-mediated antioxidant protection against doxorubicin-induced cardiac mitochondrial toxicity. *Toxicol Appl Pharmacol* 200. 2: 159-68.

Oliveira, P. J., Esteves, T. C., Seica, R., Moreno, A. J., & Santos, M. S. (2004). Calcium-dependent mitochondrial permeability transition is augmented in the kidney of Goto-Kakizaki diabetic rat. *Diabetes Metab Res Rev* 20. 2: 131-6.

Oliveira, P. J., Rolo, A. P., Seica, R., Palmeira, C. M., Santos, M. S., & Moreno, A. J. (2001). Decreased susceptibility of heart mitochondria from diabetic GK rats to mitochondrial permeability transition induced by calcium phosphate. *Biosci Rep* 21. 1: 45-53.

Oliveira, P. J., Santos, M. S., & Wallace, K. B. (2006). Doxorubicin-induced thiol-dependent alteration of cardiac mitochondrial permeability transition and respiration. *Biochemistry (Mosc)* 71. 2: 194-9.

Oliveira, P. J., Seica, R., Coxito, P. M., Rolo, A. P., Palmeira, C. M., Santos, M. S., & Moreno, A. J. (2003). Enhanced permeability transition explains the reduced calcium uptake in cardiac mitochondria from streptozotocin-induced diabetic rats. *FEBS Lett* 554. 3: 511-4.

Oliveira, P. J., & Wallace, K. B. (2006). Depletion of adenine nucleotide translocator protein in heart mitochondria from doxorubicin-treated rats--relevance for mitochondrial dysfunction. *Toxicology* 220. 2-3: 160-8.

Olson, H. M., & Capen, C. C. (1978). Chemoresponsiveness of Moloney sarcoma virus-induced osteosarcoma to adriamycin in the rat. *Cancer Res* 38. 6: 1561-7.

Palmeira, C. M., Santos, D. L., Seica, R., Moreno, A. J., & Santos, M. S. (2001). Enhanced mitochondrial testicular antioxidant capacity in Goto-Kakizaki diabetic rats: role of coenzyme Q. *Am J Physiol Cell Physiol* 281. 3: C1023-8.

Pardo Andreu, G. L., Inada, N. M., Vercesi, A. E., & Curti, C. (2009). Uncoupling and oxidative stress in liver mitochondria isolated from rats with acute iron overload. *Arch Toxicol* 83. 1: 47-53.

Parzefall, W. (2002). Risk assessment of dioxin contamination in human food. *Food Chem Toxicol* 40. 8: 1185-9.

Pereira, C. V., Moreira, A. C., Pereira, S. P., Machado, N. G., Carvalho, F. S., Sardao, V. A., & Oliveira, P. J. (2009). Investigating drug-induced mitochondrial toxicity: a biosensor to increase drug safety? *Curr Drug Saf* 4. 1: 34-54.

Pereira, G. C., & Oliveira, P. J. (2010). Pharmacological strategies to counteract doxorubicin-induced cardiotoxicity : the role of mitochondria. *Journal of Theoretical and Experimental Pharmacology* 1. 39-53.

Pereira, S. P., Pereira, G. C., Moreno, A. J., & Oliveira, P. J. (2009). Can drug safety be predicted and animal experiments reduced by using isolated mitochondrial fractions? *Altern Lab Anim* 37. 4: 355-65.

Perkins, G., Bossy-Wetzel, E., & Ellisman, M. H. (2009). New insights into mitochondrial structure during cell death. *Exp Neurol* 218. 2: 183-92.

Petersen, K. F., Krssak, M., Inzucchi, S., Cline, G. W., Dufour, S., & Shulman, G. I. (2000). Mechanism of troglitazone action in type 2 diabetes. *Diabetes* 49. 5: 827-31.

Poderoso, J. J. (2009). The formation of peroxynitrite in the applied physiology of mitochondrial nitric oxide. *Arch Biochem Biophys* 484. 2: 214-20.

Praet, M., & Ruysschaert, J. M. (1993). In-vivo and in-vitro mitochondrial membrane damages induced in mice by adriamycin and derivatives. *Biochim Biophys Acta* 1149. 1: 79-85.

Quintana, A., Kruse, S. E., Kapur, R. P., Sanz, E., & Palmiter, R. D. Complex I deficiency due to loss of Ndufs4 in the brain results in progressive encephalopathy resembling Leigh syndrome. *Proc Natl Acad Sci U S A* 107. 24: 10996-1001.

Quintana, E., Mayr, J. A., Garcia Silva, M. T., Font, A., Tortoledo, M. A., Moliner, S., Ozaez, L., Lluch, M., Cabello, A., Ricoy, J. R., Koch, J., Ribes, A., Sperl, W., & Briones, P. (2009). PDH E(1)beta deficiency with novel mutations in two patients with Leigh syndrome. *J Inherit Metab Dis*.

Rachek, L. I., Yuzefovych, L. V., Ledoux, S. P., Julie, N. L., & Wilson, G. L. (2009). Troglitazone, but not rosiglitazone, damages mitochondrial DNA and induces mitochondrial dysfunction and cell death in human hepatocytes. *Toxicol Appl Pharmacol* 240. 3: 348-54.

Rami, A. (2009). Review: autophagy in neurodegeneration: firefighter and/or incendiarist? *Neuropathol Appl Neurobiol* 35. 5: 449-61.

Reddy, P. V., Rao, K. V., & Norenberg, M. D. (2008). The mitochondrial permeability transition, and oxidative and nitrosative stress in the mechanism of copper toxicity in cultured neurons and astrocytes. *Lab Invest* 88. 8: 816-30.

Reich, E., & Luck, D. J. (1966). Replication and inheritance of mitochondrial DNA. *Proc Natl Acad Sci U S A* 55. 6: 1600-8.

Ren, X. Y., Li, Y. N., Qi, J. S., & Niu, T. (2008). Peroxynitrite-induced protein nitration contributes to liver mitochondrial damage in diabetic rats. *J Diabetes Complications* 22. 5: 357-64.

Robinson, D. S., Roberts, D. L., Smith, J. M., Stringfellow, J. C., Kaplita, S. B., Seminara, J. A., & Marcus, R. N. (1996). The safety profile of nefazodone. *J Clin Psychiatry* 57 Suppl 2. 31-8.

Rossignol, R., Faustin, B., Rocher, C., Malgat, M., Mazat, J. P., & Letellier, T. (2003). Mitochondrial threshold effects. *Biochem J* 370. Pt 3: 751-62.

Rossignol, R., Gilkerson, R., Aggeler, R., Yamagata, K., Remington, S. J., & Capaldi, R. A. (2004). Energy substrate modulates mitochondrial structure and oxidative capacity in cancer cells. *Cancer Res* 64. 3: 985-93.

Saelens, X., Festjens, N., Vande Walle, L., van Gurp, M., van Loo, G., & Vandenabeele, P. (2004). Toxic proteins released from mitochondria in cell death. *Oncogene* 23. 16: 2861-74.

Santos, D. L., Palmeira, C. M., Seica, R., Dias, J., Mesquita, J., Moreno, A. J., & Santos, M. S. (2003). Diabetes and mitochondrial oxidative stress: a study using heart mitochondria from the diabetic Goto-Kakizaki rat. *Mol Cell Biochem* 246. 1-2: 163-70.

Sardao, V. A., Oliveira, P. J., Holy, J., Oliveira, C. R., & Wallace, K. B. (2009). Morphological alterations induced by doxorubicin on H9c2 myoblasts: nuclear, mitochondrial, and cytoskeletal targets. *Cell Biol Toxicol* 25. 3: 227-43.

Sawyer, D. B., Peng, X., Chen, B., Pentassuglia, L., & Lim, C. C. (2010). Mechanisms of anthracycline cardiac injury: can we identify strategies for cardioprotection? *Prog Cardiovasc Dis* 53. 2: 105-13.

Scatena, R., Bottoni, P., Botta, G., Martorana, G. E., & Giardina, B. (2007). The role of mitochondria in pharmacotoxicology: a reevaluation of an old, newly emerging topic. *Am J Physiol Cell Physiol* 293. 1: C12-21.

Scatena, R., Bottoni, P., Martorana, G. E., Ferrari, F., De Sole, P., Rossi, C., & Giardina, B. (2004). Mitochondrial respiratory chain dysfunction, a non-receptor-mediated effect of synthetic PPAR-ligands: biochemical and pharmacological implications. *Biochem Biophys Res Commun* 319. 3: 967-73.

Scatena, R., Martorana, G. E., Bottoni, P., & Giardina, B. (2004). Mitochondrial dysfunction by synthetic ligands of peroxisome proliferator activated receptors (PPARs). *IUBMB Life* 56. 8: 477-82.

Schaars, C. F., & Stalenhoef, A. F. (2008). Effects of ubiquinone (coenzyme Q10) on myopathy in statin users. *Curr Opin Lipidol* 19. 6: 553-7.

Schug, Z. T., & Gottlieb, E. (2009). Cardiolipin acts as a mitochondrial signalling platform to launch apoptosis. *Biochim Biophys Acta* 1788. 10: 2022-31.

Seachrist, J. L., Loi, C. M., Evans, M. G., Criswell, K. A., & Rothwell, C. E. (2005). Roles of exercise and pharmacokinetics in cerivastatin-induced skeletal muscle toxicity. *Toxicol Sci* 88. 2: 551-61.

Senft, A. P., Dalton, T. P., Nebert, D. W., Genter, M. B., Hutchinson, R. J., & Shertzer, H. G. (2002). Dioxin increases reactive oxygen production in mouse liver mitochondria. *Toxicol Appl Pharmacol* 178. 1: 15-21.

Senft, A. P., Dalton, T. P., Nebert, D. W., Genter, M. B., Puga, A., Hutchinson, R. J., Kerzee, J. K., Uno, S., & Shertzer, H. G. (2002). Mitochondrial reactive oxygen production is dependent on the aromatic hydrocarbon receptor. *Free Radic Biol Med* 33. 9: 1268-78.

Shadel, G. S. (2005). Mitochondrial DNA, aconitase 'wraps' it up. *Trends Biochem Sci* 30. 6: 294-6.

Sharaf El Dein, O., Gallerne, C., Deniaud, A., Brenner, C., & Lemaire, C. (2009). Role of the permeability transition pore complex in lethal inter-organelle crosstalk. *Front Biosci* 14. 3465-82.

Shen, D., Dalton, T. P., Nebert, D. W., & Shertzer, H. G. (2005). Glutathione redox state regulates mitochondrial reactive oxygen production. *J Biol Chem* 280. 27: 25305-12.

Shenker, B. J., Guo, T. L., & Shapiro, I. M. (1998). Low-level methylmercury exposure causes human T-cells to undergo apoptosis: evidence of mitochondrial dysfunction. *Environ Res* 77. 2: 149-59.

Sheridan, C., & Martin, S. J. (2010). Mitochondrial fission/fusion dynamics and apoptosis. *Mitochondrion* 10. 6: 640-8.

Shertzer, H. G., Genter, M. B., Shen, D., Nebert, D. W., Chen, Y., & Dalton, T. P. (2006). TCDD decreases ATP levels and increases reactive oxygen production through changes in mitochondrial F(0)F(1)-ATP synthase and ubiquinone. *Toxicol Appl Pharmacol* 217. 3: 363-74.

Shi, L. M., Jiang, H., Wang, J., Ma, Z. G., & Xie, J. X. (2008). Mitochondria dysfunction was involved in copper-induced toxicity in MES23.5 cells. *Neurosci Bull* 24. 2: 79-83.

Singal, P. K., Iliskovic, N., Li, T., & Kumar, D. (1997). Adriamycin cardiomyopathy: pathophysiology and prevention. *FASEB J* 11. 12: 931-6.

Solaini, G., Baracca, A., Lenaz, G., & Sgarbi, G. (2010). Hypoxia and mitochondrial oxidative metabolism. *Biochim Biophys Acta* 1797. 6-7: 1171-7.

Son, Y. O., Lee, J. C., Hitron, J. A., Pan, J., Zhang, Z., & Shi, X. (2011). Cadmium induces intracellular Ca2+- and H2O2-dependent apoptosis through JNK- and p53-mediated pathways in skin epidermal cell line. *Toxicol Sci* 113. 1: 127-37.

Soubannier, V., & McBride, H. M. (2009). Positioning mitochondrial plasticity within cellular signaling cascades. *Biochim Biophys Acta* 1793. 1: 154-70.

Souza, M. E., Polizello, A. C., Uyemura, S. A., Castro-Silva, O., & Curti, C. (1994). Effect of fluoxetine on rat liver mitochondria. *Biochem Pharmacol* 48. 3: 535-41.
Steiner, G. (2007). Atherosclerosis in type 2 diabetes: a role for fibrate therapy? *Diab Vasc Dis Res* 4. 4: 368-74.
Stohs, S. J., Alsharif, N. Z., Shara, M. A., al-Bayati, Z. A., & Wahba, Z. Z. (1991). Evidence for the induction of an oxidative stress in rat hepatic mitochondria by 2,3,7,8-tetrachlorodibenzo-p-dioxin (TCDD). *Adv Exp Med Biol* 283. 827-31.
Stohs, S. J., & Bagchi, D. (1995). Oxidative mechanisms in the toxicity of metal ions. *Free Radic Biol Med* 18. 2: 321-36.
Sweeney, M. H., & Mocarelli, P. (2000). Human health effects after exposure to 2,3,7,8-TCDD. *Food Addit Contam* 17. 4: 303-16.
Szabados, E., Fischer, G. M., Toth, K., Csete, B., Nemeti, B., Trombitas, K., Habon, T., Endrei, D., & Sumegi, B. (1999). Role of reactive oxygen species and poly-ADP-ribose polymerase in the development of AZT-induced cardiomyopathy in rat. *Free Radic Biol Med* 26. 3-4: 309-17.
Tait, S. W., & Green, D. R. (2010). Mitochondria and cell death: outer membrane permeabilization and beyond. *Nat Rev Mol Cell Biol* 11. 9: 621-32.
Tirmenstein, M. A., Hu, C. X., Gales, T. L., Maleeff, B. E., Narayanan, P. K., Kurali, E., Hart, T. K., Thomas, H. C., & Schwartz, L. W. (2002). Effects of troglitazone on HepG2 viability and mitochondrial function. *Toxicol Sci* 69. 1: 131-8.
Tokarska-Schlattner, M., Zaugg, M., Zuppinger, C., Wallimann, T., & Schlattner, U. (2006). New insights into doxorubicin-induced cardiotoxicity: the critical role of cellular energetics. *J Mol Cell Cardiol* 41. 3: 389-405.
Turko, I. V., Li, L., Aulak, K. S., Stuehr, D. J., Chang, J. Y., & Murad, F. (2003). Protein tyrosine nitration in the mitochondria from diabetic mouse heart. Implications to dysfunctional mitochondria in diabetes. *J Biol Chem* 278. 36: 33972-7.
Twig, G., Graf, S. A., Wikstrom, J. D., Mohamed, H., Haigh, S. E., Elorza, A., Deutsch, M., Zurgil, N., Reynolds, N., & Shirihai, O. S. (2006). Tagging and tracking individual networks within a complex mitochondrial web with photoactivatable GFP. *Am J Physiol Cell Physiol* 291. 1: C176-84.
Ulivieri, C. (2010). Cell death: insights into the ultrastructure of mitochondria. *Tissue Cell* 42. 6: 339-47.
Valenti, D., Atlante, A., Barile, M., & Passarella, S. (2002). Inhibition of phosphate transport in rat heart mitochondria by 3'-azido-3'-deoxythymidine due to stimulation of superoxide anion mitochondrial production. *Biochem Pharmacol* 64. 2: 201-6.
Valenti, D., Barile, M., & Passarella, S. (2000). AZT inhibition of the ADP/ATP antiport in isolated rat heart mitochondria. *Int J Mol Med* 6. 1: 93-6.
Van Houten, B., Woshner, V., & Santos, J. H. (2006). Role of mitochondrial DNA in toxic responses to oxidative stress. *DNA Repair (Amst)* 5. 2: 145-52.
Velho, J. A., Okanobo, H., Degasperi, G. R., Matsumoto, M. Y., Alberici, L. C., Cosso, R. G., Oliveira, H. C., & Vercesi, A. E. (2006). Statins induce calcium-dependent mitochondrial permeability transition. *Toxicology* 219. 1-3: 124-32.
Vockley, J., & Whiteman, D. A. (2002). Defects of mitochondrial beta-oxidation: a growing group of disorders. *Neuromuscul Disord* 12. 3: 235-46.
Walker, U. A., Bauerle, J., Laguno, M., Murillas, J., Mauss, S., Schmutz, G., Setzer, B., Miquel, R., Gatell, J. M., & Mallolas, J. (2004). Depletion of mitochondrial DNA in liver

under antiretroviral therapy with didanosine, stavudine, or zalcitabine. *Hepatology* 39. 2: 311-7.

Wallace, D. C. (2000). Mitochondrial defects in cardiomyopathy and neuromuscular disease. *Am Heart J* 139. 2 Pt 3: S70-85.

Wallace, D. C., & Fan, W. (2010). Energetics, epigenetics, mitochondrial genetics. *Mitochondrion* 10. 1: 12-31.

Wallace, K. B. (2003). Doxorubicin-induced cardiac mitochondrionopathy. *Pharmacol Toxicol* 93. 3: 105-15.

Wallace, K. B. (2008). Mitochondrial off targets of drug therapy. *Trends Pharmacol Sci* 29. 7: 361-6.

Wallenborn, J. G., Schladweiler, M. J., Richards, J. H., & Kodavanti, U. P. (2009). Differential pulmonary and cardiac effects of pulmonary exposure to a panel of particulate matter-associated metals. *Toxicol Appl Pharmacol* 241. 1: 71-80.

Wang, C., & Youle, R. J. (2009). The role of mitochondria in apoptosis*. *Annu Rev Genet* 43. 95-118.

Warburg, O. (1930). The Metabolism of Tumors. London, Arnold Constable.

Warburg, O. (1956). On respiratory impairment in cancer cells. *Science* 124. 3215: 269-70.

Warburg, O. (1956). On the origin of cancer cells. *Science* 123. 3191: 309-14.

Wenner, C. E., & Weinhouse, S. (1953). Metabolism of neoplastic tissue. III. Diphosphopyridine nucleotide requirements for oxidations by mitochondria of neoplastic and non-neoplastic tissues. *Cancer Res* 13. 1: 21-6.

Westwood, F. R., Bigley, A., Randall, K., Marsden, A. M., & Scott, R. C. (2005). Statin-induced muscle necrosis in the rat: distribution, development, and fibre selectivity. *Toxicol Pathol* 33. 2: 246-57.

Will, Y., Hynes, J., Ogurtsov, V. I., & Papkovsky, D. B. (2006). Analysis of mitochondrial function using phosphorescent oxygen-sensitive probes. *Nat Protoc* 1. 6: 2563-72.

Wong, W. W., & Puthalakath, H. (2008). Bcl-2 family proteins: the sentinels of the mitochondrial apoptosis pathway. *IUBMB Life* 60. 6: 390-7.

Wu, W. Z., Li, W., Xu, Y., & Wang, J. W. (2001). Long-term toxic impact of 2,3,7,8-tetrachlorodibenzo-p-dioxin on the reproduction, sexual differentiation, and development of different life stages of Gobiocypris rarus and Daphnia magna. *Ecotoxicol Environ Saf* 48. 3: 293-300.

Yeung, S. J., Pan, J., & Lee, M. H. (2008). Roles of p53, MYC and HIF-1 in regulating glycolysis - the seventh hallmark of cancer. *Cell Mol Life Sci* 65. 24: 3981-99.

Yoon, S. B., Kajiyama, K., Hino, Y., Sugiyama, M., & Ogura, R. (1983). Effect of adriamycin on lipid peroxide, glutathione peroxidase and respiratory responses of mitochondria from the heart, liver and kidney. *Kurume Med J* 30. 1: 1-4.

Youle, R. J., & Narendra, D. P. (2011). Mechanisms of mitophagy. *Nat Rev Mol Cell Biol* 12. 1: 9-14.

Zhou, G., Myers, R., Li, Y., Chen, Y., Shen, X., Fenyk-Melody, J., Wu, M., Ventre, J., Doebber, T., Fujii, N., Musi, N., Hirshman, M. F., Goodyear, L. J., & Moller, D. E. (2001). Role of AMP-activated protein kinase in mechanism of metformin action. *J Clin Invest* 108. 8: 1167-74.

Zhou, S., Starkov, A., Froberg, M. K., Leino, R. L., & Wallace, K. B. (2001). Cumulative and irreversible cardiac mitochondrial dysfunction induced by doxorubicin. *Cancer Res* 61. 2: 771-7.

Zick, M., Rabl, R., & Reichert, A. S. (2009). Cristae formation-linking ultrastructure and function of mitochondria. *Biochim Biophys Acta* 1793. 1: 5-19.

Zorov, D. B., Juhaszova, M., Yaniv, Y., Nuss, H. B., Wang, S., & Sollott, S. J. (2009). Regulation and pharmacology of the mitochondrial permeability transition pore. *Cardiovasc Res* 83. 2: 213-25.

20

Electrochemical Biosensors to Monitor Extracellular Glutamate and Acetylcholine Concentration in Brain Tissue

Alberto Morales Villagrán, Silvia J. López Pérez and Jorge Ortega Ibarra
University of Guadalajara
México

1. Introduction

Glutamate (Glu) is considered the main excitatory neurotransmitter in the central nervous system and has a relevant role in several brain functions such as, synaptic plasticity, learning and memory processes (Bliss & Collingride, 1993; Fonnum, 1984; Nakanishi, 1992). Excessive release of Glu and over stimulation of its receptors has been associated with several neurological alterations including such as schizophrenia, Parkinson´s disease, stroke and epilepsy (Carlsson & Carlson, 1990; Klockgether & Turski, 1993; Dávalos et al., 2000, Morales-Villagrán, et al., 1996; Morales-Villagrán, et al., 2008). Another fast neurotransmitter; acetylcholine (Ach) has also been involved in learning and memory (Van Der Zee & Luiten, 1999), as well as a modulating agent in seizure activity, since positive stimulation of muscarinic receptor M1 could initiate generalized seizures in the basal diencephalon of the rat. (Cruickshank et al., 1994). Likewise, direct application of the agonist pilocarpine in brain tissue could produce seizures (Turski et al., 1989). To understand better the role of these fast acting neurotransmitters during normal or pathological activity, it is fundamental to precisely measure these compounds in brain tissue with high specificity and temporal resolution. Conventional analysis tools are all bulk-average-based methods, which means that the signals taken are an estimation of several physiological events that happen in a certain period of time, generally a few minutes. Microdialysis technique has been used to measure their extracellular brain concentrations; both in normal as well as in pathological conditions and these measurements are generally coupled to High performance liquid chromatography method (HPLC). However, such a technique is time consuming an especial training is required. Several methods coupled to enzymatic reactions that generate Hydrogen peroxide (H_2O_2) could be another alternative to measure some neurotransmitters, since numerous specific oxidases generate H_2O_2 as product, acting over certain neurotransmitters and avoiding the separation process. Measurement could be possible with fluorescence technique, like the use of the fluorogenic probe 10-acetyl-3,7-dihydroxiphenoxazine (AMPLEX RED), which reacts with H_2O_2 in the presence of horseradish peroxidase in 1:1 stoichiometry to produce a highly fluorescence product resorufin (Zhou, et a., 1997; Mohanty et al., 1997), which can be measured in a plate reader or in a fluorometer (In-vitrogen) but also a fraction collection of samples is required and the

time resolution will depend on the frequency of such a collection. Similarly, an alternative method to measure the H_2O_2 produced by enzymatic reactions is the use of an electrochemical detection system with about the same time resolution (Morales-Villagrán, et al., 2008a). To study the rapid neurochemical alterations during brain activity, the demand of rapid, reliable and sensitive determination of Glu and Ach is still a needing process. To overcome the necessity of fraction collection and to estimate these neurotransmitters concentration during the brain activity and near a real time resolution, the use of an enzymatic biosensor is merging.
These kind of biosensors are generally built with the same principle mentioned above, this is, they are constructed with specific enzymes that react with Glu and Ach to produce H_2O_2. In this chapter, it is described the process to built biosensors to monitor Glu and Ach during altered brain activity under the effect of 4AP.

2. Biosensor preparation

Electrochemical biosensors are prepared according to the method of Hu et al., (1994) with several modifications. A 125 μm diameter platinum (Pt) wire 13 mm in length is inserted into a fused silica tubing (175 μm i.d., 400 μm o.d.) to strengthen the wire. To accomplish an electrical component a copper wire should be soldered to one end of the platinum wire covered with epoxic glue to insulate this terminal. Two mm of Pt wire extending outside the tubing is used as an active biosensor surface. Pt wire is covered with a film of a nafion solution at 5.0 %, the tip is heated for 3 minutes (~170 ^{o}C) and after ten minutes a film of cellulose acetate 5.0 % should be applied (acetone/ethanol 2:1). Biosensors are left at room temperature before fixing the enzymes. At this point, biosensors for Glu or Ach can be prepared using different enzymes, to determine Glu, twenty μl of enzyme mixture are prepared in 20 mM of potassium buffer phosphate solution containing: 2% L-Glutamate oxidase, 0.3 % ascorbate oxidase, 5% porcine skin gelatin and albumin (2 %). This mixture was deposited on a glass surface and 5 μl of 0.0625% glutaraldehyde was added and gently shaken, the platinum wire tips were immediately immersed deep into this solution. To determine Ach, a different mixture of enzymes is prepared containing 0.4% acetycholinesterase and 0.2% choline oxidase, albumin, ascorbate oxidase and porcine skin and glutaraldehyde are at the same concentration. Theses biosensors are dried at 37 ^{o}C for 30 minutes and are kept at 4 ^{o}C before using. Biosensors kept at this temperature condition retain their activity beyond than one moth.
Biosensor calibrations are carried out in a beaker, immersing a working electrode (biosensor), reference and counter electrodes in 20 mM potassium buffer solution with continuous shaking at room temperature. In this case, the formed cell was then connected to an electrochemical detector LC 4B (Bionalytical Systems), although it can be connected to any potentiostat. The electrical analogical signal coming out from the detector (voltage) can be digitized with a regular chromatographic software. It is necessary to reach a baseline value before doing any attempt of calibration. Different aliquots of Glu or Ach are added to an individual beaker to get a calibration reference. In fig 1 (A and B) calibrations for Glu and Ach are despicted. These biosensors were calibrated in vitro by increasing the substrate concentration in the range specified. Every step represents a single addition of Glu (A) or Ach (B). A linear regression analysis was done (inset) and the R-values calculated were 0.9

and 0.99, respectively. The total voltage scale corresponds to a generated current of 20 nA for Glu and 30 nA for Ach calibrations, corresponding to 50 nA/V. These results show that biosensors are adequate for their use *in vivo* conditions.

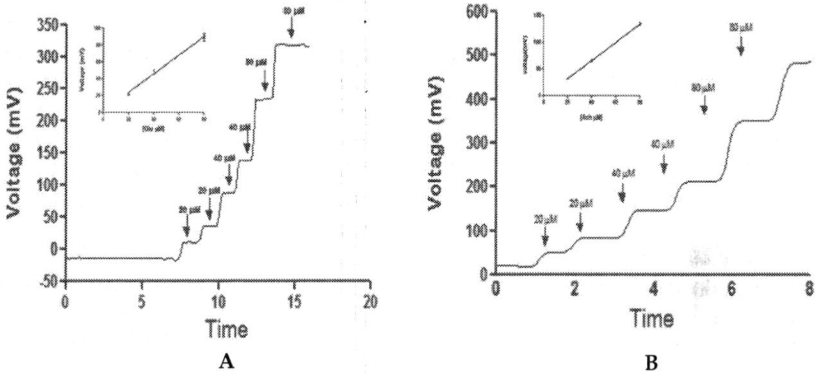

Fig. 1. Calibration curves for Glu (A) and Ach (B).

With respect to the speed of neurotransmitters measurement with these biosensors, time resolution was evaluated as the beginning of the response in each concentration until they reached a maximum value, this time was approximately of 20 seconds.

3. Animal studies

These biosensors can be used under anesthesia or in awake animals, as shown here. For Glu, biosensors were implanted into the cerebral cortex of rat pups (at three postnatal day) under anesthesia, in a three electrodes arrangement working, reference and counter, in order to accomplish an electrochemical cell *in situ*. Every biosensor must be calibrated before its use. Once the animal is recovered from anesthesia, the terminal of each electrode is connected to the potentiostat through a socket connector and after of an equilibration period to reach a baseline, the animal is ready to monitor the Glu extracellular concentration into the brain in any experimental condition. In the example showed here, the effect of subcutaneous monosodium glutamate administration in neonate rast (5mg/Kg of body weigh) was initially tested, resulting in a rise in extracelluar Glu concentration (Fig. 2A), this Glu elevation lasted approximately 20 minutes.

In previous work it has been demonstrated that in immature brain the blood brain barrier is not completely developed (Cernak, 2010) besides the high Glu concentration used is enough to disrupt the barrier due to an osmotic effect, similar effect has been found with the use of manitol (Rapoport, 2000). Additionally in our previous work, it was showed that similar dose of monosodium glutamate can induce important rise in brain extracellular Glu concentration tested by internal biosensor and HPLC methods (Lopez-Perez et al., 2010). In order to induce seizures convulsion an additional systemic injection of 4-AP (3mg/kg of body way) was used, whose effect can be seen in the right side of the fig. 2A. It can be observed that after injecting the convulsant drug (50 min after starting recording) an increase in the extracellular Glu concentration is present that could be related to the intensity of seizure activity.

To test Ach biosensors, adult rats were used; they were also implanted with three electrodes, with the only difference that the working electrode was covered with necessary enzymes to determine Ach, and in this case the area of interest was the right thalamus. After a recovery period from anesthesia that lasted at least two hours, the animal is connected in a similar way as mentioned above to monitor extracellular Ach concentration during seizure activity, characterized by strong motor alterations like tonic-clonic convulsions. In the example showed here a baseline period of twenty minutes was recorded before testing the effect of 4-AP administration at 5 mg/kg of body (intraperitoneally). After the convulsant drug administration significant increments in Ach appeared that were also related with strong seizure behavior activity, this effect lasted about one hour (Fig. 2B) and finally the animal were euthanized with an intraperitoneal injection of pentobarbital. The examples showed here represent independent animal trials for Glu and Ach, respectively.

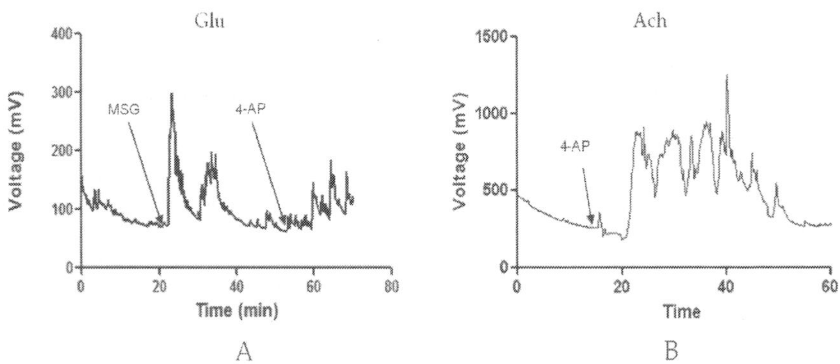

Fig. 2. Glu biosensor (A) and Ach biosensor (B) register during altered brain activity *in vivo*.

To evaluate the specificity of these biosensors, several controls can be run; one example is to test the response in vitro of these biosensors to other molecules that could produce a nonspecific signal, like monoamines and ascorbic acid, since without a good preparation a false positive result could appear. An example of such control for Ach biosensor is showed in Fig. 3A, the first two arrows represent additions of 300 μM concentration of ascorbic acid (Aa) and the two following of 80 μM Ach, they are represented by the next two arrows; it can be seen that this biosensor response specifically to Ach. Other way to test the specificity of a biosensor *in vivo* is to use one without enzymes in the cover; such naked or sentinel biosensor will not be able to sense any neurotransmitter concentration during any physiological conditions (Hascup et al., 2008) or calibration procedure. An example is showed in Fig. 3B, were a naked biosensor was inserted in the brain of an adult animal, this animal was treated with 4-AP, despite of the fact of appearance of strong seizure convulsion no any increase of Ach was detected with this biosensor. Spikes in graph B represent movement artifacts during convulsions. Similar analyses were done for Glu biosensors.

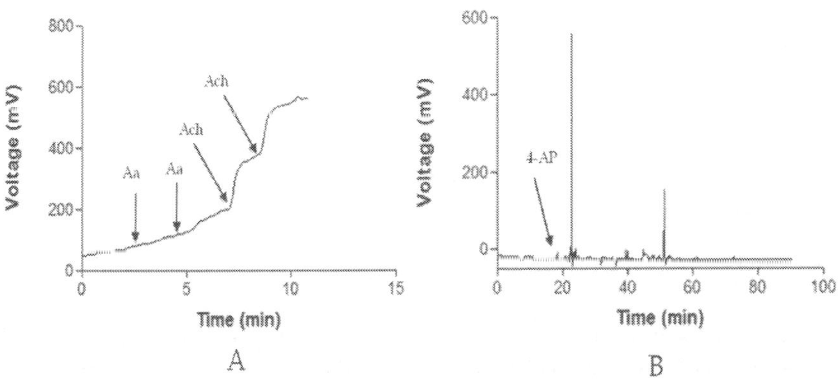

Fig. 3. Specificity test for Ach biosensor *in vitro* (A) and test of a naked or "sentinel" biosensor *in vivo* (B)

4. Conclusions

The use of electrochemical biosensors to monitor neurotransmitters concentration during normal or pathological activity in brain is an alternative approach that is gaining new users, besides, different strategies to fix enzymes over several substrates are merging, like the use of sol gel derivates or other casting materials (Sakai-Kato & Ishikura, 2009; Hyun-Jung et al., 2010). This is a very important issue; this is trying to get biosensors that last active for more prolonged periods, which could overcome the necessity to monitor the neurotransmitter concentration for prolonged time or improving the way of fixing the necessary enzymes with more molecular movements that could allow such enzymes have more activity, since in general a fixed enzyme protein decreases its activity. Recent advances in the use of gold nanoparticles due to their increased surface area to enhance interactions with biological molecules, geometric and physical properties make them another alternative to prepare biosensors (Yang et al., 2009). With the procedure used here to monitor Glu and Ach it is shown that it is possible to evaluate the role of these fast neurotransmitters during seizure activity, since the increased release of these compounds have been related with the presence of a convulsive state, these neurotransmitter alterations have been determined with other methods, like microdialysis coupled to HPLC and pharmacological studies (Morales-Villagrán & Tapia 1996; Morales-Villagrán, et al., 1996), data that match well with the results showed here, although the main difference is that using biosensors for monitoring the brain the procedure can be done during a real time and with improved resolution. This work was supported by CONACyT project # 105 807.

5. References

Bliss T. & Collingridge G. 1993. A synaptic model of memory: long-term potentiation in the hippocampus. *Nature*. Vol. 361, No. 64D7, (January 1993), pp. 31-39, ISSN 0028-0836.

Carlsson M. & Carlsson A. 1990. Schizophrenia: a subcortical neurotransmitter imbalance syndrome? *Schizophrenia Bulletin* Vol. 16, No. 3, (September 1990), pp. 425-432, ISSN 0586-7614

Cernak I., Chang T., Ahmed F., Cruz M., Vink R., Stoica B., & Faden A. 2010. Pathophysiological response to experimental diffuse brain trauma differs as a function of developmental age. *Development Neuroscience,* Vol. 32, No. 5-6, (October 2010) pp. 442-53, ISSN 0378-5866.

Cruickshank J., Brudzynski S., & McLachlan R. 1994. Involvement of M1 muscarinic receptors in the initiation of cholinergically induced epileptic seizures in the rat brain. *Brain Research,* Vol. 643, No. 1-2 (April 1994), pp. 125-129, ISSN 0006-8993.

Dávalos A., Shuaib A. & Wahlgren N. 2000. Neurotransmitters and pathophysiology of stroke: evidence for the release of glutamate and other transmitters/mediators in animals and humans. *Journal of Stroke and Cerebrovascular Disease,* Vol. 9, No. 6, (November 2000), pp. 2-8, ISSN 1532-8511.

Fonnum F. 1984. Glutamate: a neurotransmitter in mammalian brain. *Journal of Neurochemistry,* Vol. 42, No. 1, (January 1994), pp 1-11, ISSN 0022-3042.

Hascup N., Hascup E., Pomerleau F., Huettl P. & Gerhardt G. 2008. Second-by-second measures of L-Glutamate in the prefrontal cortex and striatum of freely moving mice. *The Journal of Pharmacology and Experimental Therapeutics,* Vol. 324, No. 2, (February 2008), pp. 725-731, ISSN 1521-0103.

Hu Y., Mitchell K., Albahadily F., Michaelis E. & Wilson G. 1994. Direct measurement of glutamate release in the brain using a dual enzyme-based electrochemical sensor. *Brain Research*, Vol. 659, No. 1-2, (October 1994), pp. 117-125, ISSN 0006-8993.

Kim H., Kim A. & Jeon S. 2010. Immobilization on chitosan of a thermophilic trehalose synthase from thermos thermophilus HJ6. *Journal of Microbiology and Biotechnology*, Vol. 20, No. 3, (March 2010), pp. 513-517, ISSN 1017-7825.

Klockgether T. & Turski L. 1993. Toward an understanding of the role of glutamate in experimental Parkinsonism: agonist-sensitive sites in the basal ganglia. *Annals of Neurology*, Vol. 34, No. 4, (October 1993), pp. 585-593, ISSN 0364-5134.

López-Pérez S., Ureña-Guerrero M. & Morales-Villagrán A. 2010. Monosodium glutamate neonatal treatment as a seizure and excitotoxic model. *Brain Research*, Vol. 1317, (March 2010), pp. 246-256, ISSN 1872-6240.

Morales-Villagrán A. & Tapia R. 1996. Preferential stimulation of glutamate release by 4-Aminopyridine in rat striatum in vivo. *Neurochemistry International*, Vol. 28, No. 1, (January 1996), pp. 35-40, ISSN 0197-0186.

Morales-Villagrán A., Ureña-Guerrero M. & Tapia R. 1996. Protection by NMDA receptor antagonist against seizure induced by intracerebral administration of 4-aminopyridine. *European Journal of Pharmacology*, Vol. 305, No. 1-3, (June 1996), pp. 87-93, ISSN 0014-2999.

Morales-Villagrán A., Sandoval-Salazar C. & Medina-Ceja L. 2008a. An analytical flow injection system to measure glutamate in microdialysis samples based on an enzymatic reaction and electrochemical detection. *Neurochemical Research*, Vol. 33, No. 8, (August 2008), pp. 1592-1598, ISSN 1573-6903.

Morales-Villagrán A., Medina-Ceja L. & López-Pérez S. 2008b. Simultaneous glutamate and EEG activity measurements during seizures in rat hippocampal region with the use of an electrochemical biosensor. *Journal of Neuroscience Methods*, Vol. 168, No. 1, (February 2008), pp. 48-53, ISSN 0165-0270.

Nakanishi S. 1992. Molecular diversity of glutamate receptors and implications for brain function. *Science*, Vol. 258, No. 5082, (October 1992), pp. 597-603, ISSN 0036-8075.

Rapoport S. 2000. Osmotic opening of the blood-brain barrier: principles, mechanism, and therapeutic applications. *Cellular and Molecular Neurobiology*, Vol. 20, No. 2, (April 2000), pp. 217-30, ISSN 0272-4340.

Sakai-Kato S and Ishikura K. 2009. Integration of biomolecules into analytical systems by means of silical sol-gel technology. *Analytical Science*, Vol. 25, No. 8, (August 2009), pp.969-978, ISSN 1348-2246.

Turski L., Ikonomidou C., Turski W., Bortolotto Z- & Cavalheiro E. 1989. Review: cholinergic mechanisms and epileptogenesis. The seizures induced by pilocarpine: a novel experimental model of intractable epilepsy. *Synapse*, Vol. 3, No. 2, (January 1989), pp. 154-171, ISSN 0887-4476.

Van der Zee E. & Luiten P. 1999. Muscarinic acetylcholine receptors in the hippocampus, neocortex and amygdala: a review of immunocytochemical localization in relation to learning and memory: *Progress in Neurobiology*, Vol. 58, No. 5, (August 1999), pp. 409-471, ISSN 0301-0082.

Yang M., Kostov Y., Bruck H. & Rassooly A. 2009. Gold nanoparticle-base enhanced chemiluminescence immunosensor for detection of staphylococcal enterotoxin B (SEB) in food. *International Journal of Food Microbiology*, Vol. 133, No. 3, (August 2009), pp. 265-271, ISSN 1879-3460.

21

Surface Plasmon Resonance Biotechnology for Antimicrobial Susceptibility Test

How-foo Chen[1], Chi-Hung Lin[2,3,4], Chun-Yao Su[1], Hsin-Pai Chen[5] and Ya-Ling Chiang[1]
[1]*Institute of Biophotonics, National Yang Ming University, Taipei*
[2]*Institute of Microbiology & Immunology, National Yang Ming University, Taipei*
[3]*Taipei City Hospital*
[4]*Department of Surgery, Veteran General Hospital, Taipei*
[5]*Department of Medicine, National Yang-Ming University Hospital, Yilan, Taiwan and School of Medicine, National Yang-Ming University*
Taiwan

1. Introduction

Infectious diseases are a leading cause of morbidity and mortality in hospitalized patients. This fact has placed a tremendous burden on the clinical microbiology laboratory to rapidly diagnose the agent responsible for patient's infection and to effectively provide therapeutic guidance for eradication of the microorganisms. Laboratories are expected to perform these tasks in a cost-effective and efficient manner. Two common methodologies for antimicrobial susceptibility testing in a clinical laboratory are Kirby-Bauer disk diffusion and variations of broth microdilution. The principle is based on the detection of bacterium reproduction ability under the influence of antibiotics. Therefore the testing time is determined by the doubling time of tested bacteria. These methods then usually take from one day to weeks to complete the examination. The long incubation period is inevitable for these conventional methods. Such a waiting period is not short for clinical doctors who urgently need the information to adjust the therapeutic strategy. Therefore it is important to explore new template and technology to perform an antimicrobial susceptibility test.

Surface plasmon resonance biosensing technique is well known for its characteristics of label-free, ultra-sensitive, and real-time detection capability. Thus this technique is considered as the candidate of the new platform. Surface plasmon polaritons (SPPs) was first theoretically predicted by Ritchie in 1957 (Ritchie,1957) based on the analysis of surface electromagnetic modes. The SPPs in general can be generated by electrons (Powell & Swan, 1959) or by light (Otto, 1968) under a proper excitation condition. For SPPs excited by light, in general, the dispersion characteristic of SPPs does not allow the energy of a propagation wave coupled into this surface mode: The spatial phase of a propagation wave is always smaller than that of the surface mode with the same optical frequency on a dielectric-metal interface. Thus an evanescence wave generated by a p-polarized light beam through a prism is suggested to obtain an extra spatial phase and then excite SPPs on the other surface of the metal layer. An alternative method to provide the additional spatial phase is through the aid of a grating, of which the sub-wavelength periodic structure can provide additional spatial phase. For the past two decades, SPPs excited by light has been widely applied to the study of biomaterial processes, which include biosensors, immunodiagnostics, and kinetic analysis of antibody-antigen interaction (Davies, 1996; Rich & Myszka, 2005). The main application of SPR biosensors on biomedical science is to analyze the binding dynamics between specific antibody and antigen (Davies, 1996; Rich & Myszka, 2005; Safsten et al., 2006; Misono & Kumar, 2005). Since the mode characteristics of SPPs depend on the refractive index of the material within the dielectric-metal interface of about one hundred nanometers, the refractive index of the material determines the resonance incident angle of light, the coupling efficiency, the coupling wavelength, and the optical phase of the reflected light. All the physical quantities can be measured by the reflected light, which is the uncoupled part of the incident light. Therefore, a SPR system does not require fluorescence labeling and provides real-time information with very high sensitivity (Chien & Chen, 2004). This also guarantees a very small amount of sample needed for the detection of the refractive index change through a SPR method.

Most of the biomedical applications of SPR focus on detection and identification of biomolecules. Extended applications have been applied to the detection and sorting of cells or bacteria based on the same principle (Takemoto et al., 1996). The capture of the desired biomolecules with or without cells or bacteria attached is achieved through antibodies or aptamers pre-coated on the metal thin film, where the SPR occurs. The enormous applications of SPR on biomedical science using antibody-antigen affinity can be found in Rebecca L. Rich and David G. Myszka's Survay (Rich & Myszka, 2005). For the methods using antibody-antigen binding, specific antibody is required and finding the specific antibody is usually not straight forward. This is the reason that characterization of antibody is still the main reports from utilization of SPPs. This is also an important reason that a method utilizing antibody-antigen interaction is difficult to use for antimicrobial susceptibility test. Different from the studies mentioned above, the method introduced in this chapter does not require pre-coating of specific antibodies. This method is then more versatile and can be used to detect reactions of drugs appearing on cell membranes or cell walls. While current antimicrobial susceptible testing methods take one day or more for a clinical laboratory to report the testing results (Poupard et al., 1994; Levinson & Jawetz, 1989), utilizing surface plasmon resonance significantly reduces the time duration to less than or about one hour of antibiotics treatment based on our experimental study. Antibiotics which modify or damage the cell walls of bacteria, thus, alternate the refractive index of bacterium surfaces.

Differentiation of susceptible strains of bacteria from resistant ones by using surface plasmon resonance (SPR) technique is discussed in this chapter. This technique detects the refractive index change of tested bacteria subject to antibiotics treatment in real time. Instead of detection the antimicrobial susceptibility through the cell doubling time, the SPR biosensor technology is used to detect the biochemical change of tested bacteria. A much shorter time to obtain the test result is achieved. Because of the feasibility of this antimicrobial test method using surface plasmon resonance biosensors, development of new biosensors is also very important.

Escherichia coli JM109 resistant/susceptible to ampicillin and *Staphylococcus epidermidis* resistant/susceptible to tetracycline were chosen for the antimicrobial susceptibility test in this study. Since the surface plasmon resonance is highly sensitive to the change of the refractive index of cells near the cell-metal interface, ampicillin as the antibiotic inhibiting the synthesis of cell walls was used for the examination of *Escherichia coli* JM109. This is designed for the measurement of direct effect of antibiotics on cells. Different from ampicillin, tetracycline works as an inhibitor of protein synthesis. The influence of tetracycline on cell walls and cell membranes is then indirect. Therefore, *Staphylococcus epidermidis* used as another type of bacteria susceptible/resistant to tetracycline was used for the measurement of indirect effect of antibiotics on cells.

2. Devices and methods

The detection principle can be realized on the detection of biochemical change of bacteria subject to antibiotics through the detection of their refractive index. This change on the refractive index of bacteria is achieved by an SPR biosensor. A chemical treatment of Poly-L-Lysine on the surface of the Au thin film in the SPR biosensor is used to trap bacteria. The Poly-L-Lysine layer does not provide specfic binding to select specific bacterium strain so that a pre-purification to select tested bacteria is required for the test. After the tested bacterium strain is trapped on the Poly-L-Lysine layer, antibiotic is appled to examine the antimicroial susceptibility.

2.1 Surface plasmon resonance biosensor

The experimental setup for the examination of drug resistance of the bacteria is shown in Fig. 1(a). The setup is the combination of the two parts: one is for the excitation of the surface plasmon and the other is the flow cell chamber. For the excitation of the surface plasmon, a Helium-Neon laser is used as the light source to provide the laser beam with wavelength 632.8 nm. Since surface plasmon can only be excited by p-polarized light, a polarized beam splitter is used to separate the p-polarized and s-polarized light. The s-polarized light is used as the normalization factor to eliminate the deterioration of measurement accuracy caused by the laser instability. After the polarized beam splitter, the p-polarized light is injected onto the Au thin film through a prism to generate surface plasmon. The required phase matching condition to excite the surface plasmon is provided by the proper incident angle and the prism, which provides an extra spatial phase along the gold film surface through its refractive index of the prism. Matching oil is applied between the prism and the glass substrate coated with the Au thin film to avoid occurrence of multiple reflection between the prism and the glass slide. The excitation efficiency of the surface plasmon by the p-polarized laser beam is measured through the silicon photodetector which receives the reflected p-polarized beam from the Au thin layer. When the surface plasmon resonance angle is reached, the energy of injected laser beam was transformed into the surface plasmon polaritons. Thus, the laser beam reflected from the Au layer reaches minimum. The photocurrent generated from the photodetector is amplified and transformed into a voltage signal via 16-bit A/D converter (Adventech PCI-1716). The intensity, normalized to the intensity of the s-polarized beam, of the reflected p-polarized beam as a function of the incident angle is obtained by the computer. Incident angle was controlled by a motorized rotation stage through a controller. The other arm that is for receiving reflection was controlled accordingly by another rotation stage to measure the power of the reflected beam. The resolution of the system on the change of refractive index of the dielectrics is 1.4×10^{-4} refractive index unit (RIU), which corresponds to the value of the SPR angle shift as 0.00867 degree.

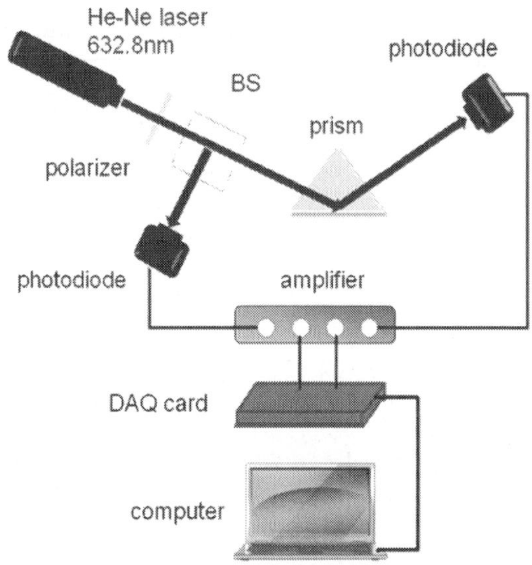

(a)

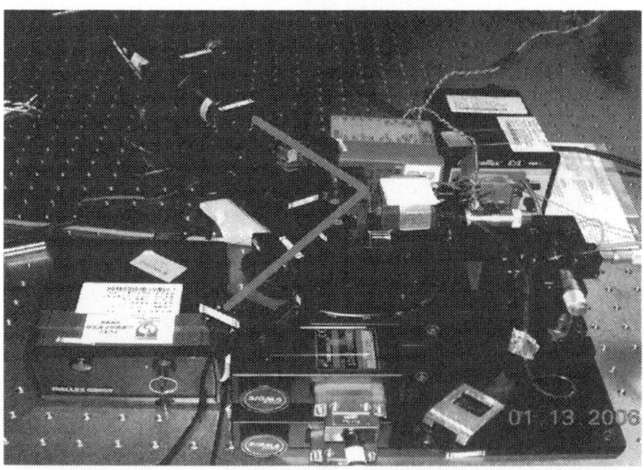

(b)

Fig. 1. SPR biosensor used for the experiment. (a) The configuration of SPR biosensor used in the study. The SPPs was excited by 632.8nm He-Ne laser. A polarizer is used to enhance the extinction of the laser beam polarization. A polarized bean splitter (BS) direct the s-polzaried light into a detector for normalization of laser intensity fluctuation. The p-polarized light is used to excite SPPs. The reflectance of the light is direct to the second detector for measurement of resonance angle, and thus measure the refractive index change of bacteria subject to antibiotics; (b) Picture of the home-made SPR biosensor. The solid red line indicates the laser beam.

2.2 Cell chamber

A flow cell chamber was constructed on the SPR system described above to provide the bacteria for testing, DI water for washing, and the antibiotics for the examination of drug resistance. An O-ring is attached to the chamber to prevent the liquid leakage. A thermister of 10KΩ is used to monitor the temperature of the chamber and a TE cooler is used to control the temperature by receiving the temperature information from the thermister. The temperature of the cell chamber was controlled with the fluctuation less than 0.1 ^{o}C, which is achieved by a temperature controller usually used for controlling the temperature of laser diodes. As is depicted in Fig 2, the target bacteria are first injected into the chamber through the flow channel and attach on the gold film by the adhesion of the Poly-L-lysine. Antibiotics are then added to test if the cell walls or membranes are affected.

2.3 Bacterium adhesive coating

Poly-L-Lysine has been demonstrated as an effective tissue adhesive for use in various biochemistry procedures. Poly-L-Lysine solution is diluted with deionized water prior to the coating procedure. The flat glass deposited with Au thin film was immersed in poly-L-lysine solution (concentration = 200 ug/ml) for from a couple of hours to 24 hours to interact with Au thin film as the preparation of the biochips. Different time intervals provide different adhesion of Poly-L-Lysine to the bacteria and antibiotics. After incubation, cells can be immobilized on the Au-coated glass.

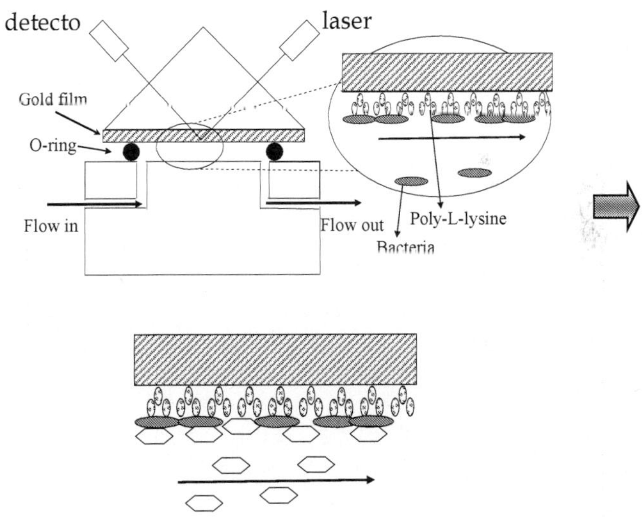

Fig. 2. Schematic illustration of the SPR device and the mechanisms of the experiment

2.4 Bacterium preparation

Preparation of Escherichia coli resistant to ampicillin Penicillin is called β-lactam drugs. An intact ting structure of β-lactam ring is essential for antibacterial activity; cleavage of the ring by penicillinases （β-lactamase）inactivates the drug (Levinson & Jawetz, 1989;

Macheboeuf et al., 2006). The antibiotics bacteria strain, *E. Coli* JM109, we use was generated by transform of ampicillin resistant plasmids to translate β-lactamase to cleave the ring of ampicillin. The *E. Coli* strain was picked out by loop and planted in 5ml LB broth over night. *Preparation of S. epidermidis resistant to tetracycline* The *S. epidermidis* were picked out by loop and were planted in 5ml LB broth over night (20 hours) and then transferred into 100ml LB broth (5 hours) for further experiment.

2.5 Scanning Electron Microscope (SEM) imaging

The glass slide with Au thin film and bacteria was placed in critical point drying (CPD) machine (Samdri-PVT) and filled with Ethanol of 100%. After that liquid CO_2 was used to replace the ethanol. The Au thin film with bacteria can then be detached from the glass slide for SEM imaging. Before taking the images, the sample was coated with Au for better conductivity. A scanning electron microscope JEOL JSM-5300 is used for the SEM images.

3. Antimicrobial susceptibility test

To test the drug resistance of bacteria using the SPR system, as depicted in Fig. 3, sterilized DI water was first injected into the flow cell chamber for 30 minutes to stabilize the system after the biochip coated with poly-L-lysine was assembled. Following the stabilization procedure, the incubated LA broth was injected into the cell chamber for the bacteria to cover the Au metal film. Another washing procedure is applied to remove the bacteria that are not bound to the poly-L-lysine coating. After that an antibiotic solution was injected. The angle of surface plasmon resonance through the entire procedure was recorded as a function of time.

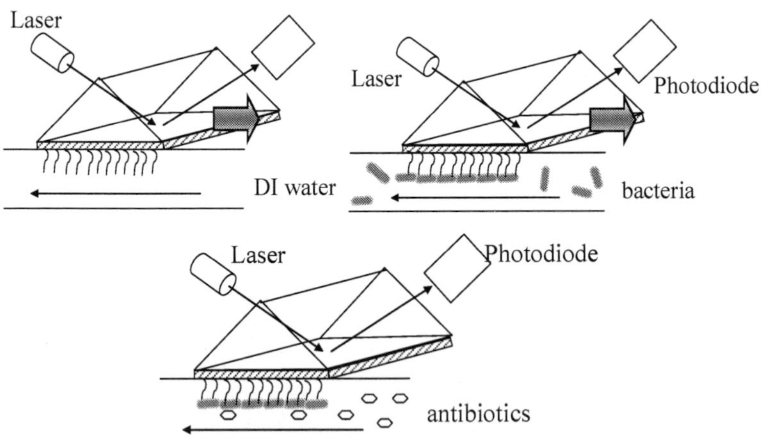

Fig. 3. Illustration of the experimental procedure. The first step is to stablize the system and make sure that the system is operated under a constant temperature; the second spet is to inject the bacteria into the cell chmaber for bacterium attachment. After the bacteria are attached on the Au thin film, a LA broth is injected into the chamber for washing out the unbound bacteria. The third step is to inject the antibiotics.

Antibiotics are classified into several categories depending on its mechanisms on the interruption of cell activities, namely cell wall synthesis, cell membrane synthesis, protein synthesis, folic acid biosynthesis, DNA gyrase, and RNA polymerase.

3.1 Gram negative bacterium – *E-Coli*

3.1.1 Injection with LB

Since surface plasmon resonance is very sensitive to the refractive index change of the cells attached on the thin gold film, ampicillin as the antibiotics interrupting cell wall synthesis is chosen in this experiment. The mechanism of ampicillin is depicted in Fig. 4. As is shown in Fig. 4(a), the cell wall and membrane of *E. Coli* consist of outer lipid bilayer and inner plasma membranes. Between the two bilayers, the peptide (peptidoglycan) and cross-link (peptide-bond) form a rigid layer to constitute cell walls. As is shown in Fig. 4(b), the generation of cross-link is achieved by the assistance of transpeptidase. The mechanism of ampicillin is to interrupt the activity of transpeptidase and then to interfere cell growth and proliferation [6], shown in Fig. 4(c). When the susceptible strain of *E. Coli* JM109 is subject to the action of ampicillin, the cell walls are modified by the antibiotics. This modification changes the resonance condition of surface plasmon. The change of the resonance condition is revealed on the detector through angular interrogation.

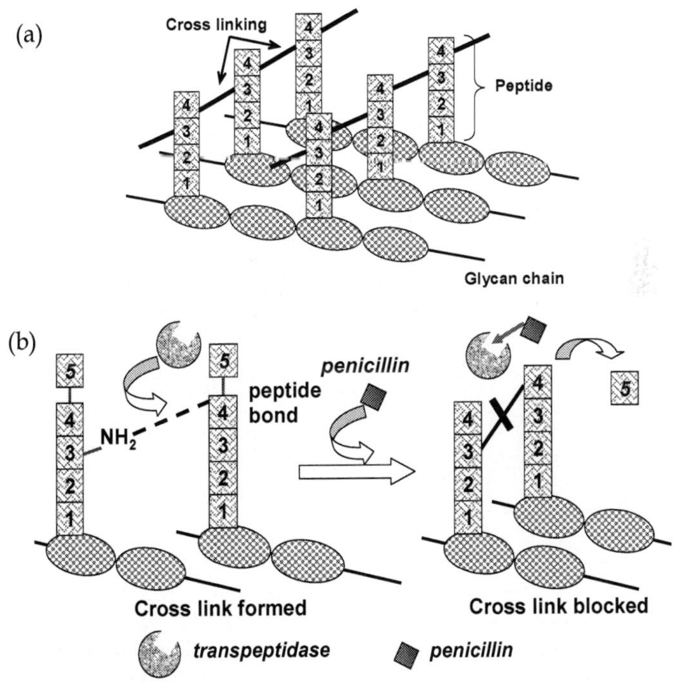

Fig. 4. (a) Cell wall structure; (b) Ampicillin mechanism

The SPR angle of antibiotic resistant strain of *E. Coli* JM109 over the operation procedures described above is shown in Fig. 5(a) and that of antibiotic susceptible strain is shown in Fig. 5(b). The shift of the SPR angle has been referred to the value of the SPR angle before the *E. Coli* was injected into the cell chamber. As shown in Fig. 5(a), the SPR angle increases when the bacteria are injected into the cell chamber. After the amount of the bacteria attached to the Au thin film coated with poly-L-lysine is saturated, DI water is injected to remove the unbounded bacteria. The SPR angle drops dramatically during this procedure. After that the 3 ug/ml ampicillin is injected to the cell chamber. The value of SPR angle, changed by the refractive index of the bacteria, is recorded over time. The same procedure is applied on the susceptible strain and the result is shown in Fig. 5(b). The result shows that, after 30 minutes treatment of ampicillin, the decrease of the SPR angle for the resistant and the susceptible strains is -0.00154 and -0.01608 in respective. The angle shift is about ten times difference between the resistant strains and the susceptible strains. It indicates that the ampicillin causes the structure of bacteria cell walls loose or even breakdown and thus decreases the refractive index of the cell wall of the susceptible *E. Coli*. Since the antibiotic resistant strain is more resistant to ampicillin, the refractive index of its cell wall does not decrease as much as the susceptible one's does.

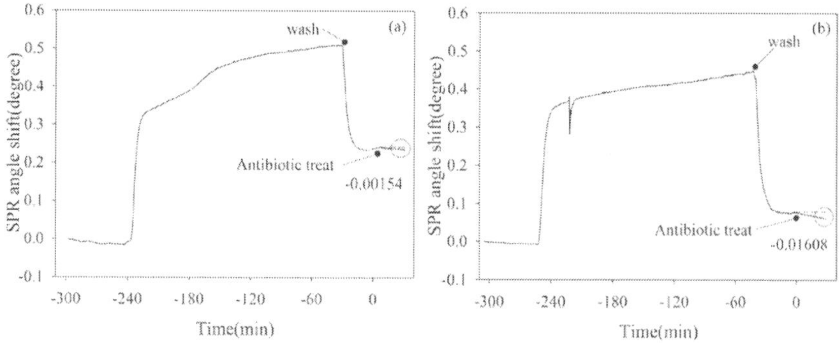

Fig. 5. Kinetic plot of SPR angle shift. The bacteria was treated by ampicillin for 30 minutes: (a) Amplicillin resistant case; (b) Ampicillin susceptible case (Chiang et al., 2009).

This difference of the resonance angle shift can be more pronounced when the concentration of the ampicillin increases to 100ug/ml. As was shown in Fig. 6, the angle shift of the ampicillin-resistant strain of *E. Coli* was almost a constant during the treatment of antibiotics. However, the angle shift of the susceptible strain increased significantly over time. This demonstrates that the angle shift in the case of susceptible strain is indeed caused by the treatment of antibiotics.

The damage degree of the ampicillin, with concentration of 3 ug/ml, on the cell walls of the antibiotic susceptible strain is examined by SEM. The *E. Coli* before the treatment of the ampicillin is shown in Fig. 7(a). The antibiotic resistant and susceptible *E. Coli* after the antibiotic treatment are shown in Fig. 7(b) and 7(c) in respective. The comparison of the SEM pictures reveals that no significant change on the appearances of the resistant strains and the susceptible strains is observed. It can be concluded that the SPR detection method is more sensitive than SEM scanning; the change detected by the SPR sensor is not shown in the SEM pictures. After 5 hours treatment of ampicillin, the susceptible strains shrank, which was verified by SEM.

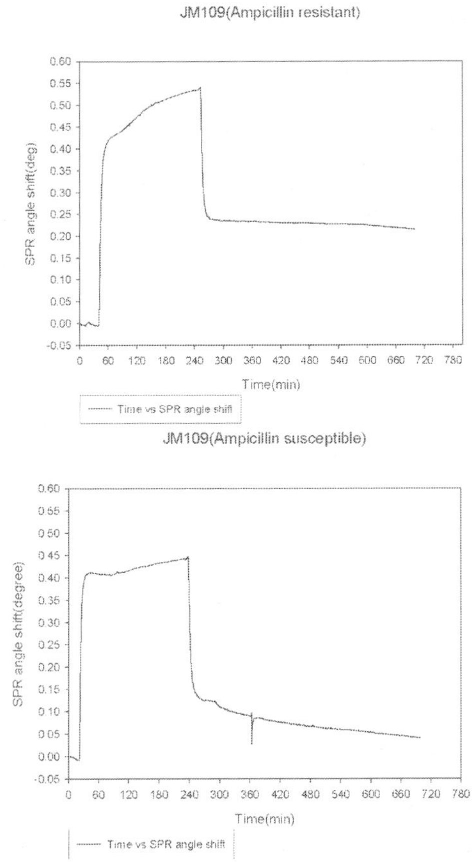

Fig. 6. Kinetic plot of SPR angle shift. The bacteria were treated with ampicillin of 100ug/ml for 300 minutes: (a) Amplicillin resistant case; (b) Ampicillin susceptible case

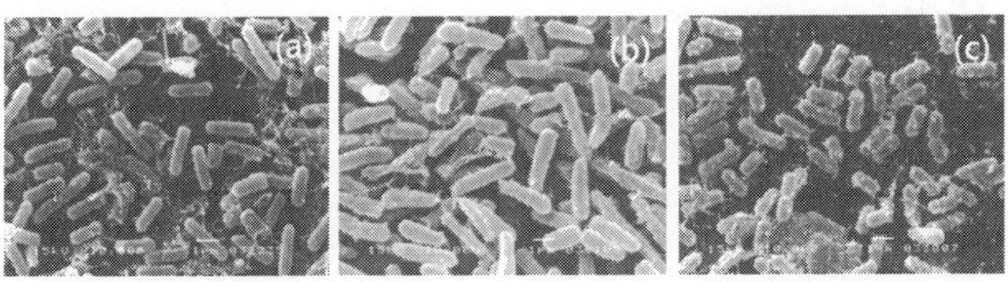

Fig. 7. SEM scanning pictures: (a) E-coli without antibiotic treating, (b) ampicillin resistant strains after 30 minutes treatment of antibiotics, (c) ampicillin susceptible strains after 30 minutes treatment of antibiotics. (Chiang et al., 2009)

In order to examine the reproducibility of the result, totally ten sets of resistant and susceptible strains of *E. Coli* JM109 were examined and the result was listed in Fig. 8. It shows that the detection of the susceptible strains is 100% correct within the limited examination number and that of the resistant strains is 90%. The incorrect set could be caused by the fall off of the gold film since gold has bad adhesion on glasses. Further verification is conducted on this issue. The angle shift difference between the resistant strains and the susceptible strains is ranged from two times to more than ten times. The variation of the result could due to the different degree of the drug resistance of the bacteria, the different distance between the prism and the Au-coated glass, and the coverage efficiency of bacteria on the surface of the thin gold film from time to time. Nevertheless an acute criterion can be set to separate these strains through the SPR scanning method proposed here.

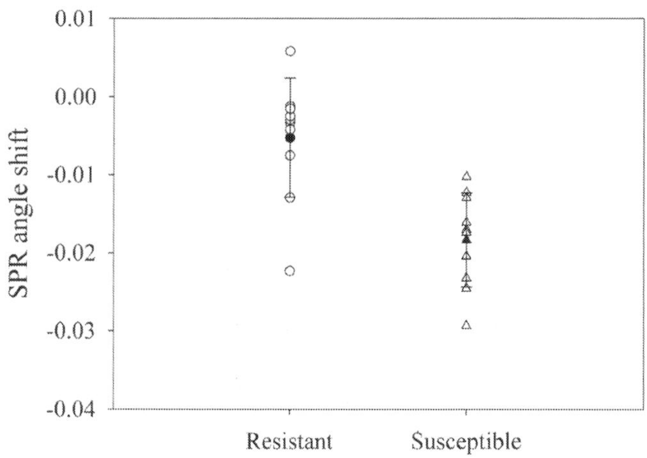

Fig. 8. Result of ten sets of resistant and susceptible strains of *E. Coli* subject to 3 ug/ml ampicillin. Solid circle indicates the average value of the angle shift in the case of resistant strain; Solid triangle indicates the average value of the angle shift in the case of susceptible strain. (Chiang et al., 2009)

3.1.2 Injection with DI water

In order to increase the accuracy of the antimicrobial susceptibility test. The coating time of Poly-L-Lysine was optimized from 24 hours to a few hours. Meanwhile, the LB injected with bacteria and for removing the unbound bacteria was replaced by DI water for reducing the interference of LB. After the adjustment, the amount of unbound or unstably bound bacteria was reduced significantly. As was shown in Fig. 9, the rinse procedure of DI water did not decrease the SPR angle from the saturation phase of bacterium adhesion as much as the situation in the injection with LB protocol. The ampicillin of 50ug/ml was applied from the time points indicated by the arrows. As shown in Fig. 9 (a), the resistant strain of *E. Coli* showed a positive angle shift right after the starting point of the ampicillin treatment and stay almost unchanged. The sudden increase on the angle shift is the result of adding ampicillin.

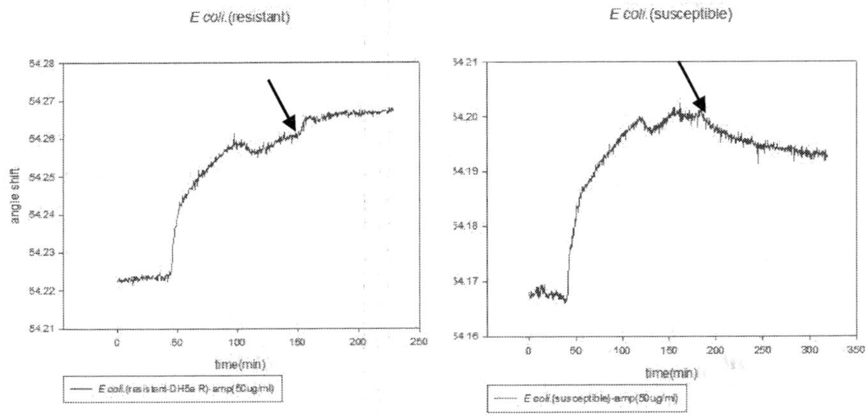

Fig. 9. Kinetic plot of SPR angle shift. The bacteria *E. Coli* were treated with ampicillin of 50ug/ml for 100 minutes: (a) Amplicillin resistant case; (b) Ampicillin susceptible case. The arrows indicate the time to start the treatment of ampicillin.

The result has demonstrated that the improved method has better accuracy in comparison with the method mentioned in the section 3.1.1. The same method using ampicillin of different concentrations, listed as 25 ug/ml, 50 ug/ml, and 100ug/ml, was also performed and the result was shown in Fig. 10. The resistant strain and susceptible strain of *E. Coli* were tested and ampicillin-only with bacteria was used as the control group. The tested groups subject to ampicillin of 25 ug/ml was marked by green solid circles; The tested groups subject to ampicillin of 50 ug/ml was indicated by red solid circles; The tested group subject to ampicillin of 100 ug/ml was indicated by blue solid circles. It revealed that the resonance angle in the resistant strain group increased because of the higher refractive index of ampicillin in comparison with that of DI water. Although the ampicillin can slightly increase the resonance angle, the resonance angle in the susceptible strain group still decreased due to the loss of cell walls, which has larger effect than that from higher refractive index of the ampicillin. This result showed that this method is suitable for the ampicillin with concentration ranged from 25 ug/ml to 100 ug/ml. We did not test ampicillin with the concentration above 100 ug/ml. For ampicillin with concentration lower than 25 ug/ml, the result became not trustable at this moment. Further study is required to push the lower limit.

3.2 Gram positive bacterium – *Enterococcus*

The protocol of DI water injection can also be used for gram positive bacteria. This tested object is *Enterococcus*. Similar result was obtained in the test, which was shown in Fig. 11. Following the same protocol, the resonance angle of SPP excitation first increased due to the higher refractive index of ampicillin in comparison with that of DI water. After the injection of the ampicillin, the angle shift of the resistant strain remained positive. However, angle shift of the susceptible strain gradually decreased to negative. The result of angle shift clearly distinguished the resistant strain from the susceptible strain.

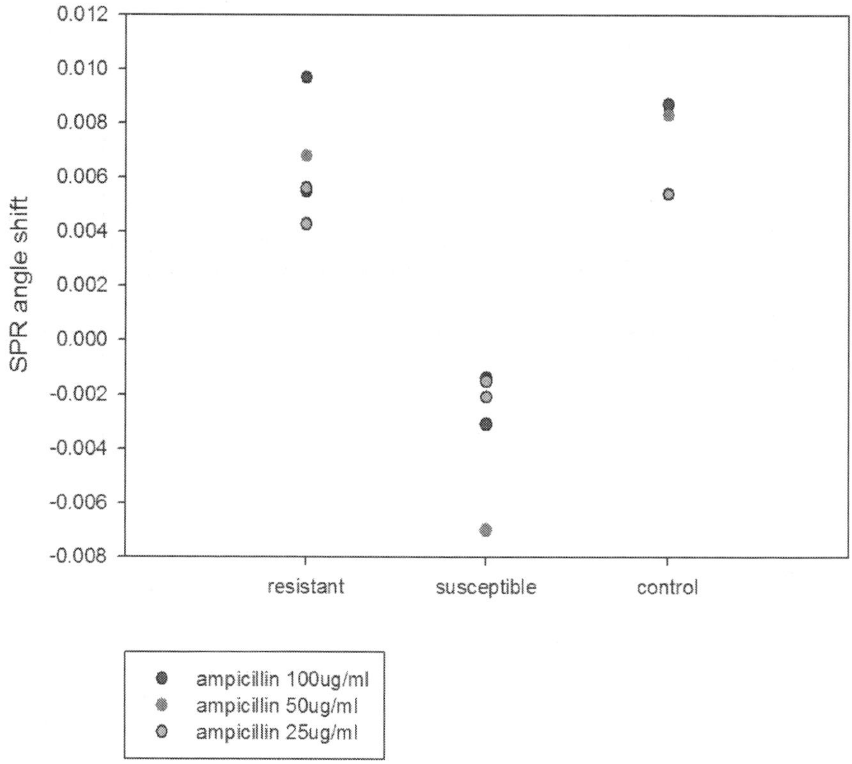

Fig. 10. Result of resistant and susceptible strains of *E. Coli* subject to ampicillin of different concentrations. Solid blue circle indicates the value of the angle shift in the case of 100 ug/ml for resistant strain, susceptible strain, and control group; Solid red circle indicates the value of the angle shift in the case of 50 ug/ml for resistant strain, susceptible strain, and control group; Solid green circle indicates the value of the angle shift in the case of 25 ug/ml for resistant strain, susceptible strain, and control group.

3.3 Different antibiotics - tetracycline

An interesting question has arisen if the same method can be used to detection antimicrobial susceptibility by antibiotic with different mechanism. For this purpose and also served as a blind test, another bacterium, *Staphylococcus Epidermidis*, is used. Tetracycline is used as the antibiotics in this test. Different from the mechanism of ampicillin, the tetracycline is a 30S inhibitor, which blocks the binding of aminoacyl-tRNA to A-site of ribosomes and then inhibits the protein synthesis (Malacinski & Freifelder, 1998). It is important to emphasize that the surface plasma wave penetrates the contacting bacteria surface of about 100 nanometers, it is only sensitive to the change of the refraction index within this depth. For the antibiotics that interrupt the synthesis of protein, SPR biosensing technique may not be able to detect any change of bacteria subject to the treatment of tetracycline since the influence of tetracycline passed to the surface of the cells is then indirect. The change of the SPR angle of the two unknown strains is shown in Fig. 12(a) and 12(b). As shown in Fig. 12, the change of the SPR angle for one of the strains is irregular after the treatment of the 10 ug/ml tetracycline and that of the other strain showed slightly monotonic decrease over time. Based on the curves shown in Fig. 12, it is judged that the strain tested in Fig. 12(b) is the susceptible strain and the other is the resistant strain. The result is consistent with the antimicrobials property of the strains. This showed that this method can also be used to detect antimicrobial susceptibility of microorganisms subject to antibiotics with mechanisms other than working on cell walls.

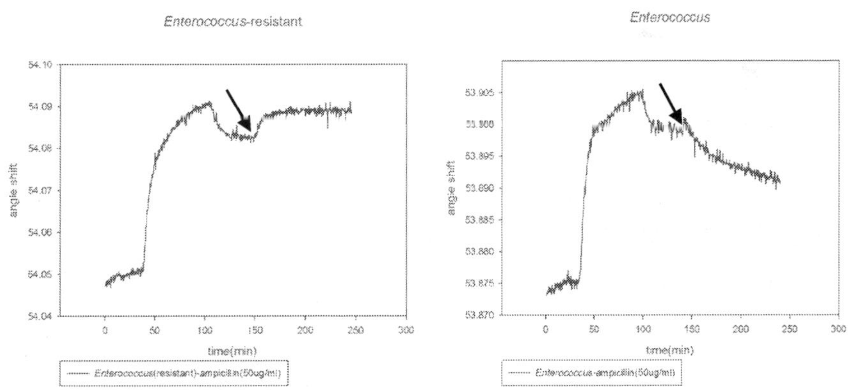

Fig. 11. Kinetic plot of SPR angle shift. The bacteria *Enterococcus* were treated with ampicillin of 50 ug/ml for 100 minutes: (a) Amplicillin resistant case; (b) Ampicillin susceptible case. The arrows indicate the time to start the treatment of ampicillin.

It is import to mention that the serum is not supplied into the system, the growth rate of *E. Coli* should not be a limited factor to generalize the potential of this method to other bacteria with longer growth time. An observation of bacteria on microscope has confirmed this point.

3. Conclusion

We have reported two innovative antimicrobial susceptible testing methods utilizing surface plasmon resonance. One is injection with LB liquid. The other is injection with DI water. In the study, the drug resistance of the gram negative bacteria, *Escherichia coli* JM109, and that of gram positive bacteria, *Enterococcus*, can be detected through the methods. This method is not limited to the antibiotics with mechanism working on the cell walls. It can be used to perform the test when antibiotics works on protein synthesis. The drug resistant of the *S. epidermidis* were successfully detected. Although the principle of the SPR testing method is based on the refractive index change of the cell-metal interface of about 100 nanometers, the resistance of the *S. epidermidis* to the tetracycline, which disturbs the protein synthesis, is still detectable by this method. This method can differentiate susceptible strain from resistant strain in a few hours and has a potential to further reduce the testing time to less than one hour if the cell adhesion time to the Au thin layer can be reduced. This method largely decreases the cost of time waste on examination and increase the chance for patient to survive.

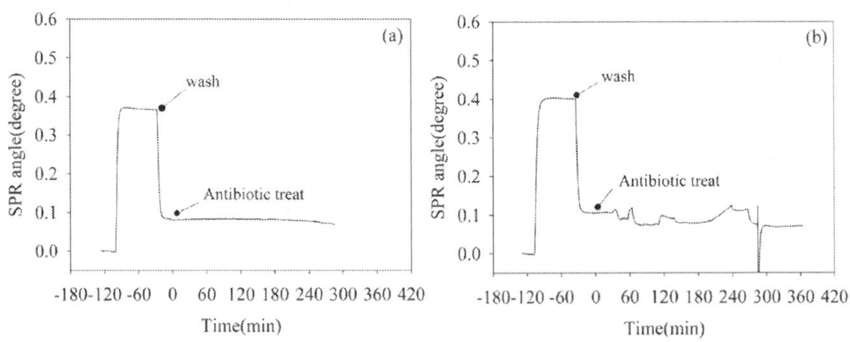

Fig. 12. Kinetic plot of SPR angle shift. The bacteria *E. Coli* were treated with ampicillin of 50 ug/ml for 100 minutes: (a) Amplicillin resistant case; (b) Ampicillin susceptible case. The arrows indicate the time to start the treatment of ampicillin. (Chiang et al., 2009)

4. Acknowledgment

This work was supported by research grant NSC 97-2627-M-010-005- and NSC 99-2112-M-010-001-MY3 from National Science Council in Taiwan and by "A grant from Ministry of Education, Aim for the Top University Plan" from National Yang Ming University.

5. References

Ritchie, R. H. (1957). Plasma Losses by Fast Electrons in Thin Films. *Physical Review*, Vol.106, No.5, (June 1957), pp. 874-881

Powell, C. J. & Swan, J. B. (1959). Origin of the Characteristic Electron Energy Losses in Aluminum. *Physical Review*, Vol.115, No.4, (August 1959), pp. 869-875

Otto, A. (1968). Excitation of nonradiative surface plasma waves in silver by the method of frustrated total reflection. *Zeitschrift für Physik A Hadrons and Nuclei*, Vol.215, No.4, (August 1968), pp. 398-410

Davies, J. (October 28, 1996). *Surface Analytical Techniques for Probing Biomaterial Processes*, CRC Press, ISBN 978-084-9383-52-6, Boca Raton, Florida, USA

Rich, R. L. & Myszka, D. G. (2005). Survey of the year 2004 commercial optical biosensor literature, *Journal of Molecular Recognition*, Vol.18, No.6, (November/December 2005), pp. 431-478

Safsten, P.; Klakamp, S. L.; Drake, A. W.; Karlsson, R. & Myszka, D. G. (2006). Screening antibody-antigen interactions in parallel using Biacore A100. *Analytical Biochemistry*, (June 2006), Vol.353, No.2, pp. 181-190

Misono, T. S. & Kumar, P. K. R. (2005). Selection of RNA aptamers against human influenza virus hemagglutinin using surface plasmon resonance. *Analytical Biochemistry*,(July 2005), Vol.342, No.2, pp. 312-317

Chien, F. C.; Chen, S. J. (2004). A sensitivity comparison of optical biosensors based on four different surface plasmon resonance modes. *Biosensors and Bioelectronics*, (October 2004), Vol.20, No. 3, pp. 633-642

Takemoto, D. K.; Skehel, J. J. & Wiley, D. C. (1996). A surface plasmon resonance assay for the binding of influenza virus hemagglutinin to its sialic acid receptor. *Virology*, (Mar 1996), Vol.217, No.2, pp. 452-458

Poupard, J. A.; Walsh L. R. & Kleger B. (1994), *Antimicrobial Susceptibility Testing: Critical Issues for the 90's*, Plenum Press, ISBN 030-6446-73-1, New York, USA

Levinson, W. E. & Jawetz E. (1989). *Medical Microbiology & Immunology*, Appleton & Lange, ISBN 978-007-1382-17-5, San Mateo, California, USA

Macheboeuf, P.; Contreras-Martel, C.; Job, V. ; Dideberg, O. & Dessen, A. (2006). Penicillin Binding Proteins: key players in bacterial cell cycle and drug resistance processes. *FEMS Microbiology Reviews*, (June 2006), Vol.30, No.5, pp. 673–691

Malacinski, G. M. & Freifelder, D. (January 15, 1998). *Essentials of Molecular Biology*, Jones & Bartlett Publishers, ISBN 978-086-7208-60-3, Sudbury, Ontario, Canada

Chiang, Y-L.; Lin, C-H.; Yen, M-Y.; Su, Y-D.; Chen, S-J. & Chen, H-F. (2009). Innovative Antimicrobial susceptibility testing method using surface plasmon resonance. *Biosensors & Bioelectronics*, (March 2009), Vol.24, No.7, pp. 1905-1910

Mammalian-Based Bioreporter Targets: Protein Expression for Bioluminescent and Fluorescent Detection in the Mammalian Cellular Background

Dan Close, Steven Ripp and Gary Sayler
Center for Environmental Biotechnology, The University of Tennessee, Knoxville
The United States of America

1. Introduction

While originally utilized primarily in prokaryotic organisms, reporter systems such as green fluorescent protein (GFP) and its variants, substrate dependent luciferase systems such as beetle and marine luciferase proteins, and substrate independent luciferase systems such as the bacterial luciferase gene cassette have now become the standards for imaging in the mammalian cellular background as well (Fig. 1). This has occurred in part because the use of cultured mammalian cells or small animal models has increased steadily over time in order to obtain more relevant human proxies for the measurement of cellular processes and bioavailability of biomedically relevant compounds of interest. However, the expression and detection of these reporter systems in eukaryotic models presents unique challenges not encountered in their prokaryotic counterparts.

The differences in gene expression and cellular compartmentalization between prokaryotic and eukaryotic cells represent the major obstacles for the efficient expression of these and other reporter systems at the cellular level, but once the line has been crossed from expression in single cells to expression in multicelluar organisms, these problems can be compounded by the increases in absorption and scattering intrinsic to whole animal imaging. As a result, much consideration must be given to the experimental design associated with bioluminescent or fluorescent detection from mammalian cells. The type of system employed, whether it be cell culture or whole animal, the depth of imaging, the relevant time period available for data collection, and even the ability to distinguish multiple reporter systems from within the same tissue must be understood and acknowledged prior to beginning any experiment.

To better prepare for selection of the most appropriate reporter protein for the detection of a bioluminescent or fluorescent signal from mammalian tissue, this chapter will highlight and compare the utility of the most commonly available reporter systems as reported in the current literature. Specifically, the chapter will focus on the green fluorescent protein (GFP) and its color shifted variants, D-luciferin based luciferase proteins (both from the firefly and from click beetles), coelenterazine based luciferase proteins (those from the *Renilla* and *Gaussia* genera), and the bacterial luciferase gene cassette (*lux*). A short background of the major reporter proteins will be given that explains the biochemical requirements of each, as well as the physical properties that make them unique (emission wavelength, quantum yield, etc.). These properties will be considered in relation to how they influence the ability to detect the resulting bioluminescent or fluorescent signal using commercially available equipment.

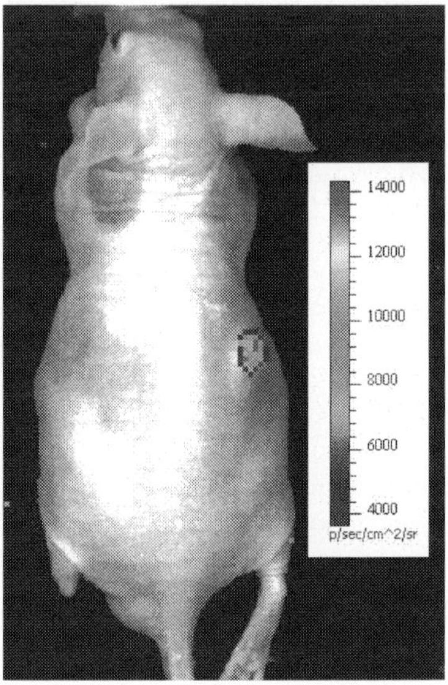

Fig. 1. Bioluminescent detection from a small animal model.
The luminescent (as shown here from cells expressing human codon-optimized bacterial luciferase genes) or fluorescent signals of a reporter cell line can be detected through the tissue of a living small animal host, allowing for localization of the cell population and estimation of its size without the need to sacrifice the host.

To provide a better understanding of the function of each of the reporter systems, relevant examples will be cited that illustrate the common use of each reporter system, as well as novel examples that show how each can be adapted to function under unique circumstances based on their biochemical requirements and physical emission properties. The relative strengths and weaknesses of each of the considered reporter systems will also be discussed, with an eye towards their role in imaging cellular processes at the level of cell culture imaging, near surface detection through tissue in small animal models, and deep tissue (beyond subcutaneous) imaging in small animal models. The overall goal is to present a fair representation of the potential uses of each of the chosen reporter systems to allow for selection of the most appropriate system for a given experimental design.

2. Imaging concerns in biological tissues

There are additional concerns when performing data collection from within a living medium that must be considered in addition to the traditional focus on experimental efficiency. The detection of a fluorescent or luminescent signal from within a tissue sample can be dependent on multiple factors, such as the total flux of photons capable of being produced by the reporter, the population size of reporter cells that are introduced into the sample, and the location of those reporter cells within the tissue sample itself (Troy et al., 2004). Subsequently, the visualization of the reporter signal is dependent on the absorption and scattering of that signal prior to its detection. One method for overcoming these detrimental conditions is to alter the emission wavelength of the reporter signal. Increasing the wavelength can serve to both reduce the amount of scattering and decrease absorption. This is possible because the majority of photon absorption is the result of signal interaction with endogenous chromophoric material within the cell. By moving to a longer, more red-shifted emission wavelength, where the level of absorption within tissue is lower, it is possible to detect a greater amount of signal intensity than would be possible from an identical reporter with a lower, more blue-shifted emission wavelength (Chance et al., 1998). Because of this, it is paramount to consider the emission wavelength of a given reporter system, along with the other desired attributes of that reporter, prior to experimental design. For example, the bioluminescent signal from the bacterial bioluminescence (*lux*) reaction is produced at 490 nm. This is relatively blue-shifted as compared to the firefly luciferase (Luc)-based bioluminescent probes that display their peak luminescent signal at 560 nm. The shorter wavelength of the *lux*-based signal has a greater chance of becoming attenuated within the tissue and therefore may not be as easily detected if it is used in deeper tissue applications such as intraperitoneal or intraorganellar injections into a small animal host. To overcome the disadvantage of increased attenuation due to the shorter, blue-shifted emission wavelength, similar detection levels using the *lux* reporter would require a longer integration time than would be expected when using the longer wavelength Luc reporter following subcutaneous injection.

It is important to remember that these effects are not specific to bioluminescent reporters and hold true when working with fluorescent reporter proteins as well. However, when introducing a fluorescent reporter system into the mammalian cellular environment, one must take into account the effect that the excitation wavelength will have on overall detectability. This is because the presence of the excitation signal can result in production of high levels of background autofluorescence under small animal imaging conditions, due to the presence of chromophoric material within the mammalian cell (Choy et al., 2003; Troy et al., 2004). This can result in difficulty distinguishing the reporter excitation signal from the background noise if the two are produced at similar wavelengths. Unlike a bioluminescent system, which does not require an excitation light signal, increasing the duration of this signal can lead to a reduction of measureable signal due to the combined results of photobleaching of the reactive photocenter of the reporter protein and the associated increase in background noise from extended excitation of endogenous chromophoric cellular material. For this reason, the photostability of a particular fluorescent protein must be considered in addition to the general concerns of efficiency and brightness that should be weighed prior to selection of any reporter protein, fluorescent or bioluminescent, when designing any experiment.

3. Green fluorescent protein (GFP)

3.1 Introduction

While the green fluorescent protein (GFP) is not the only fluorescent protein target used for visualization in the mammalian cellular background, it is certainly the most well known. Widespread familiarity with this reporter, coupled with its longstanding use in both prokaryotic and eukaryotic organisms, is perhaps the major impetus that drives investigators to select it as a target for biomarker visualization. The namesake 504 nm emission signal of GFP is relatively low (Patterson et al., 1997) in the green spectrum of visible light, making it a less than ideal candidate for high levels of fluorescent penetration through mammalian tissue (Chance et al., 1998). This disadvantage has been at least partially overcome by the introduction of mutated versions of the GFP protein that have been engineered to fluoresce at higher wavelengths where penetration is greater (Tsien, 1998; Zimmer, 2002). In addition, fluorescent proteins have since been introduced that successfully increase the emission wavelength of the fluorescent signal to a fully red-shifted wavelength for more efficient detection through tissue. This was accomplished first with the introduction of the monomeric red fluorescent protein (mRFP1), derived from the red fluorescent protein of *Discosoma* sp. (Campbell, R. et al., 2002). Further engineering was then performed to develop more efficient variants such as the popular mCherry and tdTomato proteins in use today (Shaner et al., 2004). Despite these advances in fluorescent reporter technology, GFP remains in high use, either in conjunction with or independent of these alternate reporter systems. When used properly, it can be an excellent reporter system for imaging in the mammalian cellular environment and serves as an excellent model for the function of fluorescent proteins in general.

3.2 GFP structure

Wild type GFP is composed of a single polypeptide consisting of 328 amino acids (Tsien, 1998). The mature protein forms an 11-stranded β-barrel that is roughly twice as long as it is wide (diameter of 24 Å and height of 42 Å) (Zimmer, 2002). The only exception to the β-sheet motif is the formation of two short α-helices between the 7th and 8th β-strands. These two α-helical sections act as lids to cover the open ends of the cylinder (Phillips, 1997) and support the formation of the fluorophore (Tsien, 1998). This 11-stranded β-sheet conformation is very unique and has been termed the β-can. It is hypothesized that the tight, almost seamless, structure imparted by the β-can formation is what gives the GFP protein such a high level of resistance to denaturation by heat and chemical denaturants (Ward et al., 1982).

The historical view of the mechanism suggests the fluorophore is autocatalytically formed post-translationally from the side chains of residues 65 - 67 (Phillips, 1997). Following folding into a native conformation, the carbonyl of Ser 65 undergoes a nucleophilic attack from the amide of Gly 67 leading to formation of an imidazolinone. Oxygen then dehydrogenates the α-β bond of Tyr 66 to bring its aromatic side chain into conjugation with the imidazolinone, allowing for absorbance and fluorescence to occur (Tsien, 1998). More recently this mechanism has been revisited and it has been proposed that the position of backbone residues plays a greater role than initially thought (Fig. 2). It is hypothesized that the tight β-can structure holds the residues forming the fluorophore into position, allowing Arg 96 to initiate the acid base reactions required to form an intermediate that is stabilized by Glu 222 even though it is in an energetically unfavorable state. This intermediate is then oxidized to the highly stable aromatic imidazolone and the fluorophore becomes active (Barondeau et al., 2003). It is the formation and oxidation of the fluorophore that is the limiting step in the expression of a mature GFP protein, with the process taking as little as 45 minutes following protein synthesis in optimized protein constructs (Crameri et al., 1996) or as long as 4 hours in the wild type variant (Heim et al., 1994).

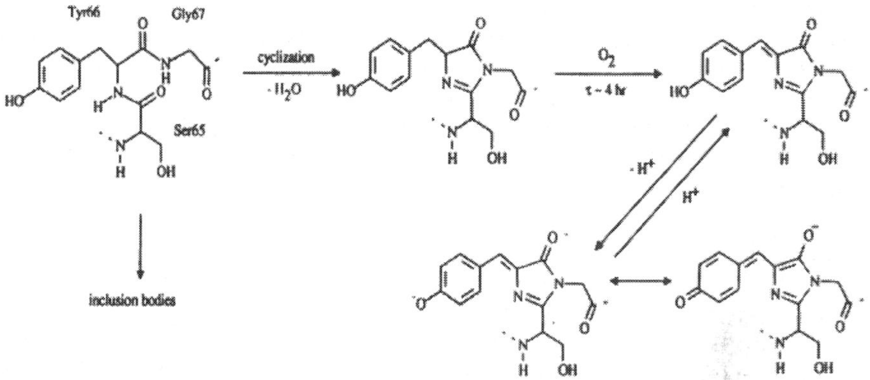

Fig. 2. The proposed biosynthetic scheme for the chromophore of GFP.
The freshly translated protein (upper left) could be trapped by inclusion bodies or remain soluable and nonfluorescent (upper center) until oxidation by O_2, which could dehydrogenate Tyr 66 to form the fluorophore (upper right). The protonated and deprotonated species (upper and lower right) may be responsible for the 394 and 470 to 475 nm excitation peaks, respectively. The excited state of phenols are much more acidic than their ground states, so that emission would come only from the deprotonated species. Originally published in (Heim et al., 1994). Copyright by the National Academy of Sciences.

While this Ser-Tyr-Gly triplet is common among known proteins, it alone is not sufficient to cause formation of a fluorophore. What makes the sequence unique in GFP is a combination of steric positioning and acid/base chemistry with the surrounding residues. It is an absolute requirement that glycine be present in position 67, as no functional GFP mutants have been isolated with any other residue at this position (Phillips, 1997). The freedom allowed by the short side chain of glycine allows for proper positioning of the fluorophore so that it can properly interact with the surrounding residues (Zimmer, 2002). These interactions provide immobilization of the fluorophore allowing for resonance stabilization under excited state conditions (Phillips, 1997).

It is possible for the native GFP protein to exist as either a monomer or a dimer, with variant fluorescent signatures in either state (Phillips, 1997). This is in contrast to homologous proteins such as GFP from *Renilla reniformis,* which is an obligate dimer (Tsien, 1998). It is generally accepted that whether or not GFP is isolated as a dimer or a monomer is dependent on the isolation conditions and not the result of any *in vivo* influences (Palm et al., 1997) and that the dissociation constant for the dimer is 100 μM (Phillips, 1997). Dimerization is localized to the hydrophobic surface formed by the Ala 206, Leu 221, and Phe 223 residues and bolstered by a host of other hydrophilic contacts (Tsien, 1998). When these contacts are made the structure of the fluorophore can be altered, presumptively because its tight immobilization relative to the backbone associated atoms of neighboring residues forces it to change orientation following bond rearrangement (Wu et al., 1996).

3.3 GFP mechanism of action

The wild type GFP protein is able to absorb light at two different wavelengths. A minor peak occurs at 475 nm with the major peak at 397 nm. Regardless of which excitation wavelength is used, emission occurs only at 504 nm (Patterson et al., 1997). The different absorption peaks have been attributed to varying protonation states of the fluorophore, with the neutral state corresponding to the major absorption peak at 397 nm and the anionic form contributing to the minor peak at 475 nm (Niwa et al., 1996). The large shift between the major absorption peak at 397 nm and the emission at 504 nm can be attributed to an excited state proton transfer from the side chain of the Tyr 66 residues of the fluorophore (Chattoraj et al., 1996) to the carboxylate oxygen of Glu 222 (Zimmer, 2002).

Based on this interconversion of the fluorophore, a three state model of photoisomerization has been put forward to explain the chemical basis for shifts in absorption. This model states that excitation of the neutral state fluorophore can cause conversion to the anionic form via an intermediate (Chattoraj et al., 1996). The intermediate is structurally similar to the neutral form of the fluorophore, but has become deprotonated at the phenol group of Tyr 66 (Zimmer, 2002). Excitation of the anionic form is capable of directly emitting fluorescence, while the neutral state must necessarily convert into an excited form of this intermediate prior to emission (Jung et al., 2005). While it is possible for the neutral form to convert to the anionic form following excitation, this is not the most favorable reaction. The majority of excited, neutral fluorophores will convert briefly to the intermediate state, where fluorescence will occur followed by reversion back to the neutral state (Chattoraj et al., 1996). Interconversion between the neutral and anionic states is possible, but requires both proton transfer and conformational change to occur (Zimmer, 2002). Similarly, the majority of anionic fluorophores will revert to the ground state following fluorescent emission, but could instead undergo a conformational change to the intermediate state and then continue on to adopt a neutral charge state (Chattoraj et al., 1996).

In a wild type population, GFP contains a 6:1 ratio of neutral to anionic fluorophores (Tsien, 1998), explaining why the major absorption peak is found at 397 nm. However, upon extended UV illumination this peak will begin to decrease and the minor peak will increase (Cubitt et al., 1995). This behavior corresponds to the photoisomerization of the neutral fluorophore form responsible for the major absorption peak being converted into the anionic form as discussed above. While the photoisomerization characteristics of GFP can prove problematic for quantification, they do allow for the study of protein movement by excitation with intense UV light at 397 nm followed by excitation at 475 nm in order to track the movement of the photoisomerized fluorophores (Yokoe & Meyer, 1996).

3.4 Color shifted GFP variants

Following the discovery of GFP it was quickly proven that amino acid substitutions were capable of altering its fluorescent characteristics. Since that time, versions of GFP have been developed that fold more efficiently at higher temperatures (Crameri et al., 1996), avoid dimerization at high concentration (Zacharias et al., 2002), or fluoresce in the blue (Heim et al., 1994), cyan (Hein & Tsien, 1996), or yellow (Ormo et al., 1996) wavelengths. The history and development of these variants has been reviewed extensively in the past (Tsien, 1998; Zimmer, 2002), and they can now all be classified by dividing the known variants into seven classes based on spectral characteristics. When applied in concert, these variants of the GFP protein have given researchers the ability to use multiple GFP-based reporters in the same environment at the same time, improving the usefulness and range of this already dynamic protein.

3.5 Red-shifted fluorescent reporter proteins for the mammalian environment

To further red-shift fluorescent emission wavelengths beyond that of the GFP variants, a fluorescent protein from an entirely new organism was used as the starting point. This protein was the red fluorescent protein (dsRed) from the *Discosoma* corals. dsRed is a 26 kDa protein that has an excitation wavelength of 558 nm and a resulting emission wavelength of 583 nm. It is capable of producing fluorescence with a quantum yield of 0.24 (Matz et al., 1999) but acts as a tetramer under wild-type conditions, making it problematic for use as an efficient reporter in its native state. To overcome the problems associated with its tetrameric quaternary structure, dsRed was engineered to functionally express fluorescence as a monomer (Campbell, R. et al., 2002) and then further refined through a process of directed evolution to produce the popular mCherry protein. While mCherry is only 27% as bright as the original dsRed protein, it has improved photostability and red-shifted excitation and emission wavelengths at 587 nm and 610 nm respectively, which allow it to function more efficiently in the mammalian cellular background (Shaner et al., 2004). These red-shifted fluorescent reporter proteins are only a few examples of the type of improved fluorescent reporter proteins that have been developed for use in mammalian imaging, but are representative of the type of mutations that must be engineered to develop additional fluorescent reporters for this unique type of imaging.

3.6 Examples of use as a mammalian biosensor

3.6.1 Steady state imaging

Steady state imaging is the classical hallmark of mammalian visualization. This process begins with transfecting the gene encoding the fluorescent reporter into a cell line. If the researcher is primarily concerned with intracellular processes, this may be all that is required. Once the reporter protein is being expressed within the host cell, its presence can be visualized using fluorescent microscopy following excitation at the appropriate wavelength. If the goal is to determine the location or population size of the cells within a small animal model, the transfected line must first be introduced and then allowed to propagate within the host until it reaches a level capable of being detected through the native host tissue. This growth period can take several days depending on the size of the initial cellular inoculum. When these types of experiments are performed, it is most important to take into consideration the wavelength and brightness of the reporter protein used to ensure efficient performance. For example, when attempting to localize a single protein within a cell, the GFP protein can be fused to the protein of interest, and then quickly and easily visualized under fluorescence microscopy. This is the strategy that was taken by Barak et. al. when they developed β-Arrestin 2/GFP fusions that were used to significantly improve detection of G-protein coupled receptor activation. Expression of the GFP-fused proteins allowed the investigators to visualize how the conjugate responded to ligand mediated receptor activation using confocal microscopy in real-time using living cells (Barak et al., 1997). This work has been instrumental in monitoring G-coupled protein receptor activation, which represents the single most important target to date for drug development and medical therapy. However, while GFP provided an excellent target for detection in single cells, when the goal is localization of a tumor cell population within a mouse model, a reporter such as mCherry should be considered because it would allow for emission in a more red-shifted wavelength, thereby improving the signal penetration through the additional host tissue and allowing for easier detection than would be expected from GFP.

3.6.2 Multi-reporter imaging

In its most basic form, multi-reporter imaging is simply an extension of steady state imaging following introduction of two or more reporter proteins. Under these conditions, the genes for the reporter proteins are introduced into the cell and, following expression, they are exposed to their respective excitation signals in a stepwise manner. The resulting emission signals can be differentiated either temporally from the staggered excitation signal applications or simultaneously based on their differential wavelength characteristics. In this type of approach the most important consideration should be the overlap of the chosen reporter excitation and emission wavelengths. Care must be used to select groupings of reporters that do not have overlapping emission and excitation signals. If multiple reporters have similar excitation wavelengths, there will be no way to separate their expression times since they will be triggered simultaneously. Likewise, if multiple reporters share overlapping emission wavelengths, it may not be possible to differentiate their locations unless they have disparate excitation wavelengths and their expression is controlled temporally. Finally, caution must be used to ensure the emission wavelength of one of the reporters is not within the excitation range of a simultaneously expressed reporter. Under these conditions the two signals cannot be differentiated and the initial signal can be partially or completely consumed during energy transfer to the second reporter in a process referred to as fluorescence resonance energy transfer (FRET).

In some cases, this type of FRET is the desired outcome. FRET is often used to boost the overall fluorescent output of the reporter system by taking advantage of a high penetration excitation wavelength of one reporter, and the resulting increased emission properties of a second. Alternatively, FRET systems can be used to visualize the interaction of proteins within a cell. By creating fusions between two proteins of interest and fluorescent proteins such as GFP and its blue-shifted variant, it is possible to visualize when the two proteins of interest are interacting at a resolution greater than that achievable using traditional optical microscopy. This is possible because these reporters display overlapping emission and excitation wavelengths, thereby allowing investigators to determine where the fused proteins are interacting by using only a single excitation wavelength and reading the opposite partner's excitation wavelength (Day, 1998).

3.6.3 Measuring changes in cellular health

There have been many examples of how fluorescent proteins can be used to monitor changes in cellular health, with an extensive review of these studies having been presented previously (Aguilera et al., 2006). In general, the methodology behind these types of experiments is fairly straightforward. The cell line of interest is first transfected with a fluorescent reporter protein, then, following determination of the baseline level of fluorescence, the cells are treated with a chemical or compound of interest and changes in fluorescent activity are monitored over time. Any resulting decrease in the fluorescent signal relative to untreated control cells indicates a reduction in cellular health. These types of experiments are beneficial because they can present a simple, high throughput method for screening large numbers of compounds prior to beginning more in depth analysis.

3.7 Summary of advantages and disadvantages

Advantages and Disadvantages of Fluorescent Reporters	
Advantages	**Disadvantages**
Diverse range of colors Quantitative correlation between signal strength and cell numbers No requirement for addition of exogenous substrate chemical Noninvasive Can be used in combination for multiple labeling	Potentially high levels of background fluorescence upon excitation signal Can be subject to photobleaching, preventing repeated imaging Non-genetic system leads to diffusion during cellular division Photoexcitation can cause tissue damage at low wavelengths

Table 1. Advantages and Disadvantages of Fluorescent Reporter Use in Mammalian Imaging

4. Luciferase proteins that require exogenous substrate addition

4.1 Introduction

At the most basic level, a luciferase protein can be defined as any protein that, upon binding to its required substrate, produces a luminescent signal as a product of the ensuing enzymatic reaction. The discovery that this signal could be generated without the requirement for introduction of an excitatory light signal has been a mainstay of the biomedical imaging community because it allows for visualization without increased production of unwanted background fluorescence. However, unlike fluorescent reporter systems, the majority of luciferase systems require the addition of an exogenous chemical substrate to elicit their bioluminescent production. While there are many different types of luciferase proteins that have been isolated to date, there are predominantly two main categories that are in common use today: luciferase proteins that utilize D-luciferin as a substrate and luciferase proteins that utilize coelenterazine as a substrate. While these two classes of luciferase proteins utilize different substrates and therefore different mechanisms of action, the end result of the reaction for each results in the production of a luminescent signal in the visible range that can often be detected at lower levels than their fluorescent counterparts due to the lack of endogenous bioluminescent production in mammalian tissue (Close, D., Xu et al., 2010). While this advantage is obvious, it is important to note that the injection of required substrate, be it either D-luciferin or coelenterazine, entails the introduction of additional concerns over the efficiency of substrate injection, the quality of the substrate being used, the rate of substrate uptake and clearing in the subject tissue, and even the cost of the substrate itself. Although each of these factors could have deleterious effects on the outcome of a particular experiment, they have not prevented the luciferase requiring proteins from becoming the most popular method for visualization in mammalian tissues because of their ease of use and high signal quality.

4.2 Luciferase proteins that utilize D-luciferin as an exogenous substrate

The chemical 2-(4-hydroxybenzothiazol-2-yl)-2-thiazoline acid is more commonly referred to simply as D-luciferin (White, E.H. et al., 1961) and is the substrate utilized by the majority of terrestrial bioluminescent organisms. The majority of these organisms are from the order Coleoptera and are best represented by the common North American firefly *Photinus pyralis* and the click beetles (Fraga, 2008). Historically, research has focused on determining the structure and mechanism of action of the firefly luciferase protein (Luc) as a model for substrate-dependent luminescent production, and recent discoveries have indicated that this mechanism is similar among all luciferase proteins that use D-luciferin as a substrate (Wood, Lam, & McElroy, 1989). Since its discovery, the Luc protein has grown into the most widely used of the bioluminescent reporter systems in mammalian imaging and therefore understanding its function is vital to interpreting the majority of published results on the subject.

4.2.1 Firefly luciferase structure

Luc is a monomeric protein composed of 550 amino acid residues with a molecular weight of 62 kDa (Conti et al., 1996). Originating from a eukaryotic organism, the genomic DNA encoding the Luc protein is comprised of seven exons and six introns that must be spliced out prior to translation in order to form the mature product (de Wet et al., 1986). The primary sequence of Luc shares extensive sequence similarity with the acyl-CoA ligases and this homology has been exploited to determine the location of the active site as well as the binding sites for its required co-factors (Conti et al., 1996). One interesting feature of the protein sequence is a C-terminal tag that directs it to the peroxisome (Viviani, 2002), although it does have some functional features of a membrane protein such as a tendency to associate with phospholipids (Ugarova, 1989).

The Luc protein can be divided into two major domains. The N-terminal domain is by far the larger of the two and comprises the first 436 residues. The C-terminal domain is formed from residues 440 to 550, and is linked to the N-terminal domain by a 4 residue long flexible loop. The large N-terminal domain is rich in secondary structure and is home to an antiparallel β-barrel and two β-sheets that are flanked by α-helices. While physically smaller, the C-terminal domain also contains a mix of secondary structures including two short antiparallel β-strands and a three-stranded mixed β-sheet associated with three α-helices arranged in an α + β structure. There are four short connecting regions in the crystal structure that are too disordered to interpret, however, these regions are all exposed to solvent and represent some of the most conserved residues in homologous proteins so their exact position is unlikely to effect structure-based predictions (Conti et al., 1996).

The N-terminal β-barrel is distorted into three distinct faces because of its interactions with the surrounding structures. Two of the three faces are formed by three-stranded antiparallel β-sheets, while the third is comprised of two strands of the neighboring major β-sheet and the disordered region connecting them. Because of this close interaction between the β-barrel and the two major β-sheets, concave depressions are formed on the surface of the protein in a "Y" shape. The two major β-sheets in the N-terminal domain are each composed of eight strands with a core of parallel strands joined to α-helices running antiparallel on either side of the sheet to form a five-layered α-β-α-β-α tertiary structure. One sheet consists of five parallel and three antiparallel β-strands with six associated helices with all but the last helix being formed from a continuous section of the polypeptide chain, while the other is split between six parallel and two antiparallel strands and six helices and is formed from two non-contiguous portions of the polypeptide (Conti et al., 1996).

There is a wide cleft between the N and C-terminal domains that is bridged by residues 436 to 440. Although the crystal structure does not include bound substrates, all of the invariant residues from the related adenylate-forming enzymes are located on the opposing faces of this cleft, sparking the hypothesis that the domains re-arranged following substrate binding (Conti et al., 1996). This hypothesis has been bolstered by the recent crystallization and X-ray analysis of the related luciferase protein from the Japanese firefly *Luciola cruciata*. This structure was obtained in the presence of bound substrates and shows a much closer association between the two domains (Nakatsu et al., 2006). It has even been proposed that the C-terminal domain changes orientation multiple times to carry out different steps in the luminescent reaction (Branchini, B.R. et al., 2005).

In order to perform its luminescent reaction, Luc must bind with the luciferin, ATP-Mg^{2+}, and oxygen (Hastings, J et al., 1953). Despite the widespread use of Luc, the actual binding sites for these components have yet to be determined conclusively. There are two current models put forth by Ugarova (Sandalova & Ugarova, 1999) and Branchini (Branchini, B. et al., 1998) that propose similar active site interactions. Both models suggest that residues Arg 218, His 245–Phe 247, Ala 313–Gly 320, and Lys 529 form the binding site for D-luciferin, with a hydrophobic surface being contributed directly by Ala 313, Ala 348, Ile 351, and Phe 247. The models differ in the importance of Arg 218, with Branchini suggesting that it interacts directly with luciferin phenolate (Branchini, B. et al., 1998) and Ugarova proposing that this interaction occurs with Arg 337. These models were bolstered by the *Luciola* crystal structure which showed association at Phe 249, Thr 253, Leu 286, Glu 311–Ser 314, Arg 337–Tyr 340, and Ala 348 (Nakatsu et al., 2006). Unfortunately, confirmation of these active site models and the determination of the exact binding locations will have to wait until a crystal structure is published showing Luc bound to its substrates.

4.2.2 Firefly luciferase mechanism of action

The Luc protein catalyzes the oxidation of the reduced D-luciferin in the presence of ATP-Mg^{2+} and oxygen to generate CO_2, AMP, PP_i, oxyluciferin, and yellow-green light at a wavelength of 562 nm. It is important to note that D-luciferin is a chiral molecule, and while both the D and L forms can bind to Luc and participate in adenylation reactions, only the D form is capable of continuing on in the reaction to generate light (Fraga, 2008). This reaction was originally reported to occur with a quantum yield of 0.88 (Seliger & McElroy, 1960), but has since been shown to actually achieve a quantum yield closer to only 0.41 (Ando et al., 2007). Because of this high quantum yield, the reaction is well suited to use as a reporter with as few as 10^{-19} mol of luciferase (2.4×10^5 molecules) able to produce a light signal capable of being detected (Gould & Subramani, 1988).

It has been known since the early 1950's that the chemical reaction underlying firefly luminescence is a two-step process that first requires adenylation of D-luciferin followed by oxidation and the production of light (Hastings, J et al., 1953). Prior to the initiation of the reaction, the Luc protein must first bind to D-luciferin. However, at this time it is not yet capable of undergoing oxidation or producing light. The first step in the generation of light is the adenylation of the bound D-luciferin with the release of pyrophosphate (Ugarova, 1989). The function of this adenylation is to increase the acidity of the C4 proton of the thiazoline ring on D-luciferin. This allows for removal of a proton from C4 causing formation of a carbanion (McCapra, F. et al., 1968). This carbanion is then attacked by oxygen, displacing AMP and driving the formation of a cyclic peroxide with an associated carbonyl group (a dioxetanone ring). As the bonds supporting this structure collapse, it becomes decarboxylated, releasing CO_2 and forming an excited state of oxyluciferin in either the enol or keto form (Fig. 3) (Ugarova, 1989).

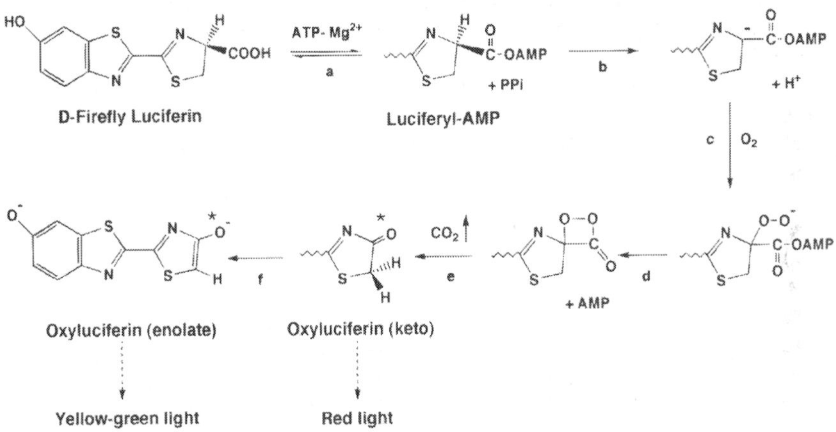

Fig. 3. The firefly luciferase bioluminescent reaction.
The luciferase protein holds the reduced luciferin to allow for adenylation (a). This process is followed by a deprotonation reaction that leads to the formation of a carbanion (b) and attack by oxygen (c), driving the formation of a cyclic intermediate (d). As this intermediate decays, carbon dioxide is released, forming the excited state luciferin in either the keto (e) or enolate (f) form. Used with permission from (Branchini, B. et al., 1998).

The kinetics of this reaction can be altered by varying the concentration of the substrates, with low concentrations (in the nM range) showing steady light production and high concentrations (μM range) producing a bright flash followed by decay to 5–10% of the maximum (DeLuca, Marlene et al., 1979). There are multiple possible inhibitory compounds that could be responsible for the kinetic profile generated under high substrate concentrations. It has previously been shown that even though oxyluciferin is a natural product of the luciferase reaction, it is capable of remaining bound as an inhibitor to enzymatic turnover (Denburg et al., 1969). The same was found to be true of another potential byproduct, L-AMP, which can account for up to 16% of the product formed during the luminescent reaction (Fontes et al., 1998). This may, in part, explain how the addition of CoA to the luminescent reaction can result in improved performance. When CoA is added during the initial steps of the reaction it prevents the fast signal decay normally observed, and when it is added following this decay it can promote re-initiation of the flash kinetics. This can be attributed to CoA's interaction with L-AMP to form L-CoA, resulting in turnover of the Luc enzyme and reoccurrence of the luminescent reaction (Airth et al., 1958).

4.2.3 Click beetle luciferase proteins

While the Luc protein from *Photinus pyralis* is the most extensively studied of the D-luciferin utilizing enzymes, it is certainly not the only example from within this order of organisms. The insects represent a large related group of bioluminescent organisms, with over 2500 species reported to be capable of generating light (Viviani, 2002). While the vast majority of these luminescent reactions remain unstudied, the main exception is in the order Coleoptera (beetles) where systems have been characterized for the click beetles (Fraga, 2008). The main advantage of the click beetle luciferase proteins are that they are available in a wider array of colors than the firefly Luc protein. Despite these differences in emission wavelength, the substrates and mechanism of action are similar to that of the more well characterized Luc system, allowing for easy substitution with the Luc system if the need arises. Another advantage of the alternate color availability of the click beetle luciferases is that they can be used in conjunction with the Luc system and imaged simultaneously if a means of differentiating the individual emission wavelengths is available.

While it was originally believed that the different colors of the click beetle luciferase proteins were the result of divergent luciferase structures, this was shown not to be the case when the sequences of four luciferase genes from *Pyrophorus plagiophthalamus* with four different emission spectra were sequenced and found that they shared up to 99% amino acid identity (Wood, Lam, Seliger et al., 1989). There are currently three mechanisms that have been proposed to explain the multiple bioluminescent colorations: the active site polarity hypothesis (DeLuca, M, 1969), the tautomerization hypothesis (White, E. & Branchini, 1975), and the geometry hypothesis (McCapra, F., Gilfoyle, DJ., Young, DW., Church, NJ., Spencer P., 1994).

The active site polarity hypothesis is based on the idea that the wavelength of light produced is related to the microenvironment surrounding the luminescent protein during the reaction. In non-polar solvents the spectrum is shifted towards blue and in polar solvents it is more red-shifted. It is questionable, however, if polarity fluctuations can account for large scale changes like those that have been observed in *P. plagiophthalamus*. The tautomerization hypothesis states that the wavelength of light produced is dependent on if either the enol or keto form of the luciferin is formed during the course of the reaction. A recent study has reported that by altering the substrate of the reaction, the keto form of the luciferin can produce either red or green light, making this hypothesis unlikely. Finally, the geometry hypothesis suggests that the geometry of the excited state oxyluciferin is responsible for determining the emission wavelength. In a 90° conformation it would achieve its lowest energy state and red light would be produced, whereas in the planar conformation it would be in its highest energy state and green light would be produced. Intermediate colors would be the result of geometries between these two extremes (Viviani, 2002).

4.2.4 Summary of advantages and disadvantages

Advantages and Disadvantages of the D-luciferin Utilizing Luciferase Proteins	
Advantages	**Disadvantages**
High sensitivity and low signal-to-noise ratio Quantitative correlation between signal strength and cell numbers Low background in animal tissues Variations of firefly luciferase (stabilized and red-shifted) and click beetle luciferases (red and green) are available Different colors allow multi-component monitoring	Requires exogenous luciferin addition Fast consumption of luciferin can lead to unstable signal ATP and oxygen dependent Currently not practical for large animal models

Table 2. Advantages and Disadvantages of Using D-luciferin Utilizing Luciferase Proteins in the Mammalian Cellular Environment

4.3 Luciferase proteins that utilize coelenterazine as an exogenous substrate

While the D-luciferin utilizing Luc system may be the most popular for mammalian imaging experiments, it is the coelenterazine utilizing luciferase proteins that are the most widely occurring. In nature there are examples of these types of luciferase proteins in cnidarians, copepods, chaetognaths, ctenophores, decapod shrimps, mysid shrimps, radiolarians, and some fish taxa as well (Greer & Szalay, 2002). The coelenterazine substrate has the chemical structure of 2-(p-hydroxybenzyl)-6-(p-hydroxyphenyl)-8-benzylimidazo-[1,2-a]pyrazin-3-(7H)-one (Bhaumik & Gambhir, 2002), and under its native function is bound to an associated protein to prevent availability to the luciferase. The strength of this bond is dependent on changes in calcium dynamics within the host cell, with increases leading to the detachment and subsequent availability of the substrate to participate in the bioluminescent reaction (Anderson et al., 1974). This system has been adapted, however, so that when the luciferase protein is expressed in a host cell, the coelenterazine substrate can be supplied exogenously, triggering the production of light without the need for changes in intracellular calcium levels. The primary example of a coelenterazine utilizing reporter is the luciferase from the sea pansy *Renilla reniformis* (RLuc). This protein interacts with its coelenterazine substrate to produce bioluminescence at 480 nm (Bhaumik & Gambhir, 2002). Because this wavelength is relatively blue-shifted compared to the D-luciferin luciferase utilizing proteins and because the two reporters require dissimilar substrates for activation, RLuc can be used either as a stand-alone reporter system or in conjunction with the Luc variants to simultaneously image multiple locations within the host. This multi-functionality has lead to an increase in the popularity of RLuc for mammalian imaging in recent years.

4.3.1 *Renilla* luciferase structure

Unlike the previously discussed luciferin proteins, those that utilize coelenterazine as a substrate have not been found to display high levels of structural similarity, even when originating from within the same family. This most likely indicates that they are predominantly the result of individual evolutionary events (Loening et al., 2007). The structure of the RLuc gene from *Renilla reniformis* will be given as an example because it is the most laboratory relevant of the coelenterazine utilizing luciferase proteins, but caution should be used when attempting to interpret the associated mechanism of action with alternate luciferase proteins without first determining their structural discrepancies.

The RLuc protein is a 37 kDa enzyme comprised of 311 amino acids that exists as a monomer in solution. Crystal structures of the RLuc protein exist (both with and without bound substrate) at a resolution of 1.4 Å, however, these were constructed using a modified version of the protein that included 8 amino acid mutations (Loening et al., 2007). These mutations were included because they allow for more efficient expression as compared to the native enzyme and have not been shown to have a deleterious effect on bioluminescent production (Loening et al., 2006). The overall structure of the RLuc enzyme can be broken down into two domains. The core domain takes the form of an α/β-hydrolase fold (Loening et al., 2007), a structure composed of 8 β-sheets connected by α-helixes. This structure is common to hydrolytic enzymes and is known to contain a catalytic triad that is responsible for carrying out their associated enzymatic reaction (Ollis et al., 1992). The cap domain is located above the core domain and consists of the residues from 146 to 330, which make up the region between α-helix "D" and β-sheet "6" (Loening et al., 2007).

The N terminal region of the protein is believed to exhibit a flexible conformation in solution, with the initial 10–15 residues capable of wrapping around the remainder of the protein towards the presumptive enzymatic pocket. However, it is not believed that these residues are absolutely required for securing the bound substrate or for proper steric positioning. To illustrate this point, RLuc proteins that have had the first 14 residues removed are still capable of producing more than 25% of their original activity. It is believed instead that a 10 amino acid flexible region corresponding to residues 153–163 within the cap domain is responsible for these actions (Loening et al., 2007). This is consistent with previously characterized, structurally similar enzymes and therefore more likely to be the case (Schanstra & Janssen, 1996).

The active site is believed to center around the catalytic triad, which is composed of the amino acids Asp 120, Glu 144, and His 285. This placement is consistent with that of other known α/β-hydrolase proteins, with the nucleophile (Asp 120) located immediately after the fifth β-sheet (Loening et al., 2006). This area is known as the "nucleophile elbow" and follows the general sequence pattern of Gly-X-(nucleophile)-X-Gly (Heikinheimo et al., 1999). In RLuc these residues are Gly 118-His 119-Asp 120-Trp 121-Gly 122. Further evidence that this is indeed the location of the active site was gathered by mutational analysis which showed that the mutations most detrimental to enzyme function occurred either in one of the three proposed catalytic triad residues or in Asn 53, Trp 121, or Pro 220, three residues that reside in the rear of the proposed active site pocket. This pocket is surrounded by a ring of hydrophobic and aromatic residues such as isoleucine, valine, phenylalanine, and tryptophan that are believed to aid in the orientation and binding of the coelenterazine substrate.

4.3.2 *Renilla* luciferase mechanism of action

In the *Renilla* luciferase bioluminescent reaction the luciferin (coelenterazine) undergoes oxidative decarboxylation in the presence of oxygen to produce CO_2, the oxidized oxyluciferin, and light at a wavelength of 480 nm (Hart et al., 1978). Under native conditions this reaction takes place within specialized subcelluar compartments called lumisomes, however, during the course of mammalian expression the protein will be located wherever the gene is targeted using common sequence tags. Activation is also simplified during mammalian expression. Unlike under native conditions when the coelenterazine substrate would be trapped by an associated binding protein until changes in local calcium concentration gradients triggered its release, making it available for binding by the RLuc protein (Anderson et al., 1974), during exogenous expression these associated binding proteins are not natively present, and therefore the injection of coelenterazine is all that is required to elicit a bioluminescent response.

The coelenterazine substrate can be thought of as containing three complex reaction sites that each serve a purpose during binding and subsequent oxidation following interaction with the RLuc protein. The first domain (R1) is a *p*-hydroxy-phenyl group, the second (R2) is a benzyl ring, and the third (R3) is a *p*-hydroxy-benzyl ring. While the exact binding locations of each region of the substrate has not been confirmed, docking simulations have suggested potential locations that can be used to support the current hypothesis for the RLuc mechanism of action. These simulations suggest that the R1 group binds in a position where it is accessible to the catalytic triad of Asp 120, Glu 144 and His 285, possibly by stabilization due to interaction between the hydroxyl of the R1 group and Asn 53 of the RLuc protein. Further stabilization would be provided by interaction of the R3 domain with the Thr 184 residue (Woo et al., 2008).

Once the substrate has been bound and localized to the active site of RLuc, the chemical reaction occurs that produces the telltale bioluminescent signal. This reaction appears to be similar to the chemical reaction that occurs in other coelenterazine utilizing luciferase proteins such as aequorin despite their structural differences (Anderson et al., 1974). Once bound to RLuc, oxygen attaches at C2 resulting in the formation of a hydroperoxide. This hydroperoxide then becomes deprotonated (presumably through interaction with the catalytic triad) and the resulting negative charge on the hydroperoxide then undergoes a nucleophilic attack on C3 of coelenterazine to irreversibly form a dioxetanone intermediate. It is this cyclization that then provides the energy required to drive the production of light from the overall reaction (Vysotski & Lee, 2004). As the bonds between newly cyclized oxygens collapse the peroxide is released as CO_2 and the excited, anionic state of coelenterazine is formed. As this form decays a photon is released, and finally the fully oxidized luciferin is formed and released (Hart et al., 1978).

4.3.3 *Gaussia* luciferase

Gaussia luciferase (GLuc) represents an interesting example of a coelenterazine utilizing luciferase protein that is naturally secreted from the cell. GLuc is a small 19.9 kDa protein consisting of only 185 amino acids that, in the presence of its substrate coelenterazine, will produce a bioluminescent signal with a peak at 480 nm similar to RLuc. However, GLuc has some interesting properties that set it apart from RLuc as an imaging target in the mammalian environment. The most unique difference is that the GLuc protein can be encoded to either remain in the cell or be naturally excreted depending on the presence or absence of an included signal peptide. This property allows the resulting luminescent signal to be used either for localization within a cell or for facile high throughput screening using spent cell culture media without the need to disturb the cells via exposure to coelenterazine. In addition to the excretable nature of the GLuc protein, it has also been shown to produce a brighter bioluminescent signal than its RLuc counterpart following substrate exposure (Tannous et al., 2005). This means that the same 480 nm bioluminescent signal can be achieved as during use with RLuc, but less of the luciferase protein is required to generate the same level of signal. Therefore GLuc, without its associated excretory signal peptide, may be a suitable alternative to RLuc if imaging is required at extremely low cell population sizes. While there are other coelenterazine utilizing luciferase proteins available, the advantages and utility of GLuc make it the main counterpart to RLuc for laboratory use today.

4.3.4 Summary of advantages and disadvantages

Advantages and Disadvantages of Coelenterazine Utilizing Luciferase Proteins	
Advantages	**Disadvantages**
High sensitivity	Requires exogenous coelenterazine addition
Quantitative correlation between signal strength and cell numbers	Low anatomic resolution
Stabilized and red-shifted *Renilla* luciferase are available	Increased background due to oxidation of coelenterazine by serum
Secretion of *Gaussia* luciferase allows for subject-independent bioluminescence measurement	Oxygen dependent
	Fast consumption of coelenterazine can lead to unstable signal
	Currently not practical for large animal models

Table 3. Advantages and Disadvantages of Using Coelenterazine Utilizing Luciferase Proteins in the Mammalian Cellular Environment

4.4 Examples of use as a mammalian biosensor

4.4.1 Steady state imaging

Steady state imaging using substrate requiring bioluminescent protein reporters is performed in a similar fashion to imaging using fluorescent reporter proteins, only with the injection of the substrate chemical performed in place of stimulation with an excitation wavelength. The main advantage offered by the use of the bioluminescent systems is that the injection of substrate does not create background luminescence because there are no native bioluminescent proteins in the mammalian tissue. This allows researchers to achieve detection with much smaller cell population sizes when using bioluminescent reporter systems. The most common use of steady state imaging using these types of reporter systems has been for the study of tumorigenesis and evaluation of tumor treatment. For example, Kim and colleagues have demonstrated this advantage with the newest generation of these reporters designed for tumor detection. These investigators were able to inject codon-optimized FLuc containing 4T1 mouse mammary tumor cells subcutaneously and then image single bioluminescent cells at a background ratio of 6:1 (Kim et al., 2010). This experiment effectively demonstrates how substrate utilizing reporters can be used to continuously monitor cancer development from a single cell all the way to complete tumor formation.

4.4.2 Multi-component bioluminescent imaging

Because the substrate requiring bioluminescent reporter systems are dependent on activation by a specific substrate, commonly either D-luciferin or coelenterazine, it is possible to use one luciferase of each type simultaneously in the same host. To trigger bioluminescent production from an individual reporter protein, its specific substrate is added. This design elicits luminescent production from the target while not activating the alternate bioluminescent reporter. This type of experimental design allows for localization of multiple cellular groups from within a single cell or host animal. It is also possible to use a bioluminescent reporter in conjunction with an associated fluorescent reporter in a manner similar to FRET, only in this case the original luminescent signal is bioluminescent in nature and not fluorescent. This type of experiment is referred to as bioluminescence resonance energy transfer (BRET) and has been used by Angers et. al. to demonstrate the presence of G-protein coupled receptor dimers on the surface of living cells. By tagging a subset of β_2-adrenergic receptor proteins with RLuc and a subset with the red-shifted variant of green fluorescent protein, YFP, it was possible to detect both a luminescent and fluorescent signal in cells expressing both variants, but no fluorescent signal in cells expressing only YFP since no fluorescent excitation signal was used (Angers et al., 2000).

4.4.3 Overall tumor load imaging

The naturally secreted nature of the GLuc protein has lead to interesting advances whereby it can be used to monitor overall tumor burden in small animal models without the requirement of directly imaging the host animal. This has been demonstrated by Chung and colleagues who induced bioluminescence from blood samples of host animals suffering from tumors that had been tagged with the gene for expression of GLuc. Since the GLuc protein was secreted into the blood it was possible to correlate bioluminescence of the blood sample with overall tumor load without ever having to introduce the coelenterazine substrate to the animal. This process was capable of reporting on tumors at lower levels than would have been possible using traditional steady state tumor imaging, and was capable of reporting on the dynamics of tumor growth in response to treatment (Chung et al., 2009).

4.5 Concerns related to substrate injection route

When working with luciferase proteins that utilize an exogenous substrate in small animal models, it will be necessary to introduce the requisite substrate through injection. However, the chosen route of substrate injection can have influential effects on the emission of a luminescent signal. As a result, although logistical concerns may be most pertinent to consideration for investigators, the method of injection should be considered in light of the proposed objectives of any study (Inoue et al., 2009). The three most common substrate injection routes are intraperitoneal, intravenous, and subcutaneous. Each results in the introduction of the substrate in a unique manner and, although each should elicit bioluminescent production of an expressed reporter protein, they will all do so on different time scales and with different expression kinetics. It is therefore important to have a basic understanding of the resulting luminescent profiles of each type of injection prior to determining which is best suited to an individual experimental design.

4.5.1 Intraperitoneal injection of substrate

The appeal of intraperitoneal injection for the majority of researchers is its convenience, however, following this route of injection the substrate must absorb across the peritoneum before reaching the luciferase expressing cell populations. Any variations in the rate of absorption can lead to variations in the resulting luminescent signal. These variations, even when subtle, can increase the difficulty of reproducing the luminescent results (Keyaerts et al., 2008). In addition, investigator error can lead to injection into the bowel, causing a weak or non-existent luminescent signal that can be confused with a negative result (Baba et al., 2007). Because of the associated diffusion, intraperitoneal injection produces lower peak luminescence levels than alternate injection techniques when inducing light production in subcutaneous tumor models, however, it has been found that it can also overestimate tumor size when used to induce luminescence from intraperitoneal or spleen-localized tumors, due to direct contact between the luciferin and the luciferase expressing cells (Inoue et al., 2009). The greater availability of the luciferin to the luciferase containing cells increases the amount of bioluminescent output by allowing them greater access to their luciferin without being limited by diffusion through non-luciferase containing tissue. This increases the influx of the luciferin compound into the cell due to the resulting increased concentration gradient.

4.5.2 Intravenous injection of substrate

Intravenous injection can be used to systematically profuse a test subject with D-luciferin or coelenterazine. It is also a facile method for exposing multiple tissue locations to the substrate on relatively similar timescales. Because the administration of the luciferin is systemic, it allows for lower doses to be administered to achieve similar luminescence intensities as would be seen using alternate injection routes (Keyaerts et al., 2008), however, studies using radio-labeled D-luciferin have indicated that the uptake rate of intravenously injected substrate is slower in the gastrointestinal organs, pancreas, and spleen than would be achieved using intraperitoneal injection (Lee et al., 2003). It is also important to note that when intravenous injection is used, the resulting luminescent signal is often of a much shorter duration than would be observed using alternate injection routes (Inoue et al., 2009).

4.5.3 Subcutaneous injection of substrate

Subcutaneous injection is often used as an alternative to intraperitoneal injection in order to avoid the signal attenuation shortcomings of the intravenous injection route. Bryant et al. (Bryant et al., 2008) have demonstrated that repeated subcutaneous injection of luciferin can provide a simple and accurate model for monitoring brain tumor growth in rats, and though there is concern that repeated injection could cause excessive tissue damage, it has been demonstrated that the repeated subcutaneous injection of D-luciferin or coelenterazine into an animal model results in minimal injection site damage while providing researchers with bioluminescent signals that correlate well with intraperitoneal substrate injection luminescent profiles, albeit with a longer lag time prior to reaching tumor models in the intraperitoneal space (Inoue et al., 2009).

5. The bacterial luciferase proteins

5.1 Introduction

Luminescent bacteria are the most abundant and widely distributed of the light emitting organisms on earth and can be found in both aquatic (freshwater and marine) and terrestrial environments. Despite the diverse nature of bacterial bioluminescence, the majority of these organisms are classified into three genera: *Vibrio*, *Photobacterium*, and *Photorhabdus*. Of these, only those from *Photorhabdus* have been discovered in terrestrial habitats (Meighen, 1991) and developed into reporters capable of functioning within the mammalian cellular environment (Close, D, Patterson et al., 2010). It is the terrestrial nature of the bacterial luciferase (*lux*) genes from *Photorhabdus* that made them suitable for adoption and use in mammalian tissues. The *lux* genes from the *Vibrio* and *Photobacterium* genera are marine in nature, and as such their protein products have been naturally adapted to function at lower ambient temperatures than those required for mammalian expression. However, even with their propensity to function efficiently at 37°C, the *Photorhabdus lux* genes required extensive modification to carry out the bioluminescent reaction in a non-bacterial host cell. Natively, the *lux* gene cassette consists of 5 genes organized sequentially in a single operon in the form *luxCDABE*. The *luxA* and *luxB* gene products form the heterodimeric luciferase enzyme, and the *luxD*, *luxC* and *luxE* gene products form a transferase, a synthase, and a reductase respectfully, that work together to produce and regenerate the required myristyl aldehyde co-substrate from endogenous myristyl groups. Because the substrates required by the *luxAB* heterodimer enzyme consist only of oxygen, $FMNH_2$, and the aldehyde that is formed by the *luxCDE* genes, this system has the unique ability to produce bioluminescence without the addition of exogenous substrate addition (Meighen, 1991). However, unlike the native, uncompartmentalized bacterial cellular environment, the mammalian intracellular environment does not contain high enough levels of reduced $FMNH_2$ to support efficient bioluminescent production. To alleviate this problem, a sixth *lux* gene must be co-expressed that is not present in all bacterial species. This sixth gene, *frp*, encodes an NAD(P)H:flavin reductase that helps to cycle endogenous FMN into the required $FMNH_2$ co-substrate (Close, D, Patterson et al., 2010).

To function properly within a mammalian host cell, the 5 *lux* genes, as well as an additional flavin reductase gene (*frp*), must be expressed simultaneously and at high levels. To accommodate these requirements the genes must be codon-optimized to the human codon preference and their expression linked via internal ribosomal entry elements or similar promoter independent intervening sequences. This allows for the relatively normalized levels of expression while reducing the overall amount of foreign DNA that must be introduced and maintained in the host genome. When expressed under these conditions, the *lux* genes are capable of producing a luminescent signal in the mammalian host cell at 490 nm without the need for any external stimulus (Close, D, Patterson et al., 2010). Although limited due to their relatively low luminescent yield compared to the luciferase-dependent reporter systems and blue-shifted luminescent signal, the unique ability of substrate-free luminescent production makes the Lux system a user friendly and attractive alternative to the D-luciferin or coelenterazine utilizing systems.

5.2 Bacterial luciferase structure

The functional bacterial luciferase enzyme is a heterodimer with a molecular weight of 77 kDa. The individual α and β subunits are the products of the *luxA* and *luxB* genes respectfully, and have molecular weights of 40 and 37 kDa. The two subunits appear to be the result of a gene duplication event owing to an approximately 30% amino acid sequence identity (Meighen, 1991). All previously characterized bacterial luciferases appear to be homologous and catalyze the same reaction, however, the majority of research has centered on the luciferase from the marine bacterium *Vibrio harveyi*, so the structure described in this review will be based on the protein from that organism along with its conventional numbering system.

Individually the α and β subunits of the luciferase heterodimer formed by the *luxA* and *luxB* genes are capable of producing a very weak bioluminescent signal, but dimerization is required for the reaction to proceed at biologically relevant levels (Choi et al., 1995). This finding, along with the similarities in structure between the two subunits would tend to implicate the dimer interface as the active site, however, the single active site has been proposed to exist only within the α subunit (Baldwin et al., 1995). Indeed, a recent crystal structure shows the oxidized FMN substrate bound to the α subunit only (Campbell, Z.T. et al., 2009).

Both of the α and β subunits have similar overall conformations, and assemble into a single-domain eight-stranded β/α barrel motif (also known as a TIM barrel after the first identified protein with that structure, triose-phosphate isomerase). The interiors of these barrels are packed with hydrophobic residues, as would be expected to aid in folding, while the N-terminal residues, which are exposed to solvent, contain hydrophilic residues. The C-terminal ends are hydrophobic, but are protected from solvent access by the presence of two antiparallel α-helices. The dimerization of the two subunits is mediated by a parallel four helix bundle centered on a pseudo two-fold axis of symmetry as it relates to the α and β subunit orientation. This region is highly populated with glycines and alanines, which allows for close contact between the two helical bundles. The majority of binding force is provided by van der Waals interactions across the 2150 $Å^2$ surface area, but twenty-two proposed hydrogen bonds, as well as forty-five water-mediated intersubunit hydrogen bonds and a series of hydrophobic interactions also aid in attachment (Fisher et al., 1996).

The active site is most probably a large, open cavity on the α subunit that is open to solvent at the C-terminal end of the barrel structure proximal to the β subunit. Crystal structures of the enzyme with an associated flavin show that it is bound here with the isoalloxazine ring in a planar conformation. The ribitol portion of the flavin extends away at an ~45° angle while the phosphate is stabilized by the side chains of Arg 107, Arg 125, Glu 175, Ser 176, Thr 179, and the backbone amide of Glu 175. The isoalloxanine ring is held in place through backbone contacts with Glu 175 and Phe 6 and the ribitol interactions cannot be clearly defined as occurring directly with the protein or being mediated by co-bound water molecules, but they can be localized to individual residues. The carbonyl oxygen at C2 of the ribitol hydrogen bonds with backbone amide hydrogen of Tyr 110, the nitrogen at position three forms a hydrogen bond with the backbone carbonyl oxygen of Glu 43, while the carbonyl oxygen at C4 hydrogen bonds to either the backbone amide proton or the enol form of the backbone carbonyl oxygen of Ala 75. It is likely, but as of yet unproven, that the aldehyde binding location is adjacent to the benzenoid portion of the isoalloxane ring because of its proximity to the FMN binding site, size, and abundance of tryptophan and phenylalanine residues (Campbell, Z.T. et al., 2009).

5.3 Bacterial luciferase mechanism of action

When the bacterial luciferase enzyme is supplied with oxygen, $FMNH_2$, and a long chain aliphatic aldehyde it is able to produce light at a wavelength of 490 nm. The natural aldehyde for this reaction is believed to be tetradecanal, however, the enzyme is capable of functioning with alternative aldehydes as substrates (Meighen, 1991). The first step in the generation of light from these substrates is the binding of $FMNH_2$ by the luciferase enzyme and until recently its active site on the enzyme was not known. It has recently been confirmed that $FMNH_2$ binds on the α subunit in a large valley on the C-terminal end of the β-barrel structure (Campbell, Z.T. et al., 2009). The nature of the interactions between $FMNH_2$ and the amino acid residues in this area is discussed in the structure section above.

In order for the reaction to proceed the luciferase must undergo a conformational change following $FMNH_2$ attachment. This movement is primarily expressed in a short section of residues known as the protease liable region: a section of 29 amino acids residing on a disordered region of the α subunit joining α-helix α7a to β-strand β7a. The majority of residues in this sequence are unique to the α subunit and have long been implicated in the luminescent mechanism (Baldwin et al., 1995). Following attachment of $FMNH_2$ this region becomes more ordered and is stabilized by an intersubunit interaction between Phe 272 of the α subunit and Tyr 115 of the β subunit. This conformational change has been theorized to stabilize the α subunit in a conformation favorable for the luciferase reaction to occur (Campbell, Z.T. et al., 2009).

NMR studies have suggested that $FMNH_2$ binds to the enzyme in its anionic state ($FMNH^-$) (Vervoort et al., 1986). With the flavin bound to the enzyme, molecular oxygen then binds to the C4a atom to form an intermediate 4a-hydroperoxy-5-hydroflavin (Nemtseva & Kudryasheva, 2007). It is important to note that this important C4a atom was determined to be in close proximity to a reactive thiol from the side chain of Cys 106 on the α subunit (Campbell, Z.T. et al., 2009), a residue that has long been hypothesized to play a role in the luminescent reaction, but since has been proven to be non-reactive through mutational analysis (Baldwin et al., 1987).

It has been shown, however, that C4a is the central atom for the luciferase reaction and, following establishment of the hydroperoxide there, it is capable of interaction with the aldehyde substrate via its oxygen molecule to form a peroxyhemiacetal group. This complex then undergoes a transformation (through an unknown intermediate or series of intermediates) to an excited state generally accepted to be a luciferase-bound 4a-hydroxy-5-hydroflavin mononucleotide, which then decays to give oxidized FMN, a corresponding aliphatic acid, and light (Fig. 4) (Nemtseva & Kudryasheva, 2007). There have classically been many theories proposed to explain the exact process required for light emission that continue to expand today as technology for detecting the intermediate complexes has improved (Hastings, JW & Nealson, 1977; Nemtseva & Kudryasheva, 2007).

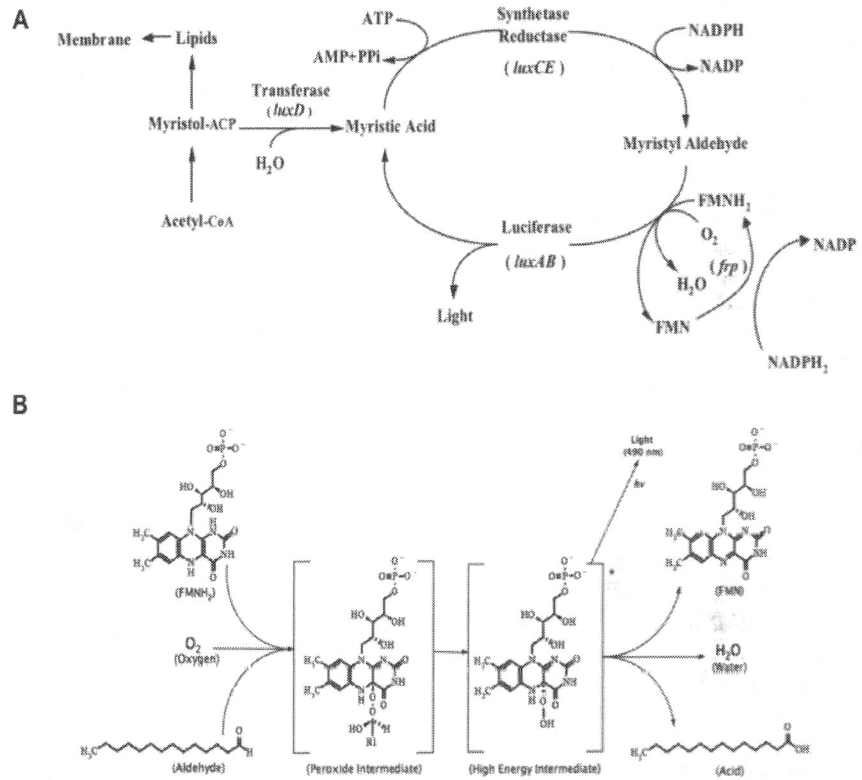

Fig. 4. Bioluminescent reaction catalyzed by the bacterial luciferase genes.
A) The luciferase is formed from a heterodimer of the *luxA* and *luxB* gene products. The aliphatic aldehyde is supplied and regenerated by the products of the *luxC*, *luxD*, and *luxE* genes. The required oxygen and reduced riboflavin phosphate substrates are scavenged from endogenous metabolic processes, however, the flavin reducatse gene (*frp*) aids in reduced flavin turnover rates in some species. B) The production of light, catalyzed by the products of the *luxAB* genes, results from the decay of a high energy intermediate (R1 = $C_{13}H_{27}$).

5.4 Use as a mammalian biosensor

Bacterial luciferase is the newest of the bioluminescent reporter proteins to be demonstrated for use with mammalian tissues. As a result, there have not been extensive publications on its use under these conditions. The initial reports, however, have been promising, with *lux*-containing cells capable of being used for steady state imaging both in culture and in small animal models (Close, D, Patterson et al., 2010). If the *lux* cassette genes undergo widespread adoption there is no reason to believe they will not become capable of functioning in roles similar to the substrate requiring bioluminescent reporter proteins. The main drawback of the *lux* genes for function in the mammalian cellular background has been their low signal strength. As a result, they may not be as well suited for small population size cellular imaging or deep tissue imaging, where their weak signal may be attenuated prior to detection. However, it is important to keep in mind that as this reporter system becomes more common it will be subjected to optimization in a process similar to the other common reporter systems. If this is the case the utility of the *lux* reporter system should continue to increase with time.

5.5 Summary of advantages and disadvantages

Advantages and Disadvantages of the Bacterial Luciferase Gene Cassette	
Advantages	**Disadvantages**
High sensitivity and low signal-to-noise ratio	Bioluminescence at 490 nm prone to absorption in animal tissues
Quantitative correlation between signal strength and cell numbers	Low anatomic resolution
Fully autonomous system, no requirement for addition of exogenous substrate	NADPH and oxygen dependent
Noninvasive	Not as bright as other luciferases
Stable signal	Currently not practical for large animal models
Rapid detection permitting real-time monitoring	Short history of use

Table 4. Advantages and Disadvantages of Using the Bacterial Luciferase Gene Cassette in the Mammalian Cellular Environment

6. Conclusions

This chapter has presented only the most basic and widely used of the mammalian reporter proteins and is by no means exhaustive. It is important to recognize that there is no universally recognized optimal reporter system and that the choice of a reporter target should be made in light of the specific demands of each experimental design. Each reporter system has its own advantages and disadvantages, and each can be adapted to work under multiple imaging scenarios. The constant introduction of improved reporter protein targets and modifications to existing reporter proteins suggest that the future of imaging in mammalian tissues should be bright for years to come.

7. Acknowledgments

Portions of this review reflecting work by the authors was supported by the National Science Foundation Division of Chemical, Bioengineering, Environmental, and Transport Systems (CBET) under award number CBET-0853780, the National Institutes of Health, National Cancer Institute, Cancer Imaging Program, award number CA127745-01, the University of Tennessee Research Foundation Technology Maturation Funding program, and the Army Defense University Research Instrumentation Program.

8. References

Aguilera, R., Montoya, J., Primm, T., & Varela-Ramirez, A. (2006). Green Fluorescent Protein as a Biosensor for Toxic Compounds. *Reviews in Fluorescence,* 2006, 463-476.

Airth, R., Rhodes, W., & McElroy, W. (1958). The function of coenzyme A in luminescence. *Biochimica et Biophysica Acta,* 27, 519-532.

Anderson, J., Charbonneau, H., & Cormier, M. (1974). Mechanism of calcium induction of *Renilla* bioluminescence. Involvement of a calcium-triggered luciferin binding protein. *Biochemistry,* 13, 6, pp. 1195-1200.

Ando, Y., Niwa, K., Yamada, N., Enomoto, T., Irie, T., Kubota, H., et al. (2007). Firefly bioluminescence quantum yield and colour change by pH-sensitive green emission. *Nature Photonics,* 2, 1, pp. 44-47.

Angers, S., Salahpour, A., Joly, E., Hilairet, S., Chelsky, D., Dennis, M., et al. (2000). Detection of B_2-adrenergic receptor dimerization in living cells using bioluminescence resonance energy transfer (BRET). *Proc. Natl. Acad. Sci. U. S .A.,* 97, 7, pp. 3684-3689.

Baba, S., Cho, S., Ye, Z., Cheng, L., Engles, J., & Wahl, R. (2007). How reproducible is bioluminescent imaging of tumor cell growth? Single time point versus the dynamic measurement approach. *Molecular imaging: official journal of the Society for Molecular Imaging,* 6, 5, pp. 315.

Baldwin, T. O., Chen, L. H., Chlumsky, L. J., Devine, J. H., Johnston, T. C., Lin, J. W., et al. (1987). Structural analysis of bacterial luciferase. *Flavins and flavoproteins. Walter de Gruyter & Co., Berlin*621-631.

Baldwin, T. O., Christopher, J. A., Raushel, F. M., Sinclair, J. F., Ziegler, M. M., Fisher, A. J., et al. (1995). Structure of bacterial luciferase. *Current Opinion in Structural Biology,* 5, 6, pp. 798-809.

Barak, L. S., Ferguson, S. S. G., Zhang, J., & Caron, M. G. (1997). A beta arrestin/green fluorescent protein biosensor for detecting G protein-coupled receptor activation. *Journal of Biological Chemistry,* 272, 44, pp. 27497.

Barondeau, D. P., Putnam, C. D., Kassmann, C. J., Tainer, J. A., & Getzoff, E. D. (2003). Mechanism and energetics of green fluorescent protein chromophore synthesis revealed by trapped intermediate structures. *Proceedings of the National Academy of Sciences of the United States of America,* 100, 21, pp. 12111-12116.

Bhaumik, S., & Gambhir, S. S. (2002). Optical imaging of *Renilla* luciferase reporter gene expression in living mice. *Proceedings of the National Academy of Sciences of the United States of America,* 99, 1, pp. 377-382.

Branchini, B., Magyar, R., Murtiashaw, M., Anderson, S., & Zimmer, M. (1998). Site-directed mutagenesis of histidine 245 in firefly luciferase: A proposed model of the active site. *Biochemistry,* 37, 44, pp. 15311-15319.

Branchini, B. R., Southworth, T. L., Murtiashaw, M. H., Wilkinson, S. R., Khattak, N. F., Rosenberg, J. C., et al. (2005). Mutagenesis evidence that the partial reactions of firefly bioluminescence are catalyzed by different conformations of the luciferase C-terminal domain. *Biochemistry,* 44, 5, pp. 1385-1393.

Bryant, M. J., Chuah, T. L., Luff, J., Lavin, M. F., & Walker, D. G. (2008). A novel rat model for glioblastoma multiforme using a bioluminescent F98 cell line. *J. Clin. Neurosci.,* 15, 5, pp. 545-551.

Campbell, R., Tour, O., Palmer, A., Steinbach, P., Baird, G., Zacharias, D., et al. (2002). A monomeric red fluorescent protein. *Proceedings of the National Academy of Sciences of the United States of America,* 99, 12, pp. 7877.

Campbell, Z. T., Weichsel, A., Montfort, W. R., & Baldwin, T. O. (2009). Crystal Structure of the Bacterial Luciferase/Flavin Complex Provides Insight into the Function of the Subunit.

Chance, B., Cope, M., Gratton, E., Ramanujam, N., & Tromberg, B. (1998). Phase measurement of light absorption and scatter in human tissue. *Review of scientific instruments,* 69, 10, pp. 3457-3481.

Chattoraj, M., King, B. A., Bublitz, G. U., & Boxer, S. G. (1996). Ultra-fast excited state dynamics in green fluorescent protein: Multiple states and proton transfer. *Proceedings of the National Academy of Sciences of the United States of America,* 93, 16, pp. 8362-8367.

Choi, H., Tang, C., & Tu, S. (1995). Catalytically active forms of the individual subunits of *Vibrio harveyi* luciferase and their kinetic and binding properties. *Journal of Biological Chemistry,* 270, 28, pp. 16813.

Choy, G., O Connor, S., Diehn, F., Costouros, N., Alexander, H., Choyke, P., et al. (2003). Comparison of noninvasive fluorescent and bioluminescent small animal optical imaging. *Biotechniques,* 35, 5, pp. 1022-1031.

Chung, E., Yamashita, H., Au, P., Tannous, B., Fukumura, D., & Jain, R. (2009). Secreted *Gaussia* luciferase as a biomarker for monitoring tumor progression and treatment response of systemic metastases. *PLoS ONE,* 4, 12, pp. e8316.

Close, D., Patterson, S., Ripp, S., Baek, S., Sanseverino, J., & Sayler, G. (2010). Autonomous Bioluminescent Expression of the Bacterial Luciferase Gene Cassette (*lux*) in a Mammalian Cell Line. *PLoS One,* 5, 8, pp. 235-260.

Close, D., Xu, T., Sayler, G. S., & Ripp, S. (2010). *In vivo* bioluminescent imaging (BLI): noninvasive visualization and interrogation of biological processes in living animals. *Sensors,* 11, 1, pp. 180-206.

Conti, E., Franks, N. P., & Brick, P. (1996). Crystal structure of firefly luciferase throws light on a superfamily of adenylate-forming enzymes. *Structure,* 4, 3, pp. 287-298.

Crameri, A., Whitehorn, E. A., Tate, E., & Stemmer, W. P. C. (1996). Improved green fluorescent protein by molecular evolution using DNA shuffling. *Nature Biotechnology,* 14, 3, pp. 315-319.

Cubitt, A., Heim, R., Adams, S., Boyd, A., Gross, L., & Tsien, R. (1995). Understanding, improving and using green fluorescent proteins. *Trends in biochemical sciences,* 20, 11, pp. 448-455.

Day, R. (1998). Visualization of Pit-1 transcription factor interactions in the living cell nucleus by fluorescence resonance energy transfer microscopy. *Molecular Endocrinology,* 12, 9, pp. 1410.

de Wet, J., Wood, K., Helinski, D., & DeLuca, M. (1986). Cloning firefly luciferase. *Methods in Enzymology,* 133, 3-14.

DeLuca, M. (1969). Hydrophobic nature of the active site of firefly luciferase. *Biochemistry,* 8, 1, pp. 160-166.

DeLuca, M., Wannlund, J., & McElroy, W. D. (1979). Factors affecting the kinetics of light emission from crude and purified firefly luciferase. *Analytical Biochemistry,* 95, 1, pp. 194-198.

Denburg, J., Lee, R., & McElroy, W. (1969). Substrate-binding properties of firefly luciferase: I. Luciferin-binding site. *Archives of Biochemistry and Biophysics,* 134, 2, pp. 381-394.

Fisher, A. J., Thompson, T. B., Thoden, J. B., Baldwin, T. O., & Rayment, I. (1996). The 1.5-A resolution crystal structure of bacterial luciferase in low salt conditions. *Journal of Biological Chemistry,* 271, 36, pp. 21956.

Fontes, R., Ortiz, B., de Diego, A., Sillero, A., & Sillero, M. A. G. (1998). Dehydroluciferyl-AMP is the main intermediate in the luciferin dependent synthesis of Ap(4)A catalyzed by firefly luciferase. *Febs Letters,* 438, 3, pp. 190-194.

Fraga, H. (2008). Firefly luminescence: A historical perspective and recent developments. *Photochemical & Photobiological Sciences,* 7, 2, pp. 146-158.

Gould, S., & Subramani, S. (1988). Firefly luciferase as a tool in molecular and cell biology. *Analytical Biochemistry,* 175, 1, pp. 5-13.

Greer, L. F., & Szalay, A. A. (2002). Imaging of light emission from the expression of luciferases in living cells and organisms: a review. *Luminescence,* 17, 1, pp. 43-74.

Hart, R., Stempel, K., Boyer, P., & Cormier, M. (1978). Mechanism of the enzyme-catalyzed bioluminescent oxidation of coelenterate-type luciferin. *Biochemical and Biophysical Research Communications,* 81, 3, pp. 980-986.

Hastings, J., McElroy, W., & Coulombre, J. (1953). The effect of oxygen upon the immobilization reaction in firefly luminescence. *Journal of cellular and comparative physiology,* 42, 1, pp. 137-150.

Hastings, J., & Nealson, K. (1977). Bacterial bioluminescence. *Annual Reviews in Microbiology,* 31, 1, pp. 549-595.

Heikinheimo, P., Goldman, A., Jeffries, C., & Ollis, D. (1999). Of barn owls and bankers: a lush variety of alpha/beta hydrolases. *Structure,* 7, 6, pp. R141-R146.

Heim, R., Prasher, D., & Tsien, R. (1994). Wavelength mutations and posttranslational autoxidation of green fluorescent protein. *Proceedings of the National Academy of Sciences of the United States of America,* 91, 26, pp. 12501.

Hein, R., & Tsien, R. Y. (1996). Engineering green fluorescent protein for improved brightness, longer wavelengths and fluorescence resonance energy transfer. *Current Biology,* 6, 2, pp. 178-182.

Inoue, Y., Kiryu, S., Izawa, K., Watanabe, M., Tojo, A., & Ohtomo, K. (2009). Comparison of subcutaneous and intraperitoneal injection of D-luciferin for in vivo bioluminescence imaging. *Eur. J. Nucl. Med. Mol. Imaging,* 36, 5, pp. 771-779.

Jung, G., Wiehler, J., & Zumbusch, A. (2005). The photophysics of green fluorescent protein: Influence of the key amino acids at positions 65, 203, and 222. *Biophysical Journal,* 88, 3, pp. 1932-1947.

Keyaerts, M., Verschueren, J., Bos, T. J., Tchouate-Gainkam, L. O., Peleman, C., Breckpot, K., et al. (2008). Dynamic bioluminescence imaging for quantitative tumour burden assessment using IV or IP administration of D-luciferin: effect on intensity, time kinetics and repeatability of photon emission. *Eur. J. Nucl. Med. Mol. Imaging,* 35, 5, pp. 999-1007.

Kim, J. B., Urban, K., Cochran, E., Lee, S., Ang, A., Rice, B., et al. (2010). Non-invasive detection of a small number of bioluminescent cancer cells *in vivo*. *PLoS ONE,* 5, 2, pp. e9364. doi:9310.1371/journal.pone.0009364.

Lee, K. H., Byun, S. S., Paik, J. Y., Lee, S. Y., Song, S. H., Choe, Y. S., et al. (2003). Cell uptake and tissue distribution of radioiodine labelled D-luciferin: implications for luciferase based gene imaging. *Nucl. Med. Commun.,* 24, 9, pp. 1003-1009.

Loening, A., Fenn, T., & Gambhir, S. (2007). Crystal structures of the luciferase and green fluorescent protein from *Renilla reniformis*. *Journal of Molecular Biology,* 374, 4, pp. 1017-1028.

Loening, A., Fenn, T., Wu, A., & Gambhir, S. (2006). Consensus guided mutagenesis of *Renilla* luciferase yields enhanced stability and light output. *Protein Engineering Design and Selection,* 19, 9, pp. 391.

Matz, M. V., Fradkov, A. F., Labas, Y. A., Savitsky, A. P., Zaraisky, A. G., Markelov, M. L., et al. (1999). Fluorescent proteins from nonbioluminescent *Anthozoa* species. *Nature Biotechnology,* 17, 10, pp. 969-973.

McCapra, F., Chang, Y., & Francois, V. (1968). The chemiluminescence of a firefly luciferin analogue. *Chemical Communications (London),* 1968, 1, pp. 22-23.

McCapra, F., Gilfoyle, DJ., Young, DW., Church, NJ., Spencer P. (1994). *The Chemical origin of color differences in beetle bioluminescence*. Chichester: Wiley.

Meighen, E. A. (1991). Molecular biology of bacterial bioluminescence. *Microbiological Reviews,* 55, 1, pp. 123-142.

Nakatsu, T., Ichiyama, S., Hiratake, J., Saldanha, A., Kobashi, N., Sakata, K., et al. (2006). Structural basis for the spectral difference in luciferase bioluminescence. *Nature,* 440, 7082, pp. 372-376.

Nemtseva, E., & Kudryasheva, N. (2007). The mechanism of electronic excitation in the bacterial bioluminescent reaction. *Russian Chemical Reviews,* 76, 1, pp. 91-100.

Niwa, H., Inouye, S., Hirano, T., Matsuno, T., Kojima, S., Kubota, M., et al. (1996). Chemical nature of the light emitter of the Aequorea green fluorescent protein. *Proceedings of the National Academy of Sciences of the United States of America,* 93, 24, pp. 13617-13622.

Ollis, D., Cheah, E., Cygler, M., Dijkstra, B., Frolow, F., Franken, S., et al. (1992). The Alpha/Beta hydrolase fold. *Protein Engineering Design and Selection,* 5, 3, pp. 197.

Ormo, M., Cubitt, A. B., Kallio, K., Gross, L. A., Tsien, R. Y., & Remington, S. J. (1996). Crystal structure of the Aequorea victoria green fluorescent protein. *Science,* 273, 5280, pp. 1392-1395.

Palm, G. J., Zdanov, A., Gaitanaris, G. A., Stauber, R., Pavlakis, G. N., & Wlodawer, A. (1997). The structural basis for spectral variations in green fluorescent protein. *Nature Structural Biology,* 4, 5, pp. 361-365.

Patterson, G., Knobel, S., Sharif, W., Kain, S., & Piston, D. (1997). Use of the green fluorescent protein and its mutants in quantitative fluorescence microscopy. *Biophysical journal*, 73, 5, pp. 2782-2790.

Phillips, G. N. (1997). Structure and dynamics of green fluorescent protein. *Current Opinion in Structural Biology*, 7, 6, pp. 821-827.

Sandalova, T. P., & Ugarova, N. N. (1999). Model of the active site of firefly luciferase. *Biochemistry-Moscow*, 64, 8, pp. 962-967.

Schanstra, J., & Janssen, D. (1996). Kinetics of halide release of haloalkane dehalogenase: evidence for a slow conformational change. *Biochemistry*, 35, 18, pp. 5624-5632.

Seliger, H., & McElroy, W. (1960). Spectral emission and quantum yield of firefly bioluminescence. *Archives of Biochemistry and Biophysics*, 88, 1, pp. 136-141.

Shaner, N., Campbell, R., Steinbach, P., Giepmans, B., Palmer, A., & Tsien, R. (2004). Improved monomeric red, orange and yellow fluorescent proteins derived from *Discosoma* sp. red fluorescent protein. *Nature Biotechnology*, 22, 12, pp. 1567-1572.

Tannous, B., Kim, D., Fernandez, J., Weissleder, R., & Breakefield, X. (2005). Codon-optimized *Gaussia* luciferase cDNA for mammalian gene expression in culture and *in vivo*. *Molecular Therapy*, 11, 3, pp. 435-443.

Troy, T., Jekic-McMullen, D., Sambucetti, L., & Rice, B. (2004). Quantitative comparison of the sensitivity of detection of fluorescent and bioluminescent reporters in animal models. *Imaging*, 3, 1, pp. 9-23.

Tsien, R. Y. (1998). The green fluorescent protein. *Annual Review of Biochemistry*, 67, 1, pp. 509-544.

Ugarova, N. (1989). Luciferase of *Luciola mingrelica* fireflies. Kinetics and regulation mechanism. *Journal of Bioluminescence and Chemiluminescence*, 4, 1, pp. 406-418.

Vervoort, J., Muller, F., Okane, D. J., Lee, J., & Bacher, A. (1986). Bacterial luciferase: A C-13, N-15, and P-31 nuclear magnetic resonance investigation. *Biochemistry*, 25, 24, pp. 8067-8075.

Viviani, V. R. (2002). The origin, diversity, and structure function relationships of insect luciferases. *Cellular and Molecular Life Sciences*, 59, 11, pp. 1833-1850.

Vysotski, E. S., & Lee, J. (2004). Ca2+-regulated photoproteins: Structural insight into the bioluminescence mechanism. *Accounts of Chemical Research*, 37, 6, pp. 405-415

Ward, W., Prentice, H., Roth, A., Cody, C., & Reeves, S. (1982). Spectral perturbations of the *Aequorea* green fluorescent protein. *Photochemistry and photobiology*, 35, 6, pp. 803-808.

White, E., & Branchini, B. (1975). Modification of firefly luciferase with a luciferin analog. Red light producing enzyme. *Journal of the American Chemical Society*, 97, 5, pp. 1243-1245.

White, E. H., McCapra, F., Field, G. F., & McElroy, W. D. (1961). The structure and synthesis of firefly luciferin. *Journal of the American Chemical Society*, 83, 10, pp. 2402-2403.

Woo, J. C., Howell, M. H., & Von Arnim, A. G. (2008). Structure-function studies on the active site of the coelenterazine-dependent luciferase from *Renilla*. *Protein Science*, 17, 4, pp. 725-735.

Wood, K., Lam, Y., & McElroy, W. (1989). Introduction to beetle luciferases and their applications. *Journal of Bioluminescence and Chemiluminescence*, 4, 1, pp. 289-301.

Wood, K., Lam, Y., Seliger, H., & McElroy, W. (1989). Complementary DNA coding click beetle luciferases can elicit bioluminescence of different colors. *Science,* 244, 4905, pp. 700.

Wu, C., Liu, Z., Rose, J., Inouye, S., Tsuji, F., Tsien, R., et al. (1996). The three-dimensional structure of green fluorescent protein resembles a lantern. *Bioluminescence and chemiluminescence; Molecular reporting with photons. Chichester: John Wiley.* pp. 399-402.

Yokoe, H., & Meyer, T. (1996). Spatial dynamics of GFP-tagged proteins investigated by local fluorescence enhancement. *Nature Biotechnology,* 14, 10, pp. 1252-1256.

Zacharias, D. A., Violin, J. D., Newton, A. C., & Tsien, R. Y. (2002). Partitioning of lipid-modified monomeric GFPs into membrane microdomains of live cells. *Science,* 296, 5569, pp. 913-916.

Zimmer, M. (2002). Green fluorescent protein (GFP): applications, structure, and related photophysical behavior. *Chem. Rev,* 102, 3, pp. 759-782.

Part 3

Biosensors for Environment and Biosecurity

23

Engineered Nuclear Hormone Receptor-Biosensors for Environmental Monitoring and Early Drug Discovery

David W. Wood and Izabela Gierach
The Ohio State University
USA

1. Introduction

Bacterial Biosensors are engineered microorganisms that can be used to detect a variety of chemicals. These chemicals can include heavy metals, toxins, hormones, hormone-like drugs and environmental endocrine-disrupting pollutants. In general, bacterial biosensors are engineered to express a biosensing protein, which can selectively bind to a target chemical (usually referred to as a "ligand"). When the target ligand is present, the biosensor protein produces an easily readable change in the cell behaviour. For example, the biosensing protein may produce a change in fluorescence or enzyme activity, or as shown in Fig. 1 & 2, may change the growth rate of the expressing cell when an appropriate ligand is present (Gillies et al, 2008; Skretas et al, 2007; Skretas & Wood, 2005a, 2005b, 2005c).

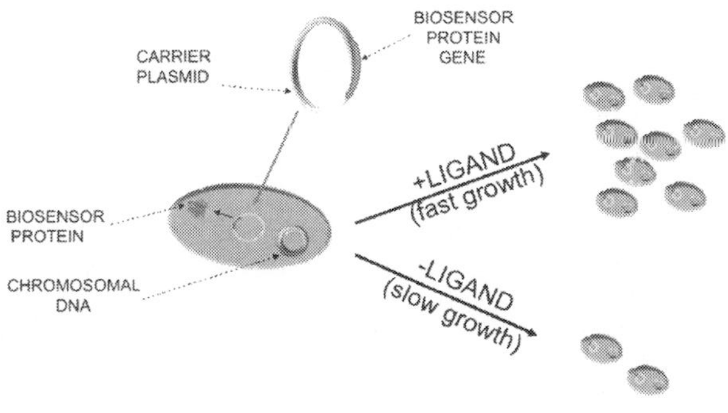

Fig. 1. Growth dependent bacterial biosensor cell. A reporter protein gene is contained on a carrier plasmid, which is transformed into a microbial strain. The expressed biosensor protein produces a ligand-sensitive growth phenotype. In this case, the presence of the appropriate ligand for the biosensor protein increases the growth rate of the biosensor cells.

The bacterial biosensors described in this chapter have been developed specifically for detecting and identifying chemicals that target human and animal nuclear hormone receptors (NHRs). As such, they can be used for identifying potentially valuable drugs for treating a variety of cancers and metabolic disorders, or they can be used to detect and identify pathogenic environmental chemicals that act through various NHRs. In drug discovery, the link between chemicals binding to NHRs and various disease states is recognized across many different metazoans (Hu et al, 2008; Jofre & Karasov, 2008).

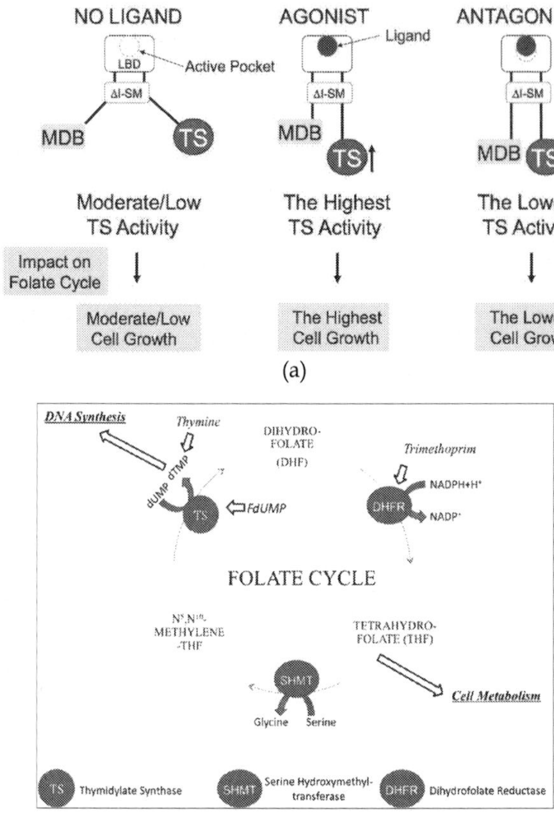

(a)

(b)

Fig. 2. (a) Schematic representation of the NHR biosensor protein and related growth phenotypes (Gillies et al, 2008; Skretas et al, 2007; Skretas & Wood, 2005a). The activity of the TS reporter enzyme is dependent on the configuration of the allosteric sensor protein, which is modulated by the binding of an NHR ligand. The activity of TS affects bacterial DNA synthesis and cellular metabolism (b). The resulting change in growth phenotype can be quantified by optical absorbance at 600 nm in liquid growth medium, allowing an indirect determination of the ligand's agonistic or antagonistic behaviour. Abbreviations: ΔI-SM (mini-intein splicing domain); MDB-maltose binding domain; TS-thymidylate synthase; dUMP- deoxyuridine monophosphate; dTMP- deoxythymidine monophosphate; FdUMP- 5-fluoro-2'-deoxyuridine 5'-monophosphate; NADP- nicotinamide adenine dinucleotide phosphate; LBD-ligand binding domain of nuclear hormone receptor.

In humans, aberrant NHR binding of native and other hormone-like compounds is associated with a wide variety of disorders (Grycewicz & Cypryk, 2008), including dyslipidemia, hypogonadism, endometriosis, cancer, obesity and diabetes, as well as reproductive organ dysfunction and infertility (Feldman et al, 2008; Fessler, 2008; Malm et al, 2007; Mattsson & Olsson, 2007; Ohno, 2008; Tancevski et al, 2009; Tokumoto et al, 2007). Mitigation of these and other disorders, however, can also be accomplished through NHR manipulation, where hormone-like compounds can reverse or otherwise treat a wide variety of diseases. Similar pathogenic NHR binding effects can be seen in animals, where hormonal imbalances arise from environmental endocrine disrupting compounds (EDCs), such as pollutants and insecticides. These imbalances can lead to infertile egg production, tissue abnormalities, degraded gonadal structure, demasculization, altered species metamorphosis patterns and abnormally fast growth (Fernandez et al, 2007; Hu et al, 2008; Katsu et al, 2007; Rempel & Schlenk, 2008). For this reason, identification of EDCs and environmental screening for endocrine disrupting activity is a critical application as well.

In humans, there are six major NHR groups, the best studied of which include the Estrogen Receptor (ER-like), Thyroid Hormone Receptor (TR-like) and Retinoid X Receptor (RXR-like) (Doweyko, 2007). Inside the cells, these NHRs bind to DNA and various transcriptional co-activators and co-repressors to regulate the transcription of large numbers of genes in response to their hormone ligands. This ability gives NHRs a tremendous impact on cell maturation, metabolism and homeostasis (Acosta-Martinez et al, 2007; Baxter & Webb, 2009; Brettes & Mathelin, 2008).

A key element of the NHRs is that, in addition to their native hormones, they can bind to a wide variety of endocrine disruptors (EDs) and complex pharmaceuticals (Fig. 3). Further, several subtypes can exist for a given NHR family (e.g., ERα or ERβ, and TRα or TRβ). Environmental pollutant EDs that target NHRs include BPA, PCBs, and dioxins, while endocrine active compounds in foods can include vitamins, phospholipids, phytoestrogens and fatty acids. Many pharmaceuticals have been developed to target NHRs, with the most important compounds typically exhibiting highly subtype-selective binding within an NHR group. Notable examples include the Selective Estrogen Receptor Modulators (SERMs; e.g. Raloxifene and Tamoxifen), and the Selective Thyroid Hormone Receptor Modulator (STRM; e.g. Eprotirome, currently in Phase II clinical trials) (Baxter et al, 2004; Leung et al, 2007). The NHR proteins can also form homo- or hetero- dimers and tetramers within the NHR subclasses (e.g., ER-ER; ER-RXR), and can form various combinations of subtype homo- and heterodimers (e.g., ERα-ERβ dimer). These aspects of NHR action can greatly complicate their function in various cells and organs, leading to a wide variety of tissue-specific effects in response to ligands of various classes.

The similar structures and functions of the NHRs makes them a perfect fit for engineering biosensors, especially since they can be expressed well in bacteria or yeast cells. Additionally, the mechanism by which ligand binding triggers gene expression is well known, which has made NHRs and NHR LBDs highly tractable for drug discovery and environmental screening in high throughput systems. There are two basic classifications for compounds that bind to NHRs: agonists and antagonists. In general, agonist compounds tend to trigger hormone-related gene transcription, while antagonists tend to suppress transcription. The exact response of a cell to a given endocrine active compound, however, depends on a variety of factors, which include the presence of various co-activators and co-repressors and aspects of the metabolic state of the cell. At the molecular level, the primary determinant for the differential response of the NHR to these two types of compounds is the

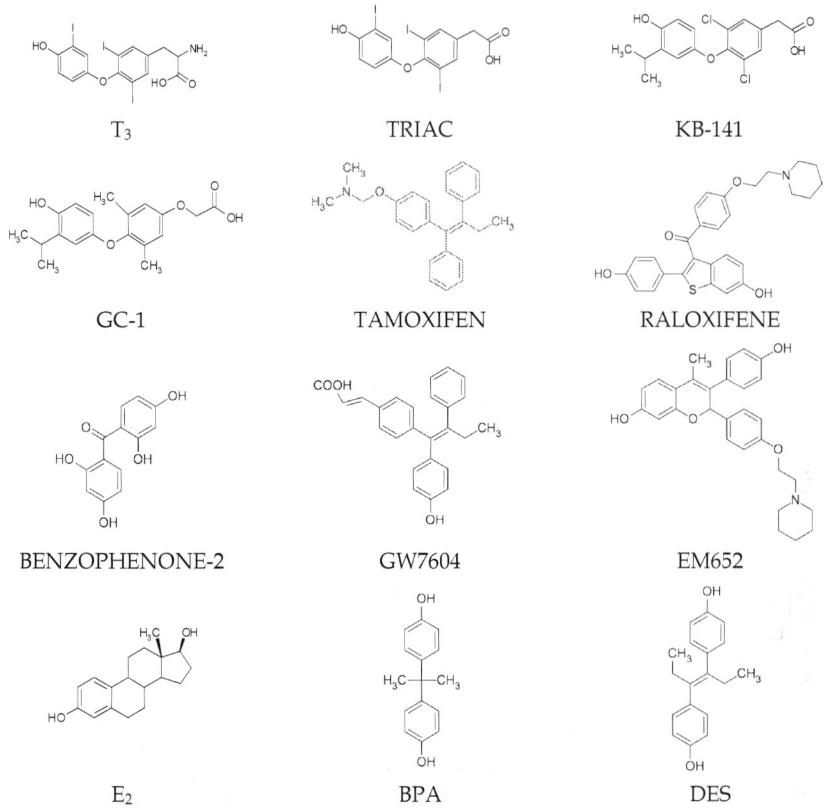

Fig. 3. Selected structures of compounds binding to NHRs. Thyroid receptor ligands include the compounds T_3 (a natural TR agonist), TRIAC (a natural TR agonist), KB-141 (a synthetic TRβ-selective agonist) and GC-1 (a synthetic TRβ-selective agonist), while estrogen receptors bind tamoxifen (a subtype-selective ER modulator), raloxifene (a subtype-selective ER modulator), benzophenone-2 (an ER agonist found in many cosmetics and perfumes), GW7604 (a synthetic selective ER downregulator), EM652 (a synthetic selective ER downregulator), E_2 (17-β-estradiol - the native ER ligand), BPA (an ER agonist and suspected ER-disruptor found in many consumer plastics), and DES (an ER agonist, formerly available small-molecule therapeutic which has been linked to cervical cancer).

repositioning of a conserved helix, generally known as helix-12 (Fig. 4a), upon ligand binding (Gulla & Budil, 2007; Shiau et al, 2002). When the bound ligand is an agonist, helix-12 tends to shift towards the NHR binding pocket, creating a charged area on the protein surface. This surface is then occupied by a co-activator, which results in initiation of transcription (MacGregor & Jordan, 1998; Schapira et al, 2000; Shiau et al, 1998). Antagonists are commonly equipped with bulky functional side group(s), causing helix-12 to rotate away from the binding pocket, which typically results in suppression of transcription (Fig. 4a; (Koehler et al, 2005)).

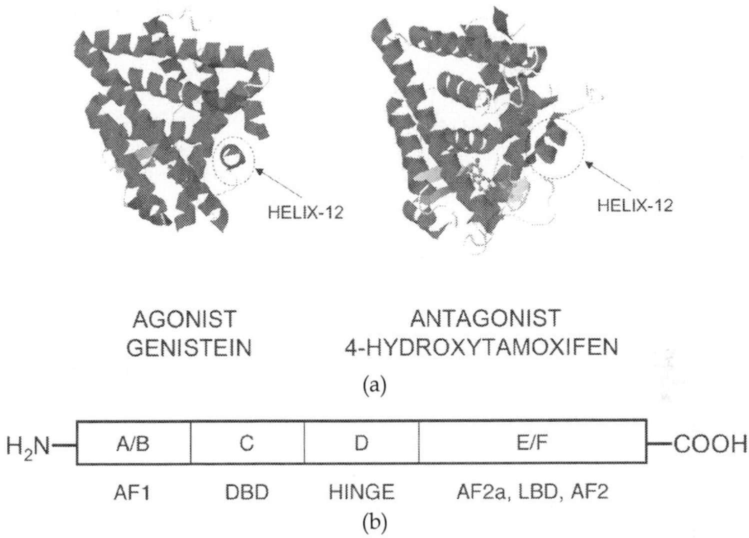

Fig. 4. (a) Comparison of ER ligand binding domain structures, with a focus on helix-12 repositioning in response to agonist binding (left; ERα bound to genistein, PDB ID: 1X7R) or antagonist (right; ERβ bound to 4 hydroxytamoxifen, or Nolvadex®, a common drug used in treatment for breast cancer patients, PDB ID: 3ERT). The solvent accessible surface around 4-hydroxytamoxifen (structure shown in Fig. 3) is underlined in yellow on the right side of the compound. Genistein is inside of the active pocket, hidden behind the α-helixes. Upon antagonist binding to ER, helix-12 rotates away from the binding pocket due to the antagonist's extended functional group. This results in a change of the protein surface, making it inaccessible to co-activators. (b) Schematic representation of the NHR domains A through F (Hewitt & Korach, 2002; Norris et al, 1997). Abbreviations: AF-1 = Activation Function-1; AF-2a = Activation Function-2a; AF2 = Activation Function-2; DBD = DNA Binding Domain.

2. Engineered allosteric bacterial biosensor

In any screening process, the success of finding unique and active compounds depends greatly on the sensitivity of the method. A large diversity of available target proteins for screening is also essential, especially when searching for subtype-selective agonistic and antagonistic behaviours. Additionally, assay limitations must also be considered, such as the impacts of solvents used for delivering the test compounds, as well as growth media or temperature. These aspects of the assay can greatly affect the numbers of false positive and false negative results, as well as the reproducibility and robustness of the assay. Finally, for high throughput applications in large library drug screening, the assay must be simple, economical, and amenable to full or partial automation.

To generate bacterial biosensors for detecting hormones and hormone-like compounds, we have engineered the ligand-binding domains of various NHR proteins into an allosteric biosensor protein scaffold. The biosensor scaffold is composed of four protein domains, including a maltose binding domain, an intein stabilization domain, an NHR ligand-binding domain (LBD), and a thymidylate synthase (TS) reporter enzyme (Fig. 2). This scaffold is designed to link ligand binding by the NHR LBD to the activity of the fused TS reporter protein. Thymidylate synthase is a critical enzyme involved in bacterial DNA synthesis, which produces a strong growth phenotype on thymineless medium based on its activity. Specifically, the TS protein is part of bacterial folate metabolism, where it consumes a single methylene tetrahydrofolate molecule as it converts a single molecule of dUMP to dTMP. The dTMP is then used for DNA synthesis, which is required for cell growth. In practice, the chimeric sensor protein undergoes a structural change when an appropriate ligand is bound to the LBD, which alters the activity of the fused TS domain, and leads to a change in growth rate of the expressing bacterial cell (Fig. 2). The involvement of TS in the folate cycle allows both positive and negative selections for TS activity. Further, the stringency of the selection can be tuned by modulating the incubation temperature and concentrations of the antibiotic trimethoprim (Belfort & Pedersen-Lane, 1984; Gillies et al, 2008; Skretas et al, 2007; Skretas & Wood, 2005a). Although there are some differences between species, NHRs share similar domain structures and sequences within the subgroups, which have allowed new NHR biosensors to be generated using the same basic sensor protein scaffold. The biosensing microbial strains expressing these proteins are referred to as "Bacterial Biosensors".

The NHR bacterial biosensors can be used to screen uncharacterized compounds for their effects on a variety of NHR targets. In particular, this method can be used for the detection and differentiation of agonistic and antagonistic compounds, and can be used to determine the half-maximal effective concentrations (EC_{50} and IC_{50} values) for a given compound (Skretas et al, 2007; Skretas & Wood, 2005a). Additionally, these bacterial biosensors can detect NHR subtype selectivity of a given compound, as well as species selectivity when used with animal-based bacterial biosensors (Gierach et al, 2011). In this case, the simple incorporation of an animal NHR ligand-binding domain generates a sensor for detecting ligands against that species.

The recognition of agonistic or antagonistic behaviour is directly correlated with TS activity of the sensor, expressed as an increase or decrease of cell growth on selective growth medium (Skretas & Wood, 2005a). In this selection system, TS activity closely depends on the conformation of the LBD-ligand complex. Reduced activity of the TS reporter enzyme, which is observed in the absence of ligands, or with non-binding or antagonistic ligands, results in lower bacterial growth. High TS activity is elicited by agonist binding and can be detected by observing the rate of increase in culture optical density at 600 nm (OD_{600}) over time. Importantly, the temperature plays an important role in the sensitivity of biosensors, and is related to the stability of TS and the cellular demand for dTMP. Therefore, bacterial cell growth is typically carried out in 96-well plates, incubated at precisely 34°C in a controlled humidity air shaker at 150 rpm (Gawrys et al, 2009; Gierach et al, 2011).

Key features of the bacterial biosensors

1. Each biosensor protein contains: Maltose Binding Protein-Intein-T4 Thymidylate Synthase Enzyme, with the NHR LBD inserted into the intein domain.
2. The activity of the fused TS enzyme is modulated by the amount and potency of the NHR ligand present.

3. TS activity can be detected qualitatively by colony formation on selective agar medium, or both qualitatively and quantitatively by observing changes in liquid growth medium optical density at 600 nm wavelength over time.
4. The LBD domain of one biosensor protein can be easily replaced with an alternate LBD, which has allowed the construction of functional biosensors for human ERα, ERβ, TRα, TRβ, PPARγ, fish (sole) ERβ and porcine (domestic pig) ERβ.
5. The assay method is non-radioactive, and has been developed for high throughput screening (HTS).
6. This method can detect strong ligands at low nM concentrations.
7. Weakly bound ligands, such as BPA and Tamoxifen for the human estrogen receptor, can be detected at low μM concentrations.
8. Three steps are required to complete a single set of assays: (a) overnight growth of fresh cells in non-selective LB medium; (b) dilution of the cells into a selective thymineless medium (-THY medium) and addition of the diluted test compounds and controls (this is done robotically in the HTS format); and (c) growth of cultures for 10 to 20 hours at 34°C, 150 rpm agitation and controlled humidity.
9. The limitations of the method are: the biosensor is sensitive to the presence of detergents, high levels of alcohols, solvents, and lipids (or any generally cytotoxic condition). Therefore, the final solvent concentration used in the assay should not exceed 1% DMSO or ethanol (test compound vehicle).

2.1 Construction of the bacterial biosensor strain

Vector and chimeric proteins

The biosensor protein is expressed from the pMal-c2 plasmid (New England Biolabs, Beverly, MA), where the plasmid backbone encodes the maltose binding protein (MBD) under control of the Ptac promoter. The biosensor gene is constructed through the following steps (Fig. 5): (1) the ΔI-SM gene, derived from the full-length *Mycobacterium tuberculosis* RecA intein (Wood et al, 1999), is fused to the C-terminus of the MBD; (2) the bacteriophage T4 *td* gene, encoding T4 TS reporter enzyme, is fused to the C-terminus of the ΔI-SM gene; (3) the native intein splicing activity is suppressed by mutation of the N- and C-terminal amino acids of the intein to alanine; (4) the NHR LBD is inserted into the ΔI mini-intein gene at the location where the original intein endonuclease domain was deleted; and (5) the Ptac promoter sequence is mutated to slightly increase basal expression of the overall fusion protein (Skretas & Wood, 2005b). The resulting plasmid names have the general form pMIT::[NHR], where pMIT stands for plasmid MBD-ΔI intein-TS reporter scaffold, and [NHR] is the inserted LBD (Fig. 5). The constructed sensor plasmids are then transformed into the *E. coli* TS knockout strain D1210Δ*thyA*::Kan^R [F-Δ(*gpt-proA*)62 *leuB6 supE44 ara*-14 *galK2 lacY*1 Δ(*mcrC-mrr*) *rpsL*20 (*Str*^{r}) *xyl*-5 *mtl*-1 *recA*13 *lacI*^{q}] (Skretas et al, 2007).
A key component of the biosensor protein is the split ΔI-SM mini-intein domain, which is thought to increase the stability of the overall fusion and transduce binding information to the TS enzyme. Mutations at the N-terminus of the mini-intein (Cys→Ala) suppresses intein splicing, while the MBD was added to assure the solubility and increase the activity of the chimeric protein. Insertion of the NHR LBD is commonly accomplished by utilizing unique *Age*I and *Xho*I restriction sites within the intein, which flank the intein-NHR insertion site (Skretas & Wood, 2005b). The constructed biosensors include two different mini-inteins for

LBD insertion: 110Δ383 and 96Δ400 (Wood et al, 1999). The 110Δ383 mini-intein was used more often, and includes the pMIT::ERβ*(h), pMIT::ERβ*(s), pMIT::ERβ*(p), pMIT::TRβ*(h) and pMIT::TRα*(h) biosensors, whereas the 96Δ400 intein was used for the pMIT::ERα*(h) fusion (Gierach et al, 2011). The specific mechanism of the biosensor action in bacterial cells is currently under investigation.

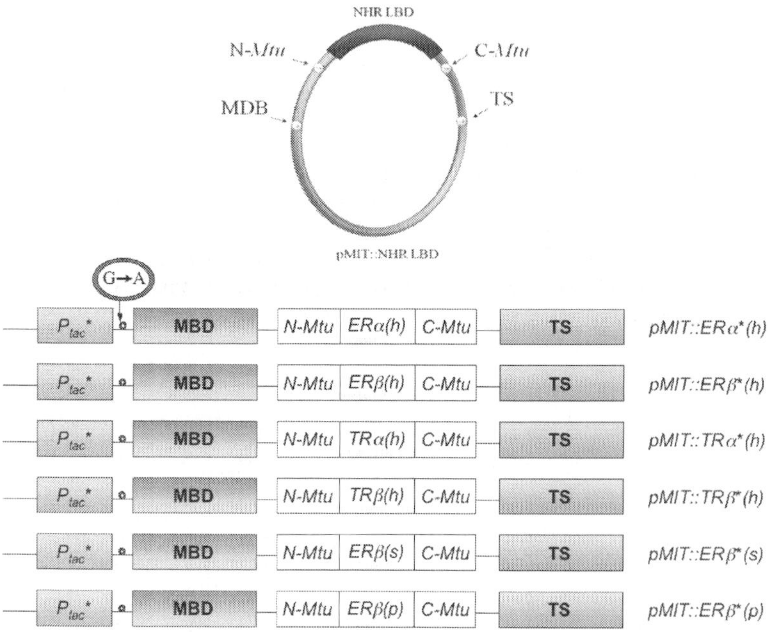

Fig. 5. Schematic representation of the plasmid vector pMal-c2 (top), which contains the MBD, intein, NHR LBD and TS genes. The swappable NHR LBD gene is inserted between the N- and C-terminal fragments of the intein. Several constructed biosensor protein fusion genes are also shown (bottom). In these diagrams, P_{tac} = Ptac promoter for controlling biosensor protein expression; MBD = Maltose Binding Domain; N-Mtu = N-terminal segment (typically amino acids 1-110) of the ΔI-SM mini-intein; ERα, ERβ, TRα, TRβ = Estrogen Receptors alpha and beta, Thyroid Receptors alpha and beta, respectively, where (h) = human, (p) = porcine and (s) = sole; C-Mtu = C-terminal segment of the ΔI-SM mini-intein; TS = Thymidylate Synthase reporter enzyme. Plasmid names are shown on the right for each of the biosensor genes, where pMIT stands for plasmid MBD-ΔI-TS and the :: symbol indicates insertion of the indicated LBD.

2.2 Usage of the NHR bacterial biosensors

2.2.1 The High Throughput Screening (HTS)

The application of bacterial biosensors in a 96-well plate HTS format (Fig. 6) is based on an earlier protocol that employed glass culture tubes. The original glass culture tube method was very labor-intensive, and the number of samples and concentrations was limited by incubator space. Most importantly, large quantities of growth medium and ligands were needed for each experiment. The HTS method in 96-well plates is approximately 100 times more sensitive, and the cells, growth medium and ligands are dispensed by a robotic liquid handler (Biomek 2000, Beckman-Coulter), which assures greater mixing quality and repeatability.

2.2.2 Agonism and antagonism detection by biosensors

There are three major tests resulting in detection of ligand agonism and antagonism, as well as toxicity of the test compounds for bacterial cells (see Table 1).

Compounds that stimulate the growth of cells in thymineless medium (-THY) are generally considered to be agonists, while antagonists can have no effect, or in some cases can decrease the growth of cells in -THY medium. Using estrogen receptor as an example, antagonist tests use competitive biosensor binding with estradiol (-THY+E_2 assay), where antagonist lowers TS activity relative to E_2 alone. However, in the TTM and TTM+E_2 assays the phenotypes are reversed, and low TS activity upon antagonist binding rescues cells. This reversal is very helpful in confirming LBD-specific effects, as opposed to more general metabolic effects. Toxicity can be determined by adding an uncharacterized compound to cells growing in non-selective medium (+THY), where cells grow freely in the presence of agonists or antagonists, but toxicity results in a loss of growth.

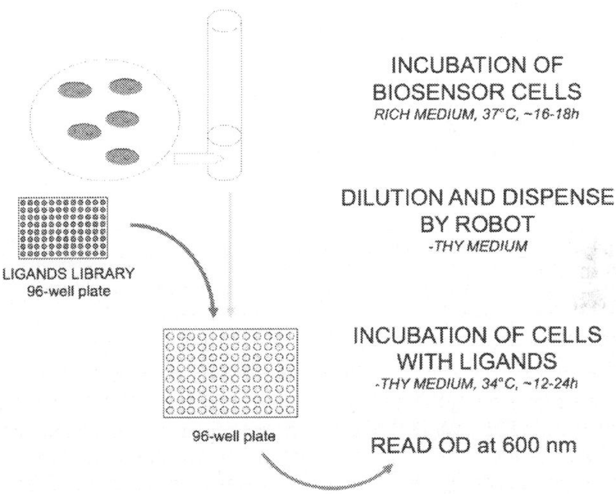

Fig. 6. Schematic representation of the intein-based biosensor method.

2.2.3 Sub-type receptor selectivity

The ligand binding domains of receptor subtypes are highly conserved (see Fig. 4), which allows multiple receptor subtypes to be used for biosensor generation. Differential binding to one biosensor subtype or another allows a quick determination of subtype selectivity for a given compound. In previous studies, we were able to confirm the subtype-selectivity of compounds bound to the estrogen receptors. Among them propylpyrazole triol (PPT) and methyl piperidinopyrazole (MPP) were found ERα selective, whereas DPN, Genistein and

Daidzein were ERβ selective. The Relative Binding Affinities (the EC_{50} ratio between ERα and ERβ) of those compounds were in correlation with the literature; PPT (593), MPP (220), DPN (0.01), Genistein (0.002) and Daidzein (0.2) (Skretas & Wood, 2005b). Additionally, the TR biosensors were able to detect Triac, GC-1 and KB-141 TRβ selectivity (unpublished results), which are also in agreement with reported results (Bleicher et al, 2008; Grover et al, 2005; Koury et al, 2009; Li et al, 2006; Marimuthu et al, 2002; Martinez et al, 2009; Scanlan, 2008; Wagner et al, 2001).

		-THY *34°C*	-THY+E_2 *34°C*	TTM *37°C*	TTM+E_2 *37°C*	+THY *37°C*
High TS Activity	**AGONISM**	+	+	-	-	+
Low TS Activity	**ANTAGONISM**	-	-	+	+	+
Low TS Activity	**TOXICITY**	n/a	n/a	n/a	n/a	-

Table 1. Summary of the NHR bacterial biosensor assays and their conditions, including temperatures and growth medium additives for optimizing results (Skretas et al, 2007). The +/- signs indicate cell growth below or above the baseline OD_{600} value obtained for cells in the presence of solvent only (which is constant throughout the sample and not higher than 1%). Abbreviations: TTM: -THY medium with 50μg/mL Thymine and 10μg/mL Trimethoprim; +THY: -THY medium with 50μg/mL Thymine; E_2 is 17-β-estradiol, typically at 0.1 to 10 μM depending on the test strain.

2.2.4 Effect of compounds across different species

We also confirmed in our studies that the effects of tested compounds varied across different species, such as sole (*Solea solea*) and human (Gierach et al, 2011). As expected, compounds expressed similar effects when bound to pig and human ERβs, but in some cases diverged for sole and human or pig. The fact that the biosensors are able to quantify differential effects across species can allow rapid screening of ED pollutants using consistent assay protocols, which will eliminate important barriers to comparing these types of data in the current literature. This creates great opportunities for understanding crosstalk of receptors in a wide range of species, and allows the selectivity of ligands across receptors and species to be explored.

2.2.5 Synergism and competition of natural hormones, pharmaceuticals and EDCs

There is a great concern that mixtures of EDCs could have stronger and more devastating effects than single compounds on health and environment. Since there is no limitation as to how many ligands can be tested simultaneously, the biosensor could detect synergistic effects acting through the NHR LBD as well.

3. Bacterial biosensors in drug discovery

The process of delivering new pharmaceuticals to the market takes approximately 10-15 years and only one compound in 10,000 has a chance to be approved by the U.S. FDA. The development cost per drug can reach $800 million on average (Brower, 2002). For these reasons, there is an urgency to discover new compounds that are more selective and have fewer side effects. Early stage discovery and pre-clinical research may take 6-7 years alone.

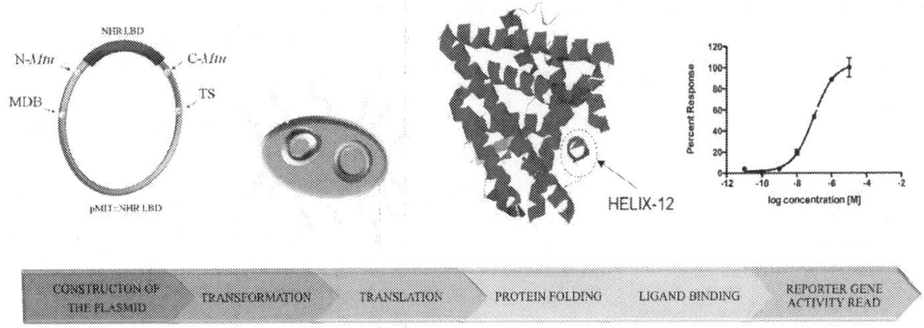

Fig. 7. The process of designing a bacterial biosensor and its utilization. First, the sequence of the plasmid is constructed computationally. The template (e.g., pMIT::**ER**α) stays intact, and the insert (N-terminal intein-**NHR LBD-**C-terminal intein) is swapped to create a new biosensor with a different LBD. Next, the plasmid is transformed into a bacterial cell, which allows the encoded gene to be transcribed and translated into the active biosensor protein. In the presence of an agonist, the activity level of the TS reporter enzyme domain is increased, leading to an increase in cellular growth rate (see the graph above). However, when antagonists are present the activity of the TS is low, which allows a distinction between these two types of the compounds. Cell growth can be quantified by OD_{600} measurements. The 3D structures of NHR LBDs proteins (such as the ER LBD shown above) can be found in the RCSB Protein Data Bank (PDB).

Therefore, the development of new methods to rapidly screen millions of ligands against new targets is essential and ongoing. The identification of ligands that bind to estrogen receptor(s) began with the development of treatments for patients with hormonal dysfunctions, cancers, and sexually transmitted bacterial infections. Several early pharmaceuticals, such as diethylstilbestrol (DES, a nonsteroidal estrogen synthesized just before World War II by Leon Golberg), failed due to their high toxicity and disastrous side effects, such as breast cancer and vaginal adenocarcinoma in second-generation girls (Birch, 1992; Jordan et al, 2008). The first human ER was discovered in 1966 by Jensen and Gorski, and it took an additional 30 years until the first mammalian ERβ sequence was cloned (Fannon et al, 2001). Interestingly, the compound tamoxifen, as well as second-generation benzothiophene derivative selective estrogen receptor modulators (SERMs) (e.g., raloxifene, known as Evista® (Pritchard, 2001; Wilkinson et al, 1982)), show unique selective action in targeted tissues. In some tissues SERMs act as an estrogen, and therefore their action is described as agonistic, but in others they block the effect of estrogen and behave as antagonists. In many cases, the mechanism of SERM action is not fully understood, and research is ongoing on the roles of the co-regulators, ligands, and cross-signaling proteins that mediate ER expression levels across the human body. For example, it was determined that ERβ is dominant in the gastrointestinal tract, whereas ERα dominates in liver. Both of these receptors are expressed in breast, bone and brain tissue, but in different ratios, allowing direct targeting of specific organs (Gustafsson, 1999). During the last 10 years, the number of targeted drug-like compounds produced in industry and academia has increased dramatically. These compounds have been developed as fertility drugs, as well as breast cancer, prostate cancer and osteoporosis therapeutics. Among them are Toremifene (Fareston® by Shire laboratories), lasofoxifene, trioxifene, droloxifene, clomifene (Clomid® by Hoechst Marion Roussel, Inc.) and ormeloxifene (originally manufactured by Torrent Pharmaceuticals), which was used as a birth control pill, and is now also prescribed to cure uterine bleeding (Blizzard, 2008; Fan et al, 2007; Musa et al, 2007; Sanceau et al, 2007). Pure antagonists were also synthesized such as ICI 182,780 (Faslodex® by AstraZeneca), which is known as a selective estrogen receptor downregulator; SERD (Abdou et al, 2008).

In previous research, we showed that bacterial biosensors could detect novel compounds and determine their behavior as agonists or antagonists (see structures of discovered compounds in Fig. 8 and Table 2) (Hartman et al, 2009; Skretas et al, 2007). Compounds **a** and **b** were found to bind to ER, and their agonistic and antagonistic effects were verified using biosensors. The new findings were confirmed by a fluorescence polarization displacement assay using extracts of human ERβ and ERα and fluorescently labeled estrogen, as well as by analyzing ERE-dependent luciferase gene activity in human embryonic kidney HEK:ERβ and breast cancer MCF-7:D5L cells. The relative binding affinities of these compounds, determined by competitive binding assays, showed the ERβ selectivity of compound **b.** Specifically, the RBA (relative binding affinities of the compound to estrogen) of compound **a** and **b** for ERα were 0.23±0.03 and 0.59±0.09, and for ERβ were 1.94±0.024 and 0.78±0.10, respectively (Skretas et al, 2007). An additional study using a luciferase reporter system revealed that compound **a** is an agonist, but compound **b** is a partial agonist and partial agonist/antagonist when bound to ERα and ERβ, respectively.

Compound	**Bacterial Biosensor**		**Compound**	**Bacterial Biosensor**	
	Agonist	Antagonists		Agonist	**Antagonists**
DES	+	-	Tamoxifen	-	+
17-β-estradiol	+	-	4-hydroxytamoxifen	-	+
Estriol	+	-	Clomiphene	-	+
17-α-estradiol	+	-	Raloxifene	-	+
Estrone	+	-	ICI182,780	-	+

Table 2. Bacterial biosensor results obtained for hormones and pharmaceuticals screened against human ERβ (Skretas et al, 2007). Concentration of the ligands was 5 μM, with the exception of tamoxifen at 2 μM. Antagonists were tested in competitive assays against 500 nM E_2. The (+/-) symbols indicate a positive/negative cell growth outcome.

The other two compounds, **c** and **d**, were originally discovered using a computational method known as Shape Signatures (Hartman et al, 2009; Nagarajan et al, 2005; Zauhar et al, 2003). Shape Signatures was created to rapidly compare chemical databases against known active compounds to detect similar bioactivity. This *in silico* method screens specifically for polarity and shape similarities by initially using a ray-tracing algorithm well known in the movie industry to computationally draw shapes of objects in 3D space. The solvent-accessible surface of each molecule is defined by a Smooth Molecular Surface Triangulator algorithm (Zauhar, 1995), and is essential for defining the volume of a molecule. The shape of the molecule, as well as the molecular electrostatic potential computed over the surface of the molecule, can be compared across large databases and scored rapidly for the most promising compounds. The two molecules **c** and **d** (Fig. 8) were derived from a Shape Signatures screening against GW7604 and EM652 (see Fig. 3).

Compounds **c** and **d** were determined to bind to the active pocket of ER using Computer-Aided Drug Design methods, and their behavior was examined using the bacterial biosensors and an ERα activation immunoassay (ELISA) containing MCF-7 cell extract (Hartman et al, 2009; Skretas et al, 2007). The predicted binding mode of compound **c** overlapped the position of Tamoxifen, which binds through weaker van der Waals interactions to the active pocket. Compound **d** showed possible hydrogen bond formation with Glu353. Overall, compounds **c** and **d** were found to be orally bioavailable by Lipinski's Rule of Five, which takes into account solubility, molecular weight, and even the number of rotational bonds and hydrogen bond donors and acceptors (Hartman et al, 2009).

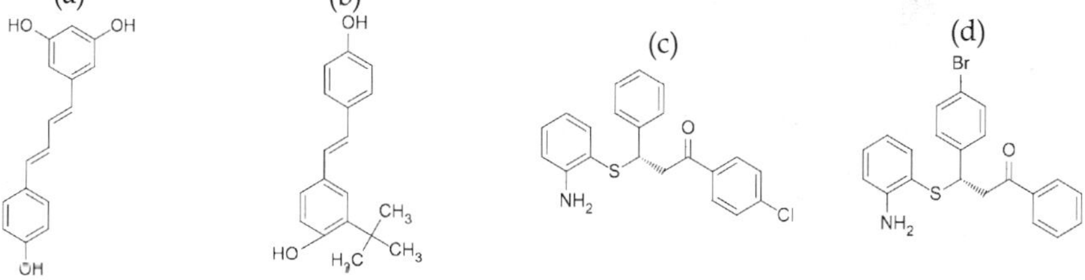

(a) AGONIST

(b) PARTIAL AGONIST/ANTAGONIST

(c) ANTAGONIST

(d) ANTAGONIST

Fig. 8. The structures of agonists and antagonists discovered and confirmed by commercial as well as conventional methods ER (Hartman et al, 2009; Skretas et al, 2007). Names of the compounds. (a) 5-[(1E,3E)-4-(4-hydroxyphenyl) 1,3 butadien-1-yl]-1,3-benzenediol; (b) 2 (1,1-dimethylethyl)-4-[(1E)-2-(4-hydroxyphenyl)ethenyl]-phenol; (c) 3-(2 aminophenyl)sulfanyl-1-(4-chlorophenyl)-3-phenyl-propan-1-one; (d) 3-(2 aminophenyl)sulfanyl-3-(4-bromophenyl)-1-phenyl-propan-1-one.

4. Environmental endocrine disruptors detection

Synthetic or natural compounds that interfere with hormonal and homeostatic systems are known as Endocrine Disruptors (EDs) (Nilsson, 2000). The targets of EDs can be NHRs, non-hormonal receptors, or numerous biological pathways involved in hormone synthesis, metabolism and excretion. Thus, EDs can cause serious disruption of the endocrine system by mimicking natural hormones, which may lead to increased or inhibited transcription of hormone-regulated genes. Some of these compounds are now associated with various cancers, genetic and reproductive diseases, as well as behavioral and developmental abnormalities. A few ED-associated disorders seen in humans are also manifest in other species, and include uterine leiomyomas, endometriosis, cancers, diabetes and obesity (Bryzgalova et al, 2008; Cook et al, 2007; Goksoyr, 2006; Koda et al, 2007; Kuiper et al, 2007;

Lee et al, 2007; Lingxia et al, 2007; Maffini et al, 2006; Negri-Cesi et al, 2008; Nilsson, 2000; Safe, 2000). EDs comprise a wide range of chemicals, including solvents, pesticides, and pharmaceuticals (e.g., DES), and even naturally occurring phytoestrogens in plants (McKinlay et al, 2008). Some EDs accumulate in the body, such as uranium from nuclear power plants, lead, mercury and cadmium, which travel to the brain and kidney (Raymond-Whish et al, 2007; Strumylaite et al, 2008; Vahter et al, 2007). Some weakly binding compounds, such as BPA, are embedded in plastic bottles used for water and soft drinks (Vandenberg et al, 2007). In particular, BPA has been shown to bind to hormone receptors across different species. Despite numerous studies on the negative effects of BPA (Vandenberg et al, 2009), to this day its impact on the body is still controversial. However, the EPA and FDA are now moving to update their disclosures on BPA in response to an internal BPA study showing negative effects of exposure on the brain and prostate, as well as on the behavior of infants and children (Keri et al, 2007).

Compound	Source
Hexestrol	Synthetic, DES derivative
Genistein	Isoflavone, found in plants e.g. soybeans
Kaempferol	Flavonoid, found in plants e.g. tea, apples
Naringenin	Flavonoid, found in plants e.g. grapefruit
Diphenylnitrosamine (DPN)	Synthetic
BPA	Plastics; e.g. bottles, caps
Apigenin	Flavonoid, found in plants e.g. parsley, celery
Zearalanols	Found in plants e.g. fungi (*Fusarium*)
Biochanin A	Flavonoid, found in plants e.g. peanuts, soy
Daidzein	Isoflavone, naturally found in plants e.g. soybeans
Phloretin	Found in plants e.g. apple leaves
Naringenin	Flavonoid, found in plants e.g. grapefruit

Table 3. Selected ER agonists detected by bacterial biosensors, including phytogestrogens and synthetic estrogen analogs. BPA, DPN and 17-β-estradiol (natural hormone, ER agonist) were additionally confirmed to be agonists in the sole and pig ERβ biosensors. BPA and Daidzein, despite the fact that they are weak ER agonists, were also detected (Breinholt & Larsen, 1998; Collins et al, 1997; Kuiper et al, 1997; Kuiper et al, 1998; Skretas et al, 2007).

One of the difficulties in determining the impact of EDs on the human body is that although a broad range of assays are available, their results are generally not directly comparable. For example, the detection limit of a given compound can vary by a factor of 1000 or more across several different *in-vivo* and *in-vitro* assays (Charles, 2004; Dobbins et al, 2008; Kramer, 1998). Measuring the impacts of these compounds on humans is also very difficult, especially when evaluating the cumulative impact of EDs over time on the body. Often, these assays cannot distinguish between high overall toxicity of EDs and their agonistic and antagonistic effects. Non-sigmoidal functions are also observed for some EDs, which exhibit U-shaped and inverted-U-shaped dual dose response curves, such as those seen for phytoestrogens and neurotransmitters. For example, at low concentrations some compounds may act as agonists, but at high concentrations they may behave more like antagonists (Li et al, 2007; Pinto et al, 2008). Additionally, EDs typically exist in the environment in mixtures, and therefore there is a need for newly developed HTS assays to assess their effects alone and in combination with other compounds (Charles et al, 2007). The effect of an ED alone or in a mixture of EDs in different assays may also vary (Benachour et al, 2007; Ramamoorthy et al, 1997).

Since EDs can be accumulated in the body, their half-life could be longer than expected, and contact with these chemicals more frequent than expected. For example, the BPA daily safe uptake is 50 μg/kg as determined by the EPA, but it accumulates in fat tissue over time. Therefore, additive daily exposure occurs, resulting from a longer than expected half-life in the human body (Diamanti-Kandarakis, 2009). Therefore, understanding the impact of these chemicals on the endocrine system and human health is challenging, especially for weakly binding EDs like BPA.

The bacterial biosensors can easily differentiate between bacterial toxicity and endocrine activity. Examples of compounds that bind to ERs, and their sources, are shown in Table 3 Some of them are naturally occurring chemicals found in plants, but others are synthetic. In each case, these compounds mimic estrogen, but their structure is not typically steroid-like (see examples of DES, BPA in Fig. 3). In some cases, the compounds could be beneficial (e.g., chemopreventive properties of Apigenin; antidepressant properties of Kaempferol) as well as harmful or epigenetic (BPA, DES and Hexestrol).

4.1 Screening of home products for estrogenic activity

The intein-based biosensors are capable of detecting small amounts of estrogenic compounds in consumer products such as perfumes, pills and plant extracts. A study using the bacterial biosensors showed that chemicals such as benzophenone-2 (see Fig. 3), which is a UV absorber used in plastic food containers and cosmetics, can be detected by this method. Benzophenone-2 (BP-2) has an agonistic effect on the human ER, and several publications suggest estrogenic effects on fish (juvenile fathead minnows) as well rats (Kunz et al, 2006; Schlecht et al, 2008; Seidlova-Wuttke et al, 2004). In other studies, BP-2 was shown to have an agonistic effect on fish (rainbow trout) and human ERs, and was found to be selective for human ERβ in an in vitro bioassay (Molina-Molina et al, 2008). BP-2 was also tested in pregnant mice to determine its impact on fetuses, where it was found that BP-2 may be a cause of hypospadia which is an abnormality in the reproductive organs of male fetuses (Hsieh et al, 2007). Additionally, BP-2 suppresses T4 (thyroid hormone), but not T3, and has estrogenic activity in rats (Seidlova-Wuttke et al, 2005). The results obtained by the bacterial biosensors also suggest an agonistic effect of BP-2 on the human ERβ. Several perfumes were tested, including Notes by Celine Dion, Amber Romance by Victoria's Secret, Roma by Laura Biagiotti and Haiku by Avon. All of the tested perfumes that contain BP-2 as an ingredient had an agonistic effect on ERβ biosensor, but no effect on the TRβ biosensor. Tests of several natural menopause-relief pills showed a weak positive effect in many cases as well, which included Black Cohosh and Dong Quai Capsules by Nature's Way, and Black Cohosh and Dong Quai Capsules by Gaia Herbs. Notably, essential oils (e.g., Lavender Oil by Plantlife) and soaps were screened but were toxic to the bacterial cells (Gawrys et al, 2009).

4.2 Testing endocrine disruptors across species

The human NHR LBDs of the biosensors can be easily exchanged for animal LBDs and the effects due to the same set of ligands can be compared. The sequences of ERβ for *Sus scrofa* and *Solea solea* were inserted in place of human ERβ in the pMIT::ERβ*, and the potencies of DES, BPA, DPN, Daidzein and E_2 were compared. The potencies across species showed that DES and E_2 have the strongest effect on all of fish, pig and human biosensors. DES was almost twice as effective on pig than on fish or human. The weakest effect was noticed for BPA in the order human>fish>pig. The half maximal effective concentrations (EC_{50}s) were compared to determine relative pseudotransactivation (RPTA, see Equation (1)). The EC_{50} values and the standard deviations of data obtained in triplicate can be presented as sigmoidal plots of OD vs. log of test compound concentration. The calculations were based on nonlinear regression with variable Hill slope (GraphPad Prism 5.01; GraphPad Software, La Jolla, CA, USA).

$$RPTA=\frac{EC_{50}^{E_2}}{EC_{50}^{ligand}}x100\% \tag{1}$$

However, the RPTA values for DPN were quite close to E_2 for human (~80%), but showed it to be less potent for pig (33%) and fish (12%). An even smaller relative effect was seen for Daidzein, commonly found in soybeans, on human ERβ (4%) ≈ pig (4%) > fish (0.9%). Similarly, BPA had very little effect on fish (5.6%) > human (0.9%) > pig (0.23%). The two-tailed p values with 95% confidence interval verified significant correlation between EC_{50} values of tested compounds on human and porcine ERβs. There was no correlation of those ERs with sole ERβ. To further examine the quality of the assay, the Z′ factor for each measurement was calculated, which is an indication of signal to noise in a measurement (see Equation (2); (Zhang et al, 1999)). In both cases the data were sufficient to distinguish ER agonists across species in HTS set up, where Z′ factor above zero is needed to robustly determine whether a given ligand is a potential EDC. In general, all of the tests produced very good Z′ factors, ranging from the strong agonist E_2 (Z′ factor of 0.4-0.6 across the three tested species), to the weaker agonist BPA (Z′ factor of 0.15-0.32) (Gierach et al, 2011).

$$Z'=1-\frac{3x(SD_{max}+SD_{min})}{|Mean_{max}-Mean_{min}|} \tag{2}$$

The data obtained here were also compared to the literature. The trends of recorded effects of ligands on human and pig ERs were similar (DES>>E_2>Daidzein>BPA). Weaker binders like Daidzein and BPA were also tested previously in a yeast transcriptional assay, and the values obtained from these studies closely correlated with our findings ($2.5x10^{-7}$ M (yeast assay) vs. $1.7x10^{-6}$ M (bacterial assay) and $1.45x10^{-7}$ M (yeast assay) vs. $3.6x10^{-7}$ M (bacterial assay), respectively; (Chu et al, 2009)). The performance of the *Solea solea* biosensor was more difficult to ascertain, due to a relative lack of available data compared to carp (*Cyprinus carpio*) and rainbow trout (*Oncorhynchus mykiss*) (Matthews et al, 2000; Matthews et al, 2001; Petit et al, 1995). In general, however, *in vivo* tests in other piscine species were less sensitive for weak binders, such as BPA. In this case, a hepatocyte vitellogenin secretion test at up to 100 μM concentration of BPA showed limited response (Smeets et al, 1999). Our studies were able to determine the binding effect of BPA in sole at lower concentrations (0.10 to 9.85 μM). In other previous assays where piscine ERs were tested, trends in the strength of binding were similar to those observed for Daidzein and DPN in the bacterial biosensors. The alternate assays included a displacement assay using a trout ER nuclear extract, or the previously mentioned hepatocyte vitellogenin secretion assay. A correlation between all of these assays was seen for strong binders, such as E_2, which closely corresponded with *in vivo* studies: 50-150 nM (vitellogenin assay) (Smeets et al, 1999) vs. 21-153 nM (bacterial biosensor assay).

Method	Detection	Bacterial Host	Reference
Heavy metals			
Green fluorescent protein (GFP)-based bacterial biosensors	Cd(II), Pb(II), and Sb(III) in sediments and soils	*Escherichia coli*	(Liao et al, 2006)
GFP bacterial biosensor	As	*Escherichia coli*	(Tani et al, 2009)
Bioluminescent bacterial biosensor	Cu, Zn, Cd, Co, Ni, Pb	*Alcaligenes eutrophus*	(Collard et al, 1994; Diels et al, 1999)
Fibre-optic luminescent bacterial biosensors	Hg and As in soils and sediments	*Escherichia coli*	(Ivask et al, 2007)
Antibiotics			
Colorimetric bacterial biosensor dipstick-based technology	Tetracycline, streptogramin and macrolide in food	*Escherichia coli*	(Link et al, 2007)
Luminescent bacterial biosensor	Tetracyclines in poultry muscle	*Escherichia coli*	(Pikkemaat et al, 2010)
Hormones, Pharmaceuticals, Endocrine Disruptors			
Cell growth based TS-deficient NHR bacterial biosensors	Wide variety of compounds e.g. estradiol, T_3, triac, tamoxifen, GC-1, diethylstilbestrol, KB-141, daidzein, DPN and genistein	*Escherichia coli*	(Gawrys et al, 2009; Hartman et al, 2009; Skretas et al, 2007; Skretas & Wood, 2005a, 2005b, 2005c)
Electrochemical bacterial biosensors	Aromatic hydrocarbons and heavy metals	*Escherichia coli*	(Paitan et al, 2003)
Fluorescent and luminescent toluene bacterial biosensors	Environmental pollution with petroleum products e.g. benzene, toluene, ethylbenzene, and xylenes	*Escherichia coli*	(Li et al, 2008)
Bioluminescent naphthalene biosensor	Naphthalene	*Pseudomonas putida*	(Werlen et al, 2004)
DNA			
Bioluminescent bacterial biosensor for DNA damage, alkylation and mutagenicity recognition	Genotoxicants included: endocrine disrupting chemicals, phenolitics and compounds causing oxidative stress (e.g. H_2O_2, CdCl)	*Escherichia coli*	(Ahn et al, 2009)
Microgravity and space radiation bacterial biosensors	Analysis of the level of radiation exposure on human body by bacterial detection	*Salmonella typhimurium*	(Rabbow et al, 2003)
Stress-responsive bacterial biosensors	DNA damage by oxidative and genotoxic conditions	*Escherichia coli*	(Mitchell & Gu, 2004)

Table 4. The review of bacterial biosensors usage.

5. Brief overview of other bacterial biosensors

The intein-NHR bacterial biosensors are useful for ED screening and drug discovery, and exhibit many advantages over conventional assays. These advantages are also observed in other bacterial biosensor systems, which have been extended into wide range of applications. These include testing for antibiotics in food, as well as detecting DNA damage by chemicals and even space radiation. Several examples of other bacterial biosensors are included in Table 4.

6. Conclusions

The bacterial biosensors presented here are an excellent tool for screening EDs, pharmaceuticals, hormones or mixtures of compounds for their agonism or antagonism against human NHRs as well as NHRs of other species. These biosensors meet the need for a method to rapidly compare the effects of NHR ligands across different species, and to estimate the potential danger of chemicals in the environment. These bacterial biosensors can be also used to rapidly and cheaply test large amounts of the unknown chemicals for possible future uses as lead compounds in pharmaceutical research, including compounds with receptor sub-type selectivity. The simplicity of the assay and very low cost are attractive key features of this method.

7. Acknowledgment

This research was supported by National Science Foundation CAREER Award BES-0348220, NIH grant 1R21ES16630 and the Nancy Lurie Marks Family Foundation.

8. References

Abdou, N. I., Rider, V., Greenwell, C., Li, X. L.,Kimler, B. F. (2008). Fulvestrant (Faslodex), an estrogen selective receptor downregulator, in therapy of women with systemic lupus erythematosus. Clinical, serologic, bone density, and T cell activation marker studies: A double-blind placebo-controlled trial. *Journal of Rheumatology,* Vol. 35, No. 5, pp. 797-803, ISSN: 0315-162X.

Acosta-Martinez, M., Horton, T.,Levine, J. E. (2007). Estrogen receptors in neuropeptide Y neurons: at the crossroads of feeding and reproduction. *Trends in Endocrinology and Metabolism,* Vol. 18, No. 2, pp. 48-50, ISSN: 1043-2760.

Ahn, J. M., Hwang, E. T., Youn, C. H., Banu, D. L., Kim, B. C., Niazi, J. H.,Gu, M. B. (2009). Prediction and classification of the modes of genotoxic actions using bacterial biosensors specific for DNA damages. *Biosens Bioelectron,* Vol. 25, No. 4, pp. 767-772, ISSN: 1873-4235 (Electronic).

Baxter, J. D.,Webb, P. (2009). Thyroid hormone mimetics: potential applications in atherosclerosis, obesity and type 2 diabetes. *Nature reviews Drug discovery,* Vol. 8, No. 4, pp. 308-320, ISSN: 1474-1784.

Baxter, J. D., Webb, P., Grover, G.,Scanlan, T. S. (2004). Selective activation of thyroid hormone signaling pathways by GC-1: a new approach to controlling cholesterol and body weight. *Trends Endocrinol Metab,* Vol. 15, No. 4, pp. 154-157, ISSN: 1043-2760 (Print).

Belfort, M.,Pedersen-Lane, J. (1984). Genetic system for analyzing *Escherichia coli* thymidylate synthase. *J Bacteriol,* Vol. 160, No. 1, pp. 371-378.

Benachour, N., Moslemi, S., Sipahutar, H.,Seralini, G. E. (2007). Cytotoxic effects and aromatase inhibition by xenobiotic endocrine disrupters alone and in combination. *Toxicology and Applied Pharmacology,* Vol. 222, No. 2, pp. 129-140, ISSN: 0041-008X.

Birch, A. J. (1992). Steroid hormones and the Luftwaffe. A venture into fundamental strategic research and some of its consequences: The Birch reduction becomes a birth reduction. *Steroids,* Vol. 57, No. 8, pp. 363-377, ISSN: 0039-128X.

Bleicher, L., Aparicio, R., Nunes, F. M., Martinez, L., Gomes Dias, S. M., Figueira, A. C., Santos, M. A., Venturelli, W. H., da Silva, R., Donate, P. M., Neves, F. A., Simeoni, L. A., Baxter, J. D., Webb, P., Skaf, M. S.,Polikarpov, I. (2008). Structural basis of GC-1 selectivity for thyroid hormone receptor isoforms. *BMC Struct Biol,* Vol. 8, No., pp. 8, ISSN: 1472-6807 (Electronic).

Blizzard, T. A. (2008). Selective Estrogen Receptor Modulator medicinal chemistry at Merck. A review. *Current Topics in Medicinal Chemistry,* Vol. 8, No. 9, pp. 792-812, ISSN: 1568-0266.

Breinholt, V.,Larsen, J. C. (1998). Detection of weak estrogenic flavonoids using a recombinant yeast strain and a modified MCF7 cell proliferation assay. *Chem Res Toxicol,* Vol. 11, No. 6, pp. 622-629, ISSN: 0893-228X (Print).

Brettes, J. P.,Mathelin, C. (2008). Dual effects of androgens on mammary gland. *Bulletin Du Cancer,* Vol. 95, No. 5, pp. 495-502, ISSN: 0007-4551.

Brower, V. (2002). Fast tracking drugs to patients. *EMBO Reports,* Vol. 3, No. 1, pp. 14-16.

Bryzgalova, G., Effendic, S., Khan, A., Rehnmark, S., Barbounis, P., Boulet, J., Dong, G., Singh, R., Shapses, S., Malm, J., Webb, P., Baxter, J. D.,Grover, G. J. (2008). Anti-obesity, anti-diabetic, and lipid lowering effects of the thyroid receptor beta subtype selective agonist KB-141. *Journal of Steroid Biochemistry & Molecular Biology,* Vol. 111, No. 3-5, pp. 262-267.

Charles, G. D. (2004). In vitro models in endocrine disruptor screening. *Ilar J,* Vol. 45, No. 4, pp. 494-501, ISSN: 1084-2020 (Print).

Charles, G. D., Gennings, C., Tornesi, B., Kan, H. L., Zacharewski, T. R., Gollapudi, B. B.,Carney, E. W. (2007). Analysis of the interaction of phytoestrogens and synthetic chemicals: An in vitro/in vivo comparison. *Toxicology and Applied Pharmacology,* Vol. 218, No. 3, pp. 280-288, ISSN: 0041-008X.

Chu, W. L., Shiizaki, K., Kawanishi, M., Kondo, M.,Yagi, T. (2009). Validation of a new yeast-based reporter assay consisting of human estrogen receptors alpha/beta and coactivator SRC-1: Application for detection of estrogenic activity in environmental samples. *Environ Toxicol,* Vol.24, No.5, pp.513-521, ISSN: 1522-7278 (Electronic).

Collard, J. M., Corbisier, P., Diels, L., Dong, Q., Jeanthon, C., Mergeay, M., Taghavi, S., van der Lelie, D., Wilmotte, A.,Wuertz, S. (1994). Plasmids for heavy metal resistance in Alcaligenes eutrophus CH34: mechanisms and applications. *FEMS Microbiol Rev,* Vol. 14, No. 4, pp. 405-414, ISSN: 0168-6445 (Print).

Collins, B. M., McLachlan, J. A.,Arnold, S. F. (1997). The estrogenic and antiestrogenic activities of phytochemicals with the human estrogen receptor expressed in yeast. *Steroids,* Vol. 62, No. 4, pp. 365-372, ISSN: 0039-128X (Print).

Cook, J. D., Davis, B. J., Goewey, J. A., Berry, T. D.,Walker, C. L. (2007). Identification of a sensitive period for developmental programming that increases risk for uterine leiomyoma in Eker rats. *Reproductive Sciences,* Vol. 14, No. 2, pp. 121-136, ISSN: 1933-7191.

Diamanti-Kandarakis, E. B., J.P.; Giudice, L.C.; Hauser, R.; Prins, G.S.; Soto, A.M.; Zoeller, R.T.; Gore, A.C. . (2009). Endocrine-disrupting chemicals: an endocrine society scientific statement. *Endocrine Reviews,* Vol. 30, No. 4, pp. 293-342, ISSN: 0021-972X (Print).

Diels, L., De Smet, M., Hooyberghs, L.,Corbisier, P. (1999). Heavy metals bioremediation of soil. *Mol Biotechnol,* Vol. 12, No. 2, pp. 149-158, ISSN: 1073-6085 (Print).

Dobbins, L. L., Brain, R. A.,Brooks, B. W. (2008). Comparison of the sensitivities of common in vitro and in vivo assays of estrogenic activity: application of chemical toxicity distributions. *Environ Toxicol Chem,* Vol. 27, No. 12, pp. 2608-2616, ISSN: 0730-7268 (Print).

Doweyko, A. M. (2007). Steroid nuclear hormone receptors: The allosteric conversation. *Drug Development Research,* Vol. 68, No. 3, pp. 95-106, ISSN: 0272-4391.

Fan, M. Y., Rickert, E. L., Chen, L., Aftab, S. A., Nephew, K. P.,Weatherman, R. V. (2007). Characterization of molecular and structural determinants of selective estrogen receptor downregulators. *Breast Cancer Research and Treatment,* Vol. 103, No. 1, pp. 37-44, ISSN: 0167-6806.

Fannon, S. A., Vidaver, R. M.,Marts, S. A. (2001). An abridged history of sex steroid hormone receptor action. *J Appl Physiol,* Vol. 91, No. 4, pp. 1854-1859, ISSN: 8750-7587 (Print).

Feldman, P. L., Lambert, M. H.,Henke, B. R. (2008). PPAR modulators and PPAR pan agonists for metabolic diseases: The next generation of drugs targeting Peroxisome Proliferator-Activated Receptors? *Current Topics in Medicinal Chemistry,* Vol. 8, No. 9, pp. 728-749, ISSN: 1568-0266.

Fernandez, M. P., Campbell, P. M., Ikonomou, M. G.,Devlin, R. H. (2007). Assessment of environmental estrogens and the intersex/sex reversal capacity for chinook salmon (Oncorhynchus tshawytscha) in primary and final municipal wastewater effluents. *Environment International,* Vol. 33, No. 3, pp. 391-396, ISSN: 0160-4120.

Fessler, M. B. (2008). Liver X receptor: Crosstalk node for the signaling of lipid metabolism, carbohydrate metabolism, and innate immunity. *Current Signal Transduction Therapy,* Vol. 3, No. 2, pp. 75-81, ISSN: 1574-3624.

Gawrys, M. D., Hartman, I., Landweber, L. F.,Wood, D. W. (2009). Use of engineered Escherichia coli cells to detect estrogenicity in everyday consumer products. *Journal of Chemical Technology & Biotechnology,* Vol. 84, No. 12, pp. 1834-1840, ISSN: 1097-4660.

Gierach, I., Shapero, K., Eyster, T. W.,Wood, D. W. (2011). Bacterial biosensors for evaluating potential impacts of estrogenic endocrine disrupting compounds in multiple species. *Environmental Toxicology and Chemistry,* (in press).

Gillies, A. R., Skretas, G.,Wood, D. W. (2008). Engineered systems for detection and discovery of nuclear hormone-like compounds. *Biotechnol Prog,* Vol. 24, No. 1, pp. 8-16, ISSN: 8756-7938 (Print).

Goksoyr, A. (2006). Endocrine disruptors in the marine environment: mechanisms of toxicity and their influence on reproductive processes in fish. *J Toxicol Environ Health A,* Vol. 69, No. 1-2, pp. 175-184, ISSN: 1528-7394 (Print).

Grover, G. J., Mellstrom, K.,Malm, J. (2005). Development of the thyroid hormone receptor beta-subtype agonist KB-141: a strategy for body weight reduction and lipid lowering with minimal cardiac side effects. *Cardiovascular Drug Reviews,* Vol. 23, No. 2, pp. 133-148.

Grycewicz, J.,Cypryk, K. (2008). Effect of sex hormones on metabolic disturbances in menopausal women. *Przeglad Menopauzalny,* Vol. 7, No. 1, pp. 29-37, ISSN: 1643-8876.

Gulla, S. V.,Budil, D. E. (2007). Ligand induced solution structure and dynamics of the helix-12 region of estrogen receptor alpha. *Faseb Journal,* Vol. 21, No. 5, pp. A253-A253, ISSN: 0892-6638.

Gustafsson, J. A. (1999). Estrogen receptor beta-a new dimension in estrogen mechanism of action. *J Endocrinol,* Vol. 163, No. 3, pp. 379-383, ISSN: 0022-0795 (Print).

Hartman, I., Gillies, A. R., Arora, S., Andaya, C., Royapet, N., Welsh, W. J., Wood, D. W.,Zauhar, R. J. (2009). Application of screening methods, shape signatures and engineered biosensors in early drug discovery process. *Pharm Res,* Vol. 26, No. 10, pp. 2247-2258, ISSN: 1573-904X (Electronic).

Hewitt, S. C.,Korach, K. S. (2002). Estrogen receptors: structure, mechanisms and function. *Rev Endocr Metab Disord,* Vol. 3, No. 3, pp. 193-200, ISSN: 1389-9155 (Print).

Hsieh, M. H., Grantham, E. C., Liu, B., Macapagal, R., Willingham, E.,Baskin, L. S. (2007). In utero exposure to benzophenone-2 causes hypospadias through an estrogen receptor dependent mechanism. *J Urol,* Vol. 178, No. 4 Pt 2, pp. 1637-1642, ISSN: 0022-5347 (Print).

Hu, F., Smith, E. E.,Carr, J. A. (2008). Effects of larval exposure to estradiol on spermatogenesis and in vitro gonadal steroid secretion in African clawed frogs, Xenopus laevis. *General and Comparative Endocrinology,* Vol. 155, No. 1, pp. 190-200, ISSN: 0016-6480.

Ivask, A., Green, T., Polyak, B., Mor, A., Kahru, A., Virta, M.,Marks, R. (2007). Fibre-optic bacterial biosensors and their application for the analysis of bioavailable Hg and As in soils and sediments from Aznalcollar mining area in Spain. *Biosens Bioelectron,* Vol. 22, No. 7, pp. 1396-1402, ISSN: 0956-5663 (Print).

Jofre, M. B.,Karasov, W. H. (2008). Effect of mono-ortho and di-ortho substituted polychlorinated biphenyl (PCB) congeners on leopard frog survival and sexual development. *Chemosphere,* Vol. 70, No. 9, pp. 1609-1619, ISSN: 0045-6535.

Jordan, V. C., Patel, R., Lewis-Wambi, J.,Swaby, R. (2008). By looking back we can see the way forward: enhancing the gains achieved with antihormone therapy. *Breast Cancer Research,* Vol. 10, No. Suppl 4, pp. S16, ISSN: 1465-5411.

Katsu, Y., Lange, A., Urushitani, H., Ichikawa, R., Paull, G. C., Cahill, L. L., Jobling, S., Tyler, C. R.,Iguchi, T. (2007). Functional associations between two estrogen receptors, environmental estrogens, and sexual disruption in the roach (Rutilus rutilus). *Environmental Science & Technology,* Vol. 41, No. 9, pp. 3368-3374, ISSN: 0013-936X.

Keri, R. A., Ho, S. M., Hunt, P. A., Knudsen, K. E., Soto, A. M.,Prins, G. S. (2007). An evaluation of evidence for the carcinogenic activity of bisphenol A. *Reproductive Toxicology,* Vol. 24, No. 2, pp. 240-252, ISSN: 0890-6238.

Koda, T., Morita, M.,Imai, H. (2007). Retinoic acid inhibits uterotrophic activity of bisphenol a in adult ovariectomized rats. *Journal of Nutritional Science and Vitaminology,* Vol. 53, No. 5, pp. 432-436, ISSN: 0301-4800.

Koehler, K. F., Helguero, L. A., Haldosen, L. A., Warner, M.,Gustafsson, J. A. (2005). Reflections on the discovery and significance of estrogen receptor beta. *Endocr Rev,* Vol. 26, No. 3, pp. 465-478, ISSN: 0163-769X (Print).

Koury, E. J., Pawlyk, A. C., Berrodin, T. J., Smolenski, C. L., Nagpal, S.,Deecher, D. C. (2009). Characterization of ligands for thyroid receptor subtypes and their interactions with co-regulators. *Steroids,* Vol. 74, No. 2, pp. 270-276, ISSN: 0039-128X (Print).

Kramer, P. J. (1998). Genetic toxicology. *J Pharm Pharmacol,* Vol. 50, No. 4, pp. 395-405, ISSN: 0022-3573 (Print).

Kuiper, G. G., Carlsson, B., Grandien, K., Enmark, E., Haggblad, J., Nilsson, S.,Gustafsson, J. A. (1997). Comparison of the ligand binding specificity and transcript tissue distribution of estrogen receptors alpha and beta. *Endocrinology,* Vol. 138, No. 3, pp. 863-870.

Kuiper, G. G., Lemmen, J. G., Carlsson, B., Corton, J. C., Safe, S. H., van der Saag, P. T., van der Burg, B.,Gustafsson, J. A. (1998). Interaction of estrogenic chemicals and phytoestrogens with estrogen receptor beta. *Endocrinology,* Vol. 139, No. 10, pp. 4252-4263, ISSN: 0013-7227 (Print).

Kuiper, R. V., Canton, R. F., Leonards, P. E. G., Jenssen, B. M., Dubbeldam, M., Wester, P. W., van den Berg, M., Vos, J. G.,Vethaak, A. D. (2007). Long-term exposure of European flounder (Platichthys flesus) to the flame-retardants tetrabromobisphenol A (TBBPA) and hexabromocyclododecane (HBCD). *Ecotoxicology and Environmental Safety,* Vol. 67, No. 3, pp. 349-360, ISSN: 0147-6513.

Kunz, P. Y., Galicia, H. F.,Fent, K. (2006). Comparison of in vitro and in vivo estrogenic activity of UV filters in fish. *Toxicol Sci,* Vol. 90, No. 2, pp. 349-361, ISSN: 1096-6080 (Print).

Lee, Y. M., Seong, M. J., Lee, J. W., Lee, Y. K., Kim, T. M., Nam, S. Y., Kim, D. J., Yun, Y. W., Kim, T. S., Han, S. Y.,Hong, J. T. (2007). Estrogen receptor independent neurotoxic mechanism of bisphenol A, an environmental estrogen. *Journal of Veterinary Science,* Vol. 8, No. 1, pp. 27-38, ISSN: 1229-845X.

Leung, F. P., Tsang, S. Y., Wong, C. M., Yung, L. M., Chan, Y. C., Leung, H. S., Yao, X. Q.,Huang, Y. (2007). Raloxifene, tamoxifen and vascular tone. *Clinical and Experimental Pharmacology and Physiology,* Vol. 34, No. 8, pp. 809-813, ISSN: 0305-1870.

Li, L., Andersen, M. E., Heber, S.,Zhang, Q. (2007). Non-monotonic dose-response relationship in steroid hormone receptor-mediated gene expression. *Journal of Molecular Endocrinology,* Vol. 38, No. 5-6, pp. 569-585, ISSN: 0952-5041.

Li, Y. F., Li, F. Y., Ho, C. L.,Liao, V. H. (2008). Construction and comparison of fluorescence and bioluminescence bacterial biosensors for the detection of bioavailable toluene and related compounds. *Environ Pollut,* Vol. 152, No. 1, pp. 123-129, ISSN: 0269-7491 (Print).

Li, Y. L., Litten, C., Koehler, K. F., Mellstrom, K., Garg, N., Garcia Collazo, A. M., Farnegard, M., Grynfarb, M., Husman, B., Sandberg, J.,Malm, J. (2006). Thyroid receptor ligands. Part 4: 4'-amido bioisosteric ligands selective for the thyroid hormone receptor beta. *Bioorg Med Chem Lett,* Vol. 16, No. 4, pp. 884-886, ISSN: 0960-894X (Print).

Liao, V. H., Chien, M. T., Tseng, Y. Y.,Ou, K. L. (2006). Assessment of heavy metal bioavailability in contaminated sediments and soils using green fluorescent protein-based bacterial biosensors. *Environ Pollut,* Vol. 142, No. 1, pp. 17-23, ISSN: 0269-7491 (Print).

Lingxia, X., Taixiang, W.,Xiaoyan, C. (2007). Selective estrogen receptor modulators (SERMs) for uterine leiomyomas. *Cochrane Database of Systematic Reviews,* ISSN: 1469-493X.

Link, N., Weber, W.,Fussenegger, M. (2007). A novel generic dipstick-based technology for rapid and precise detection of tetracycline, streptogramin and macrolide antibiotics in food samples. *J Biotechnol,* Vol. 128, No. 3, pp. 668-680, ISSN: 0168-1656 (Print).

MacGregor, J. I.,Jordan, V. C. (1998). Basic guide to the mechanisms of antiestrogen action. *Pharmacol Rev,* Vol. 50, No. 2, pp. 151-196, ISSN: 0031-6997 (Print).

Maffini, M. V., Rubin, B. S., Sonnenschein, C.,Soto, A. M. (2006). Endocrine disruptors and reproductive health: the case of bisphenol-A. *Mol Cell Endocrinol,* Vol. 254-255, No., pp. 179-186, ISSN: 0303-7207 (Print).

Malm, J., Grover, G. J.,Farnegardh, M. (2007). Recent advances in the development of agonists selective for beta1-type thyroid hormone receptor. *Mini-Reviews in Medicinal Chemistry,* Vol. 7, No. 1, pp. 79-86.

Marimuthu, A., Feng, W., Tagami, T., Nguyen, H., Jameson, J. L., Fletterick, R. J., Baxter, J. D.,West, B. L. (2002). TR surfaces and conformations required to bind nuclear receptor corepressor. *Mol Endocrinol,* Vol. 16, No. 2, pp. 271-286, ISSN: 0888-8809 (Print).

Martinez, L., Nascimento, A. S., Nunes, F. M., Phillips, K., Aparicio, R., Dias, S. M., Figueira, A. C., Lin, J. H., Nguyen, P., Apriletti, J. W., Neves, F. A., Baxter, J. D., Webb, P., Skaf, M. S.,Polikarpov, I. (2009). Gaining ligand selectivity in thyroid hormone receptors via entropy. *Proc Natl Acad Sci U S A,* Vol., No., pp., ISSN: 1091-6490 (Electronic).

Matthews, J., Celius, T., Halgren, R.,Zacharewski, T. (2000). Differential estrogen receptor binding of estrogenic substances: a species comparison. *J Steroid Biochem Mol Biol,* Vol. 74, No. 4, pp. 223-234, ISSN: 0960-0760 (Print).

Matthews, J. B., Clemons, J. H.,Zacharewski, T. R. (2001). Reciprocal mutagenesis between human alpha(L349, M528) and rainbow trout (M317, I496) estrogen receptor residues demonstrates their importance in ligand binding and gene expression at different temperatures. *Mol Cell Endocrinol,* Vol. 183, No. 1-2, pp. 127-139, ISSN: 0303-7207 (Print).

Mattsson, C.,Olsson, T. (2007). Estrogens and glucocorticoid hormones in adipose tissue metabolism. *Current Medicinal Chemistry,* Vol. 14, No. 27, pp. 2918-2924, ISSN: 0929-8673.

McKinlay, R., Plant, J. A., Bell, J. N. B.,Voulvoulis, N. (2008). Endocrine disrupting pesticides: implications for risk assessment. *Environment International,* Vol. 34, No. 2, pp. 168-183, ISSN: 0160-4120.

Mitchell, R. J.,Gu, M. B. (2004). Construction and characterization of novel dual stress-responsive bacterial biosensors. *Biosens Bioelectron,* Vol. 19, No. 9, pp. 977-985, ISSN: 0956-5663 (Print).

Molina-Molina, J. M., Escande, A., Pillon, A., Gomez, E., Pakdel, F., Cavailles, V., Olea, N., Ait-Aissa, S.,Balaguer, P. (2008). Profiling of benzophenone derivatives using fish and human estrogen receptor-specific in vitro bioassays. *Toxicol Appl Pharmacol,* Vol. 232, No. 3, pp. 384-395, ISSN: 1096-0333 (Electronic).

Musa, M. A., Khan, M. O. F.,Cooperwood, J. S. (2007). Medicinal chemistry and emerging strategies applied to the development of selective estrogen receptor modulators (SERMs). *Current Medicinal Chemistry,* Vol. 14, No. 11, pp. 1249-1261, ISSN: 0929-8673.

Nagarajan, K., Zauhar, R.,Welsh, W. J. (2005). Enrichment of ligands for the serotonin receptor using the Shape Signatures approach. *J Chem Inf Model,* Vol. 45, No. 1, pp. 49-57, ISSN: 1549-9596 (Print).

Negri-Cesi, P., Colciago, A., Pravettoni, A., Casati, L., Conti, L.,Celotti, F. (2008). Sexual differentiation of the rodent hypothalamus: Hormonal and environmental influences. *Journal of Steroid Biochemistry and Molecular Biology,* Vol. 109, No. 3-5, pp. 294-299, ISSN: 0960-0760.

Nilsson, R. (2000). Endocrine modulators in the food chain and environment. *Toxicol Pathol,* Vol. 28, No. 3, pp. 420-431, ISSN: 0192-6233 (Print).

Norris, J. D., Fan, D., Kerner, S. A.,McDonnell, D. P. (1997). Identification of a third autonomous activation domain within the human estrogen receptor. *Mol Endocrinol,* Vol. 11, No. 6, pp. 747-754, ISSN: 0888-8809 (Print).

Ohno, M. (2008). Functional analysis of nuclear receptor FXR controlling metabolism of cholesterol. *Yakugaku Zasshi-Journal of the Pharmaceutical Society of Japan,* Vol. 128, No. 3, pp. 343-355, ISSN: 0031-6903.

Paitan, Y., Biran, D., Biran, I., Shechter, N., Babai, R., Rishpon, J.,Ron, E. Z. (2003). On-line and in situ biosensors for monitoring environmental pollution. *Biotechnol Adv,* Vol. 22, No. 1-2, pp. 27-33, ISSN: 0734-9750 (Print).

Petit, F., Valotaire, Y.,Pakdel, F. (1995). Differential functional activities of rainbow trout and human estrogen receptors expressed in the yeast Saccharomyces cerevisiae. *Eur J Biochem,* Vol. 233, No. 2, pp. 584-592, ISSN: 0014-2956 (Print).

Pikkemaat, M. G., Rapallini, M. L., Karp, M. T.,Elferink, J. W. (2010). Application of a luminescent bacterial biosensor for the detection of tetracyclines in routine analysis of poultry muscle samples. *Food Addit Contam Part A Chem Anal Control Expo Risk Assess,* Vol. 27, No. 8, pp. 1112-1117, ISSN: 1944-0057 (Electronic).

Pinto, B., Bertoli, A., Noccioli, C., Garritano, S., Reali, D.,Piqelli, L. (2008). Estradiol-antagonistic activity of phenolic compounds from leguminous plants. *Phytotherapy Research,* Vol. 22, No. 3, pp. 362-366, ISSN: 0951-418X.

Pritchard, K. I. (2001). Breast cancer prevention with selective estrogen receptor modulators: a perspective. *Ann N Y Acad Sci,* Vol. 949, No., pp. 89-98, ISSN: 0077-8923 (Print).

Rabbow, E., Rettberg, P., Baumstark-Khan, C.,Horneck, G. (2003). The SOS-LUX-LAC-FLUORO-Toxicity-test on the International Space Station (ISS). *Adv Space Res,* Vol. 31, No. 6, pp. 1513-1524, ISSN: 0273-1177 (Print).

Ramamoorthy, K., Wang, F., Chen, I. C., Norris, J. D., McDonnell, D. P., Leonard, L. S., Gaido, K. W., Bocchinfuso, W. P., Korach, K. S.,Safe, S. (1997). Estrogenic activity of a dieldrin/toxaphene mixture in the mouse uterus, MCF-7 human breast cancer cells, and yeast-based estrogen receptor assays: no apparent synergism. *Endocrinology,* Vol. 138, No. 4, pp. 1520-1527, ISSN: 0013-7227 (Print).

Raymond-Whish, S., Mayer, L. P., O'Neal, T., Martinez, A., Sellers, M. A., Christian, P. J., Marion, S. L., Begay, C., Propper, C. R., Hoyer, P. B.,Dyer, C. A. (2007). Drinking water with uranium below the US EPA water standard causes estrogen receptor-dependent responses in female mice. *Environmental Health Perspectives,* Vol. 115, No. 12, pp. 1711-1716, ISSN: 0091-6765.

Rempel, M. A.,Schlenk, D. (2008). Effects of environmental estrogens and antiandrogens on endocrine function, gene regulation, and health in fish. *International Review of Cell and Molecular Biology, Vol 267,* Vol. 267, No., pp. 207-252.

Safe, S. H. (2000). Endocrine disruptors and human health-is there a problem? An update. *Environ Health Perspect,* Vol. 108, No. 6, pp. 487-493, ISSN: 0091-6765 (Print).

Sanceau, J. Y., Larouche, D., Caron, B., Belanger, P., Coquet, A., Belanger, A., Labrie, F.,Gauthier, S. (2007). Synthesis and deuterium labelling of the pure selective estrogen receptor modulator (SERM) acolbifene glucuronides. *Journal of Labelled Compounds & Radiopharmaceuticals,* Vol. 50, No. 3-4, pp. 197-206, ISSN: 0362-4803.

Scanlan, T. S. (2008). Sobetirome: a case history of bench-to-clinic drug discovery and development. *Heart Fail Rev,* Vol., No., pp., ISSN: 1573-7322 (Electronic).

Schapira, M., Raaka, B. M., Samuels, H. H.,Abagyan, R. (2000). Rational discovery of novel nuclear hormone receptor antagonists. *Proc Natl Acad Sci U S A,* Vol. 97, No. 3, pp. 1008-1013, ISSN: 0027-8424 (Print).

Schlecht, C., Klammer, H., Frauendorf, H., Wuttke, W.,Jarry, H. (2008). Pharmacokinetics and metabolism of benzophenone 2 in the rat. *Toxicology,* Vol. 245, No. 1-2, pp. 11-17, ISSN: 0300-483X (Print).

Seidlova-Wuttke, D., Jarry, H., Christoffel, J., Rimoldi, G.,Wuttke, W. (2005). Effects of bisphenol-A (BPA), dibutylphtalate (DBP), benzophenone-2 (BP2), procymidone (Proc), and linurone (Lin) on fat tissue, a variety of hormones and metabolic parameters: a 3 months comparison with effects of estradiol (E2) in ovariectomized (ovx) rats. *Toxicology,* Vol. 213, No. 1-2, pp. 13-24, ISSN: 0300-483X (Print).

Seidlova-Wuttke, D., Jarry, H.,Wuttke, W. (2004). Pure estrogenic effect of benzophenone-2 (BP2) but not of bisphenol A (BPA) and dibutylphtalate (DBP) in uterus, vagina and bone. *Toxicology,* Vol. 205, No. 1-2, pp. 103-112, ISSN: 0300-483X (Print).

Shiau, A. K., Barstad, D., Loria, P. M., Cheng, L., Kushner, P. J., Agard, D. A.,Greene, G. L. (1998). The structural basis of estrogen receptor/coactivator recognition and the antagonism of this interaction by tamoxifen. *Cell,* Vol. 95, No. 7, pp. 927-937, ISSN: 0092-8674 (Print).

Shiau, A. K., Barstad, D., Radek, J. T., Meyers, M. J., Nettles, K. W., Katzenellenbogen, B. S., Katzenellenbogen, J. A., Agard, D. A.,Greene, G. L. (2002). Structural characterization of a subtype-selective ligand reveals a novel mode of estrogen receptor antagonism. *Nat Struct Biol,* Vol. 9, No. 5, pp. 359-364, ISSN: 1072-8368 (Print).

Skretas, G., Meligova, A. K., Villalonga-Barber, C., Mitsiou, D. J., Alexis, M. N., Micha-Screttas, M., Steele, B. R., Screttas, C. G.,Wood, D. W. (2007). Engineered chimeric enzymes as tools for drug discovery: generating reliable bacterial screens for the detection, discovery, and assessment of estrogen receptor modulators. *J Am Chem Soc,* Vol. 129, No. 27, pp. 8443-8457, ISSN: 0002-7863 (Print).

Skretas, G.,Wood, D. W. (2005a). A bacterial biosensor of endocrine modulators. *J Mol Biol,* Vol. 349, No. 3, pp. 464-474, ISSN: 0022-2836 (Print).

Skretas, G.,Wood, D. W. (2005b). Rapid detection of subtype-selective nuclear hormone receptor binding with bacterial genetic selection. *Appl Environ Microbiol,* Vol. 71, No. 12, pp. 8995-8997, ISSN: 0099-2240 (Print).

Skretas, G.,Wood, D. W. (2005c). Regulation of protein activity with small-molecule-controlled inteins. *Protein Sci,* Vol. 14, No. 2, pp. 523-532, ISSN: 0961-8368 (Print).

Smeets, J. M., Rankouhi, T. R., Nichols, K. M., Komen, H., Kaminski, N. E., Giesy, J. P.,van den Berg, M. (1999). In vitro vitellogenin production by carp (Cyprinus carpio) hepatocytes as a screening method for determining (anti)estrogenic activity of xenobiotics. *Toxicol Appl Pharmacol,* Vol. 157, No. 1, pp. 68-76, ISSN: 0041-008X (Print).

Strumylaite, L., Bogusevicius, A., Ryselis, S., Pranys, D., Poskiene, L., Kregzdyte, R., Abdrachmanovas, O.,Asadauskaite, R. (2008). Association between cadmium and breast cancer. *Medicina-Lithuania,* Vol. 44, No. 6, pp. 415-420, ISSN: 1010-660X.

Tancevski, I., Eller, P., Patsch, J. R.,Ritsch, A. (2009). The resurgence of thyromimetics as lipid-modifying agents. *Current Opinion in Investigational Drugs,* Vol. 10, No. 9, pp. 912-918.

Tani, C., Inoue, K., Tani, Y., Harun-ur-Rashid, M., Azuma, N., Ueda, S., Yoshida, K.,Maeda, I. (2009). Sensitive fluorescent microplate bioassay using recombinant Escherichia coli with multiple promoter-reporter units in tandem for detection of arsenic. *J Biosci Bioeng,* Vol. 108, No. 5, pp. 414-420, ISSN: 1347-4421 (Electronic).

Tokumoto, T., Tokumoto, M.,Thomas, P. (2007). Interactions of diethylstilbestrol (DES) and DES analogs with membrane progestin receptor-alpha and the correlation with their nongenomic progestin activities. *Endocrinology,* Vol. 148, No. 7, pp. 3459-3467, ISSN: 0013-7227.

Vahter, M., Akesson, A., Liden, C., Ceccatelli, S.,Berglund, M. (2007). Gender differences in the disposition and toxicity of metals. *Environmental Research,* Vol. 104, No. 1, pp. 85-95, ISSN: 0013-9351.

Vandenberg, L. N., Hauser, R., Marcus, M., Olea, N.,Welshons, W. V. (2007). Human exposure to bisphenol A (BPA). *Reproductive Toxicology,* Vol. 24, No. 2, pp. 139-177, ISSN: 0890-6238.

Vandenberg, L. N., Maffini, M. V., Sonnenschein, C., Rubin, B. S.,Soto, A. M. (2009). Bisphenol-A and the great divide: a review of controversies in the field of endocrine disruption. *Endocr Rev,* Vol. 30, No. 1, pp. 75-95, ISSN: 1945-7189 (Electronic).

Wagner, R. L., Huber, B. R., Shiau, A. K., Kelly, A., Cunha Lima, S. T., Scanlan, T. S., Apriletti, J. W., Baxter, J. D., West, B. L.,Fletterick, R. J. (2001). Hormone selectivity in thyroid hormone receptors. *Mol Endocrinol,* Vol. 15, No. 3, pp. 398-410, ISSN: 0888-8809 (Print).

Werlen, C., Jaspers, M. C.,van der Meer, J. R. (2004). Measurement of biologically available naphthalene in gas and aqueous phases by use of a Pseudomonas putida biosensor. *Appl Environ Microbiol,* Vol. 70, No. 1, pp. 43-51, ISSN: 0099-2240 (Print).

Wilkinson, P. M., Ribiero, G. G., Adam, H. K., Kemp, J. V.,Patterson, J. S. (1982). Tamoxifen (Nolvadex) therapy-radionale for loading dose followed by maintenance dose for patients with metastatic breast cancer. *Cancer Chemother Pharmacol,* Vol. 10, No. 1, pp. 33-35, ISSN: 0344-5704 (Print).

Wood, D. W., Wu, W., Belfort, G., Derbyshire, V.,Belfort, M. (1999). A genetic system yields self-cleaving inteins for bioseparations. *Nat Biotechnol,* Vol. 17, No. 9, pp. 889-892, ISSN: 1087-0156 (Print).

Zauhar, R. J. (1995). SMART: a solvent-accessible triangulated surface generator for molecular graphics and boundary element applications. *J Comput Aided Mol Des,* Vol. 9, No. 2, pp. 149-159, ISSN: 0920-654X (Print).

Zauhar, R. J., Moyna, G., Tian, L., Li, Z.,Welsh, W. J. (2003). Shape signatures: a new approach to computer-aided ligand- and receptor-based drug design. *J Med Chem,* Vol. 46, No. 26, pp. 5674-5690, ISSN: 0022-2623 (Print).

Zhang, J. H., Chung, T. D.,Oldenburg, K. R. (1999). A Simple Statistical Parameter for Use in Evaluation and Validation of High Throughput Screening Assays. *J Biomol Screen,* Vol. 4, No. 2, pp. 67-73, ISSN: 1552-454X (Electronic).

Higher Plants as a Warning to Ionizing Radiation:Tradescantia

Teresa C. Leal[1] and Alphonse Kelecom[2]
[1]*Faculdade Paraiso*
[2]*Instituto de Biológia-UFF*
Brasil

1. Introduction

Since the 19th century, with industrial and urban development and the consequent increase in emissions from industrial activities and vehicular emissions have been observed air pollution effects on living organisms. Thus, since the beginning of the twentieth century, have been carried out several studies that include studies of the effect of pollution on plants (Chies,1983). Some features observed in these surveys are genotoxic effects, observation of falling leaves, analysis of pigments associated with photosynthetic apparatus, deposition and accumulation of chemicals in the leaves, structural and ultrastructural and effects on reproductive organs.

The need for the scientific community to understand what are the environmental agents that cause genetic damage in humans has also been since the beginning of last century and, with this concern, began to enhance the studies on the processes that cause mutations in cells. To meet these challenges, then began to be developed several bioassays Toxicogenetics, from the simplest to the most sophisticated (Ribeiro *et al.*,2003)

Each year, the amount of radioactive waste from research institutions, hospitals and nuclear power plants in Brazil and around the world is growing, and so the need to store this waste grows too. Waste storage induces questions for society concerning the amount of radiation exposure to man and the environment in the neighborhoods of waste deposit sites.

In Brazil, the organ responsible for inspecting the deposits of nuclear waste is the National Commission for Nuclear Energy (Comissão Nacional de Energia Nuclear- CNEN). The stored nuclear waste can be of low or medium activity; the material is previously compacted and maintained in steel drums. They can be stored in initial, intermediary or permanent deposits. The permanent deposits are protected by thick concrete walls and may house the materials for short or midterm intervals of time. There is, in Brazil, only one permanent deposit for waste of small to medium activity where part of the material resulting from the cesium-137 accident in Goiânia (1987) is stored. The construction of other prominent deposits is under consideration. However, selection for the location of these deposits depends on a technical analysis that includes details of different levels of data and information. There is also a need to comply with the laws nr 4.118/62 and 10.308/01 respectively and the regulations NE-6.05 - Management of Radioactive Waste in Radioactive Installations (Gerência de Rejeitos Radioativos em Instalações Radiativas), NE-6.06 - Selection and Choice of Locations for Deposits of Radioactive Waste (Seleção e Escolha de

Locais para Depósitos de Rejeitos Radioativos), NN-6.09 - Criteria of Acceptance for the Deposits of Low and Medium Levels of Radioactive Waste (Critérios de Aceitação para Deposição de Rejeitos Radioativos de Baixos e Médios Níveis de Radiação) and NE-3.01- Basic Directives for Radiological Protection (Diretrizes Básicas de Proteção Radiológica).

1.1 Effect in cell

A mutation is defined as a change in DNA sequence, which leads to a heritable change in gene function. Agents that change the sequence of DNA (mutagens) are "toxic" to the gene and are then called "genotoxic" (Ribeiro *et al.*,2003).

In order to assess and prevent the presence of genotoxic agents in the environment is necessary to use sensitive indicators to detect the action of these compounds. There are plants that are considered ideal for the study of mutagenesis, both in laboratory and in situ monitoring, thus acting as bioindicators. Among the tests with the bioindicators, the micronucleus test with Tradescantia spp. (Trad-MCN) is considered the most sensitive to genotoxic agents (Ennever *et al.*1998; Ribeiro *et al.*,2003; Saldiva *et al.*,2002). The genus Tradescantia has been used experimentally since the first studies related to gene activity with the action of compounds and chemical agents. The choice is due to a series of favorable genetic characteristics, among which stands out the fact that the cells of almost all parts of the plant provides excellent material for cytogenetic studies (Ma, 1979; Grant,1998).

The influence of chemical and physical agents (especially radiation) on the frequency of mutations has been extensively studied through analysis of changes observed in Tradescantia (Carvalho,2005). Among the features that allow the detection of agents that affect the stability of the genome in Tradescantia, some were selected as indicators in bioassays for evaluating genetic toxicity: testing the pollen tube mitosis and cell color change to pink in hair stem (Trad-SH) (Rodrigues and Campos, 2006). The evaluation of genotoxicity in Tradescantia can also be made by detecting fragments or segments of DNA induced by genotoxic agents in the air, soil and water (Carvalho, 2005), was developed as a cytogenetic test that is based on the micronucleus (Trad-MCN). Thus, the Trad-MCN test is based on the formation of micronuclei, which are a result of chromosome fragmentation, visualized in the tetrad stage of stem cells grain (Ma, 1979; Rodrigues, 1999a-b). Micronuclei are counted and the frequency in which they occur indicate the toxicity of the environment.

The micronucleus test in Tradescantia (Trad-MCN) has long been used in environmental monitoring, which is due to its effectiveness in detecting chromosomal damage, the simplicity with which it is executed and its low financial cost of its methodology. All these properties qualify it as an excellent tool for this type of monitoring (Zengh and Qingqiang, 1999). Moreover, studies over the years about the genetics and development of Tradescantia offer strong support for its use as bio-indicator for genetic toxicity testing environment (Ma, 1982). Micronuclei in stem cells of pollen grains are easily observable and tests with Tradescantia have proved valuable in studies of genotoxic agents (Rodrigues *et al.*,1997;1996; Ma and Grant, 1982).

Researchers at the International Program on Plant Bioassays with the University of Illinois (USA), were the first devised and used the micronucleus assay (Trad-MCN) in tetrads to assess the genotoxicity of certain agents. The plant used was a hybrid clone 4430 (T. Bush hirsutiflora x subacaulis T. Bush), a comparative study with tests of mutations of stem hairs (Trad-SH) to assess the effects of 1,2 - dibromoethane, a substance known to mutagenic, on the chromosomes of cells in meiosis(Ma, 1979). The basis for the development of this test was the fact that the biggest problem in the quantitative assessment of chromosomal

fragmentation was the loss of chromosomes in metaphase and his image appeared blurred in the preparations of the cells in meiosis. However, if the agent is applied at the beginning of Prophase chromosome and continues for a period of recovery, acentric fragments of chromosomes become micronuclei at the tetrad stage of meiosis, easily identified on light microscopy (Carvalho, 2005).
The use of the Trad-MCN test for monitoring environmental genotoxic agents was proposed after studies involving agents pro-mutagens (benzo-α-pyrene) in polluted cities (Ma, 1981;1982:1983;1990). In 1983, TH Ma established the protocol for the bioassay Trad-MCN [17]. The Trad-MCN with the clone 4430 was also performed to study the fitogenotoxicidade substance 2,4 - and 2,6-dinitrotoluene, intermediate in the production of toluene, explosives, propellants, among others. The tests showed positive genotoxicity of these two substances, but a greater genotoxicity of 2,4-DNT, compared to 2,6-DNT (Gong *et al.*, 2003).
At the University of Metz-Bridoux, France, studies Tradescantia exposed to 4430 ^{137}Cs indicated genotoxicity of low doses of gamma and beta radiation emitted by this radionuclide (Minouflet *et al.*, 2005). This study inspired this work in an attempt to verify the mutational effects on the response of *Tradescantia clone* 4430 (tentative) and *Tradescantia pallida* exposure to a ^{137} Cs radiation source.

2. Materials and methods

2.1 Biotesting I

The purpose of this study was to work with Tradescantia clone 4430, but this had some limitations when applied to tests that required a longer period of exposure to the source. The high temperature, humidity and variations in light intensity, here in Rio de Janeiro (Brazil) will affect the system, which favors the emergence of parasites and insects caused inhibition of flowering. These factors limit its use to a short period of time in a biomonitoring in regions of hot climates and is highly favored regions where they observed a mild climate. Although studies to establish positive results for its application in the case of ionizing radiation (Ichikawa, 1991;1992; Villalobos-Pietrini *et al.*,1999; Suyama *et al.*, 2002), there was no success in implementing this kind for long periods , as was the aim of this work. Then a new species of the same family, Comelinacea, that better fit the environmental conditions in Brazil was introduced. *Tradescantia pallida* (Rose) Hunt. variety *purpurea* Boom is a small ornamental plant from the family Comelinacea the characteristics of which make it useful for experiments involving genetic damage to cells especially those originating from exposure in a genotoxic environment.
To develop and experiment biosensors, there is a need to ensure that it meets the environmental conditions where it will be used. Hence, the choice of *T. pallida* resulted from its good adaptation to the adverse climatic conditions in the various regions around the country. This plant can be found in many streets and gardens of the cities all over the country. It is a tetraploid species that has notable resistance to both parasites and insects. It blooms all year round and needs little care and attention to grow.
T. pallida allows us to obtain response curves of biological damage *versus* dosage, based on the micronuclei methodological system developed by T.H. Ma for *Tradescantia* clone 4430 and *Vicia faba,* in 1992. This methodology has been widely used by various groups of researchers to evaluate the damaging effects of genotoxic agents and to obtain a prognosis for human health.

In this work, we evaluated the responses obtained as *Tradescantia pallida,* when exposed to a radiation source, ^{137}Cs, low activity, in order to further long-term applications. The trial established the standard for short environmental conditions of Brazil, and thereby justifies the use of plants as biosensor for environmental testing of mutagenesis at low doses of gamma radiation.

2.2 Biotesting II

Tradescantia *pallida* (Rose) Hunt. variety *purpurea* Boom is a small ornamental plant from the family Comelinacea the characteristics of which make it useful for experiments involving genetic damage to cells especially those originating from exposure in a genotoxic environment.

To develop and experiment biosensors, there is a need to ensure that it meets the environmental conditions where it will be used. Hence, the choice of *T. pallida* resulted from its good adaptation to the adverse climatic conditions in the various regions around the country. This plant can be found in many streets and gardens of the cities all over the country. It is a tetraploid species that has notable resistance to both parasites and insects. It blooms all year round and needs little care and attention to grow.

T. pallida allows us to obtain response curves of biological damage *versus* dosage, based on the micronuclei methodological system developed by T.H. Ma for *Tradescantia* clone 4430 and *Vicia faba* (Ma, 1982; 1994). This methodology has been widely used by various groups of researchers to evaluate the damaging effects of genotoxic agents and to obtain a prognosis for human health.

3. Experimental procedure

3.1 Experimental procedure I

We analyzed four groups containing vessels of Tradescantia pallida. The first group, control, and three groups, which varied the time of exposure and hence the dose absorbed by the system, including: 24 h, 36h and 48 h, exposed to the same place and the same conditions, the background rate, 0.01 mGy. Each group, 30 samples were analyzed.

The radiometry was measured at each venue in three different distance of 50 cm, 100cm and 200cm from the source, using a MRA GP500 monitor, model 7237/03.44. Once the locations had been selected, vases containing *T. pallida* were placed, in such a way that twenty samples were exposed in each group, over an interval of 24 h, 36h and 48 h. After being exposed, the samples were placed into water, for at least six to eight hours. This is enough time for the meiosis process to continue and for the mother cells of the pollen grains to reach their tetrad phase. When the tetrad phase is reached, it is possible to see the micronucleus. In the final stage, the tetrads are fixed, in a solution of acetic acid and alcohol (1:3, v/v), in agreement with the protocol published by T.H. Ma in 1979 and cited by Saldiva *et al.*, 2002.

To prepare the slides, once the inflorescences are chosen, they are mashed and treated with a drop of carmine (contrasting agent), to observe the different stages of the tetrads. The slide is squeezed slightly to visualize the tetrads under the microscope, on the same plane. The preparation is heated over a Bunsen burner at 80°C; the residuals are removed and the slides sealed with enamel. Three hundred tetrads per slide were counted, and by way of a table the number of micronuclei/slide was determined. In each selected group, 30 samples were analyzed, totaling 9000 cells per group, that were labeled as pertaining to the control group (Co), group A, group B and group C respectively, in accordance with the levels of dosage according to the distance the source.

Figure 1 shows the experimental scheme in which the samples were exposed to ^{137}Cs source, the distance of 50cm, 100cm and 200cm. For a period of 24h, 36h and 48h.

SUPERIOR VISION (source the 50cm,100cm and 200cm of height)

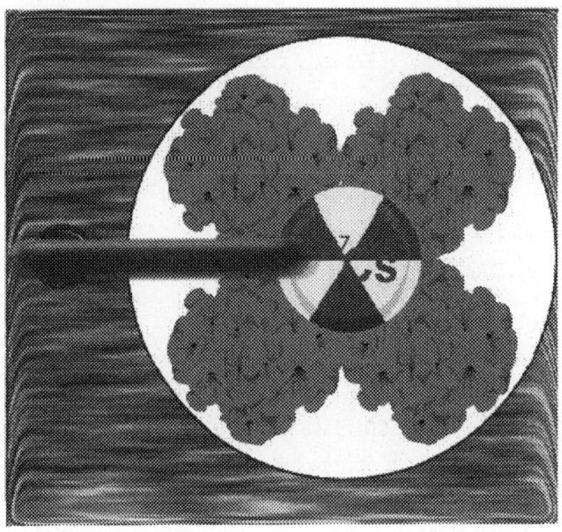

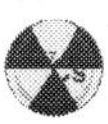 Source of Cs^{137}

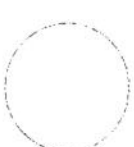 Round dish with 5 pots each

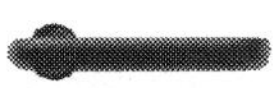 Connecting rod for support of the source

LATERAL VISION

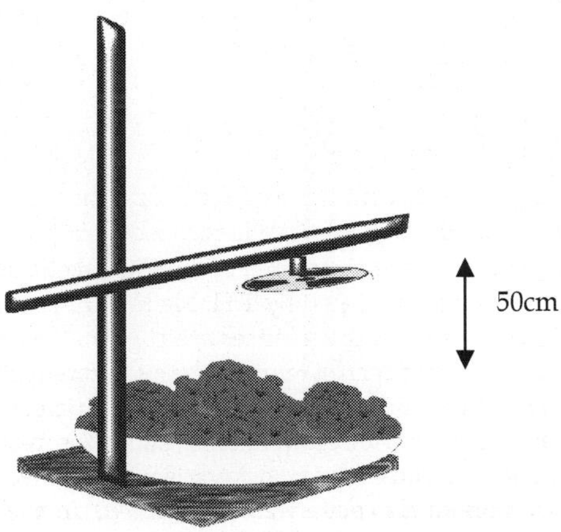

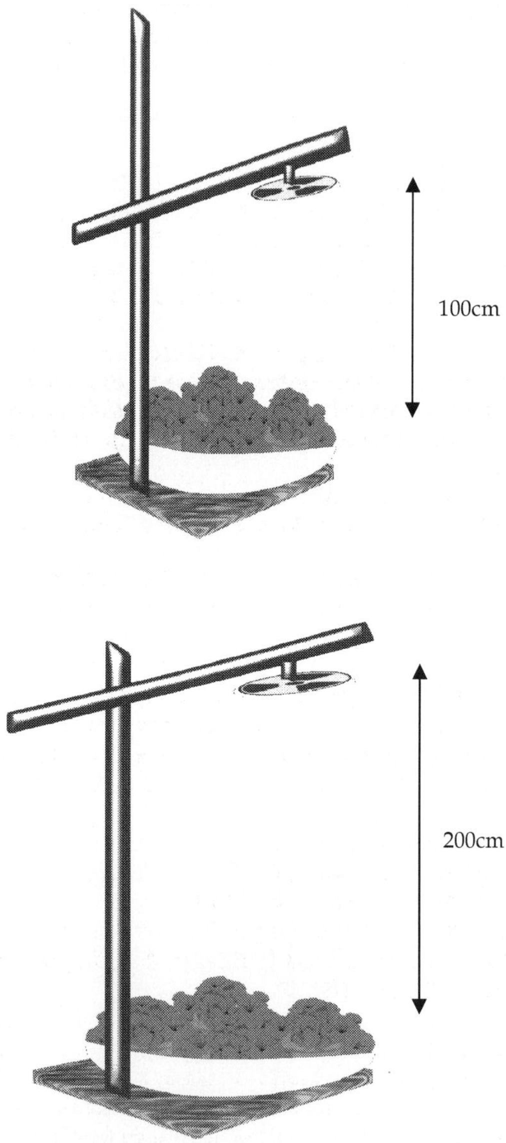

Fig. 1. Scheme of experimental exposure groups the source of ^{137}Cs, and the distances between the source and the biomarkers, 50 cm, 100cm and 200cm

3.1.1 Statistical analysis

To analyze the data the SPSS 9.0 for Windows program for statistic treatment was used (SPSS, 1999). The parameter variance was determined, in order to compare the counts in relation to the three groups from each region, to a level of significance of 0.05, the test t-Student was also used when comparing the samples (two in every two groups), in compliance with the protocol from T.H. Ma (1983).

3.2 Experimental procedure II

In this research, we have chosen four regions of merit around Brazil, because they contain nuclear waste deposits and because of their peculiar characteristics:

3.2.1 The Radioactive Waste Deposit at the Institute of Nuclear Engineering (IEN), located in the city of Rio de Janeiro: this deposit is considered of intermediate level. Some of the waste is stored for future use; others are removed to a permanent deposit.

3.2.2 The Radioactive Waste Deposit at the Nuclear Power Plant in Angra dos Reis (UNA) - located on the coastline of the state of Rio de Janeiro: it is considered to be an initial deposit; it contains richer active waste of low and medium activity. This deposit is under the custody of the Eletronuclear Corporation, and is supervised by CNEN.

3.2.3 The Radioactive Waste Deposit at the Institute for Nuclear Energy Research (IPEN) - located in the city of São Paulo: considered of intermediate level, however, it has a huge store of waste.

3.2.4 The Radioactive Waste Deposit at Abadia de Goiás (ABADIA): this is the only permanent waste deposit in Brazil, for small and medium activity.

Radiometric readings were carried out at the surroundings of each of these deposits using a MRA GP500 monitor, model 7237/03.44. At each waste deposit, three locations were selected cordance with the levels of dose rate: (1) CW (Control Waste deposit site) location where the dose rate was close to the dose rate measured at the garden where T. *pallida* was cultivated referred to as CG (Control Garden), (2) NE (nearby the entrance door of the waste deposit) and DE (along the waste deposit, but 1m distant of its entrance door).

Once the locations had been selected, vases containing T.*pallida* were placed, in such a way that 10 samples were exposed in each location, over an internal of 24h. After being exposed, the samples were placed into water, for at least 6-8hThis is time enough for the meiosis process to continue and for the mother cells of the pollen grains to reach their tetrad phase. When the tetrad phase is reached, it is possible to see the micronucleus. In the final stage, the tetrads are fixed, in a solution of acetic acid and alcohol (1:3, v/v), in agreement with the protocol published by T.H. Ma (1982).

To prepare the slides for microscope observation, chosen inflorescences are mashed and treated with a drop of carmine (contrasting agent), to observe the different stages of the tetrads. Then, the preparation is heated over a Bunsen burner at 80°C; the residuals are removed and the slides sealed with enamel. Three hundred tetrads per slide were counted, and by way of a table the number of micronuclei/slide was determined. In each radioactive waste deposit of each selected group, 100 samples were analyzed, totaling 30000 cells that were labeled as pertaining to the control negative group (Co), groups CW, NE and DE, respectively.

3.2.1 Statistical analysis

To analyze the data the SPSS 9.0 for Windows program for statistic treatment was used (SPSS, 1999). The parameter variance was determined, in order to compare the counts in relation to the three groups from each region, to a level of significance of 0.05, the test t-Student was also used when comparing the samples (two in every two groups), in compliance with the protocol from T.H. Ma (1983).

4. Results

4.1 Results and commentaries of experimental procedure I

As previously mentioned *Tradescantia* clone 4430, had some limitations when applied to tests that require a longer period of exposure to the environment. In hot climate cities such as Rio de Janeiro, was not successful in implementing this kind, and some plants died or not getting the bloom necessary.
With *Tradescantia pallida,* were analyzed 30 samples of each group and analyzed 9.000 cells per day for each of the groups, totaling 98.000 cells analyzed at the end of the experiment. Every count was compared with a control group (Co) of plants from the location of cultivation where the dosage rate measured was 0.26 μGy/h.
Table 1 presents a sample of the dosage rates resulting from each groups. The vessels with the inflorescences of *T. pallida* were placed at the site of exposure at a fixed distance of 50, 100 and 200 cm, respectively, for groups A, B and C (Table.1). The activity of the source of Cs-137 was 121KBq (2009).

Groups	Time exposure (h)	Taxa Dose	Total tetrads analyzed (cell)
*Co**	-----------	0.26 μGy/h	36000
Grup A (50 cm)	24 / 36/ 48	4.15 μGy/h	36000
Grup B (100cm)	24 / 36/ 48	9.58 mGy/h	36000
Grup C (200cm)	24 / 36/ 48	2.13 mGy/h	36000

*Co is the control group from the cultivated location.

Table 1. Exposure data of Biosensor

Equations (1) and (2) show the relation between the dose and time. The dose is directly proportional to the time of exposure, so, for the control group, it is expected that there will be an increase in micronucleus frequency of cells of pollen grains of *T. pallida.* When comparing the groups A, B and C, it is expected that there is an increase in frequency of micronuclei, proportional to the increase of exposure time.

$$dX/dt = \Gamma A / d^2 \quad (1)$$

$$dD = 0.869\ dX \text{ (in ar)} \quad (2)$$

where:
dX = the exposure rate,
dD = the dose rate,
Γ = a constant related to the specific radiation (tabulated values) of ^{137}Cs
d= distance from the source to the biosensor.

Table 2 and the graph in Figure 2 represents the number of micronuclei per hundred cells analyzed, the results of the exposure of the biosensor that relates the dosage rates to the mutational effects observed in each group. The graphic in question showed a slight growth even that load dose rates.

Temps / Groups	*Micronuclei per 100 cell*		
	24 h	36h	48h
Co	1.3	1.3	1.3
A	1.7	1.9	2.0
B	2.2	2.5	2.6
C	2.5	2.7	3.0

Note: Co is the control group from the cultivated location

Table 2. Represents data obtained from exposure of the biosensor, per group analyzed in relation to distance and time of exposure.

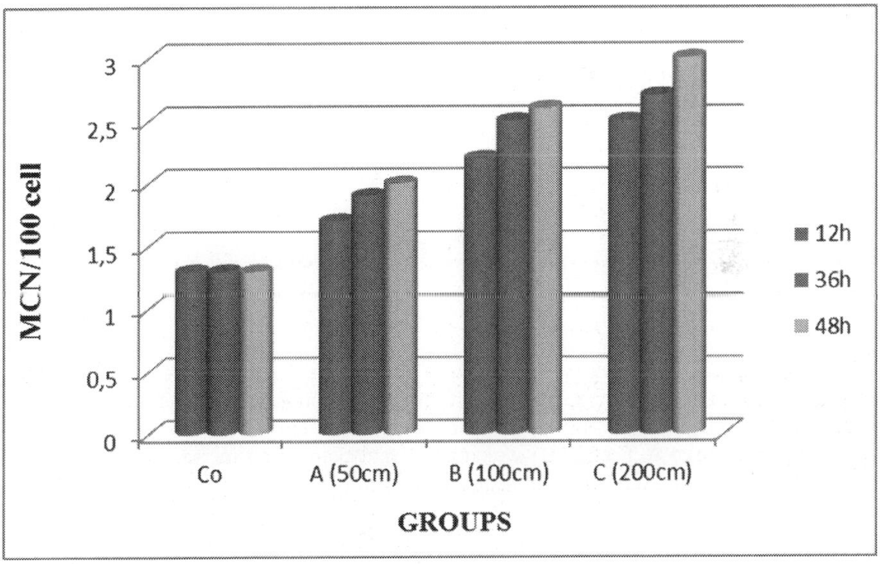

Note: Co is the control group from the cultivated location

Fig. 2. MCN/100 cell for groups Co, A, B and C

By statistical analysis it was observed that in the control group, Co, the wrapping other groups had a significant increase when exposed to a source of ^{137}Cs. When comparing the groups A and B and A and C, we also observed a significant difference between them, both for the exposed 24, 36 and 48 h. However, when comparing groups B and C, especially for times of 36 and 48 h, there were no significant differences between them. This suggests that there may have been an adaptation of the biosensor stress he underwent, or that this triggered a device to respond to stress. From the results, after comparison, we observed an increased frequency of micronuclei with a significant difference ($p<0.05$). Was also a linear relationship between absorbed dose and the response of *Tradescantia pallida,* although this has been a small increase in mutational frequency.

These results can be compared with those obtained in the literature. Villalobos-Pietrini *et al.* (1999) found a significant result, compared with the control containing the Tradescantia clone 4430, which exposed of a 800mGy with a source of Co-60 and found a response 17 MCN / 100. Suyama *et al.* (2002) reported research results that are consistent with the curve of the present study, positive response of the TRAD_MCN, for T.*pallida* when compared with the study had been validated previously for *Tradescantia* clone 4430 by Ma.

4.2 Results and commentaries of experimental procedure II

A total of 12000 cells were analyzed for each waste deposit. Every count was compared with the control group (CG) from the location of cultivation where the dose rate measured was 0.26µGy/h. Table 3 show the dose rates at each location for groups in each waste deposit.

Table 4 presents the number of micronuclei per hundred cells (MCN/100) analyzed for each group. The results tend to indicate higher micronuclei frequency per tetrads at the location of higher dose rates.

Location (Abbreviation)	Waste deposit sites Dose rates (µGy/h) IEN (Institute of Nuclear Engeneering)	UNA (Nuclear Power Plant at Angra dos Reis)	IPEN (Institute for Nuclear Energy Research)	ABADIA (Abadia of Goias)
Control garden (CG)	0.26	0.26	0.26	0.26
Control waste site (CW)	0.44	0.35	0.44	0.26
Nearby the entrance (NE)	21.9	25.4	30.0	2.20
Distant of the entrance (DE)	35.1	46.5	137	3.10

CG: negative control (garden where T.*pallida* was cultivated); CW: positive control (location of the waste deposit site where the dose rate was close to the dose rate measured at the garden); NE: location nearby the entrance door of the waste deposit; DE: location 1m distant of the entrance door of the waste deposit.

Table 3. Dose rates (µGy/h) at each location for each waste deposit site

First of all, to verify the influence suffered by the biosensors during transportation to the location of exposure, the frequencies MCN/100 tetrads were compared on the control points of the cultivation, CG (cultivation garden) with the frequencies at the positive control groups CW (radioactive waste deposit sites). From this comparison no significant difference was found ($p>0.05$), which leads one to conclude that the biosensor did not suffer any damages from stress during transportation.

Location (Abbreviation)	Waste deposit sites (MCN/100) tetrads IEN (Institute of Nuclear Engeneering)	UNA (Nuclear Power Plant at Angra dos Reis	IPEN (Institute for Nuclear Energy Research)	ABADIA (Abadia of Goias)
Control garden (CG)	1.26	1.26	1.26	1.26
Control waste site (CW)	1.37	1.73	1.43	1.20
Nearby the entrance (NE)	1.60	2.00	2.57	1.33
Distant of the entrance (DE)	1.93	2.27	5.90	1.47

Table 4. Number of micronuclei per hundred cells (MCN/100) for each location in the neighborhoods of deposits of radioactive waste as a function of dose rate

On comparing the NE and DE groups to the control group (CG), different responses could be observed. Thus, no significant difference was observed for the NE groups at IEN an ABADIA deposits. On the contrary, for groups NE at UNA and IPEN deposits (intermediate level) showed a significant increase ($p<0.05$) in mutational frequency. For group DE, a great a difference was found at the deposits of UNA, IEN and IPEN; only the deposit at ABADIA showed no significant increase when compared with the control (cultivation location).

Recent studies, using the species *Tradescantia pallida*, compare its sensitivity to the effects of exposure to radiation with those from genotoxic agents (Celebruska_Wasilewska, 1992; Ichikawa, 1991;1992 Gomes *et al.*,2001). The mutagenesis scale shown in figure 2 is coherent with that obtained by Suyama et al Suyama *et al.*(2002) when the studying a methodology of biomonitoring tests with *Tradescantia*, when exposed to x-rays. Villalobos-Pietrini *et al.*(1999) used this method with the biosensor when comparing the *Tradescantia* clone 4430, having registered and increase in the mutational frequency from 7 MCN/100 to 17MCN/100, when the plants were submitted to a dose of 0.8 Gy from a source of ^{60}Co. Recent studies have shown that the sensitivity of *Tradescantia* to the effects of radiation serve as a way of connecting gamma radiation dosage rates to which it was submitted to the mutational frequency from low dose rates , using the micronuclei a methodology (Santos leal et al., 2005;2008)

5. Conclusion

In the study of radiobiology, the system based on cells of Tradescantia *pallida* (Trad-MCN), is being considered. The sensitivity of the Tradescantia micronucleus has been used widely and has demonstrated the relation between radiation dose and frequency mutational obsevarded at low doses, looking through these studies contribute to the vexed question of the effects of low doses and their consequences for human health (Ma *et al.*,1994; Gomes *et al.*, 2002; Santos *et al.*,2005; Santos *et al.*,2008).

This system carries the advantage of observing meaningful data in a short period of time, being able to meditate effects on human health and to prevent possible accidents, when adopted as periodical monitoring.

The biosensor T. *pallida* exhibits a noticeable quantity of cell alteration in the short time following radiation exposure. Hence, the effects caused on the environment might be anticipated, and by extension on the human being, as a result of its occupation exposition level. The use of method is recommended, therefore into the environment acclimatization, and may be used, in addition, in the prevention of radiological accidents.

6. References

Carvalho, H.A. (2005). " Tradescantia as bioindicadtor plant in monitoring the clastogenic effects of ionizing radiation". Radiologia Brassileira, Vol 38, pp. 459-462.

Celebuska-Wasilewska, A. (1992). *Trandescantia* stamen hair mutation bioassay on the mutagenicity of radioisotope-contaminated air following the Chernobyl nuclear accident and one year later. Mutation Res. 270, 23-29.

Chies, JM. (1983). Integerrimine mutagenic action of the system of Tradescantia stamen hairs and root meristems of Allium cepa. UFRS. Porto Alegre.

Comissão Nacional de Energia Nuclear, (2002). "*Gerência de Rejeitos Radioativos em Instalações Radiativas*" - *Norma CNEN* NE-6.05, CNEN, Brazil.

Comissão Nacional de Energia Nuclear, (2002). "*Seleção e Escolha de Locais para Depósitos de Rejeitos Radioativos*" - *Norma CNEN* NE-6.06, CNEN, Brazil.

Comissão Nacional de Energia Nuclear, (2002). "Critérios de Aceitação para Deposição de Rejeitos Radioativos de Baixo e Médio Níveis de Radiação". *Norma CNEN* NN-6.09, CNEN, Brazil.

Comissão Nacional de Energia Nuclear, (2005). "*Diretrizes Básicas de Proteção Radiológica*" - *Norma CNEN* NN-3.01, CNEN, Brazil.

Ma, T.H. (1982). *Tradescantia* micronucleus bioassay and pollen tube aberration test for in situ monitoring and mutagen screening. Environmental Health Perspectives, 37 45-164.

Ennever, F.K.; Andreano, G. & Rosenkranz, H.S. (1998). The ability of plant genotoxicity assays to predict carcinogenicity. Mutation Research 205: 99-105.

Gomes, H.A.; Nouailhetas,Y.; Almeida, C.E.B.; Mezrahi, A. (2002). Biological response of *Tradescantia* Stamen-hair to High Levels of Natural Radiation in the Poços de Caldas Plateau. Brazilian Arquives of Biology and Technology 45, 301-307.

Gong, P.; Kuperman, R.G. & Sunahara, G.I. (2003). Genotoxicity of 2,4- and 2,6-dinitrotoluene as measured by the Tradescantia micronucleus (Trad-MCN) bioassay. Mutation Research 538: 13-18.

Grant, W.F. (1998). Higher plant assays for the detection of genotoxicity in air polluted environments. Ecosystem Health 4: 210-229.

Ichikawa, S. (1991). Validity of simplified scoring methods of somatic mutations in *Tradescantia* stamen hairs. *Environ. Exp. Bot.* 31, pp 247–252.

Ichiwaka, S. (1992). *Tradescantia* stamen-hair as an excellent botanical tester of mutagenicity; its response to ionizing radiations and chemical mutagens, and some synergistitic effects found. *Mutation Res.* 270, pp 3-22.

Ma, T.H. (1979). Micronuclei induced by X-rays and chemical mutagens in meiotic pollen mother cells of *Tradescantia* – a promising mutagen system. Mutation Research, 64 : 307-313.

Ma, T.H. (1981). *Tradescantia* micronucleus bioassay and pollen tube aberration test for in situ monitoring and mutagen screening. Environmental Health Perspectives, 37 :145-164.

Ma, T.H. (1982). Tradescantia cytogenetic tests root-tip mitosis, pollen mitosis, pollen mother-cell meiosis. Mutation Research 99: 293-302.

Ma, T.H. (1983). Tradescantia-micronucleus Trad-MCN test for environmental clastogens. In: A.R. Kolber, T.K. Wong, L.D. Grant, R.S. DeWoskin, T.J. Hughes (eds.). In vitro toxicity testing of environmental agents. Part A, Plenum, New York, pp. 191-214.

Ma, T.H. (1990). Tradescantia micronucleus test on clastogens and in situ monitoring. In: M.L.Mendelsohn, R.J. Albertini (ed.). Mutation and the Environment. New York. Wiley-Liss, pp 83-90.

Ma, T.H., Cabrera,G.L., Chen, R., Gill, B.S, Sandhu,S.S. Vandenberg,A.L. Aamone, M.F. (1994). *Tradescantia* micronucleus bioassay. Mutation Res. 310, pp 221-230.

Minouflet, M.; Ayrault, S.; Badot, P.M; Cotelle, S. & Ferard, J.F. (2005). Assessment of the genotoxicity of ^{137}Cs radiation using Vicia-micronucleus, Tradescantia-micronucleus and Tradescantia stamen-hair mutation bioassays. Journal of Environmental Radioactivity 81: 143-153.

Ribeiro L.R; Salvadori, D.M.F; & Marques, E.K. (2003). Environmental Mutagenesis. Publisher ULBRA. Canoas, RS.

Rodrigues, G.S.; Samia, A.M. & Leonard, H.W. (1996). Genotoxic activity of ozone in Tradescantia. Environmental and Experimental Botany 36: 45-50.

Rodrigues, G. S. (1999a). "Bioensaios de Toxidade Genética com Plantas Superiores: *Tradescantia (MCN, SHM), Milho e Soja*". Embrapa Meio Ambiente. Circular Técnica, 2. Jaguariúna. 30pp.

Rodrigues, G. S. (1999b). "Bioensaios de Toxidade Genética com *Tradescantia*". Embrapa Meio Ambiente. Circular Técnica, 2. Jaguariúna. 56pp.

Rodrigues, G.S.; Campos, J.M.S. (2006). An䱡ise de mutagenicidade em lodo de esgoto. EMBRAPA, Jaguarica.

Rodrigues, G.S.; Ma, T.H; Pimentel, D. & Weinstein, L.H. (1997). Tradescantia biossays as monitoring systems for environmental mutagenesis. A review. Critical reviews in Plant Sciences 16: 325-359.

Saldiva, P.H.N.; Clarke, R.W.; Coull, B.A.; Stearns, R.C.; Lawrence, J.; Murthy, G.G.K.; Diaz, E.; Koutrakis, P.; Suh, H.; Tsuda, A. & Godleski, J.J. (2002). Lung inflammation induced by concentrated ambient air particles is related to particle composition. American Journal of Respiratory and Critical Care Medicine 165: 1610-1617.

Santos, T. C.; Crispim, V.R.; Gomes, H. A.; (2005). The study of the effects of low dose level exposure to ionizing radiation using a bioindicator system. Applied Radiation and Isotopes, V.62, Issue 2,313-316.

Santos Leal, T.C. ; Silva A. X. ; Crispim, V. R. ; Frota, M ; Kelecom, A, (2008). Use of a bioindicator system in the study of the mutagenetical effects in the neighborhoods of deposits of radioactive waste. applied radiation and isotopes, v. 66, p. 535-538.

Suyama, F.; Guimarães, E.T.; Lobo, D.J.A.; Rodrigues, G.S.; Domigos, M.;Alves, E.S.; Carvalho, H.A. and Saldiva, P.H.N. (2002). Pollen mother cells of *Tradescantia* clone 4430 and *Tradescantia pallida* var. *Purpurea* are equally sensitive to the clastogenic effests of X-rays.Brasilian Journal of medical and Biologial Research, 35: 127-129.

Vilalobos-Pietrini, R.; Flores-Marques, A.R. ;Meneses, M.A.; Tavera, L.; Balcazar, M.; Gómez-Arroyo, S. (1999). Genetic effects observed in tretrads of Tradescantia induced by radon.Fundamental and Molecular Mechanisms of Mutagenesis. MutationResearch. 426: 215-219.

Zengh, D., Li, Y. & Qingqiang, L. (1999). Pollution monitoring of three rivers passing through Fuzhou City, People's Republic of China. Mutation Research 426: 159-161.

Note

1 SPSS 9.0 for Windows (SPSS Inc., Chicago, IL,1999) http://www.spss.com.br/spss.